**Drug Induced
Movement Disorders**

To Larry Corbett, Neil Lava & Bill Weiner
Three remarkable teachers
Three dear friends

SAF

To my father-in-law Arthur Racioppa.
Forever young, forever supportive,
forever tolerant, forever understanding. Forever Art.

AEL

To Lisa.

WJW

Drug Induced Movement Disorders

Second edition

Edited by

Stewart A. Factor, DO
Movement Disorders Center
Department of Neurology
Emory University
Atlanta, USA

Anthony E. Lang, MD
Movement Disorders Clinic
Toronto Western Hospital
Toronto, Canada

William J. Weiner, MD
Department of Neurology
University of Maryland School of Medicine
Baltimore, USA

Blackwell
Futura

2005

Blackwell Publishing, Inc., 350 Main Street, Malden, Massachusetts 02148-5020, USA
Blackwell Publishing Ltd, 9600 Garsington Road, Oxford OX4 2DQ, UK
Blackwell Science Asia Pty Ltd, 550 Swanston Street, Carlton, Victoria 3053, Australia

First edition 1992
Second edition 2005

ISBN: 1-4051-26191

Library of Congress Cataloging-in-Publication Data

Drug induced movement disorders / edited by Stewart A. Factor,
    Anthony E. Lang, William J. Weiner. – 2nd ed.
      p.   cm.
    Includes bibliographical references and index.
    ISBN 1-4051-2619-1
      1. Tardive dyskinesia.   2. Antipsychotic drugs – Side effects.
    3. Neuroleptic malignant syndrome.   4. Antiparkinsonian agents – Side effects.
    I. Factor, Stewart A., 1956– .   II. Lang, Anthony E.   III. Weiner, William J.
      [DNLM: 1. Dyskinesia, Drug-Induced.   2. Akathisia, Drug-Induced.
      3. Movement Disorders – classification.   4. Movement Disorders – etiology.
      WL 390 D794   2005]
    RC394.T37D78   2005
    616.8′3 – dc22   2004022596

A catalogue record for this title is available from the British Library

Acquisitions: Steve Korn
Development Editor: Katrina Chandler
Set in 9.5/12 Palatino by TechBooks
Printed and bound in India by Gopsons Papers Limited, New Delhi

For further information on Blackwell Publishing, visit our website:
www.blackwellfutura.com

The publisher's policy is to use permanent paper from mills that operate a sustainable forestry policy, and which has been manufactured from pulp processed using acid-free and elementary chlorine-free practices. Furthermore, the publisher ensures that the text paper and cover board used have met acceptable environmental accreditation standards.

Notice: The indications and dosages of all drugs in this book have been recommended in the medical literature and conform to the practices of the general community. The medications described do not necessarily have specific approval by the Food and Drug Administration for use in the diseases and dosages for which they are recommended. The package insert for each drug should be consulted for use and dosage as approved by the FDA. Because standards for usage change, it is advisable to keep abreast of revised recommendations, particularly those concerning new drugs.

Contents

List of contributors

Lenard A. Adler, MD
Departments of Psychiatry and Neurology,
NYU School of Medicine and Psychiatry
Service (116A), New York Harbor Healthcare
System,
New York, NY, USA

Karen E. Anderson, PhD
University of Maryland School of Medicine
Department of Neurology and Psychiatry
Movement Disorders Division
Baltimore, USA

Burt Angrist, MD
Department of Psychiatry, NYU School
of Medicine and Psychiatry Service (116A),
New York Harbor Healthcare System,
New York, NY, USA

Jose A. Apud, MD
Clinical Brain Disorders Branch
National Institute of Mental Health
IRP, National Institutes of Health
Bethesda, Maryland, USA

Matthew T. Avila, MA
Maryland Psychiatric Research Center
University of Maryland School of Medicine
Department of Psychiatry
Baltimore, Maryland, USA

Matthew A. Brodsky, MD
Oregon Health Sciences University
Dept of Neurology
Portland, Oregon, USA

Robert Burke, MD
Department of Neurology
Columbia University
New York, USA

Martin Cloutier, MD
Morton and Gloria Shulman
Movement Disorders Clinic
Toronto Western Hospital
Toronto, Canada

Michael F. Egan, MD
Clinical Brain Disorders Branch
National Institute of Mental Health
IRP, National Institutes of Health
Bethesda, Maryland, USA

Stewart A. Factor, DO
Movement Disorders Center
Department of Neurology
Emory University
Atlanta, Georgia, USA

Hubert H. Fernandez, MD
Movement Disorders Center
Department of Neurology
University of Florida
Gainesville, Florida, USA

Whitney C. Fisher, MD
Clinical Brain Disorders Branch
National Institute of Mental Health
IRP, National Institutes of Health
Bethesda, Maryland, USA

Joseph H. Friedman, MD
Department of Clinical Neuroscience
Brown University School of Medicine
Memorial Hospital of Rhode Island
Pawtucket, Rhode Island, USA

Madaline B. Harrison, MD
Department of Neurology
University of Virginia
Charlottesville, Virginia, USA

Elliot L. Hong, MD
Maryland Psychiatric Research Center
University of Maryland School of Medicine
Department of Psychiatry
Baltimore, Maryland, USA

Thomas M. Hyde, MD, PhD
Clinical Brain Disorders Branch
National Institute of Mental Health
IRP, National Institutes of Health
Bethesda, Maryland, USA

Shitij Kapur, MD
Canada Chair
Schizophrenia Research Scientist
PET Centre, Addiction and Mental Health
Professor of Psychiatry
University of Toronto
Toronto, Canada

Roger Kurlan, MD
University of Rochester Medical School
Department of Neurology
Rochester, New York, USA

Anthony E. Lang, MD
Morton and Gloria Shulman
Movement Disorders Clinic
Toronto Western Hospital
Toronto, Canada

James Lohr, MD
Professor and Vice Chair
Clinical Affairs
UCSD Department of Psychiatry
San Diego Director
VA VISN-22 Mental Illness Research
Education and Clinical Center
San Diego, USA

Michael F. Mazurek, MD
Division of Neurology
McMaster University Medical Centre
West Hamilton, Canada

John C. Morgan, MD, PhD
Movement Disorders Program
Department of Neurology
Medical College of Georgia and Department
   of Veterans Affairs, Medical Center
Augusta, Georgia, USA

Maria L. Moro-de-Casillas, MD
Department of Neurology
University Hospitals of Cleveland and
   Case Western Reserve
University School of Medicine
Cleveland, Ohio, USA

Anthony E. Munson, MD
Department of Neurology,
University of Maryland School
of Medicine Baltimore, Maryland, USA

John G. Nutt, MD
Oregon Health Sciences University
Dept of Neurology
Portland, Oregon, USA

Christopher O'Brien, MD
Prestwick Pharmaceuticals Inc
Washington DC, USA

Gary Remington, MD, PhD, FRCP(C)
Director
Medication Assessment Program for Schizophrenia
Schizophrenia Division
Centre for Addiction and Mental Health
Professor of Psychiatry
University of Toronto
Canada

Irene Richard, MD
University of Rochester School of Medicine
Department of Neurology
Rochester, New York, USA

David E. Riley, MD
Department of Neurology
University Hospitals of Cleveland and Case
   Western Reserve University School of Medicine
Cleveland, Ohio, USA

**Patricia I. Rosebush, MD, MScN,
FRCP (C)**
McMaster University Medical Centre
West Hamilton, Canada

John Rotrosen, MD
Department of Psychiatry, NYU School of Medicine
and Psychiatry Service (116A), New York Harbor
Healthcare System,
New York, NY, USA

Juan Sanchez-Ramos, MD, PhD
Department of Neurology, University
of South Florida, Tampa Florida

Frank Skidmore, MD
Department of Neurology
University of Maryland School of Medicine
Baltimore, Maryland, USA

Daniel Tarsy, MD
Department of Neurology
Beth Israel Deaconess Medical Center
Harvard Medical School
Boston, USA

Gunvant K. Thaker, MD
Maryland Psychiatric Research Center
University of Maryland School of Medicine
Department of Psychiatry
Baltimore, Maryland, USA

Martha E. Trieschmann, MD
Department of Clinical Neuroscience
Brown University School of Medicine
Memorial Hospital of Rhode Island
Pawtucket, Rhode Island, USA

William J. Weiner, MD
Department of Neurology
University of Maryland School of Medicine
Baltimore, Maryland, USA

Ikwunga Wonodi, MD
Maryland Psychiatric Research Center
University of Maryland School of Medicine
Department of Psychiatry
Baltimore, Maryland, USA

Acknowledgements

We would like to thank the contributors of this text. We realize that this is a complicated era in medicine and it is becoming more difficult to find the time to write book chapters. Despite that, these experts were able to put together timely, cogent and comprehensive reviews of their subject and for that we are grateful.

Our staffs have been invaluable to us as we worked toward the completion of this book. We would like to particularly thank Faith Wood, Nandy Yearwood, and Cheryl Grant Johnson for their administrative support. Finally, we are indebted to Rosalyn Newman and Victor and Marilyn Riley and Key Bank of New York for their extraordinarily generous support for our programs.

Foreword

On starting my training as a neurologist thirty years ago, Christopher Earl, one of my most influential teachers at Queen Square, told me that when he and Richard Hunter had in 1963 presented some early cases of persistent dyskinesias following phenothiazines to the Royal Society of Medicine in London, their report had been greeted with great scepticism by many of the psychiatrists present in the audience. They believed that the sort of stereotyped abnormal hyperkinetic movements Hunter and Earl were describing were an integral, if rather poorly documented, feature of chronic catatonic schizophrenia. The kinesics of major psychiatric illness remain a fascinating and inadequately explored terrain, but few would now question the sound epidemiological evidence linking either the bucco-linguo-masticatory syndrome or potentially irreversible dystonia and chorea to chronic neuroleptic usage.

In my doctoral thesis I explored the role of substituted benzamides as potential selective anti-dyskinetic agents to combat disabling chorea seen as a consequence of long-term l-dopa therapy for Parkinson's disease. This could be achieved, but only briefly, and despite scrupulous attention to delicate dose titration, breakthrough worsening of Parkinsonism inevitably occurred. Of greater concern was the apparent delay in restoring equilibrium following sulpiride and tiapride discontinuation. In contrast, useful results were seen in dopaminergic psychoses and the newer drugs clozapine and quetiapine, both reputed to have fewer extrapyramidal complications, have proved effective and useful as short-term treatments for paranoid psychosis and delirium in Parkinson's disease

It was another of my teachers, Gerald Stern, who aroused my interest in the snake-root plant (*Rauwolfia serpentina*), or Chandra as it is known in Bengali, meaning moon and suggesting a link with lunacy. Gerald pored over Sanskrit incunabula and Ayurvedic texts for long hours on lazy Sunday mornings in the libraries of Indian Universities trying to unlock some of the mysteries of this revered plant which had led to Arvid Carlsson's Nobel Prize winning work of the 1950s and put dopamine on the map as an important chemical messenger. Gerald learned that the late Mohandas Gandhi took infusions of snake-root to control his hypertension and speculated that his serene and tranquil disposition in later life could be attributed in part to the plant's ataractic properties. An under-rated paper by Degkwitz and colleagues published in 1960 which I had translated from the German when writing my thesis, reproduced Carlsson's animal experiments in man demonstrating that small doses of l-dopa combined with the non-selective mono-amine oxidase inhibitor iproniazid and vitamin B6 could counteract reserpine-induced Parkinsonism. This report paved the way for Birkmayer and Barbeau's independent but synchronous pioneering studies using l-dopa as a treatment for Parkinson's disease and strengthened my belief that the natural world had much to teach us about movement disorders. By the time Degkwitz's paper saw the light of day, the charismatic American psychiatrist Nathan Klein had already been investigating reserpine, the active alkaloid present in *Rauwolfia* for almost a decade. He showed it to have useful but modest anti-psychotic properties limited by side-effects which included depression, sedation, drooling, diarrhoea and orthostatic hypotension.

More promising, however were the phenothiazines synthesised in Europe from aniline dyes in the late nineteenth century. Paul Ehrlich prophetically had predicted that some of these, including methylene blue, might be useful to treat mental illness. Chlorpromazine, synthesised in 1949, was used by Sigwald and the group of French military psychiatrists working at Val-de Grace to treat paranoia and mania. Delay and Deniker then showed that it was a very effective antipsychotic, coining the term 'neuroleptic' to embrace the phenothiazines and the recently synthesised butyrophenone, haloperidol, and distinguishing them from narcotics, general anaesthetics and hypnotics. The impact of neuroleptics on psychiatric practice was to be colossal, allowing acute psychotic episodes to be managed in the community and freeing a multitude of chronic schizophrenics from institutional care.

Iatrogenic movement disorders occurring as a result of drugs known to modify dopamine transmission in the brain led to a new era of taxonomy in neurology and psychiatry with exotic new conditions emerging such as the Rabbit and Pisa syndromes, punding and crack dancing. More importantly, however, their occurrence stimulated a great deal of basic research on the biochemical mechanisms underlying these phenomena. This important data could be extrapolated to explain the spontaneously occurring movement disorders – hence the simplistic concepts of bradykinesia as a sign of striatal dopamine deficiency syndrome and chorea as a clinical marker for relative striatal dopamine excess. Nevertheless, clinical observation raised many conundrums. How could antipsychotic drugs already known to block striatal dopamine receptors trigger life-threatening acute dystonic reactions after just two or three exposures or provoke irreversible bucco-linguo-masticatory stereotypies after chronic exposure? How could akathisia, chorea and Parkinsonism all be induced simultaneously in different body parts and why did children with tardive dyskinesia tend to have a generalised dystonia while the elderly had a very focal chorea of the lower face? Pre-clinical attempts to answer some of these more difficult riddles using non-human primates met with partial success in the seventies and eighties but the discovery of the nigral neurotoxin MPTP and a greater interest in non-dopaminergic mechanisms in Parkinson's disease led to a reduction of movement disorder research using dopamine blocking drugs and dopamine stimulants.

Fashions change in science, and in recent years neuroleptic-induced movement disorders have been relatively neglected, receiving much less air space at biological psychiatry and movement disorder meetings. This may in part have been brought about by a perception that, with the introduction of a new wave of potentially safer anti-psychotic drugs, the problem is disappearing. This is a regrettable oversight which this book, edited by three distinguished and internationally respected North American neurologists, will help to redress. There can be no doubt that further careful clinical and scientific study of these disorders will shed light on the biochemical and molecular mechanisms which underlie basal ganglia disorders. For example, recent neuropathological studies have shown that the brains of habitual cocaine users have increased striatal dopamine transporter proteins and a threefold increase in alpha synuclein, raising the possibility that these individuals may be at greater risk of developing Parkinson's disease.

The editors of this book are to be congratulated, not only for its scholarly content but for grasping the nettle and reminding us that there is much of importance yet to discover in the field of drug-induced movement disorders. Neurologists, many of whom may have relatively little exposure to the rich panoply of odd movements seen in everyday psychiatric practice, will learn that some of the described phenomena are more than just minor inconveniences in the rehabilitation of the psychiatrically wounded, and some like the neuroleptic malignant syndrome are potentially deadly. Psychiatrists will appreciate that Parkinson's disease and the effects on it of long-term exogenous dopaminergic treatment provide a fertile and untapped natural test-bed for the investigation of many of the disorders which comprise psychiatric practice. For the committed movement disorder specialist this book will provide an essential reference source to dip into whenever one is at a loss to diagnose or manage a tricky case, may help with thorny medicolegal issues, and even act as a stimulus for fresh research.

This is a book of distinction for which Drs Factor, Lang and Weiner, together with their able team of contributors, should feel proud. I can do no more than wish it the appreciative reception it unquestionably deserves.

Andrew Lees, Director
Reta Lila Weston Institute of Neurological Studies
University College London, London, UK

Preface

When two of us (AEL and WJW) published the first edition of this book in 1992, we had assembled the first comprehensive text on Drug-induced Movement Disorders and it was well received. We succeeded in covering the entire field of pharmacologically related movement disorders in twelve well-organized chapters, which were contributed by leaders in the fields of both Neurology and Psychiatry, another first. Now, 12 years later, we thought it was time to update this work with a second edition. The fact that we are currently in the midst of a therapeutic revolution with the development of several new classes and new agents warrants this venture.

Drug-induced movement disorders continue to be a common source of morbidity in patients and appropriate recognition and diagnosis of these complex signs and symptoms remains a difficult task. The range of agents causing these problems has broadened, adding to the challenge. Antipsychotics remain the most frequently implicated class of drugs. The development of "atypical" agents, which were supposed to eliminate extrapyramidal side effects, has only added to the long list of drugs causing movement disorders even though they probably do cause movements disorders less commonly than their typical counterparts. It is well known that other agents such as dopaminergic drugs, antidepressants and antiepileptics, to name a few, are also the instigators of complex movement disorders and the development of new drugs in these classes has also added to the complexity of the field. In addition, drug-induced movement disorders continue to provide insights into the pathogenesis and pharmacology of primary neurological and psychiatric disease. With this book we have, again, tried to provide a comprehensive review of this constantly growing field. The scholarly contributions of many leaders in psychiatry and neurology have made such a text possible.

In this volume the organization and the number of chapters has changed. For many chapters, the original authors have been generous enough to revise and update their work. Several new authors were recruited for new chapters and some of the original ones. The book is comprised of four sections: General Considerations, Antipsychotics, Dopaminomimetic Drugs, and Other Drugs, with a total of 17 chapters. Chapters 1–3 discuss general considerations. The first chapter introduces the topic of movement disorders with definitions, descriptions and differential diagnosis. Chapter 2 reviews rating scales used to evaluate movement disorders in psychiatric patients and Chapter 3 provides an overview of movement disorders seen in untreated psychiatric patients, which should be helpful in recognizing the drug-induced disorders. Section 2 covers movement disorders associated with antipsychotic agents in

Chapters 4–12. In addition to those topics covered in the previous edition (and now updated), acute dystonia, parkinsonism, acute akathisia, neuroleptic malignant syndrome and tardive dyskinesia and its variants, three new chapters are added which primarily relate to atypical antipsychotic agents. Chapter 4 compares and contrasts the pharmacology of typical neuroleptics and the newer atypical agents in relation to the ability to cause movement disorders. It covers the new theories on how these drugs work and how they cause movement disorders. Chapter 11 provides a review of the literature on movement disorders caused by atypical agents. There appears to be a misconception that the development of atypical antipsychotics will lead to the disappearance of tardive dyskinesia. We have added a chapter that is more akin to an editorial to address this notion in Chapter 12, authored by a leading researcher in the field of tardive dyskinesia. Section 3, containing Chapters 13 and 14, updates the movement disorders caused by antiparkinsonian drugs and stimulants respectively. The final section contains three chapters covering antidepressants, antiepileptics and miscellaneous drugs. Substantial revisions to these topics as presented in the first edition have been required given the many additions to these classes of drugs that have occurred over the last 12 years. For example, in the first edition, antiepileptics were covered in the miscellaneous chapter but the increased reporting of movement disorders from these drugs and the addition of several new drugs in the class justifies a separate chapter on the topic.

The 17 chapters herein are scholarly, concise, up-to-date reviews that can be utilized in isolation, and they are heavily referenced for this purpose. We have also provided substantial cross-referencing so that topics of interest can be easily accessed. Finally, the book is organized to bring the chapters together in a cohesive edition. We believe that a broad spectrum of readers including medical students, neurology and psychiatry residents, clinicians, particularly primary care physicians, gerontologists, neurologists and psychiatrists, as well as clinical and basic scientists will all find something of interest here.

Stewart A. Factor, DO
Anthony E. Lang, MD
William J. Weiner, MD

PART 1

General considerations

CHAPTER 1

Movement disorders: an overview

Martin Cloutier and Anthony E. Lang

Movement disorders: an overview

Movement disorders are common and come to the attention of all physicians, but most often neurologists, psychiatrists, internists and family physicians. Prescription medications and illicit drugs are common causes for almost all types of movement disorders. Neurologists and general physicians should have an understanding of these movement disorders and an awareness of these potential complications. The common occurrence of movement disorders complicating mental illness and their treatment makes it important for psychiatrists to be able to recognize the various movement disorders as well.

Accurate diagnosis of a movement disorder complicating the use of a specific drug requires some basic understanding of the general classification of movement disorders. Too often, reports in the literature utilize terms such as chorea, tics, or myoclonus without conforming to accepted definitions of these disorders. Review of the original case report may reveal significant confusion or inaccuracy. However, the report may have been subsequently cited multiple times and the described association widely accepted despite poor or inappropriate original documentation. An appreciation of the broad differential diagnosis of movement disorders is also necessary when attempting to implicate a specific drug as causative. A lack of this awareness often accounts for case reports of a specific drug causing abnormal movements when better explanations are readily available.

Another important potential source of confusion is the possibility that certain neurological diseases can present first with nonneurological symptoms. Treatment prescribed for these symptoms may be wrongly implicated when a movement disorder eventually develops due to the primary disease process. Probably the most common example of this would be the use of neuroleptic drugs for the initial psychiatric manifestations of certain neurological disorders. We have seen this sequence of events result in significant delays in diagnosis of such disorders as Wilson's disease, Huntington's disease, and systemic lupus erythematosis. Another potential source of diagnostic error is that certain brain disorders (occult or overt) can predispose to the development of movement disorders as a consequence of specific drugs. Occasionally, the underlying disorder will require treatment in its own right quite distinct from the need for withdrawal of the agent that precipitated the obvious movement disorder.

The purpose of this introductory chapter is to define the descriptive terms that are used repeatedly in this text and to help the clinician in understanding the actual classification of the various movement disorders. Multiple tables are provided outlining the broad differential diagnoses that must be considered when faced with these clinical problems.

Definitions and differential diagnoses

The traditional approach to a neurological symptom is to address the localization of the lesion first, and then consider the possible etiologies. The neurological examination is often helpful in determining the localization of the lesion, and it is mostly the history that will determine the most likely diagnosis, depending on the abruptness of onset and the progression of the symptoms.

This approach is somewhat different when a movement disorder is the predominant problem, since for many of them, the pathophysiology is complex and often poorly understood. Many are the result of neurodegeneration affecting different circuits of the brain and it is often impossible to determine a specific anatomic localization.

The clinician must first observe and examine the patient to define the type of movement disorder that best describes the clinical picture. The age of onset, the distribution, the progression of the symptoms, a familial history of similar symptoms, and the presence of systemic signs often help to determine the most likely explanation for that movement disorder.

Movement disorders are first divided into hypokinetic versus hyperkinetic categories. Hypokinetic disorders are characterized by akinesia, bradykinesia, and rigidity. Akinesia is defined as a paucity of movement while bradykinesia refers to slowness of movement. Rigidity is an involuntary increase in muscle tone, appreciated equally in flexors and extensors. It may have a cog-wheeling component when tremor is superimposed. Parkinson's disease is the most common cause of such symptoms. Hypokinetic disorders are therefore also referred to as akinetic-rigid syndromes or parkinsonism. Hyperkinetic disorders are disorders in which there is an excess of movement, either spontaneous or in response to a volitional movement or another stimulus. They are often involuntary, but tics and some stereotyped movement (e.g., movements accompanying akathisia or restless legs syndrome) often have a voluntary component. Tremor, dystonia, tics, chorea, ballismus, and myoclonus are the most common types of hyperkinetic disorders. It is not rare for a patient to present with a combination of movement disorders, such as the resting tremor and the akinetic-rigid features of Parkinson's disease. In these cases, it is best to describe the different movement disorders as observed and then assign the broader picture according to the most prominent symptom.

Table 1.1 Differential diagnosis of parkinsonism

1. Parkinson's disease
Sporadic
Genetic
  Autosomal dominant
  Autosomal recessive

2. Secondary parkinsonism
Neurodegenerative diseases (sporadic or genetic)
  Progressive supranuclear palsy
  Multiple system atrophy
  Corticobasal degeneration
  Dementia with Lewy bodies*
  Alzheimer's disease
  ALS-parkinsonism-dementia complex of Guam
  Huntington's disease
  Spinocerebellar ataxias
  Neuroacanthocytosis
  Hallervorden-Spatz disease
  Wilson's disease
  Dopa-responsive dystonia
  Others
Drugs
  Neuroleptics, metoclopramide, prochlorperazine, tetrabenazine, cinnarizine, flunarizine, α-methyldopa, lithium
Toxic
  MPTP, manganese, carbon monoxide, mercury
Infectious
  Encephalitis lethargica
  Other encephalitis
  Subacute sclerosing panencephalitis
  Creutzfeldt-Jakob disease
Vascular
  Atherosclerosis
  Amyloid angiopathy
Neoplastic
  Brain tumor
  Other mass lesions
Normal pressure hydrocephalus
Head trauma
Others
Multiple sclerosis

*May represent the same disease as idiopathic Parkinson's disease.

Parkinsonism

Parkinsonism is a common complication of neuroleptics and occurs occasionally with the use of other medications. More commonly, it is secondary to a neurodegenerative disease such as Parkinson's disease, multiple system atrophy, progressive supranuclear palsy, or other progressive brain diseases. A more complete differential diagnosis of parkinsonism is included in Table 1.1.

Neurodegenerative causes of parkinsonism (e.g., Parkinson's disease) may be present in occult or subclinical form for several years before progressing to the point of causing overt symptoms and signs. During this time, an individual is at greater risk of developing symptoms if exposed to a drug capable of causing such symptoms, such as neuroleptics. This probably accounts for the observation that some patients with apparent drug-induced parkinsonism either fail to remit on drug withdrawal or remit only to have symptoms recur later and subsequently progress.

Bradykinesia, rigidity, resting tremor, and postural instability are the cardinal features of parkinsonism. Masked facies, micrographia, stooped posture, gait difficulties with decreased armswing, decreased amplitude of steps, festination, and freezing are additional features. A detailed history and a careful neurological examination will often reveal clues to the exact diagnosis, although sometimes only subsequent clinical evolution will lead to the correct diagnosis. A review of past and current medications might reveal the cause of parkinsonism or an aggravating factor. Neuroimaging, more commonly an MRI of the brain, and blood work-up might be useful in selected cases.

Tremor

Tremor is defined as a rhythmical, sinusoidal oscillation of a body part, produced by alternating or synchronous contractions of agonist and antagonist muscles. Tremor is classified as resting or action tremor. A resting tremor is a tremor in a limb that is in a resting position, with its weight fully supported against gravity. It is typically seen in parkinsonism, more commonly in Parkinson's disease than in other parkinsonian syndromes. Action tremor is further divided into postural, kinetic, or intention tremor. They all imply an active contraction of the muscles involved. A postural tremor is seen with the maintenance of a posture, against gravity, such as when the arms are outstretched in front of the body. A kinetic tremor is seen with a voluntary movement of the limb, such as a tremor in an upper limb during a finger-to-nose maneuver. An intention tremor is an increase in the amplitude of the tremor when approaching a target. The terms dystonic tremor and myoclonic tremor are also used in the literature. In these cases, it is understood that the authors believe that the primary underlying movement disorder is better classified as dystonia or myoclonus but there is a rhythmical or semi-rhythmical component to the movement that is worth mentioning.

A differential diagnosis of tremor is detailed in Table 1.2, along with a list of other rhythmical movement disorders.

Chorea

Chorea consists of irregular, random, brief, flowing movements that are usually distal and of low-to-moderate amplitude. They are often flitting from one body part to another in a random and purposeless sequence. Patients may incorporate them into a voluntary movement in order to mask them. Typically, chorea cannot be suppressed for any length of time and is totally involuntary.

Table 1.2 Differential diagnosis of tremor and rhythmical movement disorders

1. Physiologic tremor
Enhanced physiologic tremor
  Metabolic
    Hyperthyroidism
    Hyperparathyroidism
    Hypoglycemia
    Pheochromocytoma
  Drugs
    Caffeine
    Theophylline
    Amphetamines
    Lithium
    Valproic acid
    Antidepressants
    Amiodarone
    β-agonists
    Others
  Withdrawal of drugs
    Benzodiazepines
    Alcohol
    Others
Fever, sepsis
Anxiety, stress, fatigue

2. Primary or idiopathic
Essential tremor
Task-specific tremor
Orthostatic tremor
Idiopathic palatal tremor

3. Tremor associated with CNS diseases
Tremor with parkinsonian syndromes
  Idiopathic Parkinson's disease
  Multiple system atrophy
  Progressive supranuclear palsy
  Cortico-basal degeneration
  Neuroleptic-induced parkinsonism
Wilson's disease
Multiple sclerosis
Fragile X premutation – tremor/ataxia syndrome
Stroke
Arteriovenous malformation
Tumor
Head trauma
Midbrain tremor (Holme's tremor)

4. Tremor associated with peripheral neuropathies

5. Psychogenic tremor

6. Other rhythmical movement disorders
Rhythmical movements in dystonia
Rhythmical myoclonus
Asterixis
Clonus
Epilepsia partialis continua
Hereditary chin quivering
Spasmus nutans
Head bobbing with hydrocephalus
Nystagmus

Table 1.3 Differential diagnosis of chorea

Genetic
  Benign hereditary chorea
  Huntington's disease
  Huntington-like conditions
  Neuroacanthocytosis
  Dentatorubropallidoluysian atrophy
  Wilson's disease
  Hallervorden-Spatz disease
  Spinocerebellar ataxias
  Ataxia-telangiectasia
  Tuberous sclerosis
Infections/parainfectious causes
  Sydenham's chorea
  Acquired immunodeficiency syndrome (including complications)
  Encephalitis and post-encephalitic
  Creutzfeldt-Jakob disease
Drugs
  Levodopa, dopaminergic agonists, amphetamines, anticholinergics, anticonvulsants,
    neuroleptics, antidepressants, oral contraceptives, antihistaminics
Endocrinologic/Metabolic
  Hyperthyroidism
  Hypoparathyroidism
  Chorea gravidarum
Immunologic
  Systemic lupus erythematosus
  Antiphospholipid syndrome
  Henoch-Schonlein purpura
Vascular
  Stroke
  Hemorrhage
  Arterio-venous malformation
  Polycythemia rubra vera
Other
  Cerebral palsy
  Kernicterus
  Head trauma
  Cardiopulmonary bypass with hypothermia
  Neoplastic and paraneoplastic

Severity is quite variable, from a patient that only appears fidgety or restless, to striking, continuous movements involving the whole body. Chorea can be seen in many diseases, including some neurodegenerative conditions and metabolic diseases, and can also be the result of treatment with a number of drugs, prescribed or illicit. The causes of chorea are listed in Table 1.3.

Ballism

Ballism is defined as random flinging movements of the proximal limbs, usually violent and of wide amplitude. It is most commonly seen as a consequence of a stroke, often in the region of subthalamic nucleus, and then

Table 1.4 Differential diagnosis of ballism

Focal lesions in basal ganglia
   Vascular
      Stroke (including infarction and hemorrhage)
      Cavernous angioma
      Post-surgical complications
   Neoplastic
      Metastases
      Primary CNS tumors
   Infections
      Cryptococcosis
      Toxoplasmosis
Tuberculoma
   Inflammatory
      Multiple sclerosis
   Iatrogenic
      Subthalamotomy
      Thalamotomy
   Immunologic
      Systemic lupus erythematosus
      Scleroderma
Behcet's disease
Nonketotic hyperglycemia
Hypoglycemia
Syndenham's chorea
Head injury
Drugs
Anticonvulsants
   Oral contraceptives
   Levodopa
   Ibuprofen

these movements are acute, transient, and unilateral, hence the term hemiballism. When bilateral they will occasionally be referred to as biballism. Ballism is considered as the more severe end of the chorea spectrum. It is therefore common to see a combination of the two and this is often acknowledged in movement disorder terminology (e.g., hemichorea/hemiballismus). In addition, when ballism is treated it often slows down to become chorea before dissipating. Differential diagnosis of ballism is provided in Table 1.4.

Dystonia

Dystonia is defined as a movement disorder caused by sustained muscle contractions resulting in twisting, repetitive movements, and for abnormal postures. The movements are often slow and sustained. They can be made worse by activity, and then, in this situation, referred to as "action dystonia." The occasional patient will show a paradoxical improvement with voluntary activation of the muscles ("paradoxical dystonia"). Another common feature of dystonia is the transient improvement of the abnormal movement with the use of a sensory trick, for example, the geste antagoniste of cervical dystonia. A patient with cervical dystonia might be partially relieved by touching his or her face with a finger, or leaning into the back of a high-backed chair. Tricks are often used to mask the abnormal posture in public.

Probably more so than with other movement disorders, dystonia can be classified according to the site of involvement. Focal dystonia involves only one body part, such as blepharospasm or cervical dystonia. Segmental dystonia is used when two or more contiguous body parts are affected. Multifocal dystonia refers to the involvement of two or more noncontiguous parts of the body. Hemidystonia is unilateral, and finally generalized dystonia is reserved for dystonia affecting both legs and other body areas.

Dystonia is also classified according to etiology. Previously, it was simply divided between primary or idiopathic dystonias and secondary or symptomatic dystonias. Now, the etiologic categories of dystonia are primary dystonia, dystonia-plus, secondary dystonia, and hereditodegenerative diseases [1]. The primary dystonia are syndromes in which the only phenotypic expression is dystonia. These diseases can be hereditary or sporadic. Dystonia-plus is characterized by a combination of dystonia with other neurological signs due to a known or presumed genetic defect without an underlying progressive neurodegenerative process. Dopa-responsive dystonia and myoclonus-dystonia are examples of such diseases. Secondary dystonias are the result of acquired injury to the central nervous system, again without progressive neurodegeneration. Drug-induced dystonia would fit into this category. Hereditodegenerative diseases causing dystonia include many conditions of genetic origin but also some neurodegenerative syndromes of unknown etiology. Here dystonia is often associated with other neurological symptoms and signs.

The differential diagnosis of dystonia is given in Table 1.5.

Tics

Tics are repetitive, stereotyped movements, or vocal productions that show a striking variability in their specific nature from one patient to the next [2, 3]. Tics vary in terms of complexity, from abrupt, brief, meaningless movements or sounds to more sustained, more deliberate, almost meaningful gestures or utterances. Accordingly, they are described as simple or complex tics, although this has little if any clinical implication in itself. Tics are also described by their anatomical location, duration, and frequency. Shorter, jerky tics are often referred to as clonic, and prolonged, sustained tics are said to be dystonic or tonic tics but again these terms are simply descriptive and have no pathophysiologic significance. The frequency of the tics in an individual patient typically varies quite considerably over minutes, hours, days, weeks, and years.

There are other characteristics of tics that help to differentiate them from other abnormal movements. Although the pathophysiology of tics is not clearly understood, tics are often described by patients as being "semi-voluntary" movements or vocal productions in response to an inner, irresistible urge. Some premonitory sensory symptoms might precede the tic, generally in the

Table 1.5 Classification and causes of dystonia

1. Primary dystonias
Familial (several genetic causes and types)
Sporadic
  Usually adult onset, focal or segmental

2. Dystonia-plus
Dystonia with parkinsonism
  Dopa-responsive dystonia
  Dopamine-agonist responsive dystonia (e.g. aromatic acid decarboxylase deficiency)
Myoclonus-dystonia

3. Secondary dystonias
Perinatal cerebral injury
  Athetoid cerebral palsy
  Delayed onset dystonia
  Pachygyria
  Kernicterus
Encephalitis
  Poststreptococcal acute disseminated encephalomyelitis
  Reye's syndrome
  Subacute sclerosing leukoencephalopathy
  Wasp sting
  Creutzfeldt-Jakob disease
  Human immunodeficiency syndrome
Head trauma
Thalamotomy
Cervical cord injury
Peripheral injury
Brainstem lesion
Primary antiphospolipid syndrome
Stroke
Arteriovenous malformation
Hypoxia
Brain tumor
Multiple sclerosis
Central pontine myelinolysis
Drug-induced
Toxins
Hypoparathyroidism
Psychogenic

4. Hereditodegenerative dystonias
X-linked
  Lubag
  Pelizaeus-Merzbacher disease
Autosomal-dominant
  Rapid-onset dystonia-parkinsonism
  Huntington's disease
  Machado-Joseph disease (SCA3) and other SCAs
  Dentato-rubro-pallido-luysian atrophy
Autosomal-recessive
  Juvenile parkinsonism (e.g., due to mutations in the parkin gene)
  Wilson's disease
  Niemann-Pick type C

(Continued)

Table 1.5 *(Continued)*

GM1 gangliosidosis
GM2 gangliosidosis
Metachromatic leukodystrophy
Lesch-Nyhan syndrome
Homocystinuria
Glutaric academia
Triose-phosphate isomerase deficiency
Hartnup's disease
Ataxia-telangiectasia
Hallervorden-Spatz disease
Juvenile neuronal ceroid lipofuscinosis
Neuroacanthocytosis
Intranuclear hyaline inclusion disease
Hereditary spastic paraplegin with dystonia
Probable autosomal recessive
  Familial basal ganglia calcifications
  Progressive pallidal degeneration
  Rett's syndrome
Mitochondrial
  Leigh's disease
  Leber's disease
  Other mitochondrial cytopathies
Sporadic, with parkinsonism
  Parkinson's disease
  Progressive supranuclear palsy
  Multiple system atrophy
  Corticobasal degeneration

Adapted from Fahn, Bressman, Marsden [4].

same general anatomical area as the tic itself. There is often a relief associated with the production of the tic. Tics can be partially or completely suppressed for a variable period of time, but often at the expense of mounting inner tension and psychological discomfort. Some patients will describe an intense struggle between the perceived pressure to capitulate and let the movement happen, and the inappropriateness of these movements, especially in a social setting. Performing the tic or sometimes even substituting the socially inappropriate tic by another more acceptable behavior will alleviate the tension. Many patients will describe that some tics occur in response to a typical urge and others (either the same or different tics) are unexpected and totally involuntary.

Tic disorders are classified as primary or idiopathic, when they have no identifiable cause, or secondary, in the case of a causative underlying brain disease or environmental factor. The classification of tic disorders is presented in Table 1.6.

Myoclonus

Myoclonus comprises sudden, brief, shock-like, involuntary movements resulting from both active muscle contraction and inhibition of ongoing muscle

Table 1.6 Etiological classification of tics

---

1. Primary or idiopathic
Transient motor or phonic tics
Chronic motor or phonic tics
Adult-onset tics
Tourette Syndrome

2. Secondary tics
Genetic
    Neuroacanthocytosis
    Huntington's disease
    Hallervorden-Spatz disease
    Idiopathic dystonia*
    Duchenne's muscular dystrophy*
    Tuberous sclerosis
    Chromosomal disorders
Infections
    Sydenham's chorea
    PANDAS+
    Encephalitis and post-encephalitic
    Creutzfeldt-Jakob disease
    Neurosyphilis
Drugs
    Methylphenidate, amphetamines, cocaine, levodopa,
        carbamazepine, phenytoin, phenobarbital, lamotrigine, neuroleptics
Developmental
    Mental retardation
    Pervasive developmental disorders/Autism
Other causes
    Head trauma
    Stroke
    Carbon monoxide poisoning
    Cardiopulmonary bypass with hypothermia

3. Related disorders
Mannerisms
Stereotypies
Compulsions
Self-injurious behavior

---

*Tics have been described with these conditions but may simply be coincidental.
+Pediatric autoimmune neuropsychiatric disorders associated with streptococcal infections – the existence of this disorder remains somewhat controversial.

activity, positive or negative myoclonus, respectively [5]. The most common form of negative myoclonus is asterixis. These movements generally arise in the central nervous system (although rarely peripheral causes of myoclonus are described) and are differentiated from abnormal muscle activity associated with peripheral nervous system diseases, such as fasciculations or myokimia. They are very short, typically lasting less than 150 milliseconds.

Clinically, myoclonus can be spontaneous, action-induced, and/or reflex (induced by various sensory stimuli). Spontaneous myoclonus occurs at rest, without any provocation, and may be intermittent or repetitive. Action myoclonus occurs during volitional movement and is often very disabling. Reflex myoclonus can be triggered by visual, auditory or somesthetic stimuli. Distribution of myoclonus may be focal, segmental, multifocal or generalized. Focal reflex myoclonus will occur in response to pinprick, touch, or muscle stretch. Myoclonus can be intermittent or repetitive, and will sometimes be rhythmical. When myoclonus involves more than one body area, the movements may be synchronous or asynchronous.

Myoclonus is classified according to the anatomic site of origin or etiology.

The site of origin of myoclonus can be cortical, subcortical, or spinal. Cortical myoclonus arises from increased neuronal excitability of the cortex, probably through loss of inhibition. The myoclonus can occur spontaneously or be stimulus-sensitive. Myoclonic jerks are of short duration, and typically, though not always, electrophysiological studies demonstrate giant somatosensory evoked potentials and a cortical spike preceding the myoclonus, on backaveraged EEG. The pathology causing cortical myoclonus often does not involve the cerebral cortex, and indeed may be some distance away (e.g., in the cerebellum). Activation of muscles and spread of the myoclonic activity is in a rostrocaudal direction, down the brainstem and spinal cord, via rapidly conducting corticospinal pathways.

Subcortical myoclonus typically originates in the thalamus or particularly the brainstem (reticular myoclonus). Myoclonus can be spontaneous or reflex, and is often induced by visual or auditory stimuli. Reticular myoclonus generally begins in the mid or lower brainstem and spreads simultaneously to rostral and caudal muscles; thus multichannel EMG assessment shows activation of cranial nerve XI-innervated muscles first followed by simultaneous spread upward to facial and trigeminal innervated muscles (in that order) and downward to upper cervical muscles, etc.

Another form of myoclonus originating in the brainstem is "branchial myoclonus" or palatal myoclonus, now often referred to as palatal tremor. This rhythmical myoclonus, usually of 1–2 Hz, involves muscles of the soft palate and may be associated with abnormal movements of the eyes and similar rhythmical movements of face, limbs, and trunk. This is considered a "segmental myoclonus" of brainstem origin, comparable to spinal forms of segmental myoclonus.

Spinal myoclonus originates in the spinal cord. Two distinct forms are propriospinal and segmental. Propriospinal myoclonus typically involves the axial musculature, and it can be spontaneous or stimulus-induced. Movements usually involve axial flexion but less often extension predominates. Muscle activation spreads rostrally and caudally over many segments and speed of propagation suggests conduction over the polysynaptic propriospinal pathways rather than the more rapid conduction found in other forms of myoclonus originating from supraspinal sites (e.g., cortical myoclonus). Segmental myoclonus is often spontaneous and rhythmic, with a typical frequency of 1–2 Hz. It is generally not stimulus-sensitive. It involves muscles over one or more myotomal segments and is often caused by an underlying intramedullary lesion.

Finally, myoclonus is also classified according to etiology and it includes physiologic, essential, epileptic, and symptomatic forms. Physiologic myoclonus arises in normal healthy subjects. Examples of physiologic myoclonus are hypnic jerks and hiccups. Essential myoclonus may be sporadic or inherited. These patients often have additional postural tremor or dystonia. The condition, now known as myoclonus-dystonia, probably incorporates a variety of previously separate conditions including essential myoclonus and some forms of dystonia or tremor. Epileptic myoclonus arises in the context of seizures, including many inherited generalized epileptic syndromes and the progressive myoclonic epilepsies. Symptomatic myoclonias are seen in the context of an underlying encephalopathy, and the differential diagnosis is extensive.

The causes of myoclonus and its classification are provided in Table 1.7.

Other movement disorders

There are a variety of movement disorders that do not fit the above categories. Akathisia is relatively common and since it is often drug-induced, it deserves further consideration here. Akathisia refers to a sense of restlessness and a need to move. Typically, the patient performs a variety of purposeful or semi-purposeful, often complex, movements in response to the subjective restlessness, including pacing when standing, marching in place, rocking, shifting weight, moving legs when sitting, picking at clothing or hair, rubbing body parts with hands, and other similar movements.

Another disorder in which movements occur secondary to the subjective need to move is the restless legs syndrome. Here, unlike in akathisia, the patient typically complains of a variety of sensory disturbances in the legs, including pins and needles, creeping or crawling sensations, aching, itching, stabbing, heaviness, tension, burning, or coldness. Occasionally, similar symptoms are appreciated in the upper limbs as well. These symptoms are usually experienced during recumbency in the evening and are often associated with insomnia. This condition is commonly associated with another movement disorder, periodic leg movements of sleep (sometimes inappropriately termed nocturnal myoclonus). These periodic, slow, sustained (1–2 seconds) movements range from synchronous or asynchronous dorsiflexion of the first toes and feet to triple flexion of one or both legs. More rapid myoclonic movements or slower, prolonged dystonic-like movements of the feet and legs also may be present in these patients while awake (so called "dyskinesia while awake," DWA).

Another uncommon but well-defined movement disorder of the lower limbs has been termed painful legs and moving toes. Here, the patient typically complains of a deep pulling or searing pain in the lower limbs, associated with continuous wriggling or writhing of the toes. Occasionally, the ankle

Table 1.7 Classification and causes of myoclonus

1. Physiologic myoclonus
Sleep myoclonus
Anxiety-induced myoclonus
Exercise-induced myoclonus
Hiccups
Benign infantile myoclonus during feeding

2. Essential myoclonus
Essential myoclonus*
  Hereditary
  Sporadic
Myoclonus-dystonia*

3. Epileptic myoclonus
Fragments of epilepsy
  Isolated epileptic myoclonic jerks
  Photosensitive myoclonus
  Myoclonic absences
  Epilepsia partialis continua
  Idiopathic stimulus-sensitive myoclonus
Childhood myoclonic epilepsies
  Infantile spasms
  Lennox-Gastaut syndrome
  Cryptogenic myoclonus epilepsy
  Juvenile myoclonic epilepsy of Janz
Benign familial myoclonic epilepsy
Baltic myoclonus (Unverricht-Lundborg)

4. Symptomatic myoclonus
Storage disease
  Lafora body disease
  Lipidoses
  Neuronal ceroid lipufuscinosis
  Sialidosis
Spinocerebellar degeneration
  Friedreich's ataxia
  Ataxia-telangiectasia
  Other spinocerebellar degenerations
Basal ganglia degenerations
  Wilson's disease
  Idiopathic torsion dystonia
  Hallervorden-Spatz disease
  Progressive supranuclear palsy
  Cortico-basal degeneration
  Parkinson's disease
  Multiple system atrophy
  Huntington's disease
  Dentatorubropallidoluysian atrophy
Mitochondrial cytopathies
Dementias
  Alzheimer's disease
  Creutzfeldt-Jakob disease
  Dementia with Lewy bodies

Viral encephalopathies
  Subacute sclerosing panencephalitis
  Encephalitis lethargica
  Herpes Simplex encephalitis
  Arbovirus encephalitis
  HIV
  Postinfectious encephalitis
Metabolic
  Hepatic failure
  Renal failure
  Dialysis dysequilibrium syndrome
  Hyponatremia
  Hypoglycemia
  Nonketotic hyperglycemia
  Infantile myoclonic encephalopathy
  Multiple carboxylase deficiency
  Biotin deficiency
Toxic
  Bismuth
  Heavy-metal poisoning
  Methyl bromide, DDT
  Drugs (multiple)
Physical encephalopathies
  Post-hypoxic myoclonus (Lance-Adams)
  Post-traumatic
  Heat stroke
  Electric shock
  Decompression injury
Focal CNS damage
  Stroke
  Post-thalamotomy
  Tumor
  Trauma
  Spinal cord lesions
Paraneoplastic syndromes
Psychogenic myoclonus

*Might represent the same entity.
Adapted from Fahn, Marsden, Van Woert [6].

and less commonly more proximal muscles of the legs are involved. Rarely, a similar problem is seen in the upper limbs as well.

The term tardive dyskinesia encompasses a wide variety of abnormal movements due to chronic neuroleptic therapy. One of the most common forms of these movements involves the lower facial muscles and has been given a variety of names including "orobuccolinguomasticatory dyskinesia." The movements generally comprise repetitive chewing and smacking movements with the tongue, either briefly sticking out ("fly-catching" movements), or pushing out into the cheek ("bonbon sign"). Although the movements are somewhat choreic they are not as random as true chorea (some have used the confusing term "rhythmical chorea"). It is the more stereotypic, repetitive nature of the movements, involving not only face but limbs, that has encouraged the more recent term "tardive stereotypies."

There are a number of disorders in which abnormal or excessive startle occurs. In some patients, one simply finds an exaggerated startle response that habituates poorly after repeated stimuli. In others, there is an abnormal response to the stimuli that normally evokes startle. Hyperekplexia (or hyperexplexia), also known as "startle disease," may be more akin to certain forms of myoclonus than to a normal startle response. A variety of other unusual disorders, first described in the 19th century, manifest excessive startle. The jumping Frenchmen of Main, latah, and myriachit also demonstrate sudden striking out, echo phenomenon, automatic obedience, and several other less common features.

Some abnormal movements occur intermittently rather than in a persistent fashion. This is typical of tics and certain forms of myoclonus. Dystonia often occurs only with specific actions, but this is usually a consistent response to the action rather than periodic or unpredictable. A small group of patients with chorea and/or dystonia have bouts of sudden-onset, short-lived involuntary movements known as paroxysmal choreoathetosis. In some the episodes can be precipitated by volitional movements and are referred to as kinesigenic. These episodes are typically shorter and more frequent than nonkinesigenic forms. Response to therapy is quite different for these two types.

There are numerous abnormal movements caused by dysfunction of the peripheral nerves (e.g., fasciculations, myokimia). These are usually easily separated from the movement disorders described above. Hemifacial spasm is a common disorder in which irregular tonic and clonic movements involve the muscles innervated by the facial nerve. Eyelid twitching is usually the first symptom followed at variable intervals by lower facial muscle involvement. Rarely both sides of the face are affected, in which case the spasms are asynchronous in contrast to other pure facial dyskinesias such as cranial dystonia.

Conclusion

We have reviewed the most common movement disorders, emphasizing accurate definitions and correct characterization of phenomenology in approaching their classification. The field is rapidly evolving, especially the genetic aspect of these diseases and the classification will probably change in the future to reflect our better understanding of the pathophysiology of these disorders. In the mean time, the physician who understands this basic approach to movement disorders will be able to accurately recognize them and be able to take the appropriate steps in investigating and treating them.

References

1. Deuschl G, Bain P, Brin M. Consensus statement of the Movement Disorder Society on tremor. Mov Disord 1998; 13(suppl 3): 2–23.

2. Fahn S, Bressman SB, Marsden CD. Classification of dystonia. Adv Neurol 1998; 78: 1–10.

3. Jankovic J. Differential diagnosis and etiology of tics. Adv Neurol 2001; 85: 15–29.

4. Leckman JF, Peterson BS, King RA, et al. Phenomenology of tics and natural history of tic disorders. Adv Neurol 2001; 85: 1–14.

5. Obeso, JA. Classification, clinical features, and treatment of myoclonus. In Watts RL, Koller WC (eds) Movement Disorders – Neurologic Principles and Practice. New York, McGraw-Hill, 1997, pp. 541–550.

6. Fahn S, Marsden CD, Van Woert MH. Definition and classification of myoclonus. Adv Neurol 1986; 43: 1–5.

CHAPTER 2

Rating scales for movement disorders

Ikwunga Wonodi, Elliot L. Hong, Matthew T. Avila, and Gunvant K. Thaker

Introduction

Clinical practice and research share in common the synthesis of symptoms (subjective accounts by patients), and signs (objective observations elicited by the clinician), into diagnostic categories. A diagnosis is a hypothesis on the etiology of a disease, its pathophysiology, and a prediction of its course and outcome (prognosis).

The utilization of signs and symptoms to monitor disease progression or recovery is the hallmark of clinical medical practice or research.

In the early 1950s, the introduction of medications in the treatment of neuropsychiatric disorders led to radical and optimistic changes in the management of these disorders that otherwise were treated empirically and associated with progressive disability, and life-long institutional care of patients. One such class of medications was the neuroleptics used in the treatment of psychotic disorders, and shortly thereafter, levodopa for the treatment of Parkinson's disease. Five years after the introduction of chlorpromazine Delay and Deniker in 1952 and then Schonecker in 1957 [1, 2] described what were probably the first reported cases of extrapyramidal syndrome (EPS) and tardive dyskinesia (TD). The problem of involuntary movements, the core symptomatology in Parkinson's disease, already existed in medical practice prior to the arrival of the promising era of psychopharmacology. However, before the introduction of levodopa, the existing treatment for Parkinson's disease, pioneered in 1946 by Dr Russell Meyer, was stereotactic basal ganglia surgery. Occurring in tandem with these developments was the need to standardize observations recorded by clinicians.

The crucial need for standardized instruments for recording involuntary movements was thus defined along two lines: first to validate the claims and reproducibility of treatment efficacy of stereotactic surgery versus levodopa, in Parkinson's disease, and secondly, to monitor the emergence of neuroleptic-induced involuntary movements in temporal sequence to antipsychotic treatment. Crane is credited with the introduction of the first rating scales for recording hyperkinetic movement [3].

Today the neuropsychiatric community is attuned to several drug-induced movement disorders, and there are a growing number of assessment tools available. As with any assessment instrument, a number of factors must be considered in choosing a particular scale including item format (e.g., ordinal or interval vs. nominal scale items), factor structure (single- vs. multi-factor scales), scale and factor reliability (i.e., internal consistency), rater reliability, and the available evidence for a scale's validity (e.g., content and construct validity, predictive validity). This chapter describes a number of rating scales – focusing on those with published psychometric information, and is designed to serve as a guide to both clinicians and researchers in selecting an appropriate instrument.

Rating scales for drug-induced akathisia

The term *akathisia* was first coined by Haskovec in 1902 and may be translated literally as "not to sit" (from the Greek *"kathisia"* – "the act of sitting" and *"a"* – negative prefix); he considered akathisia to be a hysterical or neurasthenic symptom. Following the introduction of antipsychotic drugs, the term was adopted to describe features of motor restlessness occurring as a side effect of these agents. Akathisia is arguably the most common, and one of the most distressing symptoms associated with antipsychotic drugs. The syndrome is characterized by objective signs of motoric agitation, with inability to remain seated, shifting in place, shuffling from foot to foot and/or pacing, and subjective complaints of distress, and restlessness usually referable to the legs. The prevalence of drug-induced akathisia (DIA) varies widely in the literature from 12.5% to 75% with the generally accepted prevalence being approximately 20%. The wide variation is partly explained by differential ability of clinicians to recognize this syndrome, use of high- or low-potency first-generation antipsychotic (FGA) including some of the second-generation antipsychotic agents, and other medications with similar dopamine receptor antagonism, to a lack of a unified consensus between clinicians on criteria for its diagnosis. Some clinicians failed to include subjective accounts of restlessness as DIA.

Inconsistencies in the phenomenological descriptions of akathisia stemmed from the initial difficulties encountered in standardizing rating of the subjective and objective symptoms of DIA. This posed the greatest challenge for clinicians attempting to delineate DIA from other movement disorders seen in drug-treated patients. These include resting tremor, dystonia, tardive dyskinesia, tics, stereotypies, and mannerisms, a critical factor that delayed the development of specific scales to rate this disorder. The proper identification and evaluation of akathisia is of crucial importance given its widespread occurrence and its significant impact on the clinical management of psychiatric disorders.

The evaluation of akathisia initially depended on the akathisia subscales incorporated into the early combined rating scales developed to assess other movement disorders. However, recent years have witnessed the development

Table 2.1 Akathisia rating scales

Akathisia rating scales	References	Comments
Barnes Akathisia Scale	[4]	4-item scale, global impression
Hillside Akathisia Scale	[5]	Modification of Simpson/Angus scale, poor reliability in rating, arms, head and trunk, global impression
Prince Henry Hospital Akathisia Rating Scale	[6]	Similar to Barnes, no global impression, intermediate ease of use between BAS and HAS

of scales specifically designed to rate akathisia. There are several well-designed and user-friendly akathisia rating scales (see Table 2.1). However, this chapter will focus on four scales specifically designed for rating akathisia with published reliability data on their psychometric properties. In addition, the selected scales rate akathisia separately on subjective complaints and objective findings.

The Barnes Akathisia Scale (BARS, BAS) was developed by Braude and Barnes and modified by Barnes [4]. It is a 4-item scale: objective (scored "0–3"), subjective awareness of restlessness (0–3), a subscale of the subjective items which scores distress related to restlessness, and a global impression rating for overall disorder. These items are scored with the patient seated, standing, and lying. The BARS has advantages over the other scales in that (1) subjective akathisia is rated in terms of awareness and distress, (2) patients are rated in a variety of positions (sitting and standing) and settings (during formal interview and while carrying out day-to-day activities), and (3) a global assessment of akathisia is made. However, its rigorous detail (a 23-item scale) might make its application cumbersome in clinical settings.

The Hillside Akathisia Scale (HAS), a modification of the Simpson-Angus EPS Scale, has two subjective and three objective items for which anchor points are provided, resulting in good interrater reliability among trained raters (HAS) [5]. The scale also rates akathisia in a variety of positions, during activation (serial calculations and finger tapping), and has a yes-or-no response to the presence of other neuropsychiatric phenomena (objective). There is an 8-item global impression scale for akathisia. The HAS is a reliable rating scale for akathisia; however, reliability is poor when rating akathisia in head, trunk, and in the arms.

The Prince Henry Hospital Akathisia (PHHA) Rating Scale [6] is adapted from Braude et al. [7], and is similarly itemized as the BAS. The scale has three subjective and seven objective items with the objective items performed sitting (4 scores) and standing (3 scores). Unlike the BAS, there is no global score. However, the scores rated on a 4-point scale slightly differ from the structure of other scales in that point "1" is for mild but definite akathisia. The PHHA scale has undergone further standardization in its administration with a resultant improvement in its construct validity. In complexity, and ease of use, it might be considered an intermediate between the BAS and the HAS.

Rating scales for drug-induced parkinsonian bradykinesia, rigidity, and tremor

Rating scales for movement disorders were born out of the need to objectively document the treatment results for Parkinson's disease. In the 1950s, the development of stereotactic surgery and later the arrival of levodopa made it possible to effectively control disabling parkinsonian symptoms. It soon became apparent that standardized recording methods were imperative to monitor and compare treatment efficacy. For the next 20 years, more and more rating scales for Parkinson's disease were introduced. Many rating scales were developed for clinical trials by researchers conducting particular studies to record pre- and posttrial symptomatology. The most common critiques of many of the rating scales introduced in this way are their lack of internal consistency and difficulty in achieving good interrater reliabilities on individual items or the total scores.

In the 1980s, serious efforts were made to correct the problem. The result was the now most widely used Unified Parkinson's Disease Rating Scale (UPDRS). The UPDRS consists of six areas related to Parkinson's disease: Part I: Behavior, including psychiatric and motivational scores; Part II, Activity of Daily Living; Part III: Motor examination; Part IV: Additional complications of disease or treatment (e.g., dystonia, dyskinesia); Part V: Hoehn and Yahr staging; and Part VI: Schwab and England Activities of Daily Living Scale. Most pertinent to drug-induced parkinsonian symptoms is Part III, the motor examination scale. Recent data suggested a high internal consistency for bradykinesia, rigidity, and tremor factors when used in patients with Parkinson's disease of all stages [8]. Both interrater and test-retest reliability were examined and found satisfactory in large samples or multicenter studies [9, 10]. With little doubt, the collective effort in neurology had created a rating scale that has survived statistical examination and has been embraced by more and more clinicians and researchers.

In contrast, the effort to develop rating scales specific for drug-induced parkinsonian symptoms has been far less systematic. The first and once most widely used scale for neuroleptic-induced parkinsonism, the Simpson-Angus Scale [11], was also the most criticized one. The scale is composed of 10 items of objective signs, rated 0–4 in severity. Specific instructions for the examination for each item are given. However, interrater reliability varied widely among the items. Part of the reason may be due to its somewhat unconventional way of conducting the examination, which made it difficult to reach consistency among raters. The construction of the items, including one for gait/bradykinesia, six for rigidity of various body parts, and one for tremor, is oddly imbalanced.

Several efforts were made to modify the Simpson-Angus Scale [12–15]. In addition, replacement of rater's judgment with laboratory-based measures was also attempted [16]. While each rating method showed promise, few had been employed by researchers other than those who introduced them. Reliability studies of these modifications outside the developing team were also scarce. Clearly, the development of a rating scale for neuroleptic-induced parkinsonian symptoms has been stalled at the stage reminiscent of pre-UPDRS in neurology.

Therefore, there is clearly a need for instruments with consensus, either by carefully testing the existing rating scales, or constructing new ones. Meanwhile, it is not unreasonable to use the UPDRS as an instrument for neuroleptic-induced parkinsonian signs and symptoms. Recent application of UPDRS in psychiatric patients has shown an excellent quantification of parkinsonian features in neuroleptic-induced parkinsonism [17]. There is need to establish the reliability of the UPDRS or its subscales in this population.

Rating scales for drug-induced dyskinesia

A number of scales for the documentation of drug-related tardive dyskinesia have been developed and undergone comprehensive analyses of reliability and validity. In contrast, dyskinesia-rating scales used by neurologists to assess Huntington's disease or Parkinson's disease are less developed [18]. The great attention given for standardizing the assessment of tardive dyskinesia in psychiatry has several reasons. First, tardive dyskinesia is highly prevalent affecting about 25% of patients chronically treated with FGAs. Many cases of tardive dyskinesia were considered irreversible and difficult to treat – the arrival of second-generation antipsychotic (SGA) agents only moderately changed the situation. Secondly, tardive dyskinesia is often debilitating, publicly embarrassing, and in severe cases can cause secondary injury (e.g., lip ulcerations, bruises, and joint inflammation). Moreover, it is one of the most likely causes of litigation against psychiatrists.

The Abnormal Involuntary Movement Scale (AIMS) [19] is the most widely used. It is constructed only for tardive dyskinesia, and does not include drug-induced parkinsonian features such as tremor. It rates dyskinesia in seven body parts on a 5-point scale. It requires simple training and is easy to use. The interrater and test-retest reliabilities of the scale are excellent usually above 0.85. It has become a trade standard – most new scales were developed by comparing their scale's performance to that of the AIMS. It is also the most popular scale for evaluating involuntary movement among practicing clinicians.

The Dyskinesia Identification System-Coldwater (DIS-Co) has a reported interrater and test-retest reliability of 0.78 and 0.77, respectively [20]. The scale has 34 items divided for 10 body parts on a 5-point scale. The overall scheme of the scale is similar to AIMS, but gives more detailed assessment. An abbreviated version with 15 items is also available [21].

The Simpson/Rockland Tardive Dyskinesia Rating Scale [11] also contains 34 items, each being rated on a 6-point scale, plus nine unspecified items for unusual symptoms. Unlike the AIMS and DIS-Co, it contains items assessing akathisia and tremor. It is therefore not a rating scale strictly for tardive dyskinesia as the title suggests. The reported interrater reliability is excellent, although the test-retest reliability does not seem well documented in the literature [18]. An abbreviated version has also been developed.

The Smith Tardive Dyskinesia Scale [22] is a 24-item scale for drug-induced tardive dyskinesia and parkinsonism. The subscores for tardive dyskinesia and parkinsonism can be separately obtained.

Combined rating scales

Some combined rating scales have been developed with the goal of enhancing the assessment of overall drug-induced extrapyramidal symptomatology. These scales were designed as multidimensional rating scales for the evaluation of antipsychotic-induced hyperkinesias, parkinsonism, akathisia, and dystonia (see Table 2.2). While the authors of these scales had simplicity of administration in mind, some of the scales have turned out, by reason of over inclusiveness, to be cumbersome to administer.

Table 2.2 Combined rating scales

Combined rating scales	References	Comments
Maryland Psychiatric Research Center Involuntary Movement Scale (IMS)	[23]	TD and parkinsonism in 11 anatomical areas, expanded ordinal scale: Global TD, Parkinsonism, Akathisia and Dystonia scores
St. Hans Rating Scale for Extrapyramidal Syndrome (SHRS)	[24]	Dystonia scale under development 4 components that rate: dyskinesia, parkinsonism, dystonia, and akathisia. Global scores Provision for recording Dyskinesia in activated and passive states
Extrapyramidal Symptoms Rating Scale (ESRS)	[25]	Twelve questionnaire items for subjective reports. Objective scale for Parkinsonism and Dyskinesia. Sensitive to change in severity
General Akathisia Tardive phenomena & Extrapyramidal rating Schedule (GATES)	[26]	Emphasis on ease of administration. Multi-item scale convertible to AIMS, BAS, and Simpson EPS scores. Scoring guide for ESRS included Akinesia, akathisia, dystonia, dyskinesia – acute and chronic. Unpublished psychometrics

Table 2.3 Rating scales for parkinsonian signs and symptoms

Rating scales for parkinsonian signs and symptoms	References	Comments
The Unified Parkinson's Disease Rating Scale (UPDRS)	[27]	Rates six clinical areas related to Parkinson's disease. Part III: Motor examination is most relevant to apply to drug-induced Parkinsonian signs and symptoms
Simpson-Angus Neurological Rating Scale	[11]	Ten neurological signs that are rated based on specific examination procedures. Inadequate reliability.
The Scale for Targeting Abnormal Kinetic Effects (TAKE)	[15]	Rates bradykinesia, rigidity, and tremor on a 0–4 severity scale. Parallels to that of the AIMS in design

Table 2.4 Rating scales for dyskinesia

Rating scales for dyskinesia	References	Comments
Abnormal Involuntary Movement Scale (AIMS)	[19]	Sufficient reliability, most widely used
The Dyskinesia Identification System-Coldwater (DIS-Co)	[20]	34 items targeting 10 body parts. Reliability and validity were assessed. An abbreviated version (DIS-CUS) is also available [23]
The Simpson/Rockland Tardive Dyskinesia Rating Scale	[11]	Rates bradykinesia, rigidity, and tremor on a 0–4 severity scale. Parallels to that of the AIMS in design
The Smith Tardive Dyskinesia Scale	[22]	24 items divided into tardive dyskinesia and parkinsonism subscores

In this chapter, the four combined scales that meet the criteria of a composite instrument with relative ease of administration, as well as reported interrater reliability, and validity are presented. These are: the Maryland Psychiatric Research Center Involuntary Movement Scale (IMS), the St. Hans Rating Scale for extrapyramidal syndrome (SHRS), the Extrapyramidal Symptom Rating Scale (ESRS), and the recently designed General Akathisia Tardive phenomena & Extrapyramidal rating Schedule (GATES).

The IMS was primarily intended for rating the severity of tardive dyskinesia and parkinsonism in clinical and research patients (see Tables 2.3 and 2.4). It offers ratings in 11 anatomical areas as well as a rating of gait and respiratory dyskinesias. These anatomical regions are rated in a total of 28 items. Unlike the Smith scale, the IMS has an expanded ordinal scale from 5 points to 8 points (0–7), giving it advantages in the greater discrimination of anatomic place and severity in the rating of involuntary movements. This makes the IMS a valuable instrument in performing neurophysiologic and psychopharmacologic research. In addition, there are global scores for dyskinesia, parkinsonism, and akathisia. There is an IMS dystonia version, which is still under development. The scale has excellent psychometric properties [23]. The strengths of the IMS are in the rating of dyskinesias and parkinsonism. In rating akathisia, only a global scale is scored. There is no discrimination of the subjective from objective symptoms and signs of akathisia.

The SHRS rates medication-induced hyperkinesias, parkinsonism, akathisia, and dystonia. In contrast to the AIMS, the SHRS, like the IMS, contains sections for scoring of parkinsonism, akathisia, and dystonia. Like the IMS, the SHRS has mainly been used in connection with video recording. The SHRS consists of four main components; an 8-item dyskinesia subscale with a global hyperkinesias score, an 8-item Parkinsonian subscale with a global parkinsonism score, a global dystonia scale, and a global akathisia scale scoring "psychic" and "motor" symptoms of akathisia. The scores are coded on a 7-point ordinal scale (0–6). Unlike the IMS and the AIMS, the SHS has provision for recording dyskinesia in activated and passive states. In addition, the SHRS has good psychometric qualities [24].

The ESRS consists of 12 questionnaire items to identify subjective symptomatology, a clinician's examination and scoring of Parkinsonian and dyskinetic movements, and a clinical global impression of tardive dyskinesia. Parkinsonian signs are scored on an 8-item scale, under which is included akathisia (the subjective part is noted among the nine parkinsonian symptoms in the questionnaire). Psychometrically, the ESRS was found to be sensitive in its ability to detect changes in both Parkinsonian and dyskinetic symptoms and to give results consistent with those from studies using standard scales such as the AIMS [25].

The GATES, designed with a major commitment toward providing utility for research assistants and junior staff, has three components – demographics, subjective, and objective. This instrument is able to produce scores for a broad range of medication-induced involuntary movements – rigidity, akinesia, akathisia, dystonia, and dyskinesia, both in acute and chronic presentation. In addition, scores for the Simpson EPS, Barnes' akathisia scale, and the AIMS are produced due to inclusion of operationally enhanced items from these scales. A scoring guide for use with the ESRS is also produced. In keeping with the commitment in its design, only a brief training in the assessment of physical signs is required to be able to administer the GATES. However, the psychometrics of the subscales are not reported [26], and the GATES while being quite thorough in its inclusion of involuntary movements, may have the property of being too cumbersome to administer in today's brief clinical encounters. It is graphical computer-based interview, and scoring and reporting programs confer advantages for use in clinical trials research.

In summary, we have provided a brief synopsis of a few rating scales for the evaluation of medication-induced movement disorders. We are aware that we may have left some good scales out of this chapter. However, we have attempted to introduce the reader to rating scales that are unbiased, reproducible, and fairly precise. To meet these criteria, a scale should have established psychometric properties. These are thus important points to be taken into consideration when clinicians and researchers make a decision on the choice of an instrument to use. Additionally, for rater training purposes, a brief mention of the role of video recordings is in place. They offer several advantages. They offer a crucial method of establishing both test-retest and interrater reliability in relation to certain types of disorder. In doing this they provide a permanent record in a cost-effective way and are suitable for training and education. They are also very useful in conducting clinical trials for reliability maintenance and to maintain the blind.

Acknowledgments

This work is supported in part by the American Psychiatric Association/ Community Mental Health Services Minority Fellowship Training Program, and the NIMH Research Track Residency Training Program Grant MH60487, and the IRC Grant MH40279.

References

1. Delay J, Deniker, P. Trente-huit cas de psychoses traits par la cure prolongee et continue de 4568 R. Ann Med Psychol 1952; 110; 364.
2. Schonecker M. Ein eigentumliches syndrom in oralen bereich bei megaphen applikation. Nervenartz 1957; 28: 35.
3. Crane GE, Paulson G. Involuntary movements in a sample of chronic mental patients and their relation to the treatment with neuroleptics. Int J Neuropsychiatry 1967; 3: 286–291.
4. Barnes TR. A rating scale for drug-induced akathesia. Br J Pharmacol 1989; 154: 672–676.
5. Fleischhacker WW, Miller CH, Schett P, et al. The Hillside Akathisia Scale: a reliability comparison of the English and German versions. Psychopharmacology (Berl) 1991; 105: 141–144.
6. Sachdev P. Drug-induced movement disorders in institutionalised adults with mental retardation: clinical characteristics and risk factors. Austr N Z J Psychiatry 1992; 26: 242–248.
7. Braude WM, Barnes TR, Gore SM (1983): Clinical characteristics of akathisia: A systematic investigation of acute psychiatric inpatient admissions. Br J Psychiatry 143: 139–150.
8. Stebbins GT, Goetz CG, Lang AE, et al. Factor analysis of the motor section of the unified Parkinson's disease rating scale during the off-state. Mov Disord 1999; 14: 585–589.
9. Richards M, Marder K, Cote L, et al. Interrater reliability of the Unified Parkinson's Disease Rating Scale motor examination. Mov Disord 1994; 9: 89–91.
10. Siderowf A, McDermott M, Kieburtz K, et al. Test-retest reliability of the unified Parkinson's disease rating scale in patients with early Parkinson's disease: results from a multicenter clinical trial. Mov Disord 2002; 17: 758–763.

11. Simpson G, Angus JSW. A rating scale for extrapyramidal side effects. Acta Psychiatr Scand 1970; 212: 11–19.

12. Lehmann HE, Ban TA, Saxena BM. A survey of extrapyramidal manifestations in the inpatient population of a psychiatric hospital. Laval Med 1970; 41: 909–916.

13. Mindham RH, Gaind R, Anstee BH, et al. Comparison of amantadine, orphenadrine, and placebo in the control of phenothiazine-induced parkinsonism. Psychol Med 1972; 2: 406–413.

14. Perenyi A, Bagdy G, Arato M, et al. Biochemical markers in the study of clinical effects and extrapyramidal side effects of neuroleptics. Psychiatry Res 1984; 13: 119–127.

15. Wojcik JD, Gelenberg AJ, LaBrie RA, et al. Prevalence of tardive dyskinesia in an outpatient population. Compr Psychiatry 1980; 21: 370–380.

16. Caligiuri MP, Bracha HS, Lohr JB. Asymmetry of neuroleptic-induced rigidity: development of quantitative methods and clinical correlates. Psychiatry Res 1989; 30: 275–284.

17. Hassin-Baer S, Sirota P, Korczyn AD, et al. Clinical characteristics of neuroleptic-induced parkinsonism. J Neural Transm 2001; 108: 1299–1308.

18. Hoff JI, van Hilten BJ, Roos RA. A review of the assessment of dyskinesias. Mov Disord 1999; 14: 737–743.

19. Guy W. ECDEU Assessment Manual for Psychopharmacology. U.S. Department of Health, Education and Welfare NIMH 1976; 76: 338.

20. Sprague RL, Kalachnik JE, Breuning SE, et al. The Dyskinesia Identification System–Coldwater (DIS-Co): a tardive dyskinesia rating scale for the developmentally disabled. Psychopharmacol Bull 1984; 20: 328–338.

21. Sprague RL, Kalachnik JE. Reliability, validity, and a total score cutoff for the dyskinesia identification system: condensed user scale (DISCUS) with mentally ill and mentally retarded populations. Psychopharmacol Bull 1991; 27: 51–58.

22. Smith JM, Kucharski LT, Eblen C, et al. An assessment of tardive dyskinesia in schizophrenic outpatients. Psychopharmacology (Berl) 1979; 64: 99–104.

23. Cassady SL, Thaker GK, Summerfelt A, et al. The Maryland Psychiatric Research Center scale for the characterization of involuntary movements. Psychiatry Res 1997; 70: 21–37.

24. Gerlach J, Korsgaard S, Clemmesen P, et al. The St. Hans Rating Scale for extrapyramidal syndromes: reliability and validity. Acta Psychiatr Scand 1993; 87: 244–252.

25. Chouinard G, Ross-Chouinard A, Annable L, et al. Extrapyramidal symptoms rating scale. Can J Neurol Sci 1980; 7: 233.

26. Lambert T. GATES: a new instrument for the clinical and research assessment of neuroleptic-induced movement disorders. Schizophr Res 1998; 29: 177.

27. Fahn S, Elton RL. Unified Parkinson's Disease Rating Scale in Recent Developments in Parkinson's Disease. Florham Park, NJ, Macmillan Healthcare Information, 1987.

CHAPTER 3

Spontaneous movement disorders in psychiatric patients

Irene Richard, Christopher O'Brien, and Roger Kurlan

Introduction

There are a variety of movement disorders that may accompany neuropsychiatric conditions and it is important that they be differentiated from those induced by drugs. For example, the characteristic chorea or dystonia of Huntington's disease may be difficult to distinguish from tardive dyskinesias caused by neuroleptics used to treat psychiatric symptoms of the illness. Furthermore, nearly every kind of movement disorder, including chorea, dystonia, athetosis, myoclonus, tics, tremor, and parkinsonism, may also be seen in psychiatric patients as part of a conversion disorder, malingering, or Munchausen's syndrome [1–3]. They will not be discussed further. Rather, we will concentrate on a different group of disorders of excessive or reduced movement that have generally been considered to fall within the realm of psychiatric patient populations. The hyperkinetic disorders of this group consist of a variety of complex repetitive movements and include habits, mannerisms, stereotypies, and compulsions. Specific examples of each of these disorders, such as tapping, touching, or posturing, may appear identical and may be impossible to differentiate by observation from each other or from the more classic types of movement disorders such as tics or dystonia. Categorization of the movements is largely based on the setting in which they occur. For example, repetitive foot tapping might be considered a habit for a normal person, a mannerism for a schizophrenic patient, a stereotypy for a severely retarded individual, a compulsion when performed in response to an obsessive thought pattern, or a complex motor tic for an individual with Tourette's syndrome. The hypokinetic conditions, including bradykinesia, catatonia, rigidity, catalepsy, negativism, and mutism, must generally be distinguished from various forms of neurodegenerative or drug-induced parkinsonism.

Hyperkinetic disorders

Habits

Habits are repetitive, coordinated movements that are commonly seen in otherwise normal individuals, particularly during times of anxiety,

Table 3.1 Common habits

Eyes
  Eye rubbing
Ears
  Ear rubbing, pulling, and picking
Nose
  Nose picking, scratching, and rubbing
Mouth
  Thumb and finger sucking, nail biting, picking at teeth, chewing tongue
Hair
  Hair, mustache, or beard pulling, rubbing and twirling
Head
  Head or chin scratching or rubbing
Hands
  Fist clenching, popping finger joints, nail picking, twiddling thumbs, finger tapping and
    drumming, manipulation of clothing, eyeglasses, or jewelry
Genitals
  Manipulation of genitals, thigh rubbing
Legs
  Foot tapping, abduction-adduction of legs

self-consciousness, boredom, or fatigue. Common examples of habits are shown in Table 3.1. Depending on their circumstance, identical actions might be classified as compulsions or complex motor tics. A variety of habits are seen in normal children, but they tend to disappear over time as they are learned to be socially inappropriate. Some habits, such as nose picking, may be socially offensive. Chain smoking and gum or tobacco chewing could be considered to fall within this group.

Some habits are particularly common in the course of normal development [4]. Finger (usually thumb) sucking, or substituted sucking of a pacifier, blanket, or other objects, is regarded as a normal habit in early childhood. It has been estimated to occur in 80% of all infants and usually disappears by the age of 3 or 4 years. Occasional finger sucking, however, persists in up to 30% of 12-year-olds. If finger sucking persists in severe form much beyond the age of 9 years, it tends to be associated with general emotional immaturity. The cause of finger sucking is unknown, but incompleteness of the sucking phase of feeding is a theory supported by the observation that if feeding of some domestic animals is interrupted prior to satiety, licking or sucking behaviors may appear.

Nail biting is a habit that usually appears between the ages of 4 and 6 years and is reported in 40–55% of adolescents. After puberty, its frequency declines rapidly so that only 20% of young adults continue to bite their nails. Whereas finger sucking is usually seen when the child is unoccupied or getting ready for bed, nail biting is associated with times of anxiety or stress. Pencil or pen biting and chewing gum may represent substituted behaviors for nail biting.

Mannerisms

A mannerism is a peculiar or unusual characteristic mode of performing a normal activity, such as eating or walking [4]. The term is applied to odd, idiosyncratic, or bizarre variations of normal human behavior. Many normal people possess a mannerism or two that may be regarded as no more than a slight eccentricity. Mannerisms may be used to attract attention, particularly in individuals who are insecure and wish to appear more confident than they actually are. Schizophrenic patients display an astonishing number of odd, senseless variations in normal activities for which the term "mannerism" has been applied. Some examples include bizarre gaits (e.g., lifting legs like a stork), unnatural, affective flourishes incorporated into eating behavior, imitating a famous person's behavior or speech, and a variety of distorted expressive gestures. Mannerisms may remain constant for years or may be altered constantly. Some mannerisms may be so extreme as to actually interfere with the underlying action. Schizophrenic speech may also be associated with manneristic qualities, such as speaking in rhyme, telegrammatic jargon, or adding "ism" to the end of every word.

Stereotypies

A stereotypy is a coordinated, repetitive, rhythmic, and patterned movement, posture, or vocalization that is carried out virtually in the same way during each repetition and is observed in an individual with defective mentation or deprived of visual or auditory sensory input. The movements are stereotypic in their form, body distribution, and amplitude, and the timing is predictable. Stereotypies may include simple (e.g., body rocking, smiling) or more complex (e.g., walking in circles, sitting down and arising from a chair) movements (Table 3.2).

Table 3.2 Common stereotypies

Mouth
  Bruxism, lip movements, biting, grimacing, smiling, frowning, vocalizations
    (e.g., snorting, blowing, groaning, hissing, singing, screaming)
Head
  Banging, nodding, shaking, weaving, bizarre posturing
Arms and Hands
  Finger waving and flicking before the eyes, holding hand at arm's length and watching
    the fingers move, finger drumming or pill-rolling movements, hand rubbing, fist
    pounding, hand to face, mouth, or ear movements, touching or stroking parts of the
    body, fragments of common actions (e.g., smoking, combing hair)
Trunk
  Body rocking, twirling, and circling, pelvic swaying and thrusting, sitting and arising
Legs
  Jumping, hopping, lotus position, walking in circles or back and forth
Self-Injurious Behavior
  Lip manipulation, hand biting, eye poking and gouging, scratching, self-beating

Table 3.3 Conditions associated with stereotypic behavior

Mental retardation
Autism
Pervasive developmental disorder of children
Rett syndrome
Neuroacanthocytosis
Childhood encephalopathies
   Viral encephalopathies
     Ceroid lipofuscinosis
     Phenylketonuria
Schizophrenia
Severe agitated depression
Tardive stereotypies (stereotyped orofacial dyskinesia of tardive dyskinesia)
Akathisia (acute or tardive)
Congenital blindness
Congenital deafness
Development stereotypies

While the movements are usually uniform, at times incomplete forms of a given stereotypy may be seen. For example, instead of rocking the body back and forth, a patient may merely nod the head. Stereotypies are generally considered to be involuntary and non-goal-directed. However, as these movements are characteristically seen in individuals with severe cognitive impairment whose motivation cannot be assessed, the true intentional quality of these behaviors remains to be clarified. Indeed, it has been suggested that stereotypies may be purposeful in that they serve as a form of self-stimulation. When not accompanied by severe cognitive deficit, stereotypies can be temporarily suppressed. Although patients usually have little control over stereotypies, the movements often decrease when the patients engage in activities such as counting or drawing. Conditions in which stereotypies occur are listed in Table 3.3.

Mental retardation and autistic disorders are characteristically associated with stereotypies [5]. In one study of 102 institutionalized mentally retarded adults, 34% demonstrated at least one type of stereotypy, including rhythmic movements (26%), bizarre posturing (13%), and object manipulation (7%) [6]. Stereotypies, including self-stimulatory behavior, often constitute the most recognizable features of children and adults with autism of any cause [7–9]. Rett syndrome is an autistic disorder reported only in girls and associated with a mutation in the MECPZ gene at X_q 28 [10], which is characterized by stereotypic movements and other movement disorders [11]. The most common stereotypies include hand wringing, washing, clapping, clenching, patting, and rubbing. In addition, other stereotypic behaviors may be seen, such as body rocking, shifting of weight from one leg to the other, bruxism, and ocular deviations. In patients with mental retardation and autism, stereotypic self-injurious behavior may be observed. This seems particularly evident in patients with body rocking, a stereotypy most often associated with self-hitting [12]. While head banging and other self-injurious behavior may occur in normal children, this type of behavior is usually abnormal [13].

Childhood onset pervasive developmental disorder, a condition that is similar to autism but has a later age at onset and does not present with the complete clinical picture of autism, is also associated with stereotypic behavior. Children with encephalopathy caused by phenylketonuria, infantile ceroid lipofuscinosis (hand "knitting" stereotypies) [14], or a prenatal viral infection such as rubella or cytomegalovirus, may develop an autistic syndrome with stereotypies.

A variety of stereotypic behaviors were described in schizophrenic patients long before the introduction of neuroleptic drug therapy. Stereotypies are particularly characteristic of the catatonic variety [15]. Stereotypic maintenance of unusual postures, shifting position, repetitively moving mouth and jaw, tapping or touching objects, and repetitive verbalizations are typical motor features of the catatonic state. When catatonia is associated with stereotypic behavior, the diagnosis of mania should be considered [16]. Particularly strange and excessive stereotypic behavior may be seen in catatonic and other severe psychiatric disorders for which the terms "parakinesia" [17], "bizarrery," or "grotesquery" [18] have been applied.

Children with congenital deafness and blindness may also exhibit a variety of stereotypic behaviors [19]. Stereotypies are generally much more bizarre and highly repetitive in autistic children than in those with a disordered special sensory system. The stereotypies of visually disturbed children, however, may at times strongly resemble those of autism. The stereotypies of deaf children are accompanied by noises, whereas those of blind children are not. It has been suggested that severe mental retardation or autism may represent forms of sensory deprivation, analogous to congenital deafness or blindness, in that external stimuli are not processed in a cognitively appropriate fashion.

The term "stereotypy" is often employed to describe patterned and repetitive movements in other settings, although we prefer usage that is restricted to patients with severely defective mentation or severe congenital hearing or visual loss. No clear, generally accepted definition of this movement disorder has been formulated. At least some stereotyped activities, such as sucking and clasping behaviors, are associated with normal neonatal motor patterns that function to maintain close contact with the mother and that have generally been considered reflexive. With further development, other stereotypic behaviors may appear, including body rocking, bruxism, and head banging, the latter seen in up to 15% of normal children. One might consider these behaviors to represent a form of "physiological" or "developmental" stereotypy, representing a process similar to the recognized developmental chorea and dystonia of infancy and childhood [20]. Stereotypies are also commonly observed in otherwise normal children during times of emotional excitement.

The most typical form of tardive dyskinesia, the orofacial-lingual-masticatory movement, has often been classified as a choreic disorder.

However, as the movements are less random and more predictable than classic chorea, it has been labeled by some as "rhythmic" chorea or stereotypy [5]. Since all known types of involuntary movement disorders can result from the use of neuroleptic drugs, it would not be unexpected that drug-induced stereotypies may occur as well. The repetitive restless movements of patients with akathisia, such as crossing and uncrossing of legs, arising and sitting down, marching in place, and picking at clothes, have also been called stereotypic [5]. Stereotypic behavior is common in animals, particularly those housed in restraining environments with low stimulation [5, 21]. With the development of stereotypies, there is a reduction in the spectrum of behaviors normally displayed by unrestrained animals. Therefore, stereotypy has been viewed as either a self-generating sensory stimulus or a motor expression of underlying tension and anxiety [5]. Unfortunately, such animal stereotypic behavior as repetitive biting, turning, and circling are not clearly related to similar behaviors in man [22].

Developmental and behavioral theories have been proposed [23] to explain the origin of stereotypies in man. It has been suggested that social isolation may convert normal developmental stereotypic behavior into autistic stereotypies such as thumb sucking or self-clasping, a concept that has been confirmed for primates and other animals that are isolated in development [24]. The appearance of stereotypic behavior in mentally retarded children may be related to a tendency for these children to be physically isolated or for them to be effectively isolated by their mental dysfunction. Alternatively, it has been proposed that stereotypies in these children may represent an attempt to decrease what is interpreted as an overstimulating environment [25]. Others have suggested that stereotypies are an attempt to increase self-stimulation to a predetermined level [26]. One behavioral theory suggests that stereotypies arise from essentially normal behaviors that are further shaped and reinforced by a process of operant conditioning [26].

Most studies of stereotypic behavior in experimental animals have emphasized the role of dopaminergic systems in the basal ganglia and limbic structures [5, 23]. Intrastriatal injection of dopamine and systemic administration of dopaminergic drugs, such as amphetamine or apomorphine, in rats produces dose-related stereotypic behavior [27–30]. These stereotypies can be prevented by pretreatment with dopamine receptor antagonist drugs [27]. Studies indicate that the D2 dopamine receptor subtype mediates stereotypic behavior in animals and that activation of D1 receptors potentiates these D2-mediated effects [28–30]. A correlation between amphetamine-induced stereotypic behavior and striatal extracellular release of dopamine and serotonin has been demonstrated using the technique of in vivo microdialysis in freely moving rats [31]. Brain neuropeptides, such as cholecystokinin, neurotensin, and opioids, particularly in limbic sites, may play an important role in the pathogenesis of stereotypic behavior [32]. The relevance of the stereotypic behaviors seen in animals to those seen in humans remains unclear. Furthermore, stereotypies

Table 3.4 Common compulsions

Excessive or ritualistic hand washing, showering, bathing, toothbrushing, or grooming
Repeated rituals (going in/out door, up/down from chair, etc.)
Checking (doors, locks, stove, appliances, emergency brake on car, etc.)
Rituals to remove contact with contaminants
Touching
Measures to prevent harm to self or others
Ordering, arranging
Counting
Hoarding, collecting
Cleaning household or inanimate objects

appear differently in different species and the term "stereotypy" is often used in the scientific literature of animal research to describe activities that are not clearly stereotyped [21].

Compulsions

Compulsions are repetitive and seemingly purposeful behaviors that are often performed according to certain rules (i.e., are ritualistic) and are often carried out in order to ward off anticipated future harm or a dreaded event. For example, repetitive hand washing is done to prevent contamination or disease, or an individual may believe that repetitive counting of objects will prevent harm from coming to a loved one. In this respect, compulsions occur in response to an obsessive thought pattern. Obsessions are defined as recurrent, persistent ideas, thoughts, images, or impulses that are not experienced as voluntarily produced but rather as thoughts that invade consciousness and are experienced as senseless or repugnant. Attempts are made to ignore or suppress them. Obsessions are usually unpleasant and may be frightening or violent. Examples of common compulsions and obsessions are shown in Tables 3.4 and 3.5 [33].

A pervasive pattern of compulsive perfectionism and inflexibility, including excessive devotion to work, indecisiveness, restricted expression of affection,

Table 3.5 Common obsessions

Concern with dirt, germs, environmental toxins
Something terrible happening (fire, death/illness of self or loved one)
Symmetry, order, exactness
Scrupulosity (religious)
Concern or disgust with bodily wastes or secretions (urine, stool, saliva)
Lucky or unlucky numbers
Forbidden, aggressive, or perverse sexual thoughts, image, or impulses
Fear might harm others, self

From [33].

and lack of generosity, is referred to as obsessive-compulsive personality disorder. For individuals in whom obsessions and/or compulsions interfere with normal daily functioning, the diagnosis of obsessive-compulsive disorder (OCD) is made. OCD is classified as an anxiety disorder since obsessive thought patterns are associated with the development of anxiety, which may in turn be relieved by performance of compulsions. Interference with the patient's ability to carry out compulsive behavior is also anxiety-provoking. First symptoms of OCD usually occur by the early twenties, may begin suddenly or slowly, and often have an episodic course.

Obsessive-compulsive symptoms are common in other psychiatric illnesses as well. About 20% of patients with major depression have obsessive symptoms. As reviewed by Lysaker et al. [34], between 30% and 59% of those with schizophrenia experience significant obsessive or compulsive symptomatology [35, 36] and 8–23% would actually meet the criteria for OCD [37, 38]. Several investigators have suggested that schizophrenia with obsessive-compulsive symptoms may represent a unique subgroup within the schizophrenic spectrum [39–42].

There is a clear (but complex) interrelationship between OCD and tics. At least 17% of adults with OCD have tics, and increased rates of tics are reported in their relatives [43]. Approximately 50% of patients with Tourette's syndrome (TS) will show evidence of obsessive-compulsive symptoms [44, 45] and an increased prevalence of OCD is reported in first-degree relatives of TS patients independently of concurrent OCD in these probands [46]. One family study on OCD has indicated that OCD is probably heterogeneous in origin, with familial forms, one tic-related, the other not, and a form that is neither tic-related nor familial [47]. There may be some differences in the OCD symptoms between patients with tics and those without tics. Studies suggest that, in patients with tics, mental play, echophenomena, touching, symmetry behaviors, self-injurious behaviors, and aggressive and violent obsessions are more frequent, whereas OCD patients without tics report more contamination obsessions and washing behaviors [43, 48–53]. Hanna et al. [54] assessed 60 OCD patients and found that 15 had a lifetime history of tics and 45 patients had no tic history. There was no difference between the two groups in obsession categories. However, there was a significant difference between the two groups in compulsions. Ordering, hoarding, and washing compulsions were more common in those with no tic history.

Abnormalities of the central serotonergic system are thought to underlie OCD and the selective serotonin reuptake inhibitor (SSRI) antidepressants have proven to be very effective in its treatment [55, 56]. However, tic-related OCD seems to show a diminished response to SSRI treatment as compared to tic-free OCD, and treatment response is probably enhanced by the addition of dopamine-blocking agents [57, 58]. This is not surprising since abnormalities of the dopaminergic system have been strongly implicated in the development of tics [59]. Disruption of basal ganglia-frontal lobe connections with psychosurgical procedures (particularly anterior capsulotomy and cingulotomy) has been used therapeutically with same success in a limited number of patients with disabling OCD [60, 61]. Furthermore, preliminary results from recent trials [62] suggest that deep brain stimulation (DBS) in the anterior limb of the internal capsule may be of benefit for treatment-resistant OCD.

Proposed etiologies for OCD include genetic susceptibility [63], neurophysiologic abnormalities (primarily involving the neurotransmitter serotonin), and regional brain dysfunction (particularly involving the basal ganglia and frontal cortical connections) [60, 64–69]. More recently, poststreptococcal autoimmunity has been postulated as a novel etiologic mechanism for the development of childhood onset OCD and/or tics in a minority of cases. The term "pediatric autoimmune neuropsychiatric disorders associated with streptococcal infections" (PANDAS) has been applied to this subgroup of patients. There is evidence supporting an autoimmune hypothesis, which contends that strep infections trigger an abnormal immune response and subsequent inflammatory changes likely affecting the basal ganglia [70–72].

Although compulsions may at times be difficult to differentiate from complex motor tics, certain characteristics of compulsions are helpful in making this distinction. Compulsions are often associated with obsessions and/or performed in response to an obsessive thought. Furthermore, compulsions are performed according to certain rules while tics are not. The presence of such rules indicates a ritualistic disorder, and examples include performance of an action a specified number of times, in a specified order, or at a specified time of day (e.g., bedtime rituals). Thus, a patient who must tap the floor in multiples of three prior to rising from a chair is likely experiencing compulsive tapping, while patients who tap with no specified rule may be showing tapping tics. Compulsions may be performed to ward off some feared consequence, although this history is usually absent in Tourette's patients with OCD. Finally, as noted above, tics usually respond favorably to neuroleptic medications and compulsions do not, but rather often they improve following treatment with antidepressant medications that preferentially block serotonin reuptake.

Hypokinetic disorders

Motor disturbances characterized by slowness or paucity of movement are commonly encountered in psychiatric populations. Historically, patients with such hypokinetic conditions have been classified under a variety of headings. Catatonia, stupor, negativism, and catalepsy are terms that have been used, at times interchangeably [23, 73–75].

One can conceptually divide the hypokinetic disorders into active and passive types. Active immobility is brought about by increased muscle tone or effort, such as maintaining a bizarre posture against gravity. In contrast, passive immobility is related to reduced muscle tone or activation. The limp and inactive posture of a depressed person serves as an example. Active and passive

Active   Passive

Immobility   Immobility

Catatonia	Rigidity	Bradykinesia
Lethal Catatonia	Mutism	Akinesia
Catalepsy		Hypomimia
Waxy flexibility		Gagenhalten
Mitmachen		

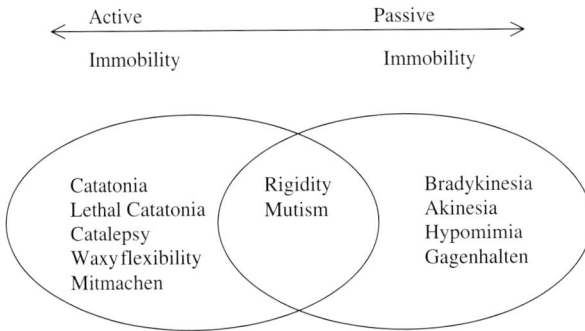

Figure 3.1 Immobility observed in patients with spontaneous hypokinesia can be viewed across a continuum ranging between active and passive types.

immobility appear to have distinct pathophysiologic correlates and therefore require different therapeutic considerations.

Most studies of hypokinesia in neurological and psychiatric populations have emphasized the role of the basal ganglia in this type of movement disorder [23, 75]. In particular, neuropharmacological manipulation of the dopaminergic system has produced the most consistent effects on hypokinesia in humans and in animal models. In general, dopaminergic stimulation ameliorates passive immobility whereas dopamine antagonism reverses active immobility. Data from animal models support the concept that passive and active immobility reflect distinct neural substrates, the former associated with dopamine underactivity, the latter with overactivity [76]. The ability of dopamine receptor antagonists to produce immobile states in animals corresponds very closely to the drug's affinity for nigrostriatal dopamine receptors [77]. For example, neuroleptics with little influence on the nigrostriatal dopamine system, such as clozapine, have little effect in this model system [78]. There also appear to be important differences in the effects on D1 and D2 receptor subtypes, as blockade of D2 receptors results in fixed postures in some animal species and this response is modulated by D1 stimulation or blockade [73]. Much study is needed to clarify the neuropharmacological basis of these phenomena. As our knowledge of pathogenesis has improved, a number of distinct etiologies of hypokinesis have been identified (e.g., tertiary syphilis) and accordingly removed from the purely psychiatric realm. Although the forms of hypokinesia in psychiatric patients may be induced by medications (e.g., drug-induced parkinsonism: see Chapter 6), a variety of hypokinetic conditions may also be observed in those who are not medicated. These will be the focus of this section (Fig. 3.1).

Bradykinesia, akinesia, and hypomimia

Although usually associated with neurological parkinsonian conditions, these terms refer to perhaps the most common form of hypokinesia observed in nonmedicated psychiatric patients, particularly those with depression or schizophrenia. Bradykinesia describes diminished velocity and amplitude of normal voluntary movement and akinesia describes poverty of all spontaneous movement. These two phenomena may be seen independently of each other and each may occur in the absence of rigidity. Diminished facial expression with a decreased rate of blinking is termed "hypomimia," a feature that is most often encountered in parkinsonian conditions and is essentially akinesia of the face. As such, hypomimia may be found, like generalized bradykinesia or akinesia, in a wide spectrum of psychiatric patients. In contrast to depressed or withdrawn patients, the hypomimic state in Parkinson's disease often does not correspond to the patient's reported emotional state.

Bradykinesia, akinesia, and hypomimia are frequently seen in psychiatric patients prior to drug therapy. Most often, slow movement and easy fatigability are encountered in patients with depression but these features have also been reported in other affective disorders, schizophrenia, and developmental disturbances.

Bradykinesia/psychomotor retardation in depression

"Psychomotor retardation" has long been recognized as a feature of major depressive episodes. In their review of psychomotor symptoms of depression, Sobin and Sackeim [79] note that it has been repeatedly shown that depressed patients differ from normal and psychiatric comparison groups with regard to objectively quantified gross motor activity, body movements, speech and motor reaction time. The similarity between the psychomotor retardation of depression and the bradykinesia and bradyphrenia (slowness of thought) of Parkinson's disease has been noted by several authors [80–86].

Sachdev and Aniss [83] studied three groups of 10 subjects each with major depression and significant motor retardation, PD with bradykinesia, and normal controls matched for age and gender. Evaluations included finger-tapping test, Purdue pegboard test, and global rating of bradykinesia on a 100-mm analogue scale designed for this study. They demonstrated a disturbance in the execution of simple and complex movements by subjects with major depression and motor retardation that resembled the disturbance seen in PD. The authors concluded that these results argue for a common pathophysiological basis for at least some aspects of motor retardation in the two disorders and suggested that reduced dopamine may partially account for these findings. Rogers et al. [80] attempted to determine whether patients with depression display the "characteristically Parkinsonian reliance on external cues," and if so, whether this is common to both melancholic and nonmelancholic types of depression. They had subjects perform a serial choice reaction time task known to be sensitive to PD movement deficits. The melancholic patients showed a parkinsonian pattern of impairment on the task, exhibiting a particular difficulty when initiating movements in the absence of external cues. The nonmelancholic patients did not show motor impairment. They suggested that the cue-dependent deficit may be due to an underlying basal ganglia dysfunction similar to that involved in PD (failure of internal cueing). Caligiuri and Ellwanger [83], using a velocity scaling measure, found that 40% of patients exhibited parkinsonian-like motor programming deficits, suggesting that a subgroup of depressed patients exhibit motor retardation that is behaviorally similar to parkinsonian bradykinesia and may stem from a similar disruption within the basal ganglia.

Overt presentations of motor slowing cannot distinguish slowness due to primary motor disturbances from slowness due to cognitive or emotional factors. It is interesting that many of the proposed explanations for psychomotor retardation in depression are that it is not a primary motor disturbance, but rather a secondary result of changes in attention, arousal, or motivation [87]. However, Sachdev and Aniss [83] commented that the motor change in melancholia should not be viewed as secondary to the mood disturbance, but rather, it should be seen as a "core" behavioral pattern, not merely a symptom.

There is some evidence to suggest that psychomotor retardation may be more common in bipolar than unipolar depression [88, 89]. More clearly, psychomotor retardation has been closely linked to melancholic depression, although there has been debate in the psychiatric literature as to whether melancholic depression is just a more severe depression or if it signifies a separate depressive syndrome with unique features.

Melancholic depression is characterized by unique emotional symptoms (anhedonia, lack of reactivity to pleasurable stimuli, a distinct quality of the depressed mood, and excessive guilt), vegetative symptoms (diurnal variation, early morning awakening, and diminished appetite) and motor features (marked psychomotor retardation or agitation) [90]. Some have suggested that the psychomotor symptoms in particular have the most discriminative validity in distinguishing depressive subtypes [79].

The distinctions drawn in the DSM-IV [90] and the majority of reports in the literature [87, 91, 92] support the notion that melancholic depression is best viewed as a unique subtype. An analysis of depressive subtypes by Florio et al. [91] supports a binary view that melancholic and nonmelancholic depression are separate clinical disorders rather than different forms of the same entity. Biochemical and molecular studies also suggest that there are two distinct subtypes. Gutierrez et al. [92] found that variability in the serotonin transporter gene was associated with an increased risk for major depression with melancholia. Wahlund et al. [93] noted that two clusters of unipolar patients appear to exist, one with low melatonin and low psychomotor retardation and another with high levels of melatonin and high psychomotor retardation. Others have cited evidence that psychomotor disturbances seem to be associated with anhedonia. In a study involving 48 depressed patients, there was a significant correlation between anhedonia and psychomotor retardation assessed by the Widocher Retardation Scale [87].

Movement disorders in schizophrenia

Limited information about the prevalence or natural history of motor disturbances in schizophrenics is available. Prior to the availability of neuroleptic drugs, abnormalities of motor function were frequently noted [73, 75]. However, interpretation of past prevalence surveys is difficult as definitions were inconsistent and many diagnosed "psychiatric" conditions would now carry a specific neurological diagnosis. Obviously, incidence and prevalence data are dependent upon precise definition of diagnostic terms, a goal not yet achieved. Diagnostic criteria [94] and rating scales [95, 96] for catatonia have recently been developed. Several recent prevalence studies are reviewed by Manschreck, who concludes that "disturbances of voluntary motor behavior (i.e., those that were not attributable to drug effects or known neurological disorder) occur in virtually all cases of conservatively defined schizophrenic disorder" [75]. He also notes that these motor phenomena may frequently be overlooked and that patients should be observed for extended periods of time.

"Negative symptoms" in schizophrenia

Schizophrenia and depression have an overlap in symptomatology, namely a slowing in both motor and mental activities, often referred to as "psychomotor retardation" in depression and "psychomotor poverty" or "poverty of movement" in schizophrenia [97].

The core symptoms of schizophrenia are divided into two categories, referred to as "positive" and "negative." The positive symptoms include the "active" phenomena, not present in normal individuals, such as hallucinations and delusions. "Negative" symptoms constitute part of a "deficit state" and, in addition to abnormally reduced levels of movement, include diminished motivation (avolition/apathy), capacity for pleasure (anhedonia), and affective expression (affective flattening). In addition to decreased spontaneous movements, patients often have diminished facial expression (hypomimia), poor eye contact, decreased speech output, and lack of vocal inflections [90, 98].

Some studies have noted that negative symptoms are more likely to be seen in males with younger onset schizophrenia and that their presence portends a poorer prognosis [98, 99]. Furthermore, negative symptoms have been correlated with "soft" neurological signs (e.g., eye tracking abnormalities) and cognitive deficits (e.g., impaired attention) [100].

Both structural and functional imaging studies have revealed a relationship between negative symptoms and prefrontal cortical abnormalities [101–103]. It has been hypothesized that the negative symptoms are related to a reduction of dopaminergic transmission in the prefrontal cortex (PFC) and that the serotonergic system (particularly via its role in modulating dopamine) may be important as well. Negative symptoms are not as responsive to treatment with classical neuroleptic antipsychotics that block D2 receptors. Atypical antipsychotics, particularly clozapine, appear to be more effective at treating the negative symptoms [104]. It has been proposed that clozapine's efficacy may result from its blockade of 5HT2A and/or 5HT1C receptors, perhaps in addition to blockade of D2 and/or D4 receptors [105]. It has also been hypothesized that clozapine's efficacy for negative symptoms may be attributable, in part, to the blockade of PFC D1 receptors, with subsequent enhancement of glutamate-facilitated dopamine activity [106].

Catatonia

Karl Ludwig Kahlbaum defined catatonia in 1868 as a condition with multiple "symptom-complexes" emerging at different times during disease progression [74]. These symptom-complexes were described as clusters of abnormal thought processes (e.g., disorientation) and motor dysfunction (e.g., increased tone). Periods of excitation and hyperkinesia as well as stupor and hypokinesia were described. Kahlbaum noted the association of catatonia with depression, mania, epilepsy, generalized paresis, and other conditions. Kahlbaum's concepts were later modified and incorporated into the theories of Kraeplin and later Bleuler within the nosologic entity of schizophrenia [107, 108]. Debates about these writings and whether or not catatonia is specific to schizophrenia have continued to the present [73, 109, 110].

As currently conceived, catatonia describes a symptom-complex with motor, affective and cognitive symptoms. Both excess movements and hypokinesia, including active and passive forms, may be part of the catatonic syndrome. Although most frequently associated with psychotic conditions (particularly schizophrenia) [111], it can also be seen in a variety of general medical disease states (e.g., hypercalcemia, hepatic encephalopathy) and neurological conditions (head trauma, encephalitis) [90], drug-induced disorders (neurologitic malignant syndrome), and has been reported to occur as a complication of autistic spectrum disorders [112].

In order to meet the diagnostic criteria for the catatonic type of schizophrenia according to DSM-IV [90], the clinical picture must be dominated by at least two of the features listed in Table 3.6.

Table 3.6 DSM-IV criteria for catatonia

---

1. Motoric immobility as evidenced by catalepsy (including waxy flexibility or stupor)
2. Excessive motor activity (that is apparently purposeless and not influenced by external stimuli)
3. Extreme negativism (an apparently motiveless resistance to all instructions or maintenance of a rigid posture against attempts to be moved) or mutism
4. Peculiarities of voluntary movement as evidenced by posturing (voluntary assumption of inappropriate or bizarre postures), stereotyped movements, prominent mannerisms, or prominent grimacing
5. Echolalia (apparently senseless repetition of a word or phrase just spoken by another person) or Echopraxia (repetitive imitation of the movements of another person)

The precise etiology of catatonia has not been elucidated. Functional imaging studies have demonstrated disturbances in hemispheric localization of activity during catatonic states [113] and persistent hypoperfusion of the basal ganglia even after achieving symptomatic remission [114]. There is evidence that schizophrenia characterized by periodic catatonia is a specific subtype transmitted in an autosomal dominant manner with evidence for genetic linkage on chromosomes 15q15 and 22q13 [115, 116].

It has been noted that the motor symptoms of catatonia can be treated with benzodiazepines [117, 118] and that lithium may be helpful in its prevention [119].

The individual signs of the catatonic syndrome (i.e., stupor, mutism, negativism, and waxy flexibility) are best considered separately as this may afford greater diagnostic precision and, in turn, more efficacious treatment. Moreover, each of these individual features has overlapping but not identical differential diagnoses, many outside the sphere of schizophrenia [73].

Lethal catatonia (see also Chapter 8)

A description of a clinical syndrome characterized by extreme physical excitement and exhaustion was provided by Stauder in 1934 [120]. These patients, all young adults, progressed from agitation to fixed postures and ultimately death. Acrocyanosis, tachycardia, and fever were usually present and autopsy revealed no obvious cause of death. The syndrome shares some clinical similarity with neuroleptic malignant syndrome (NMS), but several important differences exist [121, 122]. NMS occurs with rapid onset, often without excitatory prodrome, and is usually secondary to drug-induced dopamine receptor blockade. Lethal catatonia, on the other hand, was described long before the introduction of antipsychotic medications and often includes an excitatory prodrome. Differentiation of these two conditions is critical since very different treatment approaches are employed. Lethal catatonia is best treated with antipsychotics, benzodiazepines, and supportive care, while NMS requires immediate cessation of such drugs and treatment with dopaminergic agents and dantrolene (see Chapter 8). The true incidence of lethal catatonia, while low, remains unknown. As the early treatment of psychosis may prevent the full expression of this condition, in the current era of readily available antipsychotic therapy, NMS has become a much more common concern.

Rigidity

Three types of abnormal muscle tone have been described in psychiatric patients unexposed to psychotropic medications. Waxy flexibility is said to be present when a posture or limb position is maintained for an extended period of time after positioning by another individual.

Many unusual postures or positions have been described over the years, some with such frequency that they have earned their own names. The "psychological pillow," for example, describes a reclining patient with head held without support just above the bed surface. While these motor disturbances may still be seen in patients with affective and schizophrenic disorders, the prevalence of this phenomenon has apparently decreased over this past century for unknown reasons. Waxy flexibility is categorized as a form of active immobility since treatment with neuroleptics is the most effective therapy. ECT also has alleviated this disturbance.

Two other alterations of muscle tone may be mistaken for waxy flexibility. Mitmachen describes an immediate return to a resting or initial limb position after manipulation by the examiner. For example, a hand turned palm up by the examiner is returned to its prior pronated position. This sign is not specific to any psychiatric syndrome, although it is most commonly seen in schizophrenia. Gegenhalten (counter holding) refers to variable resistance to all passive movement. Now termed "paratonia," this sign reflects bihemispheric dysfunction and can be found in a wide range of conditions such as Alzheimer's disease, multiinfarct dementia, and metabolic encephalopathy.

Catalepsy

Most simply, catalepsy can be considered a synonym for waxy flexibility as it refers to the maintenance of an abnormal posture for prolonged periods of time following positioning by another. However, some authors use the term "waxy flexibility" in reference to a "plastic resistance" to movement and reserve "catalepsy" specifically for prolonged maintenance of an abnormal posture. In catalepsy, muscle tone is variable, ranging from marked resistance to near hypotonia. In the past, the term "catalepsy" was also employed to describe altered mental states and other motor disturbances, such as tonic seizures. Catalepsy has now, however, been placed conceptually within the spectrum of catatonia. Psychiatric patients may maintain abnormal cataleptic postures without exposure to psychotropic medications. Limbs may be held above the head, the trunk may be twisted, extended, or flexed, and the ball of one foot might support a large man for hours. Patients seem surprisingly undisturbed by these uncomfortable postures in contrast to patients with a focal dystonia, such as spasmodic torticollis, in which discomfort is often a primary feature. Catalepsy may be seen in patients with affective disturbances, both psychotic and nonpsychotic, as well as schizophrenic disorders. The true incidence of catalepsy in unmedicated patients is not known.

The term "catalepsy" is also employed frequently in the behavioral neuroscience literature in reference to animal models used to evaluate central neurochemical systems [123]. In order to assess the impact of drugs on DA, opioid, and other neurotransmitter systems, animals are placed in an unusual posture, for example, limbs on elevated bars or pegs, and the time taken to correct to normal posture is recorded. This form of catalepsy is most often induced by neuroleptic or opiate medications. A similarity between human and animal catalepsy has been inferred on the basis of neuropharmacological response, although this relationship remains speculative.

Negativism

A vaguely defined term, negativism has been applied to both observable behavior and inferred "internal" mental processes [4, 23]. As a movement disorder, negativism describes a motor activity or inactivity contrary to the intended goal. This may appear, for example, in a schizophrenic patient as an inability to shake hands due to limb withdrawal despite repeated attempts at initiating the gesture. Similar actions have also been termed motor "blocking" or "ambitendency" [4]. As a concept, negativism appears to have little diagnostic, phenomenologic, or therapeutic utility. When "negative" motor activity is observed clinically, consideration should be given to more precisely defined movement disorders or thought disturbances. For example, a patient with complex motor tics or obsessive-compulsive disorder may be similarly unable to carry out skilled actions.

Mutism

Absence of sound production in unmedicated psychiatric patients may occur without evidence for aphasia, laryngeal, or labial dysfunction. Mutism in a psychiatric patient capable of phonation is suggestive of psychosis or severe depression, but absence of sound production accompanied by akinesia raises the possibility of structural damage within the brain. Akinetic mutism has been associated with lesions of the third ventricle, thalamic nuclei, and cingulate gyrus [124]. Traumatic closed-head injury may result in a similar clinical pattern, perhaps due to the torque-induced shearing of axons in the regions surrounding the midbrain and corpus callosum. Dopaminergic medications such as dopamine agonists, levodopa/carbidopa, and amantadine may have a beneficial effect in some akinetic mute patients with or without identifiable structural abnormalities [125, 126].

References

1. Marsden CD. Hysteria-a neurologist's view. Psychol Med 1986; 16: 277–288.
2. Fahn S, Williams DT. Psychogenic dystonia. Adv Neurol 1988; 50: 431–455.
3. Ranawaya R, Riley D, Lang A. Psychogenic dyskinesias in patients with organic movement disorders. Mov Disord 1990; 5: 127–133.
4. Lee AJ (ed). Tics and Related Disorders, Edinburgh, Churchill Livingstone, 1985, pp. 104–124.
5. Jankovic J. Stereotypies. Presented at the annual meeting of the American Academy of Neurology, Miami 1990.

6. Dura JR, Mullick JA, Rasnake LK. Prevalence of stereotypy among institutionalized non-ambulatory profoundly mentally retarded people. Am J Mental Deficiency 1987; 91: 548–549.

7. Allen DA. Autistic spectrum disorders: clinical presentation in preschool children. J Child Neurol 1988; 3(suppl): S48–S56.

8. Schreibman L. Diagnostic features of autism. J Child Neurol 1988; 3(suppl): S57–S64.

9. Wing L, Attwood A. Syndromes of autism and atypical development. In Cohen DJ, Donnelan AM, Paul R (eds) Handbook of Autism and Pervasive Developmental Disorders. New York, John Wiley and Sons, 1987, pp. 3–199A.

10. Amir RE, Van den Veyver IB, Wan M, et al. Rett syndrome is caused by mutations in X-linked MECPZ, encoding methyl-CpG-binding protein Z. Nat Genet 1999; 23: 185–188.

11. Fitzgerald PM, Jankovic J, Percy AK. Rett syndrome and associated movement disorders. Mov Disord 1990; 5: 195–202.

12. Rojahn J. Self-injurious and stereotypic behavior of noninstitutionalized mentally retarded people: prevalence and classification. Am J Mental Deficiency 1986; 91: 268–276.

13. Jankovic J. Orofacial and other self-mutilations. In Jankovic J, Tolosa E (eds) Facial Dyskinesias, Advances in Neurology, Vol 49, New York, Raven Press, 1988, pp. 365–381.

14. Santavuori P, Haltia J, Raitta C. Infantile type of so-called neuronal ceroid lipofuscinosis. I. A clinical study of 15 cases. J Neurol Sci 1973; 18: 257.

15. Rogers D, Hymas N. Sporadic facial stereotypies in patients with schizophrenia and compulsive disorders. In Jankovic J, Tolosa E (eds) Facial Dyskinesias, Advances in Neurology, Vol 49. New York, Raven Press, 1988, pp. 383–394.

16. Abrams R, Taylor MA, Stolurow KA. Catatonia and mania: patterns of cerebral dysfunction. Biol Psychiatry 1979; 14: 111–117.

17. Leonhard K. In Robins E (ed) Berman R (trans), The Classification of Endogenous Psychoses. New York, Halsted Press, 1979.

18. Fish FJ. In Hamilton M (ed), Fish's Clinical Psychopathology: Signs and Symptoms in Psychiatry. Bristol, Wright, 1974.

19. Sakuma M. A comparative study by the behavioral observation for stereotypy in exceptional children. Folia Psychiatr Neurol Jpn 1975; 29: 371–391.

20. Shoulson I, Rothfield K, McBride M, et al. Physiologic chorea and dystonia of infancy. Neurology 1987; 37: 99.

21. Dantzer R. Behavioral, physiological and functional aspects of stereotyped behavior: a review and re-interpretation. J Animal Sci 1986; 62: 1776–1786.

22. Randrup A, Munkvad I. Stereotyped activities produced by amphetamine in several animal species and man. Psychopharmacologia 1967; 11: 300–310.

23. Lohr JB, Wisniewski AA (eds) Movement Disorders: A Neuropsychiatric Approach, New York, Guilford Press, 1987, pp. 91–108.

24. Berkson G. Abnormal stereotyped motor acts. In Zubin J, Hunt HF (eds) Comparative Psychopathology: Animal and Human, New York, Grune and Stratton, 1967, pp. 76–94.

25. Hutt SJ, Hutt C, Lee D, et al. A behavior and electroencephalographic study of autistic children. J Psychiatry Res 1965; 3: 181–197.

26. Baumeister AA, Forehand R. Stereotyped acts. In Ellis NR (ed), International Review of Research in Mental Retardation. Vol 6. New York, Academic Press, 1973, pp. 53–96.

27. Tschanz JT, Rebec GV. Atypical antipsychotic drugs block selective components of amphetamine-induced stereotypy. Pharmacol Biochem Behav 1988; 31: 519–522.

28. Koller WC, Herbster G. D1 and D2 dopamine receptor mechanisms in dopaminergic behaviors. Clin Neuropharmacol 1988; 11: 221–231.

29. Chipkin RE, McQuade RD, Lorio LC. D1 and D2 dopamine binding site upregulation and apomorphine-induced stereotypy. Pharmacol Biochem Behav 1987; 28: 477–482.
30. Costall B, Marsden CD, Naylor PJ, et al. Stereotyped behavior patterns and hyperactivity induced by amphetamine and apomorphine after discrete 6 hydroxydopamine lesions of extrapyramidal and mesolimbic nuclei. Brain Res 1977; 23: 89–111.
31. Kuczenski R, Segal D. Concomitant characterization of behavioral and neurotransmitter response to amphetamine using in vivo microdialysis. J Neurosci 1989; 9: 2051–2065.
32. Blumstein LK, Crawley JN, Davis LG, et al. Neuropeptide modulation of apomorphine-induced stereotyped behavior. Brain Res 1987; 404: 293–300.
33. Swedo SE, Rapoport J. Phenomenology and differential diagnosis of obsessive- compulsive disorder in children and adolescents. In Rapoport JL (ed) Obsessive-Compulsive Disorders in Children and Adolescents. Washington, DC, American Psychiatric Press, 1989, pp. 13–32.
34. Lysaker PH, Marks KA, Picone JB, et al. Obsessive and compulsive symptoms in schizophrenia: clinical and neurocognitive correlates. J Nerv Ment Dis 2000; 188: 78–83.
35. Berman I, Kalinowski A, Berman SM, et al. Obsessive and compulsive symptoms in schizophrenia. Compr Psychiatry 1995; 36: 6–10.
36. Bland RC, Newman SC, Orn H. Schizophrenia: lifetime comorbidity in a community sample. Acta Psychiatry Scand 1987; 75: 383–391.
37. Eisen JL, Beer DA, Pato MT, et al. Obsessive compulsive disorder in patients with schizophrenia or schizoaffective disorder. Am J Psychiatry 1997; 154: 271–273.
38. Proto L, Bermanzohn PC, Pollack S, et al. A profile of obsessive-compulsive symptoms in schizophrenia. CNS Spectrums 1997; 2: 21–26.
39. Hwang MY, Morgan JE, Losconzcy MF. Clinical and neuropsychological profiles of obsessive-compulsive schizophrenia: a pilot study. J Neuropsychiatry Clin Neurosci 2000; 12: 91–94.
40. Kruger S, Braunig P, Hoffler J, et al. Prevalence of obsessive-compulsive disorder in schizophrenia and significance of motor symptoms. J Neuropsychiatry Clin Neurosci 2000; 12: 16–24.
41. Reznik I, Mester R, Totler M, et al. Obsessive-compulsive schizophrenia: a new diagnostic entity? J Neuropsychiatry Clin Neurosci 2001; 13: 115–116.
42. Tibbo P, Kroetsch M, Chue P, et al. Obsessive-compulsive disorder in schizophrenia. J Psychiatric Res 2000; 34: 139–146.
43. Holzer JC, Goodman WK, McDougle CJ, et al. Obsessive-compulsive disorder with and without a chronic tic disorder: a comparison of symptoms in 70 patients. Br J Psychiatry 1994; 164: 469–473.
44. Frankel M, Cummings JL, Robertson MM, et al. Obsessions and compulsions in Gilles de la Tourette's syndrome. Neurology 1986; 36: 378–382.
45. Pitman RK, Green RC, Jenike MA, et al. Clinical comparison of Tourette's disorder and obsessive-compulsive disorder. Am J Psychiatry 1987; 144: 1166–1171.
46. Pauls DL, Raymond CL, Leckman JF, et al. A family study of Tourette's syndrome. Am J Hum Genet 1991; 48: 154–163.
47. Pauls DL, Alsobrook JP II, Goodman W, et al. A family study of obsessive-compulsive disorder. Am J Psychiatry 1995; 152: 76–84.
48. Cath DC, Hoogduin CAL, Wetering van de BJM, et al. (1992a) Tourette syndrome and obsessive-compulsive disorder: An analysis of associated phenomena. In TN Chase, AJ Friedhoff, DJ Cohen (eds) Advances in Neurology Series, Vol 58. New York, Raven Press, pp. 33–41.

49. Cath DC, Spinhoven PH, van de Wetering BJM, et al. The relationship between types and severity of repetitive behaviors in Gilles de la Tourette's syndrome and obsessive-compulsive disorder. J Clin Psychiatry 1999; 61: 505–513.

50. Cath DC, Spinhoven P, Hoogduin CA, et al. Repetitive behaviors in Tourette's syndrome and OCD with and without tics: What are the differences? Psychiatry Res 2001; 101(2): 171–185.

51. George MS, Trimble MR, Ring HA, et al. Obsessions in obsessive-compulsive disorder with and without Gilles de la Tourette's disorder. Am J Psychiatry 1993; 150: 93–97.

52. Miguel EC, Coffey BJ, Baer L, et al. Phenomenology of intentional repetitive behaviors in obsessive-compulsive disorder and Tourette's disorder. J Clin Psychiatry 1995; 56: 246–255.

53. Miguel EC, Baer L, Coffey BJ, et al. Phenomenological differences appearing with repetitive behaviors in obsessive-compulsive disorder and Gilles de la Tourette's syndrome. Br J Psychiatry 1997; 170: 140–145.

54. Hanna GL, Piacentini J, Cantwell DP, et al. Obsessive-compulsive disorder with and without tics in a clinical sample of children and adolescents. Depression & Anxiety. 2002; 16(2): 59–63.

55. Flament MF, Bisserbe J-C. Pharmacologic treatment of obsessive-compulsive disorder: comparative studies. J Clin Psychiatry 1997; 58(suppl 12): 18–22.

56. Grados M, Scahill L, Riddle MA. Pharmacotherapy in children and adolescents with obsessive-compulsive disorder. Child Adolesc Psychiatry Clin N Am 1999; 8: 617–634.

57. McDougle CJ, Goodman WK, Leckman JF, et al. Haloperidol addition in fluvoxamine-refractory obsessive-compulsive disorder: a double-blind, placebo-controlled study in patients with and without tics. Arch Gen Psychiatry 1994; 51: 302–308.

58. McDougle CJ. Update on pharmacologic management of OCD: agents and augmentation. J Clin Psychiatry 1997; 58: 11–17.

59. Jankovic J. Tourette's syndrome. New Engl J Med 2001; 345(16): 1184–1192.

60. Wise SP, Rapoport JL. Obsessive-compulsive disorders: is it basal ganglia dysfunction? In Rapoport JL (ed) Obsessive-Compulsive Disorder in Children and Adolescents. Washington, DC, American Psychiatric Press, 1989, pp. 327–344.

61. Kurlan R, Kersun J, Ballantine HT, et al. Neurosurgical treatment of severe obsessive-compulsive disorder associated with Tourette's syndrome. Mov Disord 1990; 5: 152–155.

62. Nuttin B, Cosyns P, Demeulemeester H, et al. Electrical stimulation in anterior limbs of internal capsules in patients with obsessive-compulsive disorder. Lancet 1999; 354:1526.

63. Nestadt G, Samuels J, Riddle M, et al. A family study of obsessive-compulsive disorder. Arch Gen Psychiatry 2000; 57(4): 358–363.

64. Ebert D, Speck O, Konig A, et al. H-magnetic resonance spectroscopy in OCD revealed evidence for neuronal loss in the cingulate gyrus and the right striatum. Psychiatry Res 1997; 74(3): 173–176.

65. Bartha R, Stein MB, Williamson PC, et al. A short echo 1H spectroscopy and volumetric MRI study of the corpus striatum in patients with obsessive-compulsive disorder and comparison subjects. Am J Psychiatry 1998; 155(11): 1584–1591.

66. Baxter L, Phelps M, Mazziotta J, et al. Local cerebral glucose metabolic rates of obsessive-compulsive disorder compared to unipolar depression and normal controls. Arch Gen Psychiatry 1987; 44: 211–218.

67. Saba PR, Dastur K, Keshavan MS, et al. Obsessive-compulsive disorder, Tourette's syndrome, and basal ganglia pathology on MRI. J Neuropsychiatry Clin Neurosci 1998; 10: 116–117.

68. Chacko RC, Rorbin MA, Harper RG. Acquired obsessive-compulsive disorder associated with basal ganglia lesions. J Neuropsychiatry Clin Neurosci 2000; 12: 269–272.
69. Saxena S, Brody AL, Schwartz JM, et al. Neuroimaging and frontal-subcortical circuitry in obsessive-compulsive disorder. Br J Psychiatry 1998; 35: 26–37.
70. Giedd JN, Rapoport JL, Garvey MA. MRI assessment of children with obsessive-compulsive disorder or tics associated with streptococcal infection. Am J Psychiatry 2000; 157(2): 281–283.
71. Peterson BS, Leckman JF, Tucker D, et al. Preliminary findings of antistreptococcal antibody titers and basal ganglia volumes in tic, obsessive-compulsive, and attention deficit/hyperactivity disorders. Arch Gen Psychiatry 2000; 57(4): 364–372.
72. Bottas A, Richter MA. Pediatric autoimmune neuropsychiatric disorders associated with streptococcal infections (PANDAS). Ped Infect Dis J 2002; 21(1): 67–71.
73. Gelenberg AJ. The catatonic syndrome. Lancet 1976; i: 1339–1341.
74. Barnes MP, Saunders M, Walls TJ, et al. The syndrome of Karl Ludwig Kahlbaum. J Neurol Neurosurg Psychiatry 1986; 49: 991–996.
75. Manschreck TC. Motor abnormalities in schizophrenia. In Nasrallah HA, Weinberger DR (eds) Handbook of Schizophrenia, Vol 1. 1986, pp. 65–96.
76. Klemm WR. Drug effects on active immobility responses: what they tell us about neurotransmitter systems and motor fluctuations. Progr Neurobiol 1989; 32: 403–422.
77. Campbell A, Herschel M, Cohen BM, et al. Tissue levels of haloperidol by radioreceptor assay and behavioral effects of haloperidol in the rat. Life Sci 1980; 27: 633–640.
78. Honma T, Fukushima H. Correlation between catalepsy and dopamine decrease in the rat striatum induced by neuroleptics. Neuropharmacology 1976; 15: 601–607.
79. Sobin C, Sackeim HA. Psychomotor symptoms of depression. Am J Psychiatry 1997; 154: 4–17.
80. Rogers MA, Bradshaw JL, Philips JG, et al. Parkinsonian motor characteristics in unipolar major depression. J Clin Exp Neuropsychol 2000; 22: 232–244.
81. Bermanzohn PC, Siris SG. Akinesia: a syndrome common to parkinsonism, retarded depression, and negative symptoms of schizophrenia. Compr Psychiatry 1992; 33: 221–232.
82. Flint AJ, Black SE, Campbell-Taylor I, et al. Abnormal speech articulation, psychomotor retardation, and subcortical dysfunction in major depression. J Psychiatry Res 1993; 27: 309–319.
83. Sachdev P, Aniss AM. Slowness of movement in melancholic depression. Biol Psychiatry 1994; 35: 253–262.
84. Calligiuri MP, Ellwanger J. Motor and cognitive aspects of motor retardation in depression. J Affective Disord 2000; 57: 83–93.
85. Austin MP, Mitchell P, Hadzi-Pavlovic D, et al. Effect of apomorphine on motor and cognitive function in melancholic patients: a preliminary report. Psychiatry Res 2000; 97: 207–215.
86. Rogers D, Lees AJ, Smith E, et al. Bradyphrenia in Parkinson's disease and psychomotor retardation in depressive illness – an experimental study. Brain 1987; 110: 761–776.
87. Lemke MR, Puhl P, Koethe N, et al. Psychomotor retardation and anhedonia in depression. Acta Psychiatry Scand 1999; 99: 252–256.
88. Parker G, Roy K, Wilhelm K, et al. The nature of bipolar depression: implications for the definition of melancholia. J Affective Disord 2000; 59: 217–224.
89. Mitchell PB, Wilhelm K, Parker G, et al. The clinical features of bipolar depression: a comparison with matched major depressive disorder patients. J Clin Psychiatry 2001; 62: 212–216.

90. American Psychiatric Association: Diagnostic and Statistical Manual of Mental Disorders. 4th Ed. Washington, DC, American Psychiatric Association, 1994.

91. Florio TM, Parker G, Austin MP, et al. Neural network subtyping depression. Aust N Z J Psychiatry 1998; 32: 687–694.

92. Gutierrez B, Pintor L, Gasto C, et al. Variability in the serotonin transporter gene and increased risk for major depression with melancholia. Hum Genet 1998; 103: 319–322.

93. Wahlund B, Grahn H, Saaf J, et al. Affective disorder subtyped by psychomotor symptoms, monoamine oxidase, melatonin and cortisol: identification of patients with latent bipolar disorder. Eur Arch Psychiatry Clin Neurosci 1998; 248: 215–224.

94. Peralta V, Cuesta MJ. Motor features in psychotic disorders. I. Factor structure and clinical correlates. Schizophr Res 2001; 47: 107–116.

95. Northoff G, Braus DF, Sartorius A, et al. Reduced activation and altered laterality in two neuroleptic-naive catatonic patients during a motor task in functional MRI. Psychol Med 1999; 29: 997–1002.

96. Braunig P, Kruger S, Shugar G, et al. The catatonia rating scale I–development, reliability, and use. Compr Psychiatry 2000; 41: 147–158.

97. van Hoof JJ, Jogems-Kosterman BJ, Sabbe BG, et al. Differentiation of cognitive and motor slowing in the Digit Symbol Test (DST): differences between depression and schizophrenia. J Psychiatry Res 1998; 32(2): 99–103.

98. Andreasen NC, Olsen S. Negative versus positive schizophrenia: definition and validation. Arch Gen Psychiatry 1982; 39: 789.

99. Mueser KT, Douglas MS, Bellack AS, et al. Assessment of enduring deficit and negative symptom subtypes in schizophrenia. Schizophr Bull 1991; 17: 565–582.

100. Roitman SE, Keefe RS, Harvey PD, et al. Attentional and eye tracking deficits correlate with negative symptoms in schizophrenia. Schizophr Res 1997; 26: 139–146.

101. Potkin, SG Alva G, Fleming K, et al. A PET Study of the Pathophysiology of Negative Symptoms in Schizophrenia. Am J Psychiatry 2002; 159: 227–237.

102. Vaiva G, Cottencin O, Llorca PM, et al. Regional cerebral blood flow in deficit/nondeficit types of schizophrenia according to SDS criteria. Progr Neuropsychopharmacol Biol Psychiatry 2002; 26: 481–485.

103. Andreasen NC, Rezai K, Alliger R, et al. Hypofrontality in neuroleptic-naïve patients and in patients with chronic schizophrenia. Assessment with xenon 133 single-photon emission computed tomography and the Tower of London. Arch Gen Psychiatry 1992; 49: 943–958.

104. Gaertner I, Gaertner HJ, Vonthein R, et al. Prospective 6-year trial with clozapine: negative symptoms in outpatients with schizophrenia improve despite intermittent positive symptoms [Letter]. J Clin Psychopharmacol 2002; 22(4): 437–438.

105. Kapur S, Remington G. Serotonin-dopamine interaction and its relevance to schizophrenia. Am J Psychiatry 1996; 153: 466–476.

106. Lynch MR. Schizophrenia and the D1 receptor: focus on negative symptoms. Progr Neuropsychopharmacol Biol Psychiatry 1992; 16: 797–832.

107. Kraepelin E. Dementia Praecox and Paraphrenia (Barclay RM, trans). Huntington, NY, Robert E Krieger, 1971 (facsimile 1919 edition).

108. Bleuler E. Dementia Praecox or the Group of Schizophrenias. (Zinkin J, trans), New York, International Universities Press, 1950.

109. Mazurek MF, Rosebush PI. Foundations for the classification of catatonias [reply]. Mov Disord 2000; 15: 180–181.

110. Ungvar G, Carroll BT. Foundations for the classification of catatonias [letter]. Mov Disord 2000; 15: 180.

111. Northoff G, Koch A, Wenke J, et al. Catatonia as a psychomotor syndrome: a rating scale and extrapyramidal motor symptoms. Mov Disord 1999; 14: 404–416.

112. Wing L, Shah A. Catatonia in autistic spectrum disorders. Br J Psychiatry 2000; 176: 357–362.

113. Atre-Vaidya N. Significance of abnormal brain perfusion in catatonia: a case report. Neuropsychiatry Neuropsychol Behav Neurol 2000; 13: 136–139.

114. Stober G, Franzek E, Haubitz I, et al. Gender differences and age of onset in the catatonic subtypes of schizophrenia. Psychopathology 1998; 31: 307–312.

115. Stober G, Saar K, Ruschendorf F, et al. Splitting schizophrenia: periodic catatonia-susceptibility locus on chromosome 15q15. Am J Hum Genet 2000; 67: 1201–1207.

116. Meyer J, Huberth A, Ortega G, et al. A missense mutation in a novel gene encoding a putative cation channel is associated with catatonic schizophrenia in a large pedigree. Mol Psychiatry 2001; 6: 302–306.

117. Rosebush P, Furlong B, Mazurek M. Catatonic syndrome in a general psychiatric population: frequency, clinical presentation and response to lorazepam. J Clin Psychiatry 1990; 51: 357–361.

118. Fink M, Bush G, Francis A. Catatonia: a treatable disorder occasionally recognized. Directions Psychiatry 1993; 13: 1–7.

119. Sugahara Y, Tsukamoto H, Sasaki T. Lithium carbonate in prophylaxis of reappearing catatonic stupor: case report. Psychiatry Clin Neurosci 2000; 54: 607–609.

120. Stauder KH: Die todliche katatonie. Arch Psychiatr Nervenkr 1934; 102: 614–634.

121. Mann SC, Caroff SN, Bleier HR, et al. Lethal catatonia. Am J Psychiatry 1986; 143: 1374–1381.

122. Castillo E, Rubin RT, Holsboer-Trachsler E. Clinical differentiation between lethal catatonia and neuroleptic malignant syndrome. Am J Psychiatry 1989; 146: 324–328.

123. Sanberg PR, Bunsey MD, Giordano M, et al. The catalepsy test: its ups and downs. Behav Neurosci 1988; 5: 748–759.

124. Plum F, Posner JB. The Diagnosis of Stupor and Coma, 3rd edition. Philadelphia, F.A. Davis Co., 1980.

125. Ross ED, Stewart RM. Akinetic mutism from hypothalamic damage: successful treatment with dopamine agonists. Neurology 1981; 31(11): 1435–1439.

126. Guidice MA, et al. Improvement in motor functioning with levodopa and bromocriptine following closed head injury. Neurology 1986; 36(1): 198–199.

PART 2

Antipsychotics

CHAPTER 4

The pharmacology of typical and atypical antipsychotics

Gary Remington and Shitij Kapur

The introduction of antipsychotics

The discovery of antipsychotics follows an interesting and rather circuitous path – the reader is referred to several excellent reviews of this topic [1–3]. In the first half of the 20th century, the notion that psychotic illnesses such as schizophrenia had a biological underpinning was still open to debate. The 1950s, though, heralded the introduction of effective pharmacotherapeutic agents for the treatment of schizophrenia and, in doing so, provided undisputable evidence that this illness was, at least in part, biologically mediated. Ironically, after decades without pharmacological treatment options, two appeared within several years of each other. It had been identified that the rawoulfia alkaloid, reserpine, which was being used in the treatment of hypertension, also had tranquilizing properties that proved useful in the management of various neuropsychiatric conditions. In and around the same time though, research with chlorpromazine as a possible anesthetic agent led to the serendipitous discovery that it too shared this particular feature, which became described as "artificial hibernation." It quickly became apparent that its influence was not confined to tranquilization and that there was, in fact, an antipsychotic effect. Chlorpromazine quickly established success in this regard, and interest in reserpine soon gave way to efforts intent on establishing a better understanding of chlorpromazine's clinical profile and possible mechanisms of antipsychotic action.

Herein lays one of the interesting twists that remind us of the circuitous paths drug discovery can take, and certainly one that pertains to a chapter such as this. It was noted that both reserpine and chlorpromazine induced parkinsonian-like side effects, despite the fact that they were distinctly different chemical entities. This led to the notion that this characteristic may be fundamental to their psychic benefits, and in 1957 the term "neuroleptic" (literally meaning "to take the neuron") was introduced to define this new class of agents – the criteria were outlined for inclusion, one of which required the induction of extrapyramidal symptoms (EPS) [1]. It is noteworthy that this type of definition, based on the induction of adverse events and arising out of work being done in Europe and Canada, was not well received by American psychiatry, giving rise to alternative descriptive terms, including both "major tranquilizers" and "antipsychotics" as alternatives to "neuroleptic." The definition was quickly put to use though, with the synthesis of haloperidol and its classification as a neuroleptic based on its ability to induce both catatonia and dyskinesias in preclinical animal models.

Dopamine, schizophrenia, and the D$_2$ receptor

By the early 1960s, Carlsson and his group had implicated both dopamine and postsynaptic receptor blockade as relevant to the action of antipsychotics [4, 5]. Reserpine offered an interesting variant to a drug like chlorpromazine in that it too disrupted dopamine activity, but did so through presynaptic amine depletion [1, 3, 6–8]. This work became the nidus for a biochemical model of schizophrenia, one that proposed that it was related to overactivity of certain dopamine pathways [6, 7].

Other lines of investigation provided further support for this hypothesis, including data that dopamimetic drugs like amphetamine induced psychotic symptoms [9, 10]. One of the most important breakthroughs was to come from the recognition that different dopamine receptors existed and the finding that the clinical potencies of antipsychotics relate to their affinity for the D$_2$ receptor in particular [11].

The development of antipsychotics capitalized on this information, setting as a goal the development of selective D$_2$ antagonists. The net result was a shift away from antipsychotics with a lower potency and greater pharmacological heterogeneity, for example, chlorpromazine, to higher potency, more D$_2$-selective antipsychotics, for example, haloperidol. Paradoxically, the second-generation antipsychotics reflect a move back to the development of more pharmacologically "rich" compounds, as can be seen in Table 4.1. When typical agents were being developed it was believed that the impact on receptors and systems beyond dopamine, including histamine, acetylcholine, and norepinephrine, was simply a source of side effects, without clinical benefit (see Table 4.2).

However, at the same time, thinking regarding the role of dopamine blockade began to change. No longer was it thought that the induction of EPS was necessary for antipsychotic efficacy; indeed, years of clinical experience suggested that this was to be avoided as much as possible. Unfortunately, over the years the problem had only worsened as a result of the shift to high-potency compounds that were used in increasingly higher doses in an effort to optimize clinical response [14]. That even higher doses failed to achieve this [15, 16] was a sober reminder that these drugs were not a panacea. As many as 25% of individuals with schizophrenia remain treatment-resistant, even with aggressive use of conventional antipsychotics [17], indicating substantial room for improvement (in addition to raising the possibility that other receptors and/or neurochemical systems may play a role). There also evolved the notion that while these drugs were largely effective on positive symptoms, there was

Table 4.1 Pharmacological profile of 'atypical' antipsychotics

Agent	Haloperidol	Clozapine	Risperidone	Olanzapine	Quetiapine	Ziprasidone	Aripiprazole
Chemical class	Butyrophenone	Dibenzodiazepine	Benzisoxazole	Dibenzazazepine	Dibenzothiazepine	Benzothiazolyl piperazine	Quinolinone derivative
Receptor Binding[b]							
D_1	+++	++	−	+++	+	+	−
D_2	++++	++	+++	+++	++	+++	+++
$5\text{-}HT_2$	+	++++	++++	++++	++	++++	++
α_1	++	+++	+++	+++	+++	++	+
α_2	−	+++	+	−	+	−	+
H_1	−	++++	+	++++	++++	+	++
M_1	−	++++	−	++++	+++	−	−
EPS Risk	++++	+	+++	++	+	++	+

Adapted from Kapur and Remington [12].

[b] D = dopamine; 5-HT = serotonin; α = adrenergic; H = histamine; M = acetylcholine (muscarinic).

Table 4.2 Possible adverse effects of receptor blockade by antipsychotics*

Dopamine D_2 receptors (antagonism)
  EPS: dystonia, parkinsonism, akathasia, tardive dyskinesia, rabbit syndrome
  Endocrine effects: prolactin elevation (galactorrhea, gynecomastia,
    menstrual changes, sexual dysfunction in males)
Dopamine agonism
  GI disturbance e.g., nausea
  Behavioural/cognitive symptoms
  Sleep disturbance
α_1-adrenoceptors
  Postural hypotension, dizziness
  Reflex tachycardia
  Nasal congestion
Histamine H_1 receptors
  Sedation
  Drowsiness
  Weight Gain
Muscarinic receptors
  Blurred vision
  Attack or exacerbation of narrow-angle glaucoma
  Dry mouth
  Sinus tachycardia
  Constipation
  Urinary retention
  Memory dysfunction
Serotonin 5-HT receptors
  ? weight gain
  ? sexual dysfunction

---

*This list refers to more commonly noted side effects and is not exhaustive.
Adapted from Remington and Kapur [13].

little effect on the other symptom dimensions characterizing schizophrenia. In fact, there was not a great deal of attention paid to the other symptom dimensions in the initial decades after chlorpromazine's introduction. Although it was recognized that the symptoms of schizophrenia were heterogeneous, the identification of distinct symptom clusters (and the potential benefit of the newer antipsychotics along these different dimensions), really only took hold in the 1980s with the distinction of positive and negative symptomatology [18]. Thereafter, this line of investigation flourished, particularly in the last decade as the new antipsychotics made claims regarding clinical benefits along these dimensions as well as others, for example, cognitive, affective [19, 20].

Clozapine and the concept of "atypicality"

A turning point in our understanding and expectations regarding antipsychotics occurred with the development of clozapine. Synthesized in 1960, it became apparent within the next decade that this compound, a dibenzapine, had neuoleptic-like effects *without* EPS, calling into question the notion that antipsychotic action was integrally related to the presence of EPS. Its clinical investigation received a setback in the early 1970s though, when eight deaths occurred in Finland in patients receiving clozapine (subsequently linked to a risk on the part of clozapine, albeit low, of developing agranulocytosis) [21–23].

While the drug was withdrawn from use in many countries, its use continued in others. By the 1990s, it was once again reintroduced into many others with the caveat that routine blood monitoring be carried out, given that white cell abnormalities were found to be reversible with clozapine's discontinuation. The fact that this drug would be reintroduced in the face of such restrictions spoke of the mounting evidence supporting its unique clinical profile. Not only was it largely devoid of EPS risk, it did not cause the hyperprolactinemia that characterized existing antipsychotics. Moreover, clinical experience, culminating in a seminal study comparing it to chlorpromazine, indicated its superiority in refractory schizophrenia as well as the treatment of the so-called negative symptoms of this illness [24].

In distinguishing itself from all other currently available antipsychotics, clozapine became the prototype of "atypicality" and the stimulus for the development of a new generation of agents. Interestingly, the definition of "atypical" has been somewhat of a moving target. The simplest definition, and one that all appear to agree upon, is that of a compound that effects an antipsychotic response while not inducing EPS [25]. Broader definitions include lack of prolactin elevation, lack of tardive movement disorders with chronic exposure, and a broader profile of symptom control. Suffice it to say that the criteria continue to expand as other "atypicals" are developed and clinical experience is gathered [26]. This holds true not only for clinical benefits, for example, cognition, suicide risk, but for adverse events as well, for example, weight gain (seen as more prevalent in the newer agents). This has led to the suggestion that we can no longer view antipsychotics dichotomously as either typical or atypical. With the number of criteria increasing, it is more evident that agents may differ among each other on various measures, suggesting that we take more of a dimensional approach [27].

The pharmacology of "atypical"

> *All models are wrong: some models are useful.*
> – Deming, "Guide to Stella"

Clozapine, in a sense, represented a "throwback" in antipsychotic development. With the major hypothesis of schizophrenia being one of hyperdopaminergic activity, and increased recognition regarding the role of the D_2 receptor in antipsychotic activity, focus had shifted to the development of selective D_2 antagonists, the so-called high-potency antipsychotics. Clozapine, like chlorpromazine, was a low-potency agent with a heterogeneous receptor-binding profile; moreover, it was identified as having a relatively low affinity for the D_2 receptor [22].

Given its documented efficacy though, there was reason to question if undue importance had been attributed to dopamine and its role in antipsychotic activity. Thus, clozapine turned out to be an exciting molecule at several levels. It affirmed that an antipsychotic could be effective without the induction of EPS, changing fundamentally the direction of antipsychotic development. By calling into question the importance of dopamine blockade, it also challenged the most widely held model for schizophrenia, opening up numerous possibilities in terms of alternative mechanisms of action.

In this search, a variety of hypotheses have been forwarded and it is beyond the scope of this chapter to review them all. However, certain models have garnered particular attention and, in fact, have come to provide conceptual frameworks for currently available antipsychotics. Four in particular stand out: serotonin 5-HT$_2$/dopamine D_2 binding ratio; fast dissociation from the D_2 receptor; partial dopamine agonism; and, limbic selectivity. Various aspects of this section have been detailed in earlier work by the authors [12, 26, 28].

Serotonin 5-HT$_2$/Dopamine D_2

Notable in clozapine's pharmacological profile is its serotonin 5-HT$_2$ binding – its affinity for these receptors has been shown to be twice as high as for D_2 receptors [29]. Based on preclinical work with a number of compounds, Meltzer et al. postulated that it was this profile of greater 5-HT$_2$ versus D_2 antagonism that accounted for clozapine's "atypical" clinical characteristics [30–32]. Development of putative antipsychotics embraced this model, hoping to capture clozapine's clinical benefits by incorporating this profile, while at the same time avoiding its troublesome side effects, in particular the risk of agranulocytosis. A number of such compounds were successfully brought to the market, including risperidone, olanzapine, quetiapine, ziprasidone, and zotepine (sertindole, also fitting this profile, was released briefly before being withdrawn due to identified problems related to prolonged QTc prolongation).

Numerous studies attesting to their clinical superiority on various symptom dimensions have been published [19, 20, 33, 34], although the extent and cause of these benefits have also been challenged [35–38]. One aspect that has been emphasized is a superior EPS profile, perhaps not so surprising given the established role of dopamine in such movements and evidence of serotonin's capacity to modulate dopamine at the level of the nigrostriatal pathway [39]. As a class the newer antipsychotics have been associated with a decreased risk of acute EPS, notwithstanding the issue of dose [35, 37, 40], and although long-term data are only available for clozapine [41] the preliminary evidence suggests that the benefit extends to a diminished risk of tardive movement disorders as well [42–47].

Given the heterogeneous receptor-binding profile of these different agents, the contribution of other systems to the clinical benefits of the newer antipsychotics cannot be ruled out. For example, clozapine's pharmacology includes anticholinergic activity [22], which in and of itself can mitigate against EPS. Similarly, amisulpride has also been reported to produce less EPS than conventional agents, despite being devoid of concomitant 5-HT$_2$ antagonism [48].

This last point serves as a reminder that there are limitations challenging the notion that the 5-HT$_2$/D$_2$ model represents the only explanation for "atypicality":

(a) It warrants repeating that this particular model hinges on a profile of greater 5-HT$_2$ versus D$_2$ antagonism; thus, compounds are not atypical simply because their profile includes 5-HT$_2$ binding. Loxapine, for example, *in vivo* demonstrates 5-HT$_2$ binding that approximates its D$_2$ binding curve [49–51], yet it is not atypical in the clinical setting. Moreover, the ratio of greater 5-HT$_2$ versus D$_2$ binding can be lost in a dose-dependent fashion. That is, with increasing doses 5-HT$_2$ binding approaches saturation while D$_2$ occupancy continues to rise, with the net result being loss of the differential binding. As a result, the compound can begin to look like a typical antipsychotic, for example, in terms of EPS, in a dose-dependent fashion [39, 52].

(b) Investigative trials with selective 5-HT$_2$ antagonists such ritanserin and M100906 indicated that they were not effective antipsychotics. Therefore, while the 5-HT$_2$ antagonism may have some modulatory role, or perhaps even a primary role in other symptom dimensions, it is not the critical component in antipsychotic efficacy.

(c) There are antipsychotics that have claimed atypical status, for example, amisulpride, aripiprazole [48, 53], although they are not characterized by this profile of greater 5-HT$_2$ versus D$_2$ antagonism, suggesting that this can be achieved through other mechanisms as well.

Fast dissociation from the D$_2$ receptor

A feature that *all* currently available antipsychotics, typical as well as atypical, share in common is that of D$_2$ antagonism. In contrast to selective 5-HT$_2$ antagonists, selective D$_2$ antagonists have proven to be effective antipsychotics; taken together, the evidence would suggest that D$_2$ blockade is the *sine qua non* of antipsychotic activity. At the same time, it cannot be sufficient as we can see refractory forms of psychosis even in the face of significant D$_2$ antagonism [54].

An interesting twist to the D$_2$ story has arisen more recently. That is the notion of differential dissociation from the D$_2$ receptors [55–58], and there are two aspects to this story: molecular and systemic. At a molecular level, *in vitro* studies demonstrated that antipsychotics dissociate from the D$_2$ receptor at very different rates, expressed as a k_{off} value. As a group, the atypicals appear to have higher k_{off} values, that is faster dissociation rates, than the conventionals, but they differ among themselves on this dimension as well, for example, quetiapine > clozapine > olanzapine [57, 58]. A second aspect to this story is systemic (vs. molecular). The principle is similar, but in this case other variables must be factored into the equation, for example, half-life ($t_{1/2}$) and k_{off}.

This model accounts for several features of clozapine which were, for some time, difficult to explain. Clozapine's low affinity for the D_2 receptor, in combination with its robust clinical response, challenged the notion that D_2 antagonism was necessary for antipsychotic efficacy. This was highlighted when evidence indicating that a threshold of D_2 occupancy in the range of 60–70% was required to optimize chance of clinical response – it was found that even higher doses of clozapine routinely failed to reach this level. Indeed, the dose-D_2 occupancy curve appeared relatively flat, a profile not seen with other atypicals such as risperidone and olanzapine [59]. It was subsequently established that this "glass ceiling" reflected a sampling interval that did not fully capture the occupancy curve over time. PET scans at approximately 12 hours following last administered dose did imply that the clozapine D_2 binding profile defied the existing threshold data. However, if the scans were carried out closer to the time of the last dose, that is approximately 3 hours later, this was not the case. Thus, what characterized clozapine was not its lack of D_2 binding, but rather its profile of transient D_2 binding in the 24 hours following administration. It and quetiapine, in particular, reflect a profile of higher D_2 occupancy in the initial hours after treatment, while toward the end of the 24 hours their levels are quite low [54].

While clozapine and quetiapine are similar in this regard, other atypicals like risperidone and olanzapine demonstrate higher D_2 occupancy in the initial hours following their administration, and are less transient over a 24-hour interval (although more so than what is seen with a conventional antipsychotic like haloperidol [60, 61]).

These findings dovetail nicely with what is seen in the clinical setting regarding EPS risk. An increased risk of EPS has been shown to occur with D_2 occupancy in the range of 80% or higher [62, 63]. Whereas compounds like olanzapine and risperidone will exceed this threshold as doses are increased, this is not the case for either clozapine or quetiapine. These data support the position that both of these agents do not need to call upon their concomitant 5-HT$_2$ antagonism to diminish EPS risk – their D_2 occupancy, even at higher doses does not come close to approximating the 80% threshold associated with EPS risk.

It is more difficult to reconcile the EPS data with a model based on 5-HT$_2$/D_2 ratios. For example, by most accounts the order of freedom from EPS for olanzapine, quetiapine, and risperidone is: quetiapine > olanzapine > risperidone; however, their 5-HT$_2$/D_2 ratios are in exactly the opposite order, that is, risperidone [21] > olanzapine [8.9] > quetiapine [2.6] [64].

Are there other clinical implications associated with the fast dissociation model? It is recognized that dopamine is required for a number of functions, for example, movement, affect, cognition [65], and it is possible that its role in normal functioning may be less disturbed by compounds that do not cause sustained D_2 blockade. At a molecular level, antipsychotics with higher k_{off} values are better able to decrease their occupancy in response to increased dopamine surges required for task-related activities. At a systems level, the net result includes only transient prolactin elevation and a lack of D_2 up-regulation with continued administration [12, 28, 58]. Clinically, it can be argued that many of the benefits ascribed to the second-generation antipsychotics reflect this profile of transient, rather than sustained, D_2 antagonism. This would include decreased EPS (and, therefore, secondary negative symptoms), in addition to decreased affective and cognitive disturbances.

Partial dopamine agonism

The most recent entry into the antipsychotic market in North America is aripiprazole. It has been suggested by some that it reflects a new generation of antipsychotics, that is, the third generation, since it is unlike conventional antipsychotics clinically and yet does not fit the $5\text{-}HT_2/D_2$ model. This is in contrast to all other second-generation antipsychotics available in North America.

It demonstrates both $5\text{-}HT_{1A}$ agonism and $5\text{-}HT_2$ antagonism, although its affinity for the D_2 receptors exceeds that for serotonin by an order of magnitude. Thus, it does not conform to the standard $5\text{-}HT_2/D_2$ model. What makes it particularly unique amongst the newer antipsychotics is its combined agonist/antagonist properties at the D_2 receptor [66]. Although clearly different from the fast dissociation hypothesis, a parallel can be drawn in that both are mechanisms of providing appropriate modulation of D_2 transmission at the receptor level.

Limbic selectivity

It has long been felt that the ideal antipsychotic would selectively block dopamine at the level of the mesolimbic system, since it has been hypothesized that hyperdopaminergic activity here accounts for the positive symptoms of psychosis, for example, hallucinations. In by-passing the blockade of other dopaminergic pathways, one could avoid such side effects as EPS (nigrostriatal) and hyperprolactinemia (tuberoinfundibular).

Several lines of investigation have suggested that the clinical advantages of the newer antipsychotics may, at least in part, be ascribed to a profile of limbic selectivity. One means of exploring this hypothesis has been the evaluation of early gene expression (*c-fos* and *c-jun*) as a marker of synaptic activity. Numerous reports have suggested that, as a class, the newer antipsychotics show regional differences based on these markers; for example, one of the more consistent findings has been increased *c-fos* expression in the limbic versus striatal regions, supporting the notion that the atypicals share in common the pharmacologic advantage of limbic selectivity [67–70]. Clinically, this could account for their diminished risk of dopamine-related side effects such as EPS and elevated prolactin.

The opportunity to evaluate D_2 occupancy extrastriatally has been seen as adding further support for this model, with evidence that atypicals demonstrate preferential binding for extrastriatal structures, for example, temporal cortex [71–75]. However, results have not been entirely consistent and the findings have been criticized on methodological grounds [76, 77].

Other

In the last decade, much of our attention regarding "atypicality" has been focused on dopamine and serotonin, and they continue to be the subject of intense investigation. Work involving serotonin has largely focused on the 5-HT$_{2A}$ receptor, but more recently attention has turned to the evaluation of other serotonergic receptors in terms of both clinical response and side effects [78–82]. For example, the 5-HT$_{1A}$ receptor has been implicated in anxiety, depression, and negative symptoms, while the 5-HT$_{2C}$ receptor has been linked to weight gain and improvement in EPS. In terms of dopamine, the role of the D$_3$ receptor, if for no other reason than its localization in limbic regions, remains intriguing but poorly understood [83–85]. As discussed earlier, the predominance of D$_1$, as compared to D$_2$, receptors in the prefrontal cortex, their apparent interactive roles, and the prominent D$_1$-binding properties of clozapine, all contribute to an ongoing interest in this particular receptor.

There is abundant reason to look beyond dopamine and serotonin as well, given the heterogeneous receptor-binding profile of these different compounds. Such reviews may be found in other sources [86–88].

The one system warranting comment based on the amount of attention it is currently receiving is glutamate [66, 89–91]. A strong argument for this model arises from the fact that phencyclidine (PCP), a psychotomimetic street drug, noncompetitively blocks the ion channel of the N-methyl-aspartate (NMDA) subtype of the glutamate receptor. This model does not contradict a role for dopamine; for example, one action of dopamine is to inhibit glutamate release. Thus, a state of dopaminergic hyperactivity could lead to NMDA receptor hypofunction, which in turn could produce the various symptoms linked with psychosis. To date, work with compounds acting at the level of the NMDA receptor, for example, D-cycloserine, glycine, have reported modest benefits in the treatment of positive symptoms, with more compelling evidence favoring effectiveness in negative and cognitive symptoms [92–97].

In summary, it would be inaccurate to suggest that the data convincingly support one particular model, or conversely, that we can categorically dismiss any one of these. As is the case so often, the models best offer a framework for hypothesis testing that in the end advances our understanding of how antipsychotics work.

What can be said is that the newer antipsychotics do seem to hold advantages in terms of the various movement disorders associated with conventional antipsychotic use; these include acute dystonias, parkinsonism, akathisia, and tardive movements disorders. A comment is warranted, though, regarding the issue of dose. Over the years, the dosing of conventional antipsychotics increased considerably, well beyond what is currently recommended or what has been advocated based on empirical evidence. It has been argued that the difference between the older and newer antipsychotics may be overstated, reflecting more the inappropriately high doses of conventional antipsychotics often used for comparison purposes the than fundamental differences related to pharmacology [37, 98]. While this may be true to some extent, there is now evidence that even at lower doses the risk of movements with the older drugs is higher. For example, several reports have indicated a higher risk of both parkinsonism and TD with conventional antipsychotics, even when used at doses in keeping with current guidelines [45, 99].

We are reminded as well that differences exist between the newer antipsychotics. Risperidone, and to a lesser extent olanzapine and ziprasidone, appear to invoke acute EPS in a dose-related fashion, whereas this does not appear to be the case for clozapine and quetiapine. This might best be explained by the fast dissociation model, since clozapine and quetiapine, the two atypicals identified as having the fastest k_{off} values, do not show *in vivo* the same dose-related increase in D_2 occupancy that is observed with agents such as risperidone and olanzapine [12, 59, 100].

Currently, the evidence suggesting a lower risk of tardive movement disorder is most compelling for clozapine, but this really reflects the fact that there are much more long-term data on it compared to the other newer antipsychotics. The evidence, albeit limited, that exists for these other compounds would suggest that they too are considerably better than the older antipsychotics in this regard.

In conclusion, the new compounds represent a step forward in terms of D_2-related side effects, including both EPS and hyperprolactinemia, when compared to their conventional counterparts. However, it is important to recognize that the newer antipsychotics are not equivalent to each other in this regard. Moreover, while they do seem superior to typical agents, they are not without side effects; for example, as a class they seem to be worse in terms of weight gain and an increase in diabetes has been reported that may not simply be a function of the weight increase [101, 102]. As with EPS, it appears that the new antipsychotics will differ between themselves along this dimension.

What aspects of these drugs' pharmacology account for the reduced risk of movement disorders? We have outlined here a number of theories that purport to account for this clinical benefit. That there is not a unitary explanation is not so surprising, as it is likely that "atypicality" can be achieved through a variety of pharmacological directions. In line with this thinking, it would seem simplistic to view these new antipsychotics collectively as identical, especially given their diverse pharmacology and the number of clinical dimensions we now address with respect to both outcome measures and side effects. It is more prudent to imagine that each will have its own individual profile, and it will be the "sum of the parts" that will guide a clinician's decision-making in choosing an antipsyshotic for a particular individual.

References

1. Healy D. The Creation of Psychopharmacology. Cambridge, MA, Harvard University Press, 2002.
2. Deniker P. From chlorpromazine to tardive dyskinesia (brief history of neuroleptics). Psychiatr J Univ Ottawa 1989; 14: 253–259.

3. Deniker P. The neuroleptics: a historical survey. Acta Psychiatr Scand 1990; 82(suppl 358): 83–87.
4. Carlsson A, Lindqvist M, Magnusson T, et al. On the presence of 3-hydroxytyramine in brain. Science 1958; 127: 471.
5. Carlsson A, Lindqvist M. Effect of chlorpromazine or haloperidol on formation of 3-methoxy-tyramine and normetanephrine in mouse brain. Acta Pharmacol Toxicol 1963; 20: 140–144.
6. Van Rossum J. The significance of dopamine-receptor blockade for the action of neuroleptic drugs. In Brill H, Cole J, Deniker P, Hippius H, Bradley PB (eds) Neuropsychopharmacology. Proceedings 5th Collegium Internationale Neuro-psycho-pharmacologicum. Excertica Medica, Amsterdam, 1967, pp. 321–329.
7. Matthysse S. Antipsychotic drug actions: a clue to the neuropathology of schizophrenia? Fed Proc 1973; 32: 200–205.
8. Jarvik M. Drugs used in the treatment of psychiatric disorders. In Goodman LS, Gilman A (eds) The Pharmacological Basis of Therapeutics. Macmillan, New York, 1970, pp. 151–203.
9. Fog R. On stereotypy and catalepsy: studies of the effects of amphetamines and neuroleptics in rats. Acta Neurol Scand 1972; 40: 1–66.
10. Randrup A, Munkvad I. Stereotyped activities produced by amphetamine in several animal species and man. Psychopharmacology 1967; 11: 300–310.
11. Seeman P, Lee T, Chau-Wong M, et al. Antipsychotic drug doses and neuroleptic/dopamine receptors. Nature 1976; 261: 717–719.
12. Kapur S, Remington G. Atypical antipsychotics: new directions and new challenges in the treatment of schizophrenia. In Caskey C (ed) Annual Review in Medicine: Selected Topics in the Clinical Sciences. Vol. 52. Annual Reviews, Palo Alto, 2001, pp. 503–517.
13. Remington G, Kapur S, Zipursky R. Antipsychotic drug side effects. In Csernansky J (ed) Schizophrenia: A New Guide for Clinicians. New York, Marcel Dekker, 2002, pp. 213–245.
14. Baldessarini RJ, Katz B, Cotton P. Dissimilar dosing with high-potency and low-potency neuroleptics. Am J Psychiatry 1984; 141: 748–752.
15. Baldessarini RJ, Cohen BM, Teicher MH. Significance of neuroleptic dose and plasma level in the pharmacological treatment of psychoses. Arch Gen Psychiatry 1988; 45: 79–91.
16. Bollini P, Pampallona S, Orza MJ, et al. Antipsychotic drugs: is more worse? A meta-analysis of the published randomized control trials. Psychol Med 1994; 24: 307–316.
17. Brenner HD, Dencker SJ, Goldstein MJ, et al. Defining treatment refractoriness in schizophrenia. Schizophr Bull 1990; 16: 551–561.
18. Crow TJ. Positive and negative schizophrenic symptoms and the role of dopamine. Br J Psychiatry 1980; 137: 383–386.
19. Blin O. A comparative review of new antipsychotics. Can J Psychiatry 1999; 44: 235–244.
20. Stip E. Novel antipsychotics: issues and controversies. Typicality of atypical antipsychotics. J Psychiat Neurosci 2000; 25: 137–153.
21. Hippius H. A historical perspective of clozapine. J Clin Psychiatry 1999; 60: 22–23.
22. Coward DM, Imperato A, Urwyler S, et al. Biochemical and behavioural properties of clozapine. Psychopharmacology (Berl) 1989; 99: S6–S12.
23. Baldessarini RJ, Frankenburg FR. Clozapine. A novel antipsychotic agent. N Engl J Med 1991; 324: 746–754.
24. Kane J, Honigfeld G, Singer J, et al. Clozapine for the treatment-resistant schizophrenic. A double-blind comparison with chlorpromazine. Arch Gen Psychiatry 1988; 45: 789–796.

25. Meltzer H. Atypical antipsychotic drugs. In Bloom FE, Kupfer D (eds) Psychopharmacology: The Fourth Generation of Progress. New York, Raven Press, 1995, pp 1277–1286.
26. Remington G. Understanding antipsychotic 'atypicality': a clinical and pharmacological moving target. J Psychiatry Neurosci 2003; 28: 277–285.
27. Waddington JL, O'Callaghan E. What makes an antipsychotic 'atypical'? CNS Drugs 1997; 7: 341–346.
28. Kapur S, Remingon G. Dopamine D_2 receptors and their role in atypical antipsychotic action: still necessary and may even be sufficient. Biol Psychiatry 2001; 50: 873–883.
29. Jackson DM, Mohell N, Bengtsson A, et al. What are atypical antipsychotics and how do they work? In Brunello N, Mendlewicz J, Racagni M (eds) New Generation of Antipsychotic Drugs: Novel Mechanisms of Action. Karger, Basel, 1993, pp. 27–38.
30. Meltzer HY, Matsubara S, Lee JC. Classification of typical and atypical antipsychotic drugs on the basis of dopamine D-1, D-2 and serotonin2 pKi values. J Pharmacol Exp Ther 1989; 251: 238–246.
31. Meltzer HY, Matsubara S, Lee JC. The ratios of serotonin2 and dopamine2 affinities differentiate atypical and typical antipsychotic drugs. Psychopharmacol Bull 1989; 25: 390–392.
32. Stockmeier CA, DiCarlo JJ, Zhang Y, et al. Characterization of typical and atypical antipsychotic drugs based on in vivo occupancy of serotonin2 and dopamine2 receptors. J Pharmacol Exp Ther 1993; 266: 1374–1384.
33. Fleischhacker WW, Meise U, Gunther V, et al. Compliance with antipsychotic drug treatment: influence of side effects. Acta Psychiatr Scand 1994; 89(suppl 382): 11–15.
34. Tamminga CA. The promise of new drugs for schizophrenia treatment. Can J Psychiatry 1997; 42: 265–273.
35. Leucht S, Pitschel-Walz G, Abraham D, et al. Efficacy and extrapyramidal side-effects of the new antipsychotics olanzapine, quetiapine, risperidone, and sertindole compared to conventional antipsychotics and placebo. A meta-analysis of randomized controlled trials. Schizophr Res 1999; 35: 51–68.
36. Kapur S, Remington G. Atypical antipsychotics. Br Med J 2000; 321: 1360–1361.
37. Geddes J, Freemantle N, Harrison P, et al. Atypical antipsychotics in the treatment of schizophrenia: systematic overview and meta-regression analysis. Br Med J 2000; 321: 1371–1376.
38. Carpenter WT, Gold JM. Another view of therapy for cognition in schizophrenia. Biol Psychiatry 2002; 51: 969–971.
39. Kapur S, Remington G. Serotonin-dopamine interaction and its relevance to schizophrenia. Am J Psychiatry 1996; 153: 466–476.
40. Leucht S, Wahlbeck K, Hamann J, et al. New generation antipsychotics versus low-potency conventional antipsychotics: a systematic review and meta-analysis. Lancet 2003; 361: 1581–1589.
41. Peacock L, Solgaard T, Lublin H, et al. Clozapine versus typical antipsychotics. A retro- and prospective study of extrapyramidal side effects. Psychopharmacology (Berl) 1996; 124: 188–196.
42. Beasley CM, Dellva MA, Tamura RN, et al. Randomised double-blind comparison of the incidence of tardive dyskinesia in patients with schizophrenia during long-term treatment with olanzapine or haloperidol. Br J Psychiatry 1999; 174: 23–30.
43. Glazer WM. Expected incidence of tardive dyskinesia associated with atypical antipsychotics. J Clin Psychiatry 2000; 61: 21–26.
44. Glazer WM, Morgenstern H, Pultz JA, et al. Incidence of tardive dyskinesia may be lower with quetiapine treatment than previously reported with typical antipsychotics

in patients with psychoses. 38th Annual Meeting of the American College of Neuropsychopharmacology (ACNP), Acapulco, Mexico, December 12–16, 1999.

45. Jeste DV, Lacro JP, Bailey A, et al. Lower incidence of tardive dyskinesia with risperidone compared with haloperidol in older patients. J Am Geriatr Soc 1999; 47: 716–719.

46. Jeste DV, Okamoto A, Napolitano J, et al. Low incidence of persistent tardive dyskinesia in elderly patients with dementia treated with risperidone. Am J Psychiatry 2000; 157: 1150–1155.

47. Tollefson GD, Beasley CM, Jr., Tamura RN, et al. Blind, controlled, long-term study of the comparative incidence of treatment-emergent tardive dyskinesia with olanzapine or haloperidol. Am J Psychiatry 1997; 154: 1248–1254.

48. Leucht S, Pitschel-Walz G, Engel RR, et al. Amisulpride, an unusual "atypical" antipsychotic: a meta-analysis of randomized controlled trials. Am J Psychiatry 2002; 159: 180–190.

49. Kapur S, Zipursky RB, Jones C, et al. The D_2 receptor occupancy profile of loxapine determined using PET. Neuropsychopharmacology 1996; 15: 562–566.

50. Kapur S, Zipursky R, Remington G, et al. PET evidence that loxapine is an equipotent blocker of 5-HT_2 and D_2 receptors: implications for the therapeutics of schizophrenia. Am J Psychiatry 1997; 154: 1525–1529.

51. Remington G, Kapur S. D_2 and 5-HT_2 receptor effects of antipsychotics: bridging basic and clinical findings using PET. J Clin Psychiatry 1999; 60(suppl 10): 15–19.

52. Kapur S, Remington G, Zipursky RB, et al. The D_2 dopamine receptor occupancy of risperidone and its relationship to extrapyramidal symptoms: a PET study. Life Sci 1995; 57: 103–107.

53. Kane JM, Carson WH, Saha AR, et al. Efficacy and safety of aripiprazole and haloperidol versus placebo in patients with schizophrenia and schizoaffective disorder. J Clin Psychiatry 2002; 63: 763–771.

54. Wolkin A, Barouche F, Wolf AP, et al. Dopamine blockade and clinical response: evidence for two biological subgroups of schizophrenia. Am J Psychiatry 1989; 146: 905–908.

55. Kapur S, Seeman P. Does fast dissociation from the dopamine D_2 receptor explain the action of atypical antipsychotics? A new hypothesis. Am J Psychiatry 2001; 158: 360–369.

56. Seeman P, Tallerico T. Antipsychotic drugs which elicit little or no parkinsonism bind more loosely than dopamine to brain D_2 receptors, yet occupy high levels of these receptors. Mol Psychiatry 1998; 3: 123–134.

57. Seeman P, Tallerico T. Rapid release of antipsychotic drugs from dopamine D_2 receptors: an explanation for low receptor occupancy and early clinical relapse upon withdrawal of clozapine or quetiapine. Am J Psychiatry 1999; 156: 876–884.

58. Seeman P. Atypical antipsychotics: mechanism of action. Can J Psychiatry 2002; 47: 27–38.

59. Kapur S, Zipursky RB, Remington G. Clinical and theoretical implications of 5-HT_2 and D_2 receptor occupancy of clozapine, risperidone, and olanzapine in schizophrenia. Am J Psychiatry 1999; 156: 286–293.

60. Farde L, Wiesel FA, Nordstrom AL, et al. D_1- and D_2-dopamine receptor occupancy during treatment with conventional and atypical neuroleptics. Psychopharmacology (Berl) 1989; 99(suppl): S28–S31.

61. Tauscher J, Jones C, Remington G, et al. Significant dissociation of brain and plasma kinetics with antipsychotics. Mol Psychiatry 2002; 7: 317–321.

62. Kapur S, Zipursky R, Jones C, et al. Relationship between dopamine D_2 occupancy, clinical response, and side effects: a double-blind PET study of first-episode schizophrenia. Am J Psychiatry 2000; 157: 514–520.
63. Farde L, Nordstrom AL, Wiesel FA, et al. Positron emission tomographic analysis of central D_1 and D_2 dopamine receptor occupancy in patients treated with classical neuroleptics and clozapine. Relation to extrapyramidal side effects. Arch Gen Psychiatry 1992; 49: 538–544.
64. Schotte A, Janssen PF, Gommeren W, et al. Risperidone compared with new and reference antipsychotic drugs: in vitro and in vivo receptor binding. Psychopharmacology (Berl) 1996; 124: 57–73.
65. Le Moal M. Mesocortoclimbic dopaminergic neurons: functional and regulatory roles. In Bloom FE, Kupfer D (eds) Psychopharmacology: The Fourth Generation of Progress. New York, Raven Press, 1995, pp 283–294.
66. Lawler CP, Prioleau C, Lewis MM, et al. Interactions of the novel antipsychotic aripiprazole (OPC-14597) with dopamine and serotonin receptor subtypes. Neuropsychopharmacology 1999; 20: 612–627.
67. Arnt J, Skarsfeldt T. Do novel antipsychotics have similar pharmacological characteristics? A review of the evidence. Neuropsychopharmacology 1998; 18: 63–101.
68. Fink-Jensen A, Kristensen P. Effects of typical and atypical neuroleptics on Fos protein expression in the rat forebrain. Neurosci Lett 1994; 182: 115–118.
69. Fibiger HC. Neuroanatomical targets of neuroleptic drugs as revealed by Fos immunochemistry. J Clin Psychiatry 1994; 55(suppl): 33–36.
70. Robertson GS, Matsumura H, Fibiger HC. Induction patterns of Fos-like immunoreactivity in the forebrain as predictors of atypical antipsychotic activity. J Pharmacol Exp Ther 1994; 271: 1058–1066.
71. Nyberg S, Chou YH, Halldin C. Saturation of striatal D_2 dopamine receptors by clozapine. Int J Neuropsychopharmacol 2002; 5: 11–16.
72. Stephenson CM, Bigliani V, Jones HM, et al. Striatal and extra-striatal D_2/D_3 dopamine receptor occupancy by quetiapine in vivo. [^{123}I]-epidepride single photon emission tomography (SPET) study. Br J Psychiatry 2000; 177: 408–415.
73. Bressan RA, Erlandsson K, Jones HM, et al. Optimizing limbic selective D_2/D_3 receptor occupancy by risperidone: a [^{123}I]-epidepride SPET study. J Clin Psychopharmacol 2003; 23: 5–14.
74. Xiberas X, Martinot JL, Mallet L, et al. In vivo extrastriatal and striatal D_2 dopamine receptor blockade by amisulpride in schizophrenia. J Clin Psychopharmacol 2001; 21: 207–214.
75. Xiberas X, Martinot JL, Mallet L, et al. Extrastriatal and striatal D_2 dopamine receptor blockade with haloperidol or new antipsychotic drugs in patients with schizophrenia. Br J Psychiatry 2001; 179: 503–508.
76. Olsson H, Farde L. Potentials and pitfalls using high affinity radioligands in PET and SPET determinations on regional drug induced D_2 receptor occupancy-a simulation study based on experimental data. Neuroimage 2001; 14: 936–945.
77. Talvik M, Nordstrom AL, Nyberg S, et al. No support for regional selectivity in clozapine-treated patients: a PET study with [^{11}C]raclopride and [^{11}C]FLB 457. Am J Psychiatry 2001; 158: 926–930.
78. Megens AA, Awouters FH, Schotte A, et al. Survey on the pharmacodynamics of the new antipsychotic risperidone. Psychopharmacology (Berl) 1994; 114: 9–23.
79. Leonard BE. Serotonin receptors-where are they going? Int Clin Psychopharmacol 1994; 9(suppl 1): 7–17.

80. Lucki I. Serotonin receptor specificity in anxiety disorders. J Clin Psychiatry 1996; 57: 5–10.
81. Roth BL. Multiple serotonin receptors: clinical and experimental aspects. Ann Clin Psychiatry 1994; 6: 67–78.
82. Sussman N. The potential benefits of serotonin receptor-specific agents. J Clin Psychiatry 1994; 55(suppl): 45–51.
83. Griffon N, Sokoloff P, Diaz J, et al. The dopamine D_3 receptor and schizophrenia: pharmacological, anatomical and genetic approaches. Eur Neuropsychopharmacol 1995; 5: 3–9.
84. Healy D. D_1 and D_2 and D_3. Br J Psychiatry 1991; 159: 319–324.
85. Sokoloff P, Martres MP, Giros B, et al. The third dopamine receptor (D_3) as a novel target for antipsychotics. Biochem Pharmacol 1992; 43: 659–666.
86. Jones HM, Pilowsky L. New targets for antipsychotics. Expert Rev Neurotherap 2002; 2: 61–68.
87. Kilts CD. The changing roles and targets for animal models of schizophrenia. Biol Psychiatry 2001; 50: 845–855.
88. Kinon BJ, Lieberman JA. Mechanisms of action of atypical antipsychotic drugs: a critical analysis. Psychopharmacology (Berl) 1996; 124: 2–34.
89. Javitt DC, Zukin SR. Recent advances in the phencyclidine model of schizophrenia. Am J Psychiatry 1991; 148: 1301–1308.
90. Olney JW, Farber NB. Glutamate receptor dysfunction and schizophrenia. Arch Gen Psychiatry 1995; 52: 998–1007.
91. Tamminga CA, Holcomb HH, Gao XM, et al. Glutamate pharmacology and the treatment of schizophrenia: current status and future directions. Int Clin Psychopharmacol 1995; 10(suppl 3): 29–37.
92. Leiderman E, Zylberman I, Zukin SR, et al. Preliminary investigation of high-dose oral glycine on serum levels and negative symptoms in schizophrenia: an open-label trial. Biol Psychiatry 1996; 39: 213–215.
93. Heresco-Levy U, Javitt DC, Ermilov M, et al. Double-blind, placebo-controlled, crossover trial of D-cycloserine adjuvant therapy for treatment-resistant schizophrenia. Int J Neuropsychopharmacol 1998; 1: 131–135.
94. Heresco-Levy U, Javitt DC, Ermilov M, et al. Efficacy of high-dose glycine in the treatment of enduring negative symptoms of schizophrenia. Arch Gen Psychiatry 1999; 56: 29–36.
95. Heresco-Levy U. N-methyl-D-aspartate (NMDA) receptor-based treatment approaches in schizophrenia: the first decade. Int J Neuropsychopharmacol 2000; 3: 243–258.
96. Heresco-Levy U, Ermilov M, Shimoni J, et al. Placebo-controlled trial of D-cycloserine added to conventional neuroleptics, olanzapine, or risperidone in schizophrenia. Am J Psychiatry 2002; 159: 480–482.
97. Goff DC, Tsai G, Levitt J, et al. A placebo-controlled trial of D-cycloserine added to conventional neuroleptics in patients with schizophrenia. Arch Gen Psychiatry 1999; 56: 21–27.
98. Green MF, Marder SR, Glynn SM, et al. The neurocognitive effects of low-dose haloperidol: a two-year comparison with risperidone. Biol Psychiatry 2002; 51: 972–978.
99. Zimbroff DL, Kane JM, Tamminga CA, et al. Controlled, dose-response study of sertindole and haloperidol in the treatment of schizophrenia. Am J Psychiatry 1997; 154: 782–791.

100. Kapur S, Zipursky R, Jones C, et al. A positron emission tomography study of quetiapine in schizophrenia. Arch Gen Psychiatry 2000; 57: 553–559.

101. Henderson DC. Atypical antipsychotic-induced diabetes mellitus: how strong is the evidence? CNS Drugs 2002; 16: 77–89.

102. Allison DB, Casey DE. Antipsychotic-induced weight gain: a review of the literature. J Clin Psychiatry 2001; 62: 22–31.

CHAPTER 5

Acute drug-induced dystonia

Michael F. Mazurek and Patricia I. Rosebush

Introduction

Antipsychotic medications are used to treat a wide range of neuropsychiatric disorders, including schizophrenia, acute mania, drug-induced psychosis, Tourette's syndrome, and Huntington's disease. Since shortly after the introduction of chlorpromazine in the early 1950s, it has been recognized that antipsychotic agents are associated with a number of acute and subacute neurological side effects, one of which is dystonia. Recent experience has shown that many of the newer "atypical" antipsychotic drugs, once thought to be relatively free of neurological complications, are in fact fully capable of provoking acute dystonic reactions. Other types of medication, particularly antiemetic compounds and selective serotonin reuptake inhibitors, can also induce dystonia.

The present review starts with conventional antipsychotic drugs, since most of the data regarding the clinical features, incidence, and risk factors for drug-induced dystonia are derived from the study of patients taking these agents. This is followed by an outline of the evidence linking various other medications with dystonia. The final sections discuss pathophysiology, treatment issues, and emerging research developments.

Conventional antipsychotic drugs

Clinical features
Signs and symptoms

Drug-induced dystonia may involve any part of the body. The most commonly affected muscles tend to be those of the neck, resulting in a turning of the head to one side (torticollis) or a pulling of the head straight back (retrocollis). In the retrospective series reported by Swett [1], torticollis accounted for about 30% of cases, while in our own prospective series [2–5] 42% of the dystonic reactions involved torticollis/retrocollis (Fig. 5.1).

Another common site of drug-induced dystonia is the jaw, which was affected in 39% of the patients in our series. In milder cases this may manifest as grimacing and a sense of tightness in the jaw muscles, but some patients (almost 15% in the Swett study) develop masseter spasm sufficiently severe to produce jaw closure (trismus). The most clinically worrisome site of

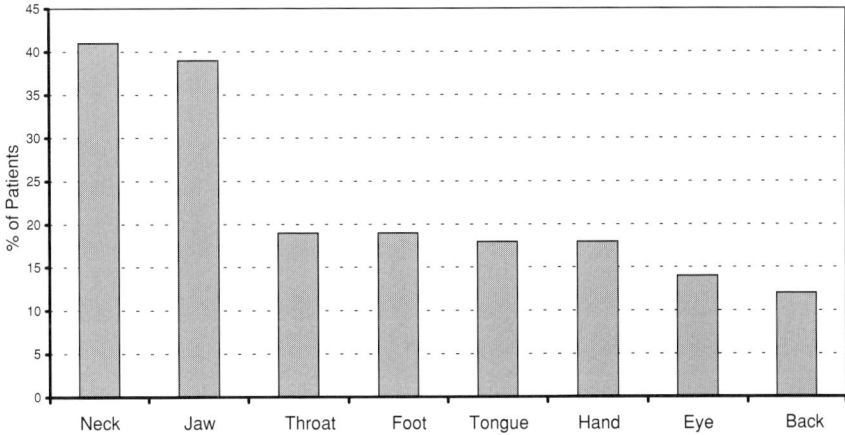

Figure 5.1 Anatomical targets of dystonic reactions in patients taking antipsychotic drugs for the first time.

drug-induced dystonia is the throat, which was involved in 19% of our cases and an unspecified number in the Swett series. This typically begins with a sense of tightness in the throat, often accompanied by difficulty in swallowing. If not treated immediately, the problem can progress to laryngospasm and/or supraglottic pharyngeal dystonia, with potentially fatal consequences [6, 7].

One of the more bizarre but surprisingly common forms of drug-related dystonia is the "swollen tongue." This phenomenon was present in 17% of cases in the Swett series and in 18% of ours. It has generally been assumed that the symptom of tongue swelling is simply a subjective sensation, but our experience suggests that this may not be the case. In several patients we have witnessed what appears to be actual swelling of the tongue, though we have unfortunately never managed to obtain photographic documentation of this observation.

Perhaps the most spectacular manifestation of drug-induced dystonia is the oculogyric crisis, in which the eyeballs appear to roll up into the head. This unforgettable clinical scenario represented 6% of the dystonic reactions reported by Swett and 14% in our series. Oculogyric crisis was well known to neurologists in the first half of the 20th century, being observed in up to 20% of patients who had recovered from the acute phase of encephalitis lethargica [8]. By description, the postencephalitic cases of oculogyric dystonia appear to have been very similar to those that develop in the context of antipsychotic drug treatment. It is not clear why, in both clinical settings, the rotation of the eyes is almost invariably upward.

Dystonia of the facial muscles can result in curling of the upper lip, producing a sneering appearance and eyelid closure manifesting as blepharospasm. These distributions are rarely seen with conventional antipsychotic medications.

While a majority of drug-induced dystonic reactions target the muscles of the head and neck, the trunk and limbs can also be affected. Truncal dystonia manifested as a bizarre arching of the back (opisthotonus) in 3.5% of the cases described by Swett and in 12% of our cases. In our experience, opisthotonus and oculogyric dystonia have often been misinterpreted as willful posturing or attention seeking on the part of the psychiatric patient, with unfortunate consequences for treatment.

Dystonic reactions involving the upper limbs, seen in 18% of our cases, typically manifest as wrist flexion along with extension of the forefinger and flexion of the other fingers, as if the patient were pointing with the forefinger. In the lower limbs, the dystonia most commonly presents as a foot cramp, although proximal muscles may on occasion be involved. Unlike opisthotonus, dystonic spasms in the hands and feet tend not to be misinterpreted as voluntary posturing.

Emotional accompaniments
Many episodes of dystonia develop in the context of situational stress. One interpretation of this is that a heightened emotional state may play a role in precipitating an attack, such as was proposed to have occurred with postencephalitic dystonic attacks [9]. Alternatively, the state of emotional arousal may represent the prodrome or the initial symptoms of the developing dystonic episode [10]. The fairly abrupt onset of acute distress, particularly in a newly treated patient, warrants a careful examination for incipient dystonia.

Whatever the role of antecedent stress in precipitating or heralding a dystonic reaction, there is unanimous recognition that the dystonic reaction itself is associated with a great deal of anxiety on the part of the patient (and also, not uncommonly, on the part of the staff).

Timing
The vast majority of acute dystonic reactions occur very early in the course of antipsychotic drug treatment [2, 3, 11–13] (Fig. 5.2). The attacks begin suddenly, often building to full intensity within a minute or two of onset.

An intriguing aspect of antipsychotic drug-induced acute dystonia is the circadian pattern in the timing of the attacks. In a study of 196 consecutive reactions, episodes of acute dystonia were four times more likely to occur during the afternoon or evening (between the hours of 12 noon and 11 p.m.) than during the night or morning (i.e., the period 11 p.m. to 12 noon [4] Fig. 5.3). Analysis of the data indicated that the observed circadian pattern could not be accounted for by sleep, fatigue, changing blood levels of medication, or time elapsed from the last dose. This suggested that the circadian pattern of dystonic reaction might be related to endogenous diurnal rhythms [4]. A similar pattern of diurnal variation, with dystonia more likely to occur later in the day, was observed in patients with postencephalitic oculogyric crises [9, 10, 14].

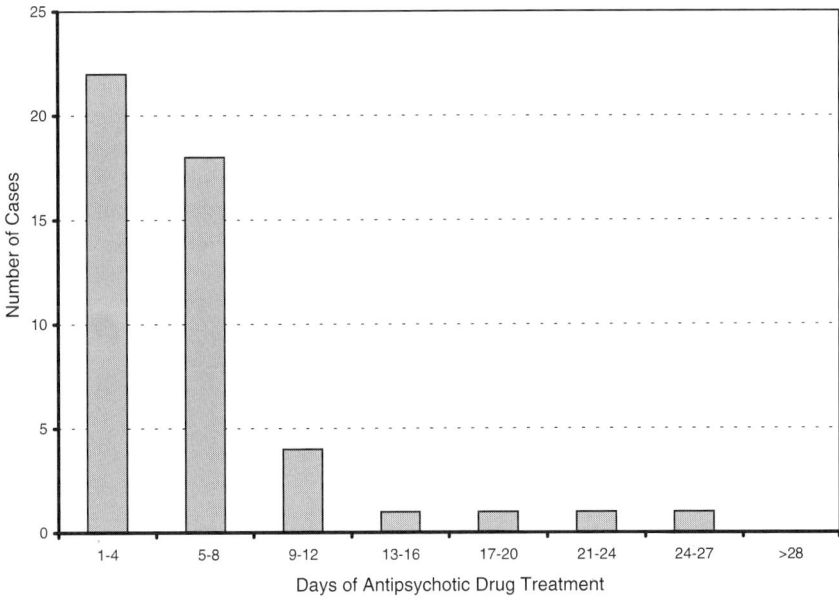

Figure 5.2 Timing of first dystonic reaction after initiation of antipsychotic medication in patients with no previous exposure to neuroleptic drugs.

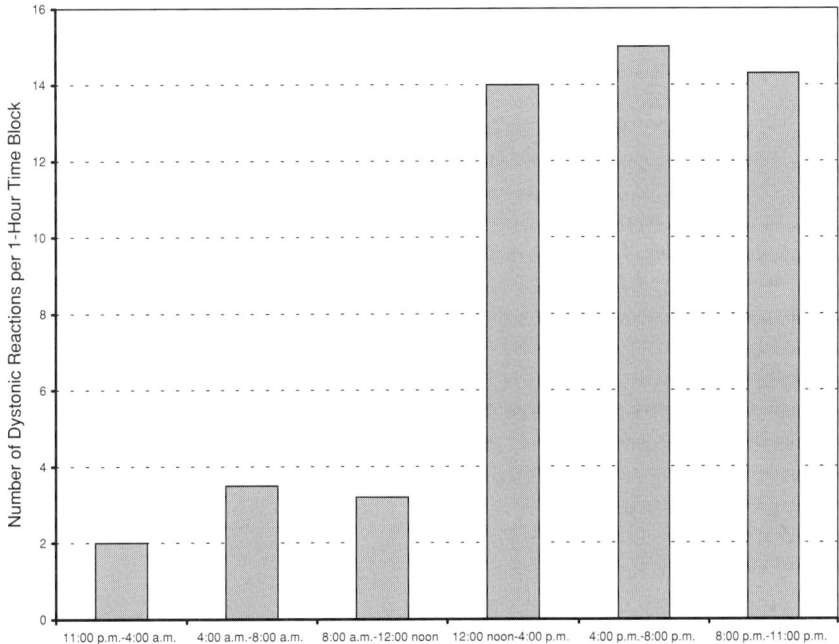

Figure 5.3 Circadian pattern of acute dystonic reactions in patients taking antipsychotic medication for the first time.

Epidemiology
Incidence
Estimates of the incidence of acute dystonic reaction after treatment with antipsychotic medication are dependent on a number of factors, including the patient population being studied, the type and dosage of drug being administered, and the concurrent use of prophylactic medication. Since most dystonic episodes occur within the first week of drug treatment, the figure of greatest interest is the risk of acute dystonia among patients taking antipsychotic drugs for the first time. Studies focusing on patients with first-onset psychosis treated with conventional neuroleptics have reported the risk of drug-induced acute dystonia to be in the range of 34–60% [4, 13, 15–17]. Among those with chronic illness on maintenance doses of medication, the incidence of dystonia is much lower, with one study reporting a figure of 1.7% over a 2-month period [18]. The precise figures for both first-onset and chronic patients will be strongly influenced by some of the factors outlined below.

Risk factors
Age
There is a strong negative correlation between the age of the patient and the risk of suffering a dystonic reaction upon exposure to antipsychotic medication. Keepers and Casey [19] reported a linear reduction of risk between the ages of 10 and 40 years, with the risk falling from over 60% among those younger than 20 years to almost zero after the age of 40 years. This agrees with general clinical experience as well as with data from our own prospective series (Fig. 5.4).

Sex
Early data from retrospective studies suggested that males may be at a higher risk of developing drug-induced dystonic reactions [1, 11]. More recent prospective investigations, however, have failed to confirm this association, finding instead either no sex difference [13, 17] or a higher risk for females [16]. Our own prospective study of drug-naïve patients indicates that, once age is taken into account, men and women are at equal risk of developing dystonic reactions when exposed to antipsychotic medication (Fig. 5.4).

Cocaine
Among the various drugs abused by psychiatric patients, cocaine has emerged in recent years as an important risk factor for drug-induced acute dystonia. A small study of cocaine addicts found that a high percentage (86%) developed dystonic reactions when exposed to the antipsychotic medication, haloperidol [20]. This was followed by two further studies that reported a three-fold increase in dystonic reactions among cocaine users [21, 22]. A more recent prospective investigation confirmed that cocaine is a significant risk factor for the development of drug-induced dystonia, with a relative risk of 4.4 [23]. Case reports suggest that cocaine may, even without concurrent administration of antipsychotic drugs, be capable of triggering a dystonic reaction [24, 25].

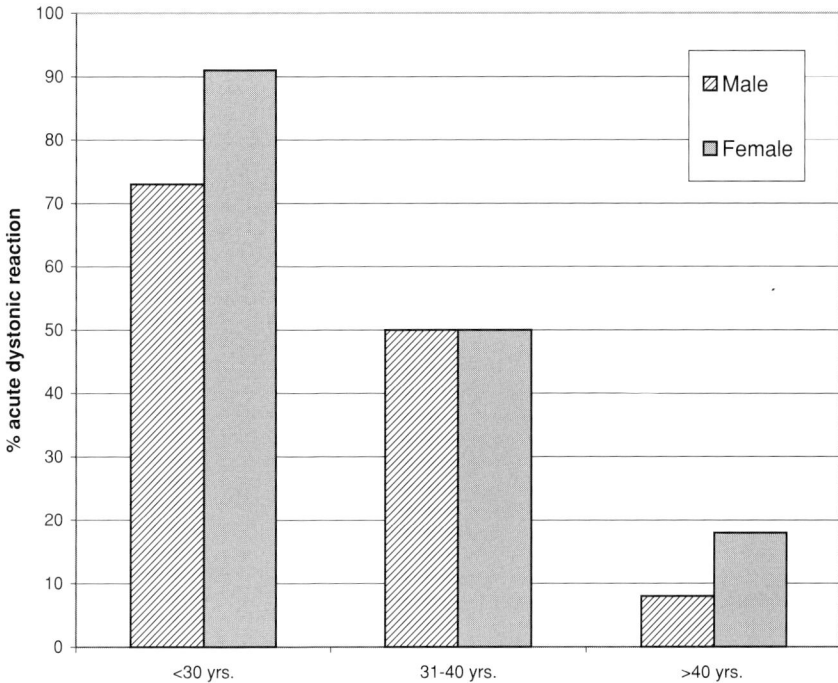

Figure 5.4 Incidence of acute dystonic reaction as a function of age and sex in patients receiving antipsychotic medication for the first time.

Previous dystonic reaction

A substantial fraction of patients who experience a dystonic reaction when treated with antipsychotic medication will go on to experience further episodes as treatment is continued [4, 19]. Among the first 89 patients in our prospective series who suffered an initial episode of dystonia, 51 (57%) had at least one more dystonic reaction during their in-patient hospitalization [4]. Those with recurrent episodes almost invariably had more widespread dystonia, with involvement of multiple body parts [2, 3].

Dosage of antipsychotic medication

The relationship between drug dosage and the risk of acute dystonia is not as straightforward as might be supposed. While one study reported a positive correlation between dosage and rates of dystonia [26], other evidence suggests an inverted U-shaped curve, with middle-range doses more likely to produce dystonia than very low or very high dosing schedules [19]. Our prospective investigation of drug-naïve patients showed that, even at very low dosages (mean daily dose of haloperidol 3.7 mg, which translates roughly into 175 mg of chlorpromazine equivalents), the risk of dystonia is substantial in this population [5]. It may be that dosage is related to neuroleptic-induced dystonia more as an epiphenomenon than as a direct risk factor.

High-potency versus low-potency medication

Epidemiological studies indicate that the risk of inducing dystonia is related to the potency with which the antipsychotic drug blocks D_2 dopamine receptors. High-potency agents, such as fluphenazine or haloperidol, have been associated with a much higher rate of dystonic reaction than lower-potency medications, such as thioridazine or chlorpromazine [27, 28], while drugs with intermediate levels of affinity for the D_2 receptor, such as perphenazine, fall somewhere in between. It is not clear, however, that this relationship between potency and dystonia is directly related to the receptor binding properties of the drugs. Baldessarini and colleagues [29] found that when antipsychotic equivalency was taken into account, there is a tendency for high-potency medication to be used in substantially higher doses than lower-potency agents. Others have pointed out that the lower-potency agents tend to have greater anticholinergic actions [30]. In other words, the higher risk of dystonia observed with high-potency antipsychotics may be attributable, at least in part, to differences in effective dosage and associated anticholinergic properties.

Concurrent AIDS infection

It has been recognized for some time that patients with acquired immunodeficiency syndrome (AIDS) are prone to developing neurological side effects, including parkinsonism, dystonia, and catatonia, when treated with antipsychotic medication [31–36]. A retrospective study estimated the risk of drug-induced extrapyramidal problems to be 2.4 times higher in AIDS patients than in age-matched psychotic patients without AIDS [32]. This AIDS-related vulnerability is consistent with increasing evidence that the AIDS virus may preferentially target the nuclei of the basal ganglia [37–39].

Atypical antipsychotic drugs

Clozapine

Originally developed in 1960 as a potential antidepressant, the dibenzodiazepine compound clozapine went almost 30 years before its antipsychotic properties came to attention. The landmark clinical trial [40], which demonstrated the efficacy of clozapine focused on patients with chronic schizophrenia who were resistant to standard antipsychotic drugs. Because of its propensity to cause agranulocytosis, clozapine continues to be used almost exclusively for patients who do not respond to, or who cannot tolerate, other medications.

From the beginning, it has been clear that clozapine has a much different side effect profile than conventional antipsychotics. This includes an almost negligible tendency to induce acute dystonic reactions, with only the occasional isolated case report appearing in the literature [41]. This may, in part, reflect the fact that clozapine is used only for those with previous, and generally rather prolonged, exposure to antipsychotic medications. As noted earlier, the vast majority of dystonic reactions occurs very early in the course of treatment. Even in chronically treated patients, however, the incidence of dystonia is in the range of 2–3% with conventional antipsychotic drugs [11, 18], but close to zero with clozapine, suggesting that the lack of dystonia with clozapine requires some other explanation. The most likely reason for the "atypical" side effect profile of clozapine lies in its pharmacology, with very low binding to the D_2 dopamine receptor accompanied by strong anticholinergic action.

Risperidone
The breakthrough discovery with clozapine was that the antipsychotic efficacy of a drug is not inextricably linked to neurological toxicity. This insight has given rise to a search for other "atypical" agents that might share the benign neurological profile of clozapine without producing its unwanted hematological side effects. The first of these newer drugs was risperidone, which was proclaimed in the early 1990s to have a side effect profile comparable to that of a placebo [42–44]. This putative lack of neurological toxicity was ascribed to the high affinity of the medication for the 5-HT_{2a} serotonin receptor [45], the notion being that this antiserotonergic action might, through some unclarified mechanism, nullify the potent D_2 receptor blockade that risperidone is known to produce in the striatum [46]. Other pharmacological properties of risperidone include antagonism at the α-1 and α-2 adrenergic receptors, but only very low affinity for the muscarinic acetylcholine receptor [47].

Contrary to initial expectations, the currently available literature suggests that the risk of acute dystonia with risperidone is roughly comparable to what is observed with older antipsychotic drugs [48]. In a prospective study of 246 consecutive acutely psychotic, neuroleptic-naïve patients treated with either low-dose risperidone (mean daily dosage 3.2 mg) or low-dose haloperidol (mean dosage 3.7 mg), dystonic reactions were recorded in 26.4% of the risperidone-treated patients, a figure which did not differ significantly from the rate of 34.5% among patients treated with haloperidol [5] (Fig. 5.5). An earlier multicenter trial involving patients with chronic schizophrenia reported dystonic reactions in 1.7% of risperidone-treated patients compared with 2.4% in those receiving haloperidol [49], figures that are in the range of what has been reported in other chronically treated patient populations [11, 18]. There is controversy about the incidence of dystonic reactions when risperidone is used to treat behavioral disturbances in children with autism. Some authors reported no dystonia when using doses ranging from 0.5 to 3.5 mg per day [50] while others found "frequent" dystonic side effects on doses of 3 mg per day [51].

Just as the incidence of acute dystonia with risperidone is similar to what is observed with other antipsychotic drugs, so too is the range of clinical manifestations (Table 5.1). In the aforementioned prospective study [5] of patients with

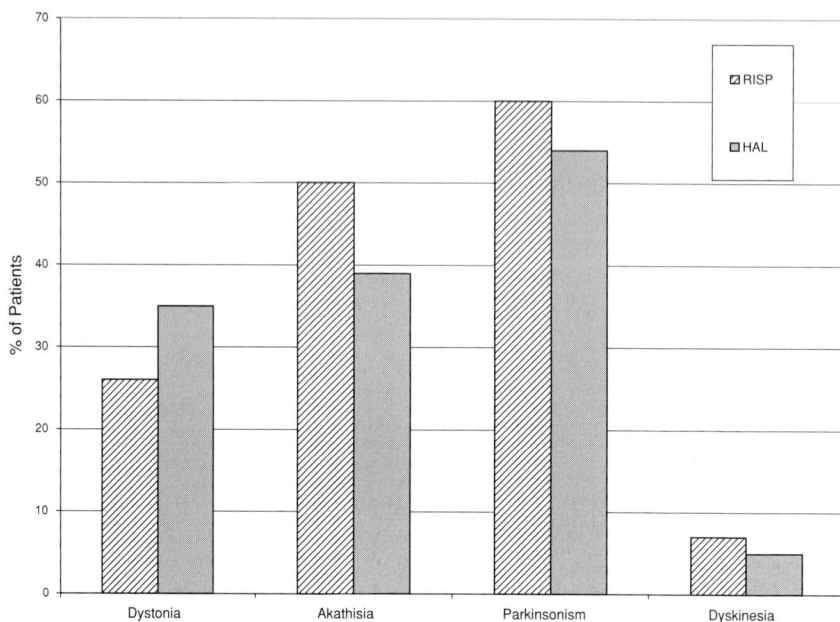

Figure 5.5 Comparative incidence of neurological side-effects in neuroleptic-naïve patients treated with risperidone or haloperidol. Reprinted with permission [5].

Table 5.1 Sixteen case reports of risperidone-induced dystonia

Authors	Case	Treatment day	RISP dosage (mg)	Nature of reaction
Dickson [52]	36 M	3	6	Trismus
Lombroso [53]	17 M	Not given	2	Acute dystonia
Radford [54]	21 M	2	2	Not specified – repeated reactions
Mandoki [55]	8 F	3	2	Tongue protrusion
	16 F	10	6	Tongue protrusion; oculogyric crisis
Anand [56]	23 M	4	8	Neck and back stiffness;
			4	thick tongue
Brody [57]	34 M	4	6	Laryngospasm, lingual impairment
Cheslik [58]	3 M	1	4	Oculogyric crisis
Faulk [59]	33 M	4	6	Oculogyric crisis; torticollis
Sanderson [60]	31 M	3	6	Laryngospasm; oculogyric crisis; retrocollis
Takhar [61]	17 M	2	2	Laryngospasm
Brown [62]	26 M	2	2	Laryngospasm; lingual impairment
Rosebush [63]	6 M	7	1	Oculogyric crisis
	24 F	3	2	Laryngospasm
	58 M	14	2	Trismus
Factor [36]	40 F	Unclear	6	Torticollis

no previous exposure to antipsychotic medication, the risperidone-induced dystonic reactions included trismus, torticollis, laryngospasm, and lingual impairment. Among the individual additional case reports in the literature for which sufficient clinical information is provided [36, 52–63], the profiles of risperidone-induced dystonic reactions included the following: laryngospasm (N = 5), oculogyric crisis (N = 5), torticollis/retrocollis (N = 3), trismus (N = 2), and lingual dysfunction including stiffness and/or thickening of the tongue (N = 5); some patients had involvement of more than one body part. Most of the dystonic reactions described in these case reports occurred within 7 days of starting treatment, with the dose of risperidone in all cases but one being 6 mg per day or less.

Olanzapine

Like risperidone, the thienobenzodiazepine compound, olanzapine, has potent affinity for the serotonergic (5 HT_2, 5 HT_6, and to a lesser extent 5 HT_3), dopaminergic (D_2, D_3 and D_4), and adrenergic (α-1) receptors [64, 65]. Unlike risperidone, olanzapine has strong anticholinergic effects, reflecting its high affinity for the M_{1-5} muscarinic receptors [64, 65].

As was the case with clozapine and risperidone, the initial clinical trials of olanzapine were conducted in patients with chronic schizophrenia who had prolonged prior exposure to antipsychotic medication [66, 67]. In these trials, however, the risk associated with olanzapine tended to be even lower than with haloperidol (1.1–1.4% vs. 3.6–5.3%) [66, 67]. A study of acutely agitated patients with chronic schizophrenia-type illness found that none of the 131 who were treated with 1–3 doses of intramuscular olanzapine (10 mg) developed dystonia, compared with 9 of the 126 who received intramuscular haloperidol [68]. Unfortunately, none of these reports includes useful details regarding the nature of the dystonia or the criteria for diagnosis, making it difficult to judge whether the events described with haloperidol were indeed dystonic reactions.

While the available literature suggests that olanzapine may be less likely than most antipsychotic drugs to provoke dystonia, the risk is not zero, even in chronically treated patients, as illustrated by some clear case reports from the literature (Table 5.2). A 50-year-old man with chronic schizophrenia and a previous history of drug-induced torticollis developed neck stiffness on olanzapine (15 mg) and frank torticollis when the dose was later increased from 20 to 25 mg per day [69]. A 68-year-old woman with long-standing schizoaffective disorder and an earlier history of severe parkinsonism on haloperidol developed acute lingual dystonia and dysarthria 2 days after switching from risperidone to olanzapine 10 mg, with the recurrence of the lingual dystonia after the olanzapine was increased from 10 to 15 mg per day [69]. A third case involved a 56-year-old woman with chronic schizophrenia and a previous history of oculogyric crisis in response to antipsychotic drugs. When switched to olanzapine (5 mg) she presented with torticollis and "oculogyric signs," followed by lingual dystonia and dysarthria when the dose was

Table 5.2 Seven case reports of olanzapine-induced dystonia

Authors	Case	Diagnosis	Duration of illness	Olanzapine Rx Dose (mg)	Olanzapine Rx Duration of Rx	Nature of dystonia
Landry and Cournoyer [69]	50 M	Schizophrenia	15 yrs.	15–25	~14 wks.	Torticollis
	68 F	Schizophrenia	45 yrs.	10	2 days	Lingual dystonia with dysarthria
Alevigos et al. [70]	56 F	Schizophrenia	20 yrs.	5	<5 days	Torticollis and oculogyric crisis
	50 M	Schizophrenia	17 yrs.	5	2–3 hrs.	Severe torticollis, lingual dystonia with dysarthria
Rosebush and Mazurek	44 F	Bipolar	6 yrs.	5	2–3 hrs.	Throat tightness with laryngospasm
	27 M	Bipolar	First onset	6	2 days	Torticollis
	32 M	Atypical psychosis	First onset	10	4 days	Torticollis, limb dystonia

increased to 10 mg per day [70]. Another report described a 50-year-old man with long-standing treatment-resistant schizophrenia and sensitivity to previous antipsychotic medication. Within a few hours of starting on olanzapine (5 mg) he suffered an acute dystonic reaction characterized by severe torticollis and lingual dystonia with dysarthria [70]. We recently consulted on another patient who developed dystonia on a very low dose of olanzapine. This 44-year-old woman with a 6-year history of bipolar disorder was taking valproic acid but no other medications at the time of admission to hospital. She was given olanzapine (5 mg) at bedtime for treatment of agitation and insomnia. Within a few hours of receiving her initial dose she developed throat tightness/laryngospasm, promptly relieved by benztropine (2 mg) (Rosebush and Mazurek, unpublished observation).

With the recent emphasis on early intervention strategies in psychosis, it has become important to determine the risk of dystonic reactions for patients with no prior exposure to antipsychotic medication. We recently completed data collection from a prospective randomized controlled trial comparing olanzapine with haloperidol in drug-naïve patients with first-onset psychosis. Early data from the study show the rate of acute dystonia in olanzapine-treated patients to be about 12% compared with a rate of approximately 35% among those receiving haloperidol (Rosebush and Mazurek, unpublished data). Two cases from this series illustrate the phenomenon. One was a 27-year-old man with bipolar disorder who developed torticollis a few days after starting on olanzapine 5 mg per day. The second involved a 32-year-old man with a diagnosis of atypical psychosis who suffered torticollis and limb dystonia while taking olanzapine (10 mg/day). These observations indicate that olanzapine can indeed provoke dystonic reactions in first-onset patients, but apparently at a lower rate than is observed with haloperidol.

Quetiapine

Another of the newer "atypical" antipsychotic drugs to be released in the past decade is the dibenzothiazepine compound, quetiapine. Like risperidone and olanzapine, it blocks the $5HT_{2a}$ subtype of serotonin receptor, a pharmacological property that is presumed to reduce the risk of neurological toxicity. Quetiapine also exerts potent antagonism at the H_1 subtype of histamine receptor, an effect that may be responsible for the sedation and weight gain that have been associated with its use. Like clozapine, quetiapine has less affinity for striatal D_2 dopamine receptors than do most other antipsychotic medications [71, 72].

Several case reports have documented the ability of quetiapine to induce acute dystonic reactions. A 20-year-old man with treatment-resistant schizophrenia but no past history of dystonia developed lingual dystonia, torticollis, and oculogyric crisis within 2 days of starting quetiapine 25 mg b.i.d [73]. A 30-year-old woman with long-standing bipolar illness and no recent exposure to antipsychotic medication reported neck tightness and difficulty swallowing within 2 days of starting quetiapine [73]. Both patients responded promptly to treatment with diphenhydramine. An unusual case involved an 18-year-old woman who was diagnosed with Meige syndrome, completely responsive to biperiden, within a month of beginning quetiapine [74]. The relative risk of dystonia with quetiapine compared with other antipsychotic medications is not known. While the general clinical impression is that acute dystonic reactions may be less likely with quetiapine than with therapeutically equivalent doses of older drugs, such as chlorpromazine and haloperidol, comparative studies offer little direct evidence for this [75, 76].

Ziprasidone

The benzothiazolyl piperazine derivative, ziprasidone, shares with many other recently developed antipsychotic drugs a greater affinity for the $5\,HT_{2a}$ serotonin receptor than for the D_2 dopamine receptor. An early pilot study found one case of severe akathisia but no acute dystonic reactions among the 14 children and adolescents who received ziprasidone in doses up to 40 mg per day for treatment of Tourette syndrome [77]. A recent case report, however, suggests that ziprasidone, like most other antipsychotic medications, can induce dystonic reactions under at least some circumstances. A 10-year-old boy of borderline intelligence developed intense muscle rigidity and tongue protrusion shortly after starting on ziprasidone for treatment of disruptive behavior disorder; the dystonia resolved quickly with benztropine [51].

Other drugs that can induce dystonia

Antiemetics

Dopaminergic stimulation of the area postrema, which lies in the floor of the 4th ventricle, produces nausea. It is therefore not surprising that many drugs used as antiemetic agents are potent antagonists of the D_2 dopamine receptor. Because the area postrema is physiologically outside the blood brain barrier, antiemetic drugs are usually selected for their poor CNS penetrance. This ideally would allow them to block dopamine receptors of the chemoreceptor trigger zone in the area postrema while exerting relatively little effect on regions protected by the blood brain barrier. Despite this, several antiemetic agents have been reported to produce neurological side effects, particularly in patients with AIDS [78–80]. One suspects that AIDS-related impairment of the blood brain barrier might allow the drugs greater access to striatal dopamine receptors than would normally be anticipated. Even patients with an apparently intact blood brain barrier, however, can occasionally suffer acute dystonic reactions with antiemetic medication. A study reviewing the side effects of metoclopramide estimated the prevalence of acute dystonic/dyskinetic reactions to be 109 per million prescriptions among patients in the 12–19-year age range [81]. It is likely that a prospective study with specific attention to the emergence of dystonia would find the prevalence to be considerably higher.

Antidepressants
Conventional tricyclic antidepressants (TCAs)
After nearly a half-century of use, tricyclic antidepressant medications are recognized to be associated only rarely with acute dystonic reactions. A 30-year-old depressed woman developed what may have been an oculogyric crisis after a single 75-mg dose of amitriptyline, then later reported two further episodes of apparent dystonia, including oculogyric crisis, limb dystonia, and lingual dystonia, shortly after starting on another tricyclic medication, doxepin [82]; there was no mention in the report of whether the patient had recent exposure to cocaine. A second case involved a 30-year-old man who developed retrocollis after taking his second dose of amitriptyline (25 mg), followed by another episode of retrocollis the following day after amitriptyline (75 mg) [83]. A third patient was a 20-year-old man who abruptly developed opisthotonos, retrocollis, lingual dystonia, and orofacial dystonia after having taken amitriptyline 50 mg per day for 3 months [84]. As with the other two cases there was no specific mention of whether the patient may have recently used cocaine. The overall experience is that tricyclic-induced dystonia is an extremely rare phenomenon.

Monoamine oxidase inhibitors (MAOIs)
Like the tricyclic drugs, monoamine oxidase inhibitors (MAOIs) have been used to treat depression for almost 50 years. Tranylcypromine has been implicated in a single case of acute truncal dystonia, but even that case was complicated by concurrent withdrawal from antipsychotic medication and two recent courses of electroconvulsive therapy [85]. The paucity of reported cases in the literature would suggest that the overall rate of MAOI-induced dystonia is essentially negligible.

Selective serotonin reuptake inhibitors (SSRIs)
In contrast to the other categories of antidepressant medication, SSRI-type drugs have a well-established tendency to induce dystonic reactions. The initial case report of SSRI-induced dystonia appeared in 1979, very shortly after the drugs were first introduced [86]. By 1996, pharmaceutical records had documented 383 cases of dystonia associated with the use of fluoxetine, sertraline, or paroxetine [87]. The range of dystonic phenomena associated with SSRIs includes torticollis [86, 88, 89], jaw stiffness/trismus [86, 88–91], lingual dystonia [90, 92], truncal dystonia/opisthotonos [89, 93, 94], oculogyric crisis [95, 96], throat tightness/laryngospasm [97], limb dystonia [89, 98], blepharospasm [94], and facial dystonia [99]. Most of the reported dystonic reactions occurred early in the course of treatment or after a dosage increase.

Men and women appear to be at equal risk of suffering SSRI-induced dystonia [100]. One review identified 20 cases of SSRI-related dystonia, half of which occurred in men. Another retrospective review found that over two-thirds of reported cases of SSRI-induced dystonia developed in women [101]. This relative preponderance of women in the latter review may be related to the two-fold greater prevalence of depression, and therefore of antidepressant therapy, in women [102].

The incidence of SSRI-induced dystonia has probably been underappreciated. A short-term study undertaken to evaluate the efficacy of a new SSRI medication found that 4 of 41 patients treated with fluvoxamine developed evidence of dystonia within 7 days of beginning treatment, compared with none in the placebo-treated group [103].

Serotonin and noradrenaline reuptake inhibitors (SNRIs)

Venlafaxine is a prototype of the recently introduced subtype of antidepressant medication known as SNRIs. While venlafaxine is ostensibly distinct from other forms of antidepressants, early clinical experience suggests a side effect profile similar to that of the SSRIs, including an ability to induce dystonic reactions. We recently encountered a 44-year-old man who, after unsuccessful trials of buproprion and paroxetine, was started on venlafaxine for treatment of his depressive symptoms. Over the next 13 months, while taking venlafaxine (150 mg/day), he suffered seven episodes of apparent oculogyric crisis and recurrent episodes of limb dystonia involving his hands, forearms, and calves. The episodes abated after venlafaxine was discontinued. It turned out that the patient had been abusing cocaine during the entire time he was receiving antidepressant medication, but it was only on the venlafaxine that he experienced the apparent dystonic reactions.

Pathophysiology

Dystonia in relation to motor programs: the role of the basal ganglia

At a conceptual level, dystonia, like other movement disorders, can be seen as resulting from defective "readout" or "playback" of a motor program. According to this theory, repertoires of various movements are encoded in the brain in much the same way that a music program, for example, is encoded and stored on a compact disc. Activation of a particular motor program results in an exquisitely orchestrated coordination of neural activity which, in turn, produces a precise pattern of stimulation/inhibition involving specific muscle groups.

While various neuronal structures are involved in the storage and activation of motor programs, the basal ganglia, and especially the striatum, appear to be of particular importance. Inadequate dopaminergic signaling in the striatum, for example, such as occurs in Parkinson's disease, results in the impaired volitional activation of the motor program. The clinical consequences of this are the akinesia (difficulty initiating movement) and bradykinesia (slowness in carrying out the movement) that we recognize as the core features of parkinsonism. Degeneration of the GABAergic output neurons of the striatum, as happens in Huntington's disease, leads to impaired selectivity in the activation of motor programs. The resulting dyskinetic movements can in this sense be viewed as reflecting the "intrusion" of related but unselected repertoires into the "chosen" motor program. Dystonia, being a form of dyskinesia, can be understood as a defect of selectivity, whereby the "selected" motor action is accompanied by abnormally prolonged contraction of agonist muscles and defective reciprocal inhibition of antagonists. Not surprisingly, the lesions most commonly associated with dystonia are in the putamen [104], the "motor" portion of the striatum. It has been proposed that aberrant striatal output may result in the abnormal sensorimotor coordination in the cerebral cortex that is thought to be the physiological substrate of dystonia [105, 106]. It therefore makes sense to try to understand drug-induced dystonia in terms of the effects exerted by the responsible medications on striatal function.

The neurochemical anatomy of the striatum

The striatum contains two morphologically and functionally distinct subpopulations of neurons: (1) spiny projection cells that carry output signals from the striatum to other basal ganglia structures and that comprise about 90% of all striatal neurons; and (2) aspiny interneurons that project locally within the striatum. There are two subgroups of spiny output cells: those that preferentially project to the internal globus pallidus and the reticular portion of the substantia nigra contain GABA colocalized with substance P and dynorphin [107–112]; those projecting to the external globus pallidus contain GABA colocalized with met-enkephalin [111–112]. The locally projecting aspiny neurons can likewise be divided into chemically distinct subgroups: large aspiny cholinergic interneurons that comprise 1–4% of all striatal neurons [113]; medium-sized aspiny interneurons containing the neuropeptides somatostatin and neuropeptide Y, colocalized with the neuronal isoform of nitric oxide synthase [114, 115]; various subpopulations of aspiny parvalbumin-positive GABAergic interneurons [116–118]; and multiple subtypes of calretinin-containing interneurons [117]. The major afferent projections to the striatum are the massive glutamatergic pathways from cerebral cortex and thalamus, which together account for almost 80% of all afferent terminals [119–122]; and the dopaminergic input from substantia nigra pars compacta, which constitutes another 15–20% of striatal afferents [122]. Less prominent afferent systems include the serotonergic input from the dorsal raphe nucleus [123] and glutamatergic fibers from the hippocampus and amygdala [119, 124]. In addition to these exogenous inputs, the various subpopulations of intrinsic striatal neurons make extensive synaptic connections with each other [125–127].

Drug-induced dystonia: antipsychotic medications

The most important cause of drug-induced acute dystonia is antipsychotic medication. The propensity of any particular antipsychotic drug to induce dystonia correlates strongly with its pharmacological affinity for D_2 dopamine receptors in the striatum [128]. An understanding of how these agents cause dystonia should focus on the ways that dopamine, and in particular D_2-receptor-mediated signaling, influences the intricate neuronal circuitry of the striatum.

Direct actions on spiny "output" neurons of the striatum

The dopaminergic input to the striatum originates in the compact part of the substantia nigra, with some additional contribution from the retrorubral area. A majority of the dopaminergic fibers of the nigrostriatal tract converge with the glutamatergic terminals of the corticostriatal pathway on individual dendritic spines of the medium spiny projection neurons in the striatum [129, 130]. This provides an anatomical basis for the electrophysiological, neurochemical, and behavioral evidence that dopamine acts in the striatum to modify glutamatergic signaling [131–133]. The precise mechanism by which this happens is not clear. The conventional notion is that dopamine acts through D_1 receptors to exert a net excitatory influence on the GABA/substance P/dynorphin-containing neurons that project in the "direct" pathway from striatum to the internal globus pallidus and the pars reticulata of substantia nigra [127]. The model further posits that dopaminergic activation of D_2 receptors results in a net inhibitory effect on the GABA- and enkephalin-containing neurons that give rise to the "indirect" pathway from striatum to the external globus pallidus [127]. The model is complicated, however, by the finding that D_1 and D_2 receptors, instead of being segregated to neurons of the direct and indirect pathways, as originally suggested [111], are colocalized on individual projection neurons [134–136].

Actions mediated by aspiny interneurons
Cholinergic interneurons
In addition to its direct effects on the medium spiny output neurons, dopamine acts on the various subpopulations of striatal interneurons. Of particular interest in this regard are the large aspiny cholinergic cells, which are sensitive to minute changes in membrane potential and which have extensive axonal and dendritic fields [137]. Widely dispersed populations of these tonically active neurons develop synchronous firing patterns in response to context-specific sensory cues, thereby forming what amounts to a "neuronal grid" that can coordinate signaling among the wide range of striatal neurons with which they made synaptic contact [138–140]. In other words, the network of cholinergic interneurons may serve as a mediator of sensorimotor integration in the striatum. This leads to the hypothesis that dysfunction of the cholinergic system might give rise to the aberrant sensorimotor processing that is thought to be the fundamental impairment in dystonia. Consistent with this notion, a recent study using positron emission tomography showed a reduction of markers for cholinergic nerve terminals and cholinergic interneurons in the striatum of patients with cervical dystonia [141]. These same cholinergic interneurons in striatum express D_2 dopamine receptors [142] and D_2 receptor

stimulation modulates acetylcholine release in the striatum [143, 144]. The tendency of antipsychotic drugs to induce dystonia may therefore relate to altered dopaminergic control of cholinergic signaling in the striatum.

GABAergic interneurons

Another population of striatal interneurons that has been implicated in dystonia is the network of fast-spiking parvalbumin-immunoreactive aspiny GABAergic cells. These constitute only 3–5% of striatal neurons but are thought to represent the main source of inhibitory signaling in the striatum [145, 146]. Like their cholinergic counterparts, the parvalbumin-containing GABAergic interneurons make extensive synaptic connections with striatal projection neurons, and are linked to each other through electrotonic coupling [146, 147]. This allows them, too, to function as a sort of neuronal signal "grid" and to exert widespread influences on striatal output. The potential relevance of these GABAergic interneurons to dystonia was underlined by the finding that they are markedly depleted in a genetic hamster model of paroxysmal dystonia [148]. Dopamine acts through D_2 receptors to inhibit GABA release in the striatum [149–151], an effect that would be expected to produce the same functional result as the loss of GABAergic interneurons in the dystonic mutant hamster.

NOS-positive interneurons

A third population of striatal interneurons that may participate in antipsychotic drug-induced dystonia is the subgroup of medium-sized aspiny cells that contain somatostatin (SS), neuropeptide Y (NPY), and the neuronal isoform of nitric oxide synthase (NOS), in many cases colocalized with GABA [115, 118, 145, 152]. Like other interneuron families in the striatum, the SS/NPY/NOS/GABA cells may be electrotonically linked, allowing them to operate as a system or grid. Unlike the cholinergic and parvalbumin-positive populations, however, the SS/NPY/NOS/GABA neurons do not rely exclusively on axonal ramifications to communicate with other cells. Because they contain NOS, this group of interneurons can produce the gaseous transmitter, nitric oxide, which can then diffuse radially in all directions, much as a sound wave propagates outward from the point of origin. This means that the SS/NPY/NOS/GABA cells have properties that would be well suited to functions of sensorimotor integration, such as have been proposed for the cholinergic and parvalbumin-immunoreactive populations. In addition, the somatostatin released by these interneurons alters dopaminergic adenylate cyclase activity [153] and acts through the sst_2 subtype of somatostatin receptor to stimulate dopamine release in the striatum [154–156]. While SS/NPY/NOS/GABA cells have few D_1 receptors and virtually no D_2 receptors [157–158], pharmacological manipulation of D_2 receptors can modulate the somatostatinergic function in the striatum [159, 160], presumably through indirect connections.

Actions on striatal afferents

The pharmacological effects of antipsychotic drugs in the striatum are not limited to their actions on the various subpopulations of spiny projection neurons and aspiny interneurons. Dopamine has been reported to inhibit glutamatergic transmission in the striatum, ostensibly through a D_2-receptor-mediated action on cortical-striatal terminals [161]. Dopamine also acts through D_2 autoreceptors to inhibit transmitter synthesis and release from the terminals of the nigral-striatal tract. Blockade of these D_2 receptors by antipsychotic medication would thus be expected to produce a short-term increase in the release of both glutamate and dopamine, with corresponding effects on neural signaling in the striatum.

Effects on dopaminergic neurons in substantia nigra

It has long been recognized that the neurological side effects of antipsychotic drugs cannot be adequately explained on the basis of D_2 receptor blockade alone. Tardive dyskinesia, for example, typically develops months or even years after the start of therapy and may persist long after the drug has been discontinued. Similarly, drug-induced parkinsonism usually does not appear until several days after the start of antipsychotic treatment, even though the D_2 receptors are pharmacologically blocked within hours. This temporal dysjunction between the pharmacological and clinical effects of the medication suggests that antipsychotic drugs do more than simply block D_2 dopamine receptors. This notion was recently confirmed with the demonstration that neuroleptic medications have profound effects on the dopaminergic cell bodies of the nigrostriatal tract, dramatically downregulating the biosynthetic enzyme tryosine hydroxylase and inducing apoptotic changes [162–166]. The time course for some of these actions was surprisingly rapid, with highly significant changes evident within 10 minutes of the initial dose [166]. The implications of these emerging observations for dopaminergic signaling in the striatum, and for the understanding of drug-induced dystonia, have not yet been determined.

Drug-induced dystonia: SSRI medications

The other category of medication that has shown some propensity to induce acute dystonia is that of SSRIs. As indicated by their name, SSRIs block the transporter responsible for taking synaptically released serotonin back into the presynaptic terminal. The precise effects of this on serotonergic transmission are not entirely clear. At first glance, this pharmacological action would appear to increase synaptic and extrasynaptic levels of serotonin, thereby promoting serotonergic stimulation of postsynaptic receptors. On the other hand, the short-term rise in extraneuronal serotonin levels will activate the 5-HT_1 families of presynaptic and somatodendritic autoreceptors, resulting in a *reduction* of serotonin release. Furthermore, preliminary studies suggest that SSRI medications induce a marked downregulation of tryptophan hydroxylase, the rate-limiting enzyme for serotonin biosynthesis, in the dorsal raphe neurons that project to the cortex and the striatum [167] (Mazurek MF and Rosebush PI, unpublished observations). The ultimate effect of these competing influences on serotonergic transmission is thus likely to be rather complicated.

The serotonergic innervation of the basal ganglia arises principally from the dorsal raphe nucleus, with a lesser contribution from the median raphe [168]. As with dopamine afferents, the primary synaptic targets of serotonergic terminals in the striatum are the dendrites of medium-sized spiny output neurons [169]. In addition to the actions mediated by these direct synaptic relationships with striatal projection neurons, serotonin can influence dopaminergic and cholinergic transmission in the striatum, presumably through axo-axonic appositions and release from nonsynaptic terminals [130, 170, 171].

The effects of serotonin are mediated by a multiplicity of receptor subtypes, at least 14 of which have thus far been identified. The 5-HT_{1A}, 5-HT_{1B}, and 5-HT_{1D} subtypes function as autoreceptors, providing feedback inhibition of both firing rate and release from serotonergic projections arising from the dorsal and median raphe [172–175]. 5-HT_{1B} receptors are also found on axon terminals of the striatonigral projection neurons, where they serve to regulate GABA release [176, 177]. While receptors of the 5-HT_2 family are generally associated with actions in the cerebral cortex [178], binding sites for some classes of 5-HT_2 receptors have been identified in the striatum [179, 180]. 5-HT_3 receptors have the unique property among monoaminergic receptors of being linked to a ligand-gated ion channel [181] and appear to be expressed throughout the striatum [182, 183]. Other classes of serotonin receptors that have been localized to striatum are the 5-HT_4 [184], 5-HT_6 [185], and 5-HT_7 [186] subtypes. The functional interactions among these numerous receptor subgroups and their various signal transduction mechanisms are inevitably complex. It is therefore not surprising that a clear model has yet to emerge regarding the ways that serotonergic transmission contributes to neural signaling in the striatum. While it seems likely that the pathophysiology of SSRI-induced dystonia in some way involves the effects of these drugs on basal ganglia function, the mechanisms by which this might occur remain obscure.

Treatment

The acute episode

Acute dystonia demands immediate therapeutic intervention. Most episodes resolve within 15–20 minutes following a single intramuscular dose of an anticholinergic/antihistaminergic compound such as benztropine (Cogentin; 1–2 mg) or diphenhydramine (Benadryl; 25–50 mg). Equally efficacious are benzodiazepine medications such as diazepam (Valium; 2–5 mg), or lorazepam (Ativan; 1–2 mg) [187]. For acute laryngospasm, which is a potentially life-threatening condition, intravenous administration of a benzodiazepine is the treatment of choice.

If an episode of acute dystonia persists after an initial dose of parenteral medication, a second dose of the same drug can be given about 30 minutes later. Should that prove unsuccessful, one should switch to a different medication. Any case that fails to respond in the usual way should prompt consideration of an alternative diagnosis. The persistence of trismus, for example, might point beyond dystonia to a dislocated jaw.

Prophylaxis following the acute episode

There is no clear consensus about the use of prophylactic medication in the patient who has suffered an acute dystonic reaction. A substantial fraction of those who experience an initial episode of dystonia will go on to have further episodes unless preventive measures are instituted [4]. A reasonable recommendation might be to follow treatment of the initial dystonic reaction with regular doses of a suitable prophylactic medication such as benztropine. Since most dystonic reactions occur in the first week of antipsychotic drug treatment, it should be sufficient to continue with benztropine, or a suitable alternative, for 4–7 days following the initial episode, after which time the prophylactic agent can be withdrawn.

Primary prophylaxis

The decision of whether to use prophylactic medication at the *start* of antipsychotic drug therapy – that is, prior to any episodes of dystonia – depends on the relative risk of the possible dystonic reaction compared with the projected side effects of the prophylactic agent. A high-risk individual, for example, such as a young patient with no prior exposure to antipsychotic medication and recent exposure to cocaine, would probably warrant a 1-week course of prophylactic benztropine. An elderly person, on the other hand, is at much lower risk of drug-induced dystonia and at the same time considerably more susceptible to the visual blurring, cognitive impairment, and other side effects that can accompany benztropine treatment.

Routine use of prophylactic agents, particularly on a prolonged basis, is discouraged [188]. The side effects of anticholinergic compounds typically include dry mouth, which in a psychotic patient who may already have poor personal hygiene, can easily lead to oral candidiasis. Another potentially serious complication is constipation, which can lead to bowel obstruction. Furthermore, most of the medications used for dystonia prophylaxis, such as benztropine and benzodiazepines, are themselves potential drugs of abuse. Finally, there is some evidence that anticholinergic/antihistaminergic agents might increase the risk of tardive dyskinesia [188].

There is one situation in which primary prophylaxis should *always* be used. Patients who are receiving antipsychotic drugs and who require seclusion must receive prophylactic medication to reduce the risk of laryngospasm, which could prove fatal in such a situation.

Future directions

Acute drug-induced dystonia generally responds well to pharmacological intervention. This places a premium on the accurate recognition of cases. Unfortunately, the early literature on the newer "atypical" antipsychotic drugs gave rise to a perception that these agents were virtually free of neurological side effects. This led to an underappreciation of the abilities of these newer drugs to induce dystonic reactions. An important goal in the coming years will be to obtain an accurate profile of the dystonia risk associated with each of the newer antipsychotic medications, particularly in patients with no prior exposure to antipsychotic drugs. A related need is for accurate data regarding the propensity of other agents, such as SSRI medications, to induce dystonic reactions.

The judicious use of prophylactic drugs requires an ability to identify those individuals that are at the highest risk of dystonia when challenged with a particular medication. An especially promising development in this regard is the emerging field of pharmacogenomics. With the rapid advances in molecular genetics that have taken place in recent years, there is good reason to expect progress in the identification of gene markers that are associated with specific drug-induced side effects, including dystonia. This will allow a more precise targeting of prophylactic strategies to individuals at risk of experiencing a dystonic reaction when given a particular medication.

References

1. Swett C, Jr. Drug-induced dystonia. Am J Psychiatry 1975; 132: 532–534.
2. Mazurek MF, Rosebush PI. A prospective study of neuroleptic-induced dystonia: incidence and relationship to age, sex, medications and concurrent parkinsonism. Neurology 1991; 41(suppl 1): 274.
3. Mazurek MF, Rosebush PI. Drug-induced dystonia in patients taking neuroleptic medication for the first time. Mov Disord 1992; 7(suppl 1): 54.
4. Mazurek MF, Rosebush PI. Circadian pattern of acute, neuroleptic-induced dystonic reactions. Am J Psychiatry 1996; 153: 708–710.
5. Rosebush PI, Mazurek MF. Neurologic side effects in neuroleptic-naive patients treated with haloperidol or risperidone. Neurology 1999; 52: 782–785.
6. Flaherty JA, Lahmeyer HW. Laryngeal-pharyngeal dystonia as a possible cause of asphyxia with haloperidol treatment. Am J Psychiatry 1978; 135: 1414–1415.
7. Newton-John H. Acute upper airway obstruction due to supraglottic dystonia induced by a neuroleptic. Br Med J 1988; 297: 964–965.
8. Wilson SAK. Epidemic encephalitis. In Bruce AN (ed) Neurology. London, Edward Arnold, 1940, pp. 99–144.
9. Jelliffe SE. Psychologic components in postencephalitic oculogyric crisis. Arch Neurol Psychiatry 1929; 21: 491–532.
10. Owens DGC. A guide to the extrapyramidal side-effects of antipsychotic drugs. Cambridge UK, Cambridge University Press, 1999.
11. Ayd FJ. A survey of drug-induced extrapyramidal reactions. JAMA 1961; 175: 1054–1060.

12. Keepers GA, Clappison VJ, Casey DE. Initial anticholinergic prophylaxis for neuroleptic-induced extrapyramidal syndromes. Arch Gen Psychiatry 1983; 40: 1113–1117.
13. Singh H, Levinson DF, Simpson GM, et al. Acute dystonia during fixed-dose neuroleptic treatment. J Clin Psychopharmacol 1990; 10: 389–396.
14. McCowan PK, Cook LC. Oculogyric crises in chronic epidemic encephalitis. Brain 1928; 51: 285–309.
15. Remington GJ, Voineskos G, Pollock B, et al. Prevalence of neuroleptic-induced dystonia in mania and schizophrenia. Am J Psychiatry 1990; 147: 1231–1233.
16. Chakos MH, Mayerhoff DI, Loebel AD, et al. Incidence and correlates of acute extrapyramidal symptoms in first episode of schizophrenia. Psychopharmacol Bull 1992; 28: 81–86.
17. Aguilar EJ, Keshavan MS, Martinez-Quiles MD, et al. Predictors of acute dystonia in first-episode psychotic patients. Am J Psychiatry 1994; 151: 1819–1821.
18. Tan CH, Chiang PC, Ng LL, et al. Oculogyric spasm in Asian psychiatric in-patients on maintenance medication. Br J Psychiatry 1994; 165: 381–383.
19. Keepers GA, Casey DE. Prediction of neuroleptic-induced dystonia. J Clin Psychopharmacol 1987; 7: 342–345.
20. Kumor K, Sherer M, Jaffe J. Haloperidol-induced dystonia in cocaine addicts. Lancet 1986; 2(8519): 1341–1342.
21. Choy-Kwong M, Lipton RB. Cocaine withdrawal dystonia. Neurology 1990; 40: 863–864.
22. Hegarty AM, Lipton RB, Merriam AE, et al. Cocaine as a risk factor for acute dystonic reactions. Neurology 1991; 41: 1670–1672.
23. van Harten PN, van Trier JC, Horwitz EH, et al. Cocaine as a risk factor for neuroleptic-induced acute dystonia. J Clin Psychiatry 1998; 59: 128–130.
24. Merab J. Acute dystonic reaction to cocaine. Am J Med 1988; 84: 564.
25. Choy-Kwong M, Lipton RB. Dystonia related to cocaine withdrawal: a case report and pathogenic hypothesis. Neurology 1989; 39: 996–997.
26. Khanna R, Das A, Damodaran SS. Prospective study of neuroleptic-induced dystonia in mania and schizophrenia. Am J Psychiatry 1992; 149: 511–513.
27. National Institute of Mental Health Psychopharmacology and Service Center Collaborative Study Group. Phenothiazine treatment in acute schizophrenia. Arch Gen Psychiatry 1964; 10: 246–261.
28. Cole JD, Davis JM. Antipsychotic Drugs. New York, Grune and Stratton, 1969.
29. Baldessarini RJ, Katz B, Cotton P. Dissimilar dosing with high-potency and low-potency neuroleptics. Am J Psychiatry 1984; 141: 748–752.
30. Snyder S, Greenberg D, Yamamura HI. Antischizophrenic drugs and brain cholinergic receptors: affinity for muscarinic sites predicts extrapyramidal effects. Arch Gen Psychiatry 1974; 31: 58–61.
31. Kieburtz KD, Epstein LG, Gelbard HA, et al. Excitotoxicity and dopaminergic dysfunction in the acquired immunodeficiency syndrome dementia complex: therapeutic implications. Arch Neurol 1991; 48: 1281–1284.
32. Hriso E, Kuhn T, Majdeu JC, et al. Extrapyramidal symptoms due to dopamine blocking agents in patients with AIDS encephalopathy. Am J Psychiatry 1991; 148: 1558–1561.
33. Factor SA, Podskalny GD, Barron KD. Persistent neuroleptic induced rigidity and dystonia in AIDS dementia complex: a clinico-pathological case report. J Neurol Sci 1994; 127: 114–120.
34. Manji H, Sweeney B, Connolly S, et al. Movement disorders in AIDS: infective, neoplastic and iatrogenic causes. Parkinsonism Relat Disord 1995; 1: 13–19.

35. Scamvougeras A, Rosebush PI. AIDS-related psychosis with catatonia responding to low-dose lorazepam. J Clin Psychiatry 1992; 53: 414–415.
36. Factor SA, Troche-Panetto M, Weaver SA. Dystonia in AIDS: Report of four cases. Mov Disord 2003; 18: 1492–1498.
37. Berger JR, Nath A. HIV dementia and the basal ganglia. Intervirology 1997; 40: 122–131.
38. Nath A, Anderson C, Jones M, et al. Neurotoxicity and dysfunction of dopamine systems associated with AIDS dementia. J Clin Psychopharmacol 2000; 14: 222–227.
39. Wiley CA, Soontornniyomkij V, Radhakrishnan L, et al. Distribution of brain HIV load in AIDS. Brain Pathol 1998; 8: 277–284.
40. Kane J, Honigfeld G, Singer J, et al. Clozapine for the treatment-resistant schizophrenic. A double-blind comparison with chlorpromazine. Arch Gen Psychiatry 1988; 45: 789–796.
41. Kastrup O, Gastpar M, Schwarz M. Acute dystonia due to clozapine. J Neurol Neurosurg Psychiatry 1994; 57: 119.
42. Chouinard G, Jones B, Remington G, et al. A Canadian multicenter placebo-controlled study of fixed doses of risperidone and haloperidol in the treatment of chronic schizophrenic patients. J Clin Psychopharmacol 1993; 13: 25–40.
43. Marder SR, Meibach RC. Risperidone in the treatment of schizophrenia. Am J Psychiatry 1994; 151: 825–835.
44. Peuskens J. Risperidone in the treatment of patients with chronic schizophrenia: a multinational, multi-centre, double-blind, parallel-group study versus haloperidol. Br J Psychiatry 1995; 166: 712–726.
45. Abi-Dargham A, Laruelle M, Aghajanian GK, et al. The role of serotonin in the pathophysiology and treatment of schizophrenia. J Neuropsychiatry Clin Neurosci 1997; 9: 1–17.
46. Busatto GF, Pilowsky LS, Ell PJ, et al. Dopamine D2 receptor occupancy in vivo and response to the new antipsychotic risperidone. Br J Psychiatry 1993; 163: 833–834.
47. Leysen JE, Gommeren W, Eens A, et al. Biochemical profile of risperidone, a new antipsychotic. J Pharmacol Exp Ther 1988; 247: 661–670.
48. Rosebush PI, Mazurek MF. The neurological side-effects of risperidone. Essent Psychopharmacol 1999; 3: 43–64.
49. Simpson GM, Lindenmayer JP. Extrapyramidal symptoms in patients treated with risperidone. J Clin Psychopharmacol 1997; 17: 194–201.
50. McCracken JT, McGough J, Shah B, et al. Risperidone in children with autism and serious behavioral problems. N Engl J Med 2002; 347: 314–321.
51. Sathpathy S, Winsberg B. Extrapyramidal symptoms in children on atypical antipsychotic drugs. J Clin Psychopharmacol 2003; 23: 675–677.
52. Dickson R, Williams R, Dalby D. Dystonic reaction and relapse with clozapine discontinuation and risperidone initiation. Can J Psychiatry 1994; 39: 184.
53. Lombroso PJ, Scorhill L, King RA, et al. Risperidone treatment of children and adolescents with chronic tic disorders. A preliminary report. J Am Acad Child Adolesc Psychiatry 1995; 34: 1147–1152.
54. Radford JM, Brown TM, Borison RL. Unexpected dystonia while changing from clozapine to risperidone. J Clin Psychopharmacol 1995; 15: 225–226.
55. Mandoki MW. Risperidone treatment of children and adolescents: increased risk of extrapyramidal side effects? J Child Adolesc Psychopharmcol 1995; 5: 49–67.
56. Anand HS. Re: Acute dystonic reaction with risperidone. Can J Psychiatry 1996; 41: 412.
57. Brody AL. Acute dystonia induced by rapid increase in risperidone dosage. J Clin Psychopharmacol 1996; 16: 461–462.

58. Cheslik TA, Erramouspe J. Extrapyramidal symptoms following accidental ingestion of risperidone in a child. Ann Pharmacother 1996; 30: 360–363.
59. Faulk RS, Gilmore JH, Jensen EW, et al. Risperidone-induced dystonic reaction. Am J Psychiatry 1996; 153: 577.
60. Sanderson DR. Drug interaction between risperidone and phenytoin resulting in extrapyramidal symptoms. J Clin Psychiatry 1996; 57: 177.
61. Takhar J, Manchanda R. Acute dystonic reaction with risperidone. Can J Psychiatry 1996; 41: 61–62.
62. Brown ES. Extrapyramidal side effects with low-dose risperidone. Can J Psychiatry 1997; 42: 325–326.
63. Rosebush PI, Mazurek MF. Extrapyramidal side-effects of risperidone. Neurology 1997; 48: 325–326.
64. Bymaster FP, Calligaro DO, Falcone JF, et al. Radioreceptor binding profile of the atypical antipsychotic olanzapine. Neuropsychopharmacology 1996; 14: 87–96.
65. Bymaster F, Perry KW, Nelson DL, et al. Olanzapine: a basic science update. Br J Psychiatry 1999; 174 (suppl 37): 36–40.
66. Tollefson GD, Beasley CM, Jr., Tran PV, et al. Olanzapine versus haloperidol in the treatment of schizophrenia and schizoaffective and schizophreniform disorders: results of an international collaborative trial. Am J Psychiatry 1997; 154: 457–465.
67. Gomez JC, Sacristan JA, Hernandez J, et al. The safety of olanzapine compared with other antipsychotic drugs: results of an observational prospective study in patients with schizophrenia (EFESO Study). J Clin Psychiatry 2000; 61: 335–343.
68. Wright P, Birkett M, David SR, et al. Double-blind, placebo-controlled comparison of intramuscular olanzapine and intramuscular haloperidol in the treatment of acute agitation in schizophrenia. Am J Psychiatry 2001; 158: 1149–1151.
69. Landry P, Cournoyer J. Acute dystonia with olanzapine. J Clin Psychiatry 1998; 59: 384.
70. Alevizos B, Papageorgiou C, Christodoulou GN. Acute dystonia caused by low dosage of olanzapine. J Neuropsychiatry Clin Neurosci 2003; 15: 241.
71. Hagberg G, Gefvert O, Bergstrom M, et al. N-[11C]methylspiperone PET, in contrast to [11C]raclopride, fails to detect D2 receptor occupancy by an atypical neuroleptic. Psychiatry Res 1998; 82: 147–160.
72. Gefvert O, Bergstrom M, Langstrom B, et al. Time course of central nervous dopamine-D2 and 5-HT2 receptor blockade and plasma drug concentrations after discontinuation of quetiapine (Seroquel) in patients with schizophrenia. Psychopharmacology 1998; 135: 119–126.
73. Jonnalagada JR, Norton JW. Acute dystonia with quetiapine. Clin Neuropharmacol 2000; 23: 229–230.
74. Nishikawa T, Nishioka S. A case of Meige dystonia induced by short-term quetiapine treatment. Hum Psychopharmacol Clin Exp 2002; 17: 197.
75. Arvanitis LA, Miller BG. Multiple fixed doses of "Seroquel" (quetiapine) in patients with acute exacerbation of schizophrenia: a comparison with haloperidol and placebo. Biol Psychiatry 1997; 42: 233–246.
76. Peuskens J, Link CG. A comparison of quetiapine and chlorpromazine in the treatment of schizophrenia. Acta Psychiat Scand 1997; 96: 265–273.
77. Sallee FR, Kurlan R, Goetz CG, et al. Ziprasidone treatment of children and adolescents with Tourette's syndrome: a pilot study. J Am Acad Child Adolesc Psychiatry 2000; 48: 292–299.
78. Hollander H, Golden J, Mendelson T, et al. Extrapyramidal symptoms in AIDS patients given low-dose metoclopramide or chlorpromazine. Lancet 1985; 2 (8465): 1186.

79. Edelstein H, Knight RT. Severe parkinsonism in two AIDS patients taking prochlorperazine. Lancet 1987; 2 (8554): 341–342.
80. Der Kleij FG, de Vries PA, Stassen PM, et al. Acute dystonia due to metoclopramide: increased risk in AIDS. Arch Int Med 2002; 162: 358–359.
81. Bateman DN, Rawlins MD, Simpson JM. Extrapyramidal reactions with metoclopramide. Br Med J Clin Res Ed 1985; 291: 930–932.
82. Lee HK. Dystonic reactions to amitriptyline and doxepin. Am J Psychiatry 1988; 145: 649.
83. Finder E, Lin KM, Ananth J. Dystonic reaction to amitriptyline. Am J Psychiatry 1982; 139: 1220.
84. Ornadel D, Barnes EA, Dick DJ. Acute dystonia due to amitriptyline. J Neurol Neurosurg Psychiatry 1992; 55: 414.
85. Pande AC, Max P. A dystonic reaction occurring during treatment with tranylcypromine. J Clin Psychopharmacol 1989; 9: 229–230.
86. Meltzer HY, Young M, Metz J, et al. Extrapyramidal side effects and increased serum prolactin following fluoxetine, a new antidepressant. J Neural Transm 1979; 45: 165–175.
87. Leo RJ. Clinical manifestations of dystonia and dyskinesia after SSRI administration. J Clin Psychiatry 1997; 58: 403–404.
88. Shihabuddin L, Rapport D. Sertraline and extrapyramidal side effects. Am J Psychiatry 1994; 151: 288.
89. Coulter DM, Pillans PI. Fluoxetine and extrapyramidal side effects. Am J Psychiatry 1995; 152: 122–125.
90. Reccoppa L, Welch WA, Ware MR. Acute dystonia and fluoxetine. J Clin Psychiatry 1990; 51: 487.
91. George MS, Trimble MR. Dystonic reaction associated with fluvoxamine. J Clin Psychopharmacol 1993; 13: 220–221.
92. Berk M. Paroxetine induces dystonia and parkinsonism in obsessive compulsive disorder. Hum Psychopharmacol Clin Exp 1993; 8: 444–445.
93. Brod TM. Fluoxetine and extrapyramidal side effects. Am J Psychiatry 1989; 146: 1352–1353.
94. Dave M. Fluoxetine-associated dystonia. Am J Psychiatry 1994; 151: 149.
95. Horrigan JP, Barnhill LJ. Paroxetine-pimozide drug interaction. J Am Acad Child Adolesc Psychiatry 1994; 33: 1060–1061.
96. Gill HS, DeVane CL, Risch SC. Extrapyramidal symptoms associated with cyclic antidepressant treatment: a review of the literature and consolidating hypotheses. J Clin Psychopharmacol 1997; 17: 377–389.
97. Ketai R. Interaction between fluoxetine and neuroleptics. Am J Psychiatry 1993; 150: 836–837.
98. Metz A. Interaction between fluoxetine and buspirone. Can J Psychiatry 1990; 35: 722–723.
99. Stanislav SW, Childs NL. Dystonia associated with sertraline. J Clin Psychopharmacol 1999; 19: 98–100.
100. Leo RJ. Movement disorders associated with the serotonin selective reuptake inhibitors. J Clin Psychiatry 1996; 57: 449–454.
101. Gerber PE, Lynd LD. Selective serotonin-reuptake inhibitor-induced movement disorders. Ann Pharmacother 1998; 32: 692–698.
102. Wells BG, Hayes PE. Depressive illness. In DiPiro JT, Talbert RL, Hayes PE, et al. (eds) Pharmacotherapy: A Pathophysiologic Approach. New York, Elsevier, 1989, pp. 748–764.

103. Porro V, Fiorenzoni S, Menga C, et al. Single-blind comparison of the efficacy of fluvoxamine versus placebo in patients with depressive syndrome. Curr Ther Res 1988; 43: 621–629.

104. Chuang C, Fahn S, Frucht SJ. The natural history and treatment of acquired hemidystonia: report of 33 cases and review of the literature. J Neurol Neurosurg Psychiatry 2002; 72: 59–67.

105. Dauer WT, Burke RE, Greene P, et al. Current concepts on the clinical features, aetiology and management of idiopathic cervical dystonia. Brain 1998; 121: 547–560.

106. Tamburin S, Manganotti P, Marzi CA, et al. Abnormal somatotopic arrangement of sensorimotor interactions in dystonic patients. Brain 2002; 125: 12–30.

107. Gerfen CR, Young WS, III. Distribution of striatonigral and striatopallidal peptidergic neurons in both patch and matrix compartments: an in situ hybridization histochemistry and fluorescent retrograde tracing study. Brain Res 1988; 460: 161–167.

108. Bolam JP, Smith Y. The GABA and substance P input to dopaminergic neurones in the substantia nigra of the rat. Brain Res 1990; 529(1–2): 57–78.

109. Parent A, Charara A, Pinault D. Single striatofugal axons arborizing in both pallidal segments and in the substantia nigra in primates. Brain Res 1995; 698: 280–284.

110. Parent A, Cicchetti F, Beach TG. Striatal neurones displaying substance P (NK1) receptor immunoreactivity in human and non-human primates. Neuroreport 1995; 6721–6724.

111. Gerfen CR, Engber TM, Mahan LC, et al. D1 and D2 dopamine receptor-regulated gene expression of striatonigral and striatopallidal neurons. Science 1990; 250: 1429–1432.

112. Parent A, Cote PY, Lavoie B. Chemical anatomy of primate basal ganglia. Progr Neurobiol 1995; 46: 131–197.

113. Calabresi P, Centonze D, Gubellini P, et al. Acetylcholine-mediated modulation of striatal function. Trends Neurosci 2000; 23: 120–126.

114. Kowall NW, Ferrante RJ, Beal MF, et al. Neuropeptide Y, somatostatin, and reduced nicotinamide adenine dinucleotide phosphate diaphorase in the human striatum: a combined immunocytochemical and enzyme histochemical study. Neuroscience 1987; 20: 817–828.

115. Garside S, Woulfe J, Mazurek MF. The ontogeny of NADPH-diaphorase neurons in serum-free striatal cultures parallels in vivo development. Neuroscience 1997; 78: 615–624.

116. Cowan RL, Wilson CJ, Emson PC, et al. Parvalbumin-containing GABAergic interneurons in the rat neostriatum. J Comp Neurol 1990; 302: 197–205.

117. Prensa L, Gimenez-Amaya JM, Parent A. Morphological features of neurons containing calcium-binding proteins in the human striatum. J Comp Neurol 1998; 390: 552–563.

118. Kubota Y, Kawaguchi Y. Dependence of GABAergic synaptic areas on the interneuron type and target size. J Neurosci 2000; 20: 375–386.

119. Fuller TA, Russchen FT, Price JL. Sources of presumptive glutamergic/aspartergic afferents to the rat ventral striatopallidal region. J Comp Neurol 1987; 258: 317–338.

120. Dube L, Smith AD, Bolam JP. Identification of synaptic terminals of thalamic or cortical origin in contact with distinct medium-size spiny neurons in the rat neostriatum. J Comp Neurol 1988; 267: 455–471.

121. McGeorge AJ, Faull RL. The organization of the projection from the cerebral cortex to the striatum in the rat. Neuroscience 1989; 29: 503–537.

122. Smith AD, Bolam JP. The neural network of the basal ganglia as revealed by the study of synaptic connections of identified neurones. Trends Neurosci 1990; 13: 259–265.

123. Soghomonian JJ, Descarries L, Watkins KC. Serotonin innervation in adult rat neostria-tum. II. Ultrastructural features: a radioautographic and immunocytochemical study. Brain Res 1989; 481: 67–86.

124. McDonald AJ. Topographical organization of amygdaloid projections to the caudatop-utamen, nucleus accumbens, and related striatal-like areas of the rat brain. Neuroscience 1991; 44: 15–33.

125. Takagi H, Somogyi P, Somogyi J, et al. Fine structural studies on a type of somatostatin-immunoreactive neuron and its synaptic connections in the rat neostriatum: a correlated light and electron microscopic study. J Comp Neurol 1983; 214: 1–16.

126. Pickel VM, Chan J. Spiny neurons lacking choline acetyltransferase immunoreactiv-ity are major targets of cholinergic and catecholaminergic terminals in rat striatum. J Neurosci Res 1990; 25: 263–280.

127. Smith Y, Bevan MD, Shink E, et al. Microcircuitry of the direct and indirect pathways of the basal ganglia. Neuroscience 1998; 86: 353–387.

128. Farde L, Nordstrom AL, Wiesel FA, et al. Positron emission tomographic analysis of central D1 and D2 dopamine receptor occupancy in patients treated with classical neu-roleptics and clozapine. Relation to extrapyramidal side effects. Arch Gen Psychiatry 1992; 49: 538–544.

129. Freund TF, Powell JF, Smith AD. Tyrosine hydroxylase-immunoreactive boutons in synaptic contact with identified striatonigral neurons, with particular reference to den-dritic spines. Neuroscience 1984; 13: 1189–1215.

130. Parent A, Hazrati LN. Functional anatomy of the basal ganglia. I. The cortico-basal ganglia-thalamo-cortical loop. Brain Res Rev 1995; 20: 91–127.

131. Halpain S, Girault JA, Greengard P. Activation of NMDA receptors induces dephospho-rylation of DARPP-32 in rat striatal slices. Nature 1990; 343: 369–372.

132. Cepeda C, Buchwald NA, Levine MS. Neuromodulatory actions of dopamine in the neostriatum are dependent upon the excitatory amino acid receptor subtypes activated. Proc Natl Acad Sci USA 1993; 90: 9576–9580.

133. Garside S, Furtado JC, Mazurek MF. Dopamine-glutamate interactions in the striatum: behaviourally relevant modification of excitotoxicity by dopamine receptor-mediated mechanisms. Neuroscience 1996; 75: 1065–1074.

134. Lester J, Fink S, Aronin N, et al. Colocalization of D1 and D2 dopamine receptor mRNAs in striatal neurons. Brain Res 1993; 621: 106–110.

135. Surmeier DJ, Song WJ, Yan Z. Coordinated expression of dopamine receptors in neos-triatal medium spiny neurons. J Neurosci 1996; 16: 6579–6591.

136. Aizman O, Brismar H, Uhlen P, et al. Anatomical and physiological evidence for D1 and D2 dopamine receptor colocalization in neostriatal neurons. Nat Neurosci 2000; 3: 226–230.

137. Di Chiara G, Morelli M, Consolo S. Modulatory functions of neurotransmitters in the striatum: ACh/dopamine/NMDA interactions. Trends Neurosci 1994; 17: 228–233.

138. Aosaki T, Tsubokawa H, Ishida A, et al. Responses of tonically active neurons in the primate's striatum undergo systematic changes during behavioral sensorimotor condi-tioning. J Neurosci 1994; 14: 3969–3984.

139. Graybiel AM, Aosaki T, Flaherty AW, et al. The basal ganglia and adaptive motor control. Science 1994; 265: 1826–1831.

140. Blazquez PM, Fujii N, Kojima J, et al. A network representation of response probability in the striatum. Neuron 2002; 33: 973–982.

141. Albin RL, Cross D, Cornblath WT, et al. Diminished striatal [^{123}I]iodobenzovesamicol binding in idiopathic cervical dystonia. Ann Neurol 2003; 53: 528–532.

142. Aubry JM, Schulz MF, Pagliusi S, et al. Coexpression of dopamine D2 and substance P (neurokinin-1) receptor messenger RNAs by a subpopulation of cholinergic neurons in the rat striatum. Neuroscience 1993; 53: 417–424.

143. Chang HT. Dopamine-acetylcholine interaction in the rat striatum: a dual-labeling immunocytochemical study. Brain Res Bull 1988; 21: 295–304.

144. Abercrombie ED, DeBoer P. Substantia nigra D1 receptors and stimulation of striatal cholinergic interneurons by dopamine: a proposed circuit mechanism. J Neurosci 1997; 17: 8498–8505.

145. Kawaguchi Y, Wilson CJ, Augood SJ, et al. Striatal interneurones: chemical, physiological and morphological characterization. Trends Neurosci 1995; 18: 527–535.

146. Koos T, Tepper JM. Inhibitory control of neostriatal projection neurons by GABAergic interneurons. Nat Neurosci 1999; 2: 467–472.

147. Martina M, Vida I, Jonas P. Distal initiation and active propagation of action potentials in interneuron dendrites. Science 2000; 287: 295–300.

148. Gernert M, Hamann M, Bennay M, et al. Deficit of striatal parvalbumin-reactive GABAergic interneurons and decreased basal ganglia output in a genetic rodent model of idiopathic paroxysmal dystonia. J Neurosci 2000; 20: 7052–7058.

149. Girault JA, Spampinato U, Glowinski J, et al. In vivo release of [3H]gamma-aminobutyric acid in the rat neostriatum – II. Opposing effects of D1 and D2 dopamine receptor stimulation in the dorsal caudate putamen. Neuroscience 1986; 19: 1109–1117.

150. Harsing LG, Jr., Zigmond MJ. Influence of dopamine on GABA release in striatum: evidence for D1-D2 interactions and non-synaptic influences. Neuroscience 1997; 77: 419–429.

151. Delgado A, Sierra A, Querejeta E, et al. Inhibitory control of the GABAergic transmission in the rat neostriatum by D2 dopamine receptors. Neuroscience 2000; 95: 1043–1048.

152. Beal MF, Mazurek MF, Ellison DW, et al. Somatostatin and neuropeptide Y concentrations in pathologically graded cases of Huntington's disease. Ann Neurol 1988; 23: 562–569.

153. Moser A, Cramer H. Somatostatin acts through G-proteins on dopaminergic adenylate cyclase in the caudate-putamen of the rat. Neurochem Res 1990; 15: 1085–1087.

154. Thermos K, Radke J, Kastellakis A, et al. Dopamine-somatostatin interactions in the rat striatum: an in vivo microdialysis study. Synapse 1996; 22: 209–216.

155. Hathway GJ, Emson PC, Humphrey PP, et al. Somatostatin potently stimulates in vivo striatal dopamine and gamma-aminobutyric acid release by a glutamate-dependent action. J Neurochem 1998; 70: 1740–1749.

156. Hathway GJ, Humphrey PP, Kendrick KM. Evidence that somatostatin sst2 receptors mediate striatal dopamine release. Br J Pharmacol 1999; 128: 1346–1352.

157. Le Moine C, Normand E, Bloch B. Phenotypical characterization of the rat striatal neurons expressing the D1 dopamine receptor gene. Proc Natl Acad Sci USA 1991; 88: 4205–4209.

158. MacLennan AJ, Lee N, Vincent SR, et al. D2 dopamine receptor mRNA distribution in cholinergic and somatostatinergic cells of the rat caudate-putamen and nucleus accumbens. Neurosci Lett 1994; 180: 214–218.

159. Engber TM, Boldry RC, Kuo S, et al. Dopaminergic modulation of striatal neuropeptides: differential effects of D1 and D2 receptor stimulation on somatostatin, neuropeptide Y, neurotensin, dynorphin and enkephalin. Brain Res 1992; 581: 261–268.

160. Izquierdo-Claros RM, Boyano-Adanez MC, Larsson C, et al. Acute effects of D1- and D2-receptor agonist and antagonist drugs on somatostatin binding, inhibition of adenylyl cyclase activity and accumulation of inositol 1,4,5-trisphosphate in the rat striatum. Mol Brain Res 1997; 47: 99–107.

161. Flores-Hernandez J, Galarraga E, Bargas J. Dopamine selects glutamatergic inputs to neostriatal neurons. Synapse 1997; 25: 185–195.
162. Mazurek MF, Savedia SM, Bobba RS, et al. Persistent loss of tyrosine hydroxylase immunoreactivity in the substantia nigra after neuroleptic withdrawal. J Neurol Neurosurg Psychiatry 1998; 64: 799–801.
163. Levinson AJ, Garside S, Rosebush PI, et al. Haloperidol induces persistent down-regulation of tyrosine hydroxylase immunoreactivity in substantia nigra but not ventral tegmental area in the rat. Neuroscience 1998; 84: 201–211.
164. Mazurek MF, Krasnik C, Rosebush PI, et al. Evidence that antipsychotic drugs and 3-nitroproprionic acid independently induce cell death in mid-brain dopamine neurons by activation of the apoptosis cascade. Ann Neurol 2002; 52: S85–S86.
165. Xu Y, Krasnik C, Bell V, et al. Differential effects of typical vs. atypical antipsychotic drugs on midbrain dopamine neurons. Neurosci Abst 2003; 948.7.
166. Mazurek MF, Krasnik C, Xu Y, et al. Rapid induction of pro-apoptotic proteins in nigral dopamine neurons by antipsychotic medication. Ann Neurol 2003; 54 (suppl 7): S42.
167. Harrison SJ, Mazurek MF. Comparative effects of antipsychotic and antidepressant drugs on dopaminergic, noradrenergic and serotonergic cell groups in the rat. Neurosci Abst 1998; 24: 2179.
168. Lavoie B, Parent A. Immunohistochemical study of the serotoninergic innervation of the basal ganglia in the squirrel monkey. J Comp Neurol 1990; 299: 1–16.
169. Snyder AM, Zigmond MJ, Lund RD. Sprouting of serotoninergic afferents into striatum after dopamine-depleting lesions in infant rats: a retrograde transport and immunocytochemical study. J Comp Neurol 1986; 245: 274–281.
170. De Simoni MG, Dal Toso G, Fodritto F, et al. Modulation of striatal dopamine metabolism by the activity of dorsal raphe serotonergic afferences. Brain Res 1987; 411: 81–88.
171. Jackson D, Bruno JP, Stachowiak MK, et al. Inhibition of striatal acetylcholine release by serotonin and dopamine after the intracerebral administration of 6-hydroxydopamine to neonatal rats. Brain Res 1988; 457: 267–273.
172. Middlemiss DN, Bremer ME, Smith SM. A pharmacological analysis of the 5-HT receptor mediating inhibition of 5-HT release in the guinea-pig frontal cortex. Eur J Pharmacol 1988; 157: 101–107.
173. Hoyer D, Pazos A, Probst A, et al. Serotonin receptors in the human brain. I. Characterization and autoradiographic localization of 5-HT$_{1A}$ recognition sites: apparent absence of 5-HT$_{1B}$ recognition sites. Brain Res 1986; 376: 85–96.
174. Limberger N, Deicher R, Starke K. Species differences in presynaptic serotonin autoreceptors: mainly 5-HT$_{1B}$ but possibly in addition 5-HT$_{1D}$ in the rat, 5-HT$_{1D}$ in the rabbit and guinea-pig brain cortex. Naunyn-Schmiedebergs Arch Pharmacol 1991; 343: 353–364.
175. Starkey SJ, Skingle M. 5-HT$_{1D}$ as well as 5-HT$_{1A}$ autoreceptors modulate 5-HT release in the guinea-pig dorsal raphe nucleus. Neuropharmacology 1994; 33: 393–402.
176. Boschert U, Amara DA, Segu L, et al. The mouse 5-hydroxytryptamine1B receptor is localized predominantly on axon terminals. Neuroscience 1994; 58: 167–182.
177. Stanford IM, Lacey MG. Differential actions of serotonin, mediated by 5-HT$_{1B}$ and 5-HT$_{2C}$ receptors, on GABA-mediated synaptic input to rat substantia nigra pars reticulata neurons in vitro. J Neurosci 1996; 16: 7566–7573.
178. Gellman RL, Aghajanian GK. Serotonin$_2$ receptor-mediated excitation of interneurons in piriform cortex: antagonism by atypical antipsychotic drugs. Neuroscience 1994; 58: 515–525.
179. Pazos A, Palacios JM. Quantitative autoradiographic mapping of serotonin receptors in the rat brain. I. Serotonin-1 receptors. Brain Res 1985; 346: 205–230.

180. Ward RP, Dorsa DM. Colocalization of serotonin receptor subtypes 5-HT$_{2A}$, 5-HT$_{2C}$, and 5-HT$_6$ with neuropeptides in rat striatum. J Comp Neurol 1996; 370: 405–414.

181. Maricq AV, Peterson AS, Brake AJ, et al. Primary structure and functional expression of the 5HT$_3$ receptor, a serotonin-gated ion channel. Science 1991; 254: 432–437.

182. Davies PA, Pistis M, Hanna MC, et al. The 5-HT$_{3B}$ subunit is a major determinant of serotonin-receptor function. Nature 1999; 397: 359–363.

183. Waeber C, Dixon K, Hoyer D, et al. Localisation by autoradiography of neuronal 5-HT3 receptors in the mouse CNS. Eur J Pharmacol 1988; 151: 351–352.

184. Waeber C, Sebben M, Nieoullon A, et al. Regional distribution and ontogeny of 5-HT$_4$ binding sites in rodent brain. Neuropharmacology 1994; 33: 527–541.

185. Monsma FJ, Jr., Shen Y, Ward RP, et al. Cloning and expression of a novel serotonin receptor with high affinity for tricyclic psychotropic drugs. Mol Pharmacol 1993; 43: 320–327.

186. Heidmann DE, Szot P, Kohen R, et al. Function and distribution of three rat 5-hydroxytryptamine$_7$ (5-HT$_7$) receptor isoforms produced by alternative splicing. Neuropharmacology 1998; 37: 1621–1632.

187. Rosebush PI, Mazurek MF. Do benzodiazepines modify the incidence of neuroleptic-induced dystonia? Am J Psychiatry 1993; 150: 528.

188. World Health Organization. Prophylactic use of anticholinergics in patients on long-term neuroleptic treatment: a consensus statement. Br J Psychiatry 1990; 156: 412.

CHAPTER 6

Drug-induced parkinsonism

**Joseph H. Friedman, Martha E. Trieschmann,
and Hubert H. Fernandez**

> The emergence of parkinsonism during chlorpromazine and reserpine therapy constitutes undoubtedly one of the most fascinating developments in psychiatric therapy.
>
> Freyhan, 1957 [1]

Introduction

Drug-induced parkinsonism (DIP) would appear to be the most straightforward of the drug-induced movement disorders [2]. In the most simplistic model, drugs that either block dopamine receptors [2, 3] or deplete dopamine stores [3] cause a functional dopaminergic deficiency and produce a condition that mimics idiopathic Parkinson's disease (IPD), a known dopamine deficiency state [2]. This model is heuristically valuable, but it does not explain many observations. Since the first edition of this book was published, clozapine and several other atypical antipsychotic (AA) drugs have become available. While DIP has become much less common, it is less often looked for and therefore less frequently recognized. It may also be missed in patients treated with nonpsychiatric dopamine blockers such as metoclopromide and prochlorperazine. DIP still occurs and still constitutes a clinically important disorder.

History

Historically, the importance of DIP in understanding IPD cannot be overemphasized [4]. Although the neuropathology of IPD was relatively well understood by the 1920s, the biochemistry was not, until 1960 [5]. Animal studies demonstrated that reserpine acted by depleting catecholamine stores and that sufficiently high but nontoxic doses induced an akinetic syndrome [4]. It was later noted in human studies that reserpine, when used for treating psychiatric disorders, often induced a syndrome identical to IPD [3]. This observation led to the momentous discovery that catecholamine stores were depleted in IPD and that dopamine, in particular, was drastically reduced [5]. Understanding of this deficiency led directly to the development of levodopa and its use in treating IPD [4, 6].

For many years, it was debated whether parkinsonism was required for an antipsychotic effect [3, 7] or whether it was an untoward toxic effect of all neuroleptic drugs. It was even suggested that IPD protects against schizophrenia and vice versa. It has become clear in recent years that antipsychotic effects do not require the imposition of parkinsonism and that IPD and schizophrenia do not preclude each other [8].

While many physicians believe that the atypical antipsychotics have made these concerns of historical interest only, this is not the case. The increasing population of elderly patients has resulted in a dramatically increased number of demented patients who have a wide spectrum of associated behavioral problems, often requiring treatment with antipsychotic drugs. Thus, virtually all physicians who see adult patients are confronted with those suffering from dementia and behavioral problems. As a result, antipsychotic medications are among the most commonly prescribed drugs in North America.

While DIP occurs mainly in patients treated for psychiatric disorders, the antiemetics prochlorperazine (Compazine) and droperidol (Inapsine), and the gastric motility enhancer, metoclopramide (Reglan), have made recognition of DIP important in nonpsychiatric patients. Furthermore, though not approved in the United states, certain calcium channel-blocking drugs (e.g., Flunarizine) are common causes of DIP in other parts of the world [9–11]. The antihypertensive agent, alpha-methyldopa, also has the potential to cause parkinsonism, but it is rarely used.

Clinical aspects

The DIP syndrome

Drug-induced parkinsonism cannot be clinically distinguished from IPD [12]. It is defined as an akinetic-rigid syndrome induced by pharmacological agents. The cardinal features are rigidity, akinesia, bradykinesia, tremor at rest, and postural instability. Minor features include abnormal posture, micrographia, seborrhea, and changes in speech. The *rigidity* is often described as cogwheeling in nature but is not always. Cogwheel rigidity is not pathognomonic of parkinsonism and may be difficult to distinguish from "gegenhalten" or paratonia, a resistance to passive movement caused by frontal lobe dysfunction. The rigidity can be best appreciated by the examiner passively flexing and extending the elbows, wrists, and neck, but it may also be found at other joints. It can often be brought out by reinforcement maneuvers such as opening and closing the nonexamined hand. The rigidity is not uniform and often affects one limb more than another and one side more than the other.

Akinesia refers to a relative paucity of spontaneous, generally automatic and unconscious movements that are part of the normal resting repertoire. The "masked facies" of parkinsonism, or facial hypomimia, is the result of akinesia and rigidity of the facial muscles. Akinetic patients blink less than normals, thus appearing to stare. They swallow less than normals, causing pooling of saliva and a tendency to drool. They exhibit fewer unconscious movements at rest such as crossing their legs while sitting or touching their hands to their face. The lack of such "natural" movements is often overlooked by inexperienced observers but is as obvious as tremor to trained observers.

Bradykinesia refers to slowness of movement. We often rate bradykinesia by asking the patient to tap fingers together or open and close a hand as fast as possible. More demanding tasks such as buttoning a shirt or putting on a coat reveal how severely compromised a patient may be in activities of daily living. In IPD, bradykinesia is one of the most debilitating features of the illness. It is important to note that akinesia and bradykinesia, while often thought to be synonymous, are not. Frequently, patients will perform remarkably well on timed tasks, indicating only a mild degree of bradykinesia, while being profoundly akinetic. Rarely, patients may exhibit "kinesia paradoxica," a condition in which severely akinetic subjects respond more quickly than expected when faced with startling or threatening stimuli.

The *tremor* of DIP may be mild or severe. It typically involves the fingers or the hands but may involve the jaw, feet, or tongue. Head tremor is uncommon, although a severe tremor that emanates from the elbow or shoulder can often cause a conducted movement that passively involves the head. The tremor is present at rest and often with the arms held in a fixed posture, but usually resolves with movement. The "pill rolling" tremor of parkinsonism refers to a finger tremor, in which the thumb and opposing fingers appear to be rolling a pill back and forth in the hand. It is less common than hand tremor and is often absent. Because the tremor is often present in sustained postures, it can severely interfere with important functions of everyday living such as eating and writing. The tremor, present at rest, resolves as the patient picks up the utensil but recurs as the hand is positioned over the target, whether a pile of peas, a bowl of soup, or a writing pad. It resolves as the hand moves but then recurs as the fork or spoon stops to deliver its contents to the mouth. Patients also taking lithium may have a more prominent action tremor in addition to the neuroleptic-induced resting and postural tremor, complicating the clinical picture.

Postural instability refers to a diminished response to postural displacements resulting in loss of balance. When a normal subject is pulled backward, the arms go up in front and the person steps backward. If a backward fall is imminent, the knees buckle to allow a cushioned landing on the buttocks. If the fall is forward or to the side, the arms go up to break the fall. In parkinsonism, these responses are impaired. Subjects may take many steps, often increasing in frequency as they decrease in amplitude (*festination* if forward) (*retropulsion* if pulled or falling backward) and they may entirely fail to put out their arms. Thus, a parkinsonian may fall like a stiff board when knocked off balance and strike the occiput or the face.

The *posture* of parkinsonism probably in part reflects truncal rigidity. Parkinsonian patients have a flexed posture, both sitting and standing. Their shoulders are stooped. In advanced disease, patients are flexed at all joints. While in part due to rigidity, this posture can also represent an aberrant orientation that may even result in tilting to one side in addition to being flexed. The gait has a normal-to-narrow base but the stride is reduced. Arm swing is reduced or absent. In severe cases, the arms are flexed at the elbows, producing an appearance much like that of hemiparetic patients after a stroke. Tremor in the hands and fingers may become evident or more pronounced with walking. Shuffling is common, and some patients develop a tendency to run forward with increasingly small steps: the "festinating gait" of Parkinson's disease. Patients may turn "en bloc," requiring several steps rather than a pivot, and turning is commonly associated with falls. In contrast, mild stooping and decreased arm swing may be the only gait abnormalities in younger DIP patients, and these may be so minor as to escape detection on routine exam.

Toxic and metabolic derangements generally cause symmetric, nonfocal deficits. In DIP, however, asymmetry is common and should not be misconstrued as evidence against that diagnosis. Tremor, stiffness, akinesia, and bradykinesia may all be more prominent on one side, and are occasionally present only on one side. A patient may have more facial hypomimia on one side and may therefore appear to have unilateral facial muscle weakness. Thus, DIP cannot be distinguished from IPD on the basis of asymmetry. If there is, indeed, a difference between the distribution of parkinsonian signs in DIP and IPD, a large study with age-matched groups would be necessary to demonstrate it.

Although DIP may exactly mimic IPD, there tends to be less tremor in DIP patients [13]. In a study [12] of 26 DIP patients with a median age of 61 years, the major sign of parkinsonism was rigidity in 18 patients, bradykinesia in 14 patients, tremor in 13 patients, and gait abnormality in 5 patients. The signs were asymmetrical in 14 patients, and 11 had associated tardive dyskinesia (TD). In comparison, tremor is thought to be present in 80% of cases of IPD. This difference in tremor could be due to the younger age of most DIP patients or to other poorly defined differences between the two conditions.

Some parkinsonian features may be intrinsic to the psychiatric illness and may not necessarily represent medication effect [14]. For example, depressed and catatonic patients may be akinetic and bradykinetic. This was noted in a large double-blind study [14] comparing neuroleptics and placebo in treating psychosis. Signs of parkinsonism were identified as part of the screening for adverse effects. Since the age of the patients was very young (mean age 28.2 years), the incidence of parkinsonism was low. Of particular notice, however, was the incidence of parkinsonian features in placebo-treated subjects (Table 6.1). This finding could be explained either by poor assessment techniques or the natural occurrence of parkinsonian signs among psychotic

Table 6.1 Incidence in percent of parkinsonian features in NIMH study

	Chlorpromazine	Fluphenazine	Thioridazine	Placebo
Facial rigidity	12.5	14.3	8.8	5.4
Tremors	5.7	12.1	13.2	5.4
Loss of associated movements	3.4	19.8	0.0	2.7

patients. The youth of the subjects makes it unlikely that IPD was the explanation for the placebo-associated parkinsonism. In general, patients with less severe disease are often unaware of their parkinsonian signs [15, 16]. In DIP, patients are aware mainly of their tremor [16]. When tremor is absent, there are frequently no symptoms to correlate with the signs of rigidity and akinesia.

A rare form of DIP is the aptly named *rabbit syndrome* [17]. It does not look like typical IPD. Patients exhibit "perioral muscular movements strikingly imitating the rapid chewing-like movements of a rabbit's mouth" [17]. The syndrome is typically due to a tremor of the lips and perioral region without involvement of the tongue. It is generally believed that this is a restricted form of DIP that responds to anticholinergic medications in the same fashion as the more typical resting limb tremor. Irregular lip movements and nasal flaring in some patients with TD may cause diagnostic confusion. The syndrome was initially reported with conventional neuroleptics but has more recently been described in a patient on risperidone [18].

Differential diagnosis

When all the features of parkinsonism are present and a history of drug exposure is obtained, the diagnosis is simple. Mild parkinsonism is more difficult to diagnose. Screening surveys searching for DIP in at-risk populations commonly observe only asymptomatic facial hypomimia or a mildly stooped posture with diminished arm swing. On the other hand, IPD patients generally seek help only when symptomatic or when an outside observer notes some abnormality, and their presenting signs are therefore more obvious.

When patients are evaluated for parkinsonism, a complete drug history is mandatory. The effects of neuroleptics can persist for surprisingly long periods, and sensitivity to the extrapyramidal effects of these drugs is surprisingly varied.

There are a few clinical settings in which the differential diagnosis of DIP is important. Most commonly encountered is the older patient who develops signs of parkinsonism on a chronic, stable dose of antipsychotic that he or she has tolerated well for years without apparent adverse effects. The question then arises as to whether the patient has IPD or DIP. The dopamine receptor blockade may have prematurely "unmasked" IPD [9, 19, 20], or, alternatively, the patient may have simply become more sensitive to the drug [21] with age. In either case, discontinuation of the antipsychotic should ameliorate the syndrome, although the time course for improvement may be well over a year [12, 22]. If the antipsychotic is stopped, DIP should improve significantly and eventually resolve, whereas IPD always worsens after the improvement gained by stopping the neuroleptic recedes. With new techniques that measure dopamine or dopamine-secreting cells in the brain, it may be possible to distinguish DIP from IPD using PET or SPECT scans [23].

Less common but more important is the clinical distinction between catatonia and severe DIP. Quite clearly, the treatment is very different. While the obvious diagnostic differences include waxy flexibility versus cogwheeling rigidity, muteness versus dysarthria, absence of tremor in catatonia, and parkinsonian gait in DIP, these distinctions may prove difficult to elicit in practice. The catatonic may not keep his arms in a statuesque posture and probably will not attempt to walk. In addition, the catatonic patient is likely to have received neuroleptics, further complicating the picture. On the other hand, the patient with DIP may be psychotic and uncooperative and refuse to allow a full examination, leaving the examiner uncertain as to what degree of akinesia is drug-induced and how much is catatonia. Luckily, catatonia is rare and the history will hopefully help clear up the dilemma.

Depression can also mimic DIP with decreased facial expression and bradykinesia. Though the two conditions can present together, the typical DIP patient does not have symptoms of depression. When the patient is depressed, the clinician must depend more on physical signs such as tremor, rigidity, and gait changes. Similarly, severe obsessive compulsive disorder may produce slowness and akinesia that are very suggestive of parkinsonism [24].

The differential diagnosis must also include causes of parkinsonism other than IPD. A long list of disorders including degenerative diseases, toxins, tumors, and hydrocephalus may cause parkinsonism. Certain of these may also cause psychiatric disorders early in the course. Progressive parkinsonism may then be mistakenly ascribed to the neuroleptic treatment of these psychiatric features rather than to a primary brain disorder causing both problems. Wilson's disease is probably the most important condition with potential to cause this scenario in view of its treatability and universally fatal outcome if the diagnosis is missed. In young people, Huntington's disease may occur in the "rigid form," which can be mistaken for IPD. Hypothyroidism is another rare consideration.

Psychogenic parkinsonism is rare. To make the diagnosis, the examiner must attempt to distract the patient or to observe the patient when the subject is unaware of the surveillance. A sodium amytal interview may also be considered. Depending on the underlying psychiatric problem, neuroleptics may even be helpful!

Clinical course

In the largest survey of extrapyramidal drug side effects Ayd [21] looked at 3775 patients and reported that DIP generally occurs later than akathisia and dystonia: 90% of cases developed within the first 72 days, but that the time of onset varied with the mode of drug administration (Fig. 1.1). He noted that patients complained of prodromal symptoms such as weakness, paresthesias, and joint pains, mainly in limbs later affected by parkinsonism. Patients with the syndrome were "constantly aware of fatigue" in affected limbs. These descriptions are in contrast to other observations [15, 16] and may reflect differences in the populations under study. Akinetic patients were apathetic and less active.

The initial signs of DIP were rigidity and impaired arm swing in 65% of patients, and tremor in about 35%. The tremor usually began asymmetrically in one arm. Tremor eventually developed in 60% of patients (vs. 80% in IPD).

Freyhan [25] reported earlier that the great majority of patients developed parkinsonism before the 20th day, whereas Medinar et al. [26] found that the majority of patients developed parkinsonism within the first week. One study [27] reported that the time of onset of parkinsonism was dose related in patients on haloperidol, with higher doses producing akinesia within 2 weeks.

With continued drug exposure, the natural course of DIP is unknown. Patients successfully treated for DIP with antiparkinson drugs can often have these drugs discontinued without a recurrence of DIP. This suggests that DIP is often a temporary phenomenon that ameliorates with time. Animal data [28, 29] show that chronic exposure to dopamine receptor-blocking agents causes an increase in dopamine turnover and alters the sensitivity of dopamine receptors. Thus, compensatory mechanisms occur in animals that, if present in humans, could explain a decline in parkinsonism in people chronically exposed to receptor-blocking drugs.

There are conflicting reports regarding the decline in DIP over time. One study [30] reported resolution within 2 months. In another study of patients on trifluoperazine for over 3 years, 27 of 63 continued to have tremor and 24 had rigidity. This DIP prevalence of almost 50% was seen despite concurrent anticholinergic therapy in most cases [31]. Another report, however, found that chronic antiparkinsonian therapy was rarely required, with only 9 out of 1000 chronic patients receiving it [32]. This, of course, only implies that severe, chronic DIP is uncommon, but it does not help in assessing the actual prevalence of the syndrome.

In order to gauge the long-term course of DIP as well as tardive dyskinesia, Fernandez et al. examined 53 chronic schizophrenic residents of a state psychiatric hospital in 1984 and again in 1998 [33]. Remaining on high-dose neuroleptic therapy over the 14-year interval, these patients experienced a significant decrease in tardive dyskinesia but a significant increase in parkinsonism, as measured by the Rating Scale for Extrapyramidal Signs (REPS). These results suggest that DIP progresses over time.

Special aspects

Drug-induced parkinsonism in the elderly

The elderly may be at increased risk for DIP [15, 23]. A study of parkinsonism in Olmsted County, Minnesota indicated that the rate of DIP in ages 70 to 99 years actually increased over three 5-year periods between 1976 and 1995 [34]. If there is a higher risk of DIP in the elderly, it could relate to the increasing likelihood of IPD in this age group, or it could simply be due to the diminished number of nigral dopaminergic neurons [35]. Both of these changes would increase the sensitivity to dopamine antagonists that occurs with normal aging. If DIP is more common in women [21, 36], as is reported in some studies (but not all [31]), then the increased incidence of DIP in the elderly would only be partly explained by subclinical IPD, as most studies (but not all [37, 38]) show IPD to be more common in men [35, 36, 39].

In a prospective study, 9% of all new cases referred to a geriatrics unit had parkinsonism. Of this total of 95 cases, 51% were drug-induced [40]. Interestingly, only 25% of referring physicians had recognized the parkinsonism. The most common offending agent was prochlorperazine (Compazine), an antiemetic, which the authors felt was not indicated in even a single case. The clinical features of DIP were similar to those encountered in IPD. Twenty-five percent of the DIP patients could not walk, 60% gave a history of falls, and 45% required hospital admission. The DIP persisted for a mean of 7 weeks (range 1–36) before resolution in the two out of three who resolved during the study. Of note was the later development of parkinsonism, presumably due to IPD, in five patients (11%) within 18 months, a higher number than anticipated in an age-matched control population.

The prognostic implications of recognizing DIP in the elderly are great since the disorder may not be benign [41]. In one study, 54% of the elderly with DIP died within 41 months of diagnosis, a far higher rate than expected for healthy, age-matched controls. Whether the mortality rate is higher for age in medically matched controls is unknown. This study also found that 25% of DIP patients developed IPD within 41 months of drug discontinuation.

These studies emphasize the problems associated with parkinsonism in the elderly. The diagnosis of IPD cannot be made in a patient who has received dopamine antagonists within the past year or more unless the parkinsonism has slowly worsened off the drug. IPD develops in up to 25% of the elderly with DIP, presumably reflecting the extra sensitivity to dopamine blockade in preclinical IPD. And finally, the presence of DIP forewarns of a poor prognosis. It is associated with gait dysfunction, falling, prolonged hospitalization, and increased mortality. Undoubtedly, the indications for neuroleptic use also play a role in determining this prognosis.

DIP and tardive dyskinesia

The coexistence of DIP and tardive dyskinesia is a relatively common although not well-known fact. The heuristic concept of parkinsonism representing a dopamine deficiency state and tardive dyskinesia representing a dopamine excess state is clearly violated in its most simple formulation by the concurrence of these syndromes.

Richardson and Craig [42] surveyed 132 patients at a state psychiatric hospital of whom 91% were on neuroleptics and found that 28% had TD only, and 19.7% had DIP only, while 17.4% had both. There were no significant differences in neuroleptic dose, duration of exposure, or antiparkinson drug use. Crane [43] had similar results in a population that was probably comparable (chronic state psychiatric in-patients). At the Institute of Mental Health [44], the only state psychiatric hospital in Rhode Island, a survey of the entire in-patient population, acute and chronic patients, revealed a smaller percentage of patients with both syndromes, but the combination was not rare.

The coexistence of TD and DIP is analogous to the situation of the IPD patient with levodopa-induced dyskinesias. In such a case, the patient may still be bradykinetic and rigid while showing obvious chorea. The explanation presumably lies in the differences in altered biochemistry occurring simultaneously in different regions of the brain. Thus in TD, the presumed receptor alterations have a predisposition, for unknown reasons, to affect neurons controlling the oral and facial regions (see Chapter 5). With an increase in dopamine blockade, the TD usually decreases (is masked) and parkinsonism develops [33]. The relative balance between the receptor supersensitivity (hypothesized to account for TD) in certain brain regions involved in generating TD versus dopamine receptor blockade in those controlling other body segments may determine whether or not the TD is suppressed before DIP appears. On the other hand, this cooccurrence could be considered a further argument against the dopamine receptor supersensitivity hypothesis for TD.

Withdrawal emergent parkinsonism

An unexplained and rarely reported [34, 35] form of DIP is that caused by neuroleptic withdrawal ("withdrawal emergent parkinsonism"). The first patient reported with this syndrome developed rigidity, drooling, and shuffling gait over a 2-week interval as thioridazine 100 mg, chlorpromazine 150 mg, and flurazepam 30 mg daily were tapered to a final schedule of chlorpromazine 50 mg daily [45]. The syndrome rapidly improved with the addition of benztropine.

A second report [46] concerned a prospective study of abrupt neuroleptic withdrawal in 15 chronically hospitalized schizophrenics on long-term neuroleptic therapy (mean dose 1081 chlorpromazine equivalents). Those taking anticholinergics had them withdrawn 5 to 7 days before the neuroleptic. Six patients developed new or worsened parkinsonism within 1 to 4 days of neuroleptic withdrawal. Three had not been on anticholinergics, and the other three had not worsened when the anticholinergics were stopped. All six had rest tremor, two were hypokinetic, two had excess salivation, and four had seborrhea. Of special note was the transient nature of the syndrome in one patient, lasting only for a few hours, and the remarkable responsiveness to treatment of the DIP with either anticholinergics or neuroleptics.

The authors of these reports provide no adequate explanation for their observations. This phenomenon certainly contradicts the simplistic theory that neuroleptics act primarily by blocking dopamine receptors and suggests a more complex set of actions for these drugs. It is troubling, however, that a syndrome that occurred in 40% of an unselected group of subjects is not recognized more often. Abrupt discontinuation of neuroleptics is common among psychiatric patients, yet withdrawal emergent parkinsonism is almost unknown. No reports confirming these observations have been published since 1989. There has been, however, one report of withdrawal emergent rabbit syndrome in a patient on a tapering dose of risperidone [47]. The patient improved with anticholinergic therapy.

Epidemiology

Risk factors

While a number of risk factors have been tentatively identified for the development of DIP, few have been confirmed by later studies, and contradictory reports are common. Only one fact is unambiguous. All studies have demonstrated a rather remarkable individual variation in susceptibility to the extrapyramidal effects of dopamine-blocking drugs. This fact was noted as early as 1957 [1] "...our observations reveal that neither drug quantity nor treatment duration can account for the severity of extrapyramidal symptoms." The author then went on to suggest that DIP subjects may have had an increased incidence of neurological disorders, brain injury, and subnormal intellect in family members, but he lacked sufficient data to compare this information on DIP patients to non-DIP patients.

The purported major risk factors for the development of DIP are female sex, old age, high drug potency, and increased drug dose [36, 48, 49]. Several studies have also indicated that, not surprisingly, preexisting extrapyramidal signs increase the risk of DIP [49]. However, one has to wonder if what the authors called "normal" levels of EPS signs were really evidence of mild, presymptomatic IPD. These are potential risk factors only and individual patients with all of these predispositions may not develop any extrapyramidal syndromes (EPS).

Ayd conducted the first major study of the clinical epidemiology of DIP [21]. He identified three risk factors for DIP: female gender, old age, and the use of high-potency neuroleptics. Ayd surveyed 3775 phenothiazine-treated patients for all identifiable extrapyramidal reactions. Since he used a classification system that allowed only one adverse effect per patient, his numbers may be artificially low. He observed (1) that women were almost twice as likely to suffer DIP than males in all age groups except for those below 10 and above 80 years old (both groups had small numbers of patients); (2) that DIP was related to drug potency with trifluoperazine causing a 42% higher incidence than chlorpromazine (chlorpromazine equivalent doses for the drugs were not given); and (3) that older patients were at greater risk than the younger in both sexes (Fig. 2.1). However, like Freyhan [1], he noted that 61% of the patients had no extrapyramidal signs and that many of these were on larger doses of neuroleptics than those suffering from EPS. The NIMH study of 1964 [14] also documented the relationship between DIP and potency of neuroleptic with thioridazine and chlorpromazine causing less DIP than fluphenazine. This study did not comment on age or sex factors. A study of parkinsonism in Olmsted County, Minnesota from 1976 to 1990 [36] found DIP to account for 20% of all parkinsonian patients. The incidence increased with age and was higher in women across all age groups, though the incidence of both parkinsonism and IPD was higher in men.

These observations, although generally accepted [48], are not universally supported. Other studies have found no sex differences [31] and even age as a risk factor has been contested [50, 51]. Most (but not all) [37, 38] studies of IPD show a male predilection [35, 36, 39], so the reversal of sex predominance in DIP, if true, is surprising.

Many other potential risk factors have been explored. Myrianthopoulos et al. [52] evaluated family history of parkinsonism as a potential risk factor. Detailed family histories on psychiatric patients taking neuroleptics were obtained, 59 of whom had moderate-to-severe DIP and 67 of whom were without any signs of parkinsonism (controls), despite being on neuroleptics. They found a history of parkinsonism in 15 relatives of patients in the first group but in only three relatives of the controls, concluding that there may be a familial susceptibility to DIP. Unfortunately, although the patients and controls were matched for age, gender, and drug exposure, the identification of affected family members was based solely on history. The authors repeated their study [53] and again found similar results but only for American Caucasian patients, not for African Americans. This racial discrepancy may be real since there is some evidence that African Americans are less prone to IPD than American Caucasians [39], although no data exist on the relative risks of race on DIP.

Pursuing the possibility of a hereditary predisposition to DIP, one group of investigators [54] performed HLA typing in 52 chronically hospitalized schizophrenic white men on neuroleptics. They found a single antigen, B44, significantly more common in the group with DIP than in the group without. This antigen had not been associated with IPD in previous HLA studies. Although the authors speculated on a variety of potential mechanisms to explain this association, the possibility of a chance association in one of 80 antigens tested must be considered. A comparable study from a different center will be required to confirm these results.

A puzzling risk factor cited for DIP is taste sensitivity for quinine. One study found that more sensitive tasters had a greater sensitivity to DIP at low doses of trifluoperazine yet less sensitivity at high doses [55].

Some studies have implicated brain damage as a risk factor for DIP. Eleven of 18 lobotomized schizophrenics [56] suffered from DIP whereas only 3 of the 11 nonlobotomized had DIP despite their use of lower doses of anticholinergics. This result, however, was not found in another group of lobotomized patients [56]. In a separate study looking at the effects of structural brain damage, lateral ventricule size was found to correlate with DIP in patients taking the same doses of chlorpromazine [57]. However, DIP was defined as the ward physicians' use of antiparkinson medication. In addition, there was no one-to-one correlation between ventricular size and DIP: some normal controls and non-DIP neuroleptic-treated patients had larger ventricles than did some patients with DIP.

Several studies indicate that the presence of dementia increases the risk of developing DIP, especially in the elderly [49]. A study by Chakos et al. showed an association between severity of psychiatric disease and risk of DIP [51].

Serum levels of neuroleptic have been shown to correlate only variably with DIP [54, 58, 59]. However, the question of a relationship between DIP and serum levels of neuroleptic is somewhat misleading since DIP may persist for months after a drug is discontinued [22]. In such cases, the serum drug level may be zero but the dopamine receptors in the brain may remain strongly blocked.

The question of a correlation between DIP and psychiatric response has been debated. Alpert et al. [60] found that DIP, as measured by tremor in a single finger, was dose related and negatively correlated with psychiatric response. This has not been confirmed with repeat studies, and such studies are complicated by the dissociation between the temporal motor and psychiatric responses to neuroleptics.

Neuroleptic potency and neuroleptic dose are unequivocal risk factors for DIP. Increasing age, preexisting EPS signs, dementia, severe psychiatric disease, and brain damage are possible predisposing factors. However, the development of DIP is notoriously unpredictable. In one study, a patient receiving 480 mg trifluoperazine had no DIP [61], and we have seen a patient on long-term haloperidol 200 mg per day without parkinsonism.

Pathophysiology

Pharmacology

The term "neuroleptic," literally meaning "that which grips the nerve," was coined by Delay and Deniker and is used in a somewhat arbitrary fashion. Originally introduced to describe the effects of chlorpromazine and reserpine on animals and humans, the term referred to a unique constellation of qualities that included both the tranquilizing and antipsychotic effects of the drugs as well as characteristic EPS effects. Eventually, the term came to be synonymous with "antipsychotic" and became less associated with the dopamine-depleting drugs. With the advent of atypical antipsychotic drugs, "neuroleptic" has taken on the connotations of the neurologic profile it originally described and is now primarily associated with the conventional antipsychotics and other dopamine-blocking drugs that cause extrapyramidal side effects [62]. In common neurological parlance, the term "neuroleptic" is used to mean a dopamine receptor-blocking drug, including the antipsychotics, the antiemetics, and metoclopramide. The latter drugs, if used in high doses, also possess some antipsychotic efficacy. There are five general categories of neuroleptic drugs: phenothiazines (thioridazine, prochlorperazine), butyrophenones (haloperidol, droperidol), thioxanthenes (thiothixene), dibenzaepines (loxapine, clozapine), and substituted benzamides (metoclopramide). Dopamine-depleting drugs are usually considered separately.

Clozapine and the newer antipsychotics are not usually described as "neuroleptics," but are instead referred to as "atypical antipsychotic" (AA) drugs. Though poorly defined, the term "atypical antipsychotic" is usually used to describe antipsychotics associated with a low incidence of EPS. In addition to clozapine, these medications include risperidone, olanzapine, quetiapine, and ziprasidone These drugs first came to attention because they did not induce catalepsy or antagonize amphetamine stereotypies in animals at doses comparable to conventional antipsychotics. Other characteristics include a high

Table 6.2 Characteristics of atypical antipsychotics

Characteristics	Clozapine	Risperidone	Olanzapine	Quetiapine
Fails to induce catalepsy or antagonize amphetamine stereotypy	+	−	−	+
5HT/D_2 ratio	+	+	+	+
No prolactin elevation	+	−	+/−	+
Improves negative symptoms	+	+	+	+
Decreased EPS	+	−	−**	+/−**

*Modified from Friedman JH, Meltzer H. Atypical antipsychotics. In: Factor SA, Weiner WJ (eds.) Parkinson's Disease: Diagnosis and Clinical Management. New York: Demos Medical Publishing, 2002: 412; and Friedman JH, Factor SA. Atypical antipsychotics in the treatment of drug-induced psychosis in Parkinson's disease. Mov Disord 2000; 15(2):201–211.
**EPS reported in parkinson-sensitive/vulnerable populations.

ratio of $5HT_2$-to-D_2 receptor activity and failure to cause increases in prolactin levels. These factors have been found to correlate well with the clinical effects of these drugs in humans, namely, better efficacy than conventional antipsychotics, especially on negative symptoms, with less risk of EPS effects and tardive dyskinesia (see Chapter 12) [63]. The most purely atypical antipsychotic, clozapine has all of these qualities, but its use is limited by rare agranulocytosis and the need for weekly blood monitoring. The other AAs have varying degrees of atypical features and carry more risk of EPS (Tables 6.2 and 6.3) In order of atypicality, from greatest to least, the AAs can be ranked as follows: clozapine, quetiapine, ziprasidone and olanzapine, risperidone. Risperidone, in particular, is a controversial member of this group because it has few atypical features, and some authors believe that it should not be included in this category at all [63–66].

Clozapine

The first AA, clozapine, opened a new era in the treatment of schizophrenia because it offered no extrapyramidal side effects in addition to better efficacy than conventional neuroleptics, especially on negative symptoms. The drug was

Table 6.3 Receptor binding of atypical antipsychotics

Drug	D_1	D_2	5HT-2A	α_1	α_2	H_1	M_1
Clozapine	++	++	+++	+++	+++	+++	++++
Risperidone	+	+++	++++	++	+++	++	0
Olanzapine	++	++	++++	+++	0	++++	++++
Quetiapine	+	+	+	+++	+	++++	+

D = Dopamine, 5HT-2A = Serotonin, α = alpha adrenergic, H = Histamine, M = Muscarinic.
*Taken from Friedman JH, Meltzer H. Atypical antipsychotics. In: Factor SA, Weiner WJ (eds.) Parkinson's Disease: Diagnosis and Clinical Management. New York, Demos Medical Publishing, 2002: 412.

first released in Europe, but initial enthusiasm cooled after several patients developed agranulocytosis and some died [63]. In 1988 the Clozaril Collaborative Study Group published a large trial [67] comparing clozapine with chlorpromazine in refractory, chronically hospitalized schizophrenics and found the drug to be significantly more efficacious than chlorpromazine. Furthermore, after switching from haloperidol, EPS symptoms improved significantly more in the clozapine-treated group than in the chlorpromazine group. Based on this study, the FDA approved clozapine for the treatment of refractory schizophrenia, and use of the drug has since broadened to include treatment of psychosis in patients at high risk for developing extrapyramidal side effects.

Many consider a drug's effect in parkinsonian populations to be the true "litmus test" of its propensity to cause parkinsonism in the general population. Initial reports of clozapine in parkinsonian patients were, for the large part, positive, describing good efficacy in the treatment of psychosis without worsening of motor symptoms [68]. The 1999 PSYCLOPS trial [69] and the French Clozapine Parkinson Study Group trial [69] were two major multicenter, double-blind, placebo-controlled trials of low-dose clozapine for the treatment of drug-induced psychosis in Parkinson's disease. Both trials found clozapine to be effective without worsening parkinsonism. Moreover, the drug actually improved tremor. Unfortunately, its potential to cause agranulocytosis limits its use, and patients in the United States are required to have weekly blood monitoring. Agranulocytosis occurs in less than 1% of patients, and this reaction is idiosyncratic and unrelated to dose.

Risperidone
Risperidone was the next AA to be approved in the United States. The North American trials [70, 71] and the International trial [72] were multicenter double-blind studies evaluating the safety and efficacy of multiple doses of risperidone in the treatment of schizophrenia. Although the North American trials showed no significant difference in the EPS effects of risperidone 6 mg per day compared to placebo (based on ESRS score and use of antiparkinsonian meds) [70, 73, 74] they did show an increase in EPS effects at higher doses of the drug [70, 74]. A study of risperidone in dementia over 12 weeks showed no significant EPS difference from placebo [75], and a comparison of clozapine and risperidone in 86 patients with chronic schizophrenia showed similar EPS effects in both drug groups [76].

Other reports, however, revealed an increased risk of EPS in patients on risperidone [73]. In a comparison trial of clozapine, risperidone, and conventional antipsychotics, patients on risperidone scored significantly higher on the Simpson-Angus Scale than clozapine patients, and there was no significant difference between the scores associated with risperidone and those associated with conventional antipsychotics [73]. On the Subjective Extrapyramidal Rating Scale, patients on conventional antipsychotics actually scored significantly better than patients on risperidone [73]. Similarly, a study of risperidone and haloperidol in neuroleptic-naïve patients showed no significant difference between EPS effects of risperidone and those of haloperidol [64].

Based on these results in the schizophrenia population, one would expect risperidone's EPS effects to be problematic in parkinsonian patients. Results to date have been mixed [68]: although some studies have reported risperidone to be safe in PD patients [77, 78], other studies have shown that many patients are unable to tolerate the drug due to motor worsening [65, 66]. Moreover, the studies supporting the safety of risperidone in PD [77, 79, 80] are controversial, and their conclusions have been contested [68, 81]. In 2001, Factor et al. found 82 cases in the literature of PD patients treated with risperidone, 23 of which (33%) described motor worsening [81].

Overall, risperidone's EPS effects appear to fall somewhere between those of clozapine and the conventional antipsychotics [73], with higher doses carrying greater risks of DIP and other extrapyramidal signs. Many believe its risk of EPS to be closer to that of the typical antipsychotics than the other AAs [64, 73, 81], and DIP remains a concern.

Olanzapine

There were four pivotal trials of olanzapine for the treatment of schizophrenia: the U.S. clinical trial [82] and the North American trial [83] were placebo controlled, while the Eastern Hemisphere [84] and International trials [85] compared olanzapine to haloperidol. All four pivotal trials showed improvement from baseline EPS symptoms in olanzapine-treated patients as measured by the Simpson-Angus scale [86]. The two placebo-controlled trials, however, also showed EPS improvement in patients on placebo [82, 83, 86], and there was no significant difference between the improvements in EPS seen with olanzapine and placebo [82, 83]. In the three trials that included haloperidol, olanzapine was associated with fewer EPS side effects than haloperidol [83–85]. In a separate trial comparing olanzapine to risperidone, olanzapine had a lower incidence of EPS effects based on both patient report and objective assessment [86, 87]. The trials that included multiple fixed doses of olanzapine did not show a dose-dependent increase in EPS symptoms with olanzapine [86].

The drug's seemingly low EPS profile in schizophrenia raised the hope that it could be used to treat psychosis in IPD, and there have been several studies of olanzapine in Parkinsonian patients. Despite an initial open study [88] that showed no motor worsening in PD patients, subsequent reports have demonstrated a deleterious effect of the drug on motor functioning in PD [63, 89–95]. Two multicenter, double-blind, placebo-controlled trials of olanzapine in parkinsonian patients have been published [96], as well as a third, single-center study [97]. Both reports described no benefit of olanzapine over placebo in the treatment of psychosis, but olanzapine did cause significant worsening of motor function. Although olanzapine's EPS profile is certainly better than that of conventional neuroleptics, and probably better than that of risperidone, DIP remains a risk in olanzapine-treated patients.

Quetiapine

Two double-blind, placebo-controlled trials of quetiapine in schizophrenia found its EPS effects to be no different from those of placebo [98, 99]. Although unrelated to clozapine pharmacologically, its low potential to produce catalepsy in animals and its effects on apomorphine-induced stereoptypies are similar to those of clozapine. Furthermore, it does not cause elevations in prolactin levels and has a high $5HT_2/D_2$ receptor ratio [68] (Table 6.2). Thus, the "atypicality" of its pharmacologic profile is second only to that of clozapine.

Although there have not been any double-blind trials of quetiapine in PD patients, experience with the drug in parkinsonian populations has been consistent with the above data [68]. Numerous reports have described good efficacy without worsening parkinsonism [68]. Even in those studies that showed motor worsening in significant numbers of patients, the symptoms were not severe enough to cause discontinuation of the drug in most patients. It is possible that most of the increased parkinsonism could be due to disease progression rather than quetiapine, especially in long-term trials [68].

Based on the available data, only clozapine carries a lower risk of DIP than quetiapine. Although quetiapine is inferior to clozapine in terms of DIP and antipsychotic potency, it does not carry the life-threatening risk of agranulocytosis.

Ziprasidone

A newer AA, ziprasidone, was approved for use in the United States in February, 2001. As a result, experience with the drug is not as extensive as with the other atypical antipsychotics. Ziprasidone was approved for the treatment of schizophrenia based on two major double-blind, placebo-controlled trials [100, 101]. Both studies showed no notable difference in the EPS effects of ziprasidone and placebo, but more ziprasidone patients required treatment with benztropine. However, patients not treated with benzotropine had similar Simpson-Angus scores regardless of their treatment arm. In one of the studies [101], there appeared to be a slight trend toward increasing the incidence of patient-reported EPS with higher ziprasidone doses, but only one patient on ziprasidone discontinued the study because of a movement disorder.

In addition to these two trials, a number of short-term (4–6 weeks) studies were conducted during late-stage development of the drug, most of which were published in abstract form [102, 103]. A review of these short-term, placebo-controlled trials showed similar results to the two pivotal trials [103]. A more recently published, longer trial compared ziprasidone with haloperidol in the long-term treatment of schizophrenia [104]. Not surprisingly, patients on ziprasidone had significantly less parkinsonism on exam than patients on haloperidol. Despite these objective data, 15% of patients reported experiencing a movement disorder on ziprasidone, though only one of these patients discontinued the trial for this reason [104].

Overall, ziprasidone appears to be associated with a low incidence of DIP, and its EPS effects have been found to be comparable with placebo in several trials [100–103, 105, 106]. Although these trials have not shown any relationship between dose and EPS symptoms [100, 102], many experts believe that EPS is more likely to occur in patients on higher doses of the medication and in patients who are already at risk for movement disorders [101, 105]. This has been the case with several other atypical antipsychotics, and their true propensities for EPS effects have been revealed when the drugs were used in high-risk populations such as parkinsonian patients. As ziprasidone use has yet to be reported in PD patients, the actual extent of its EPS effects remains unclear. The trials in schizophrenia and the drug's minimal effect on prolactin levels suggests that its EPS profile may be similar to that of olanzapine [105].

Nonneuroleptic DIP

Lithium

Several nonneuroleptic drugs have also been reported to cause DIP. Lithium-associated EPS was first described in 1975 when Shopsin and Gershon described cogwheel rigidity in 15 out of 27 outpatients on chronic lithium without concomitant neuroleptic use [107]. Subsequent reports have described tremor, rigidity, and other EPS symptoms in lithium-treated patients, but many of these patients were also on neuroleptic medication. A cross-sectional study [108] evaluated 130 outpatients for EPS, 110 of whom were treated with lithium. Of these, 19 were also on neuroleptics, and another 40 had been on neuroleptics in the past 6 months. The study found tremor to be significantly associated with both lithium and neuroleptics, but no association was found between lithium and hypokinesia or akathisia. There was a trend toward more EPS symptoms (as rated by the ESRS) in patients on the combination of lithium plus a neuroleptic. Thus, the risk of DIP with lithium remains unclear, the combination of lithium and neuroleptics may carry greater risk than either drug alone. We have seen lithium induce a syndrome identical to IPD that reversed upon lithium's discontinuation.

Valproic acid

DIP has also been reported in patients on valproic acid (VPA). A study of 36 patients [109] on VPA for 12 months or more revealed 75% of them as having parkinsonism, defined as three or more of the following: 4–7 Hz resting tremor, rigidity or cogwheeling, posture and gait abnormalities, decreased motion rates of alternating movements, or hypokinetic speech. Of these, 96% experienced a mean improvement of 19.6 points on the Unified Parkinson's Disease Rating Scale (UPDRS) after stopping VPA. Patients were also found to have cognitive and hearing impairment, and these deficits improved as well. The authors concluded that chronic VPA therapy can cause a reversible syndrome of parkinsonism and cognitive impairment that is characterized by an insidious onset over several years, often accompanied by hearing impairment. Although this study was not blinded, other case reports have described similar patients as well as a more acute syndrome associated with short-term therapy [110, 111]. Given the potential for resolution of symptoms, DIP should be considered in parkinsonian patients on VPA.

The pathophysiology of VPA-induced parkinsonism is unclear. Interestingly, VPA does not affect dopamine receptors [112]. Some authors suggest that VPA may cause mitochondrial dysfunction, specifically defective NADH CoQ reductase, which leads to reversible parkinsonism. The drugs GABAergic activity may also play a role [109].

Calcium channel blockers

Although not approved in the United States, the calcium channel blockers, cinnarizine and its derivative, flunarizine, have been shown to cause DIP. Both drugs have antihistaminic, antiserotinergic, and antidopaminergic activity, but flunarizine is more potent and has a longer half-life. Looking for evidence of EPS, Micheli et al. [10] examined 101 patients treated with either flunarizine or cinnarizine without a history of exposure to neuroleptics. Ninety-three of these patients had parkinsonism. After withdrawal of the medication, all 93 patients experienced a full recovery over a range of 7–270 days.

A more recent Spanish study [9] of 306 parkinsonian patients revealed DIP to be the diagnosis in 172 patients, of whom 74 had been taking cinnarizine for an average of 33 months. In 45 patients cinnarizine was the offending drug. After discontinuation of cinnarizine, 89% of patients recovered completely over 1–16 months, a higher rate of recovery than seen with the other DIP patients in this study.

Despite the good outcome in this series, other reports suggest that flunarizine- and cinnarizine-induced parkinsonism may not be so reversible. A study [113] of 13 such patients found that they continued to exhibit parkinsonian signs over a period of ≥ 7 years after the discontinuation of the offending drug.

Several studies suggest that susceptibility increases with advanced age, female gender, and a background of familial essential tremor [9, 10, 113]. The Negrotti study also suggested that calcium blocker-induced parkinsonism may be associated with preferential involvement of the arms and a longer latency of onset compared to neuroleptic-induced parkinsonism, but other studies have not shown such differences [9].

The mechanism of action behind the EPS effects of these calcium channel blockers is unclear. It has been postulated that calcium channel blockade may influence calcium-mediated neurotransmitter release from the presynaptic terminal [10], thereby decreasing the amount of neurotransmitter available in the synapse. Since EPS is not seen with other calcium channel blockers, this explanation does not seem entirely adequate, but presynaptic influences on dopamine may still play a role. Cinnarizine has also been shown to block postsynaptic dopamine receptors in the striatum, and flunarizine acts at these receptors as well [9, 11].

Selective serotonin reuptake inhibitors

The most commonly prescribed antidepressants, selective serotonin reuptake inhibitors (SSRIs), can also cause parkinsonism. Though this side effect is uncommon, the widespread use of these drugs makes it important to recognize their association with DIP.

In a 1996 review [114], Leo identified 71 cases of SSRI-induced movement disorders, 10 of which were categorized as parkinsonism. This series also identified seven cases of preexisting parkinsonism made worse by the addition of an SSRI. Fluoxetine was the most commonly implicated drug, with a few cases also attributed to paroxetine and fluvoxamine. Sertraline was not linked with any cases of parkinsonism. Prescribing frequencies are most likely primarily responsible for these different rates of association, Although different pharmacologic properties of the various SSRIs may also contribute. For example, fluoxetine has a longer half-life than many other SSRIs, while sertraline has a negative effect on dopamine reuptake. More recent reports have described DIP in patients on sertraline [115] as well as in patients on other SSRIs.

In a 1998 review [116], Gerber and Lynd identified 127 published cases of SSRI-induced movement disorders, 25 of which were categorized as parkinsonism, and 15 of which were mixed. Industry reports provided 516 reports of parkinsonism in patients on SSRIs.

Despite these reports, more recent studies of SSRI effects in parkinsonian patients have been mixed. Several reports have described motor worsening with SSRI use in these patients [117, 118] and there have been reports of SSRI-induced parkinsonism in patients who later developed IPD [119, 120] suggesting that the SSRI "unmasked" the underlying disease. Other studies suggest that SSRIs are safe in parkinsonian patients [121–123]. It should be noted, however, that two of these negative studies described patients with increased off-time and/or tremor, both of which reversed with discontinuation of the SSRI [122, 123]. In a retrospective chart review, Richard and Maughn [124] identified 58 parkinsonian patients who received treatment with SSRIs. Of these, only five experienced possible motor worsening related to SSRI therapy, and in each case the authors found possible alternative explanations for the worsening.

The mechanism behind SSRI-induced DIP is unclear but likely involves serotinergic inhibition of dopaminergic pathways [114, 125]. SSRIs may also affect the metabolism and availability of other drugs with DIP potential, thereby increasing the risk of DIP in patients on multiple medications. The reverse is also possible: other drugs may alter the effects of SSRIs and increase the risk of DIP. For example, one patient on fluoxetine developed DIP only after the addition of cimetidine [126].

Catecholamine-depleting agents

Reserpine is a naturally occurring substance derived from the rauwolfia shrub. It acts to deplete intraneuronal catecholamines by blocking their reuptake. Tetrabenazine also acts to deplete intraneuronal catecholamine stores but is less potent than reserpine. The action of tetrabenazine is considerably shorter than reserpine, so that adverse effects reverse more readily and the onset of action is quicker. However, tetrabenazine, in addition to depleting catecholamines, also may block dopamine receptors [127]. Alphamethyltyrosine (metyrosine) is a competitive inhibitor of tyrosine hydroxylase, the rate-limiting enzyme that converts tyrosine to diorthophenylalanine (levodopa) in the synthesis of dopamine, norepinephrine, and epinephrine. It depletes catecholamine stores by reducing synthesis.

Mechanisms of action (see also Chapter 3)

All neuroleptics (if one excludes the catecholamine depletors) block dopamine receptors [128] (see also Chapter 3). All of the conventional antipsychotics induce similar biochemical, physiological, and behavioral changes in animals and presumably in humans. In animals, they induce catalepsy (the prolonged maintenance of abnormal postures), reduce aggressive and hostile behavior, and decrease normal exploratory and locomotor behavior. In humans, they lessen emotions and interest in the environment in normal controls, and they reduce psychotic symptoms in psychiatric patients. They inhibit the actions of dopamine agonists in animals such as apomorphine-induced motor and stereotypic behaviors, vomiting, and climbing. The neuroleptics have diverse profiles with respect to which dopamine agonist actions they antagonize most.

There are several dopaminergic systems within the brain, but the one that is particularly important in understanding parkinsonism is the nigrostriatal pathway. Within this and the other dopamine systems there have been at least five classes of identified dopamine receptors. These are classified into two groups, the D_1 family (D_1 and D_5 receptors) and the D_2 family (D_2, D_3, and D_4 receptors). The D_1-type receptors are linked to G-proteins that stimulate adenylate cyclase and lead to an increase in cAMP. The D_2-like receptors are coupled to G-proteins that either inhibit adenylate cyclase, are inactive, or link with phospholipase C [129]. Both families of receptors influence various ion channels as well. The D_2 receptor has been most closely linked to both the parkinsonian side effects of neuroleptics and to the antipsychotic properties of these drugs.

Different regions of the brain have different ratios of the various dopamine receptors. For example, the caudate, putamen, and nucleus accumbens contain a higher density of D_1 receptors than the thalamus and cortex. D_2 receptors are concentrated in the striatum and substantia nigra, but D_4 receptors are more concentrated in the cortex and limbic areas [129]. Different antipsychotics have different affinities for the various receptors. For example, among the conventional neuroleptics, butyrophenones and benzamides have a low affinity for the D_1 family and a high affinity for receptors in the D_2 family. Clozapine has a uniquely high affinity for the D_4 receptor. It was postulated that the different affinities of various antipsychotics for different receptors concentrated in different areas of the brain helped to explain their variable extrapyramidal profiles, with D_4 receptors mediating antipsychotic effects and D_2 receptors mediating extrapyramidal symptoms. Thus, the conventional neuroleptics cause EPS effects because of their action at D_2 receptors in the basal ganglia, with high D_2 affinity drugs such as fluphenazine causing more EPS than drugs with lower D_2 affinities. According to this thinking, clozapine is free of EPS risks because of its high affinity for D_4 rather than D_2 receptors.

This model does not, however, adequately explain the mechanism of action of the AAs. Both typical and atypical antipsychotics bind to D_2 receptors, yet only the conventional neuroleptics cause EPS effects. Moreover, typical neuroleptics bind to D_4 receptors with an even greater affinity than clozapine [130]. Clozapine itself acts on other receptors, sometimes with affinities greater than its affinity for the D_4 receptor. Thus, it is unlikely that D_4 properties fully explain the effects of antipsychotics, either typical or atypical.

In addition to dopamine receptors, the AAs bind to several other sites as well (Table 6.3), and these other receptors may help explain their atypical effects. Atypical antipsychotics have been shown to have a higher $5HT_2/D_2$ ratio than typical antipsychotics [131, 132], and it has been suggested that this 5HT activity is responsible for atypicality. Proponents argue that the combination of 5-HT and D_2 receptor blockade influences dopamine release in the striatum, cortex, and limbic system. Several drugs selected for development based on this theory subsequently proved to be clinically atypical (risperidone, olanzapine, quetiapine, and ziprasidone) [133].

Other neurotransmitter systems may also be important, but their role remains unclear. In IPD, the degeneration of dopaminergic pathways releases cholinergic neurons from dopaminergic inhibition, and these neurons become hyperactive [134]. In DIP, dopamine blockade produces a similar effect. By decreasing the cholinergic hyperactivity, antipsychotics with anticholinergic properties may balance some of their antidopaminergic effects. However, this concept does not adequately explain the different EPS profiles of antipsychotics or even the difference between the typical and atypical drugs. Clozapine has a high affinity for muscarinic receptors and therefore has anticholinergic properties [135], but this alone is clearly insufficient to explain its lack of EPS. The two-drug combination of an anticholinergic and a typical neuroleptic does not mimic clozapine's lack of extrapyramidal effects, and low-potency neuroleptics such as thioridazine have relatively similar antimuscarinic properties [136] yet do not have clozapine's extrapyramidal profile. Conversely, other AAs do not display prominent anticholinergic activity.

More recently, attention has returned to the D_2 receptor. It has been theorized that a drug's extrapyramidal and antipsychotic effects depend not on the type of receptors bound, but rather on the time bound to a single receptor, specifically the D_2 receptor. Drugs dissociate from the D_2 receptor at different rates, thereby resulting in different occupancy rates for each drug. At equivalent doses, drugs with slow dissociation rates reach higher receptor occupancy levels than drugs with fast dissociation rates and can be described as having a higher affinity for the receptor; conversely, low-affinity drugs dissociate faster. According to this theory, antipsychotic effects occur above a certain threshold occupancy rate, and EPS effects appear only above an even higher occupancy rate. Thus, fast dissociation drugs achieve occupancy rates above the threshold required for antipsychotic effects without reaching the level associated with extrapyramidal symptoms, while slow dissociation drugs push occupancy rates above the EPS threshold and cause unwanted side effects [130]. Haloperidol and other conventional antipsychotics are slow dissociating, clozapine and quetiapine are fast dissociating, and risperidone and olanzapine are in between, with dissociation rates that are dose dependent. Proponents of this theory argue that low affinity for the D_2 receptor is both necessary and sufficient for atypicality and that other receptors are only of secondary importance. Critics point out that this theory does not adequately explain the actions of certain AAs and that it has not led to the development of any new agents [133, 137].

As ascending serotinergic pathways inhibit dopaminergic pathways in the basal ganglia [134], the role of serotonin may also be important. Simply put, antipsychotics with a high $5HT_2/D_2$ receptor ratio could increase dopamine transmission by blocking inhibitory serotinergic influences, thereby counteracting some of the effects of dopamine receptor blockade: the higher the $5HT_2/D_2$ ratio, the less overall effect on dopamine motor systems. While some authors believe that $5HT_2$ receptor activity is central to explaining the mechanism of AAs, others have questioned this theory.

Antipsychotics may also affect noradrenergic and GABAergic pathways as well as neuropeptide systems, but less is known about drug interactions with these systems. Moreover, the role of these pathways in parkinsonism is still unclear [134].

Treatment of DIP

Introduction
Problems in the treatment literature

Ideally, the treatment for DIP is discontinuation of the offending agent, but this is often not possible. Alternatively, the patient can switch to a medication with a lower risk of DIP; the advent of AAs has opened a new field of therapeutic alternatives to conventional neuroleptics. In some cases, however, an alternate drug is not an option. When additional treatment is required, DIP is usually treated with anticholinergics or amantadine. Diphenhydramine is another possible option. However, the data to support these choices are scanty. Few double-blind trials have been performed to prove efficacy, and even fewer have compared active drug to placebo. Most have compared one drug with another. The problems inherent in this area have been well reviewed by Mindham [138], including problems with rating instruments, the natural tendency of untreated DIP to improve over time, the reporting of results that strain credibility, the occasional failure to obtain baseline measurements, the use of nonblinded raters, the use of untrained raters, and the use of different populations. Treatment studies for DIP fall into three categories: treatment of symptomatic DIP, prophylaxis against DIP, and chronic treatment/prophylaxis of

DIP while on neuroleptics. The last category refers to the questionable need for continued long-term antiparkinsonian medication in view of the fact that DIP can resolve spontaneously even though the patient remains on a neuroleptic. Some of these issues have resolved over time and with the advent of AAs, but others remain.

Rating scales

Although it was evident quite early that DIP and IPD appeared to be clinically similar, the two Parkinson syndromes were evaluated differently. As was the case with investigations of IPD, psychiatric papers used a variety of rating instruments to score parkinsonian severity. In neurological trials in IPD, however, there has been an increasing trend to use the UPDRS [139]. Similarly, over the past 10 years, psychiatric trials have moved toward use of the Simpson-Angus Scale (SAS) to evaluate DIP. This standardization has significantly improved the ability to compare data from different studies.

The Simpson-Angus scale [140] uses a 5-point scale to rate each of nine different items. It is readily apparent that scoring is heavily weighted toward rigidity. Seven of nine items are measures of rigidity. Glabellar tapping to measure akinesia and gait analysis for posture and arm swing are the only other items analyzed. Tremor, bradykinesia, and postural instability are notably absent from the scale. Furthermore, the tests advocated for rigidity are extremely difficult to perform because of limited patient compliance.

Other tests employed to rate EPS signs include the Rating Scale for Extrapyramidal Symptoms (REPS) [141], the Extrapyramidal System Rating Scale (ESRS) [142], and Mindham's scale [138]. The REPS fails to rate bradykinesia but is useful for patients whose parkinsonism is not severe. It does not assess subjective symptoms and is easy to use. The ESRS scores DIP signs in each limb so that measures of tremor or rigidity acquire extra weight by being multiplied by the number of limbs involved. Thus, a severely disabled person "barely able to walk" may have the same score as a patient with occasional low-amplitude tremors in multiple limbs. The objective portion of the scale is brief, and the ESRS is therefore vulnerable to bias. Mindham's scale includes the useful concept of a global assessment of parkinsonism rather than a sum of scores.

While objective measures provide clearly defined and easy-to-compare results, they require consistent cooperation from the subject. This is readily achievable with some subjects but can be virtually impossible in severely affected psychiatric patients. Diminished attention for any reasonimpairs reliability of the results, and since individual patients act as their own controls, the tests must be reliable.

Treatment of symptomatic DIP
Anticholinergics
Negative reports. Simpson [143] treated patients with advanced phenothiazine-induced parkinsonism with single boluses of intravenous anticholinergics and

found no difference compared to placebo. He then treated six patients with oral biperiden in standard doses for 5 weeks. Only one patient improved. The surprising conclusion of the study was that it is exceedingly difficult to measure DIP. "As benztropine and biperiden are widely used for the treatment of parkinsonism, we may be justified in rejecting" the conclusion that there is no difference between active drug and placebo. This study exemplifies the problems of clinical trials in this area.

In looking at individual variations in response to neuroleptics, Simpson et al. [61] treated those who developed DIP with benztropine and reported benefit "in a small number of cases" only.

In one of the only double-blind, placebo-controlled studies, amantadine and orphenadrine were compared to placebo in a crossover fashion [142], and no differences from placebo were found.

Positive reports. An open study [26] of phenothiazine-induced DIP used biperiden in doses of up to 18 mg daily. The majority responded well to 6 mg per day. In another double-blind controlled trial [142] comparing procyclidine, piribedil, and placebo, procyclidine was found to be more effective than placebo on clinical evaluations, yet timed tasks (which are presumably more objective or measure different functions than the clinical assessment) showed no differences. Using young male patients as their own controls, Kelly et al. [144], found in a double-blind controlled study of DIP that benztropine at 2–4 mg per day was able to induce virtually total clinical remission. However, here too, objective scores using timed tasks showed no changes. Amantadine, though helpful, was less effective. DiMascio et al. [141] also reported benefit from anticholinergics in a blinded study without placebo.

Amantadine

The mechanism of action of amantadine is thought to be glutamate antagonism via inhibition of the NMDA receptor subtype. In addition, amantadine may work through the dopamine system by increasing dopamine release, acting as a dopamine receptor agonist, and blocking dopamine reuptake. It may also possess some anticholinergic activity [145].

In an open study of DIP patients, amantadine produced moderate-to-marked benefit in 9 of 10 cases [74]. In a double-blind comparison of benztropine and amantadine [141], both were found to be equally effective in DIP, but amantadine was better tolerated. Greenblatt et al. [146] reported that amantadine was beneficial and that, in general, improvement paralleled serum levels of amantadine. Stenson et al. [147] reported benefit in 100% of patients on amantadine and found that it was as effective as benztropine, with a similar incidence of adverse effects. Pacific et al. [148] found that amantadine led to a rapid and marked improvement within 4 to 6 days in rigidity and tremor in 15 patients whose DIP had been unresponsive to anticholinergics. There was no relationship found between individual responses and serum amantadine levels. Only the placebo-controlled study of Mindham et al. [142] has reported negative results using amantadine. Thus, the results for amantadine are somewhat less conflicting than for anticholinergics.

Treatment with levodopa

Treating DIP with levodopa initially seems somewhat counterintuitive. On one hand, since dopamine receptors are blocked, increasing dopamine should not have any effect. On the other, it is known that dopamine receptor blockade in animals produces a reactive increase in dopamine turnover and an increase in dopamine receptors. Thus, one could argue that DIP occurs when there are too few available receptors or the reactive dopamine increase has been insufficient. This might justify a trial of levodopa in order to increase dopamine production. Whether levodopa actually increases available dopamine in neuroleptic-treated patients is unknown. In reserpinized rodents [149], it does not reverse locomotor changes that are due to catecholamine depletion.

Several reports have been published concerning both the mental and the motoric effects of levodopa in neuroleptic-treated psychiatric patients. As with other treatment aspects of DIP, the published results are contradictory both for the psychiatric and for the parkinsonian aspects.

In a nonblinded study [150] comparing single intravenous boluses of levodopa given at 2 mg per kg over 5 minutes to placebo in treating DIP, all 40 patients improved in terms of akinesia and rigidity, with tremor being the least responsive. The mildest cases of DIP responded best. Men and women responded equally, but the patients taking chlorpromazine benefited more than those taking haloperidol. Improvement began within 5 to 20 minutes. The maximum effect occurred between 1 and 2 hours and was lost by 3 hours. Psychiatrically, there was a "trend toward euphoria." There was no response to the placebo. Angrist et al. [151] reported behavioral worsening in 10 of 10 schizophrenics treated with 3–6 gm of levodopa, possibly because they had discontinued ongoing neuroleptic therapy.

Twenty patients taking neuroleptics and "standard" antiparkinson medication for observed extrapyramidal syndromes were taken off their antiparkinson drugs and then placed on increasing doses of levodopa [152]. Sixteen subjects failed to tolerate removal of their antiparkinson medications and the four who received levodopa (maximum daily doses 1400–2600 mg for 8–23 days) all worsened psychiatrically without motor improvement. Resumption of the previous medications resulted in improvement.

A study [153] involving 84 chronic schizophrenics given levodopa up to 1200 mg daily reported a moderate-to-marked improvement in the "negative" symptoms of the disease such as rapport, emotional blunting, and autism. However, no comments were made on the response of DIP.

From a referred population of patients with disabling DIP, Hardie and Lees [12] treated 15 patients (5 maintained on neuroleptics and 10 withdrawn from them) with levodopa plus benserazide in doses of 300–1000 mg of levodopa. Seven had a moderate (41–75%) and two had a complete response to levodopa while the rest had no (<20%) or slight (20–40%) benefit. However, this was a highly selected population referred to a movement disorders clinic. These patients had been on anticholinergics and therefore may have been referred precisely because they were unresponsive to typical antiparkinson medications. Thus, they may have constituted a refractory population.

Other levodopa studies in small populations have also produced conflicting results. While some investigators have found it extremely effective in the management of young patients with severe, disabling DIP persisting after neuroleptic withdrawal (A. Lang, personal communication), it would seem that there is a limited role for levodopa in the routine treatment of DIP. It appears to be ineffective in most cases where anticholinergics fail and possibly less effective than anticholinergics in cases where the latter work. The reports of levodopa's beneficial effects on psychiatric symptoms are counterbalanced by negative reports. It is, therefore, not recommended for treatment of typical DIP.

Electroconvulsive therapy (ECT)

ECT has been helpful in IPD for treating depression and paranoid psychosis and has been reported to ameliorate the motoric features as well. In two studies, ECT [154, 155] was used to treat "on-off" clinical fluctuations in subjects who had no psychiatric problems and was found to improve parkinsonism for periods of time lasting from hours to several weeks. Moellentine et al. [156] described improved motor functioning in 14 of 25 parkinsonian patients receiving ECT for psychiatric purposes. Moreover, several reports have described motor improvement with maintenance (repeated) ECT specifically for IPD [157, 158].

Isolated case reports have documented similar effects in DIP but few prospective studies have been performed. One study [159] found that bilateral ECT given at the rate of three shocks weekly progressively improved parkinsonism beginning within the first week and continuing until therapy was concluded, after which the DIP began to worsen again. By the end of the second week post-ECT, the DIP was still improved compared to baseline, but anticholinergics had been increased, making interpretation difficult. In a separate series, 35 schizophrenics receiving treatment with both neuroleptics and ECT were examined for EPS signs and found to have no evidence of DIP [160]. This finding led the investigators to speculate that ECT may protect against DIP.

ECT's effect on parkinsonism may influence a decision on whether or not to use ECT for psychiatric purposes. For example, depressed patients with DIP unresponsive to anticholinergics might benefit from ECT for treatment of both problems. However, negative aspects of ECT also need to be kept in mind since they can offset the benefits. In the elderly especially, transient delirium and memory dysfunction may occur. There has been one case report of ECT worsening DIP and dystonia [161]. The duration of the antiparkinson effect is measured in days to weeks, so the potential motor benefit should be considered only secondarily.

How ECT works in ameliorating parkinsonism is unknown but it appears to be independent of improvement in mood and thinking ability. In animal models, ECT has been shown to enhance dopaminergic transmission and the sensitivity of dopamine receptors, but its biochemical effects are so manifold that a definitive explanation for its antiparkinson action is lacking.

Other treatments
Other treatments for DIP have been tried without much success. A 1993 study of propranolol in DIP [162] showed no benefit over placebo. Spivak et al. [163] reported improvement of EPS symptoms in refractory schizophrenic patients treated with clozapine. However, the patients had previously been on neuroleptics and underwent a washout period of only 2 weeks. Thus, the improvement in DIP and other EPS signs was likely due more to the discontinuation of neuroleptic therapy than to the addition of clozapine [164].

Management of coexistent DIP and TD
Management of these coexistent conditions is extremely difficult and is usually quite unsatisfactory. In a double-blind, placebo-controlled study [165], both amantadine and trihexiphenidyl worsened TD as they improved DIP. DeFraites et al. [166] demonstrated in a single patient that benztropine improved DIP and worsened TD, while physostigmine, a centrally acting muscarinic agent, did the opposite. Aggravation of dyskinesias was dose-limiting in two patients whose DIP was treated with 1000 mg of levodopa and benserazide, while there was no mention of change in TD in another six patients treated with 300–1000 mg [12].

Fahn and Mayeux [167] argued that dopamine-depleting drugs such as reserpine and alpha-methyltyrosine ameliorate TD without worsening parkinsonism. Jankovic and Casabona [168] reported beneficial response of the combined syndromes to catecholamine-depleting agents and levodopa. Their patients had all been off neuroleptics for at least 6 months. Treatment of these patients depends on a careful analysis of each symptom's contribution to disability: the DIP, the various features of the TD, and the underlying psychiatric illness. One is then faced with balancing potential benefit with complications of drug intervention. Ideally, prolonged neuroleptic withdrawal may allow both DIP and TD to resolve, but this may not be feasible. There may be a role for ECT in the management of difficult or refractory cases. Amantadine may improve parkinsonism while exerting its purported antiglutaminergic effect, thereby improving dyskinesias as well. However, reports on amantadine improving TD are lacking.

Prophylaxis
The issue of whether patients started on a neuroleptic should be treated simultaneously with an antiparkinsonian drug is controversial. On one hand, these

drugs do reduce the risk of extrapyramidal adverse reactions, but the trade-off is the potential for other adverse effects. The introduction of AAs has made this debate almost irrelevant.

Several studies, both prospective and retrospective, have supported the use of prophylactic treatment for DIP [50, 169, 170]. These studies showed that significantly fewer patients receiving prophylaxis developed DIP compared to patients not treated with prophylaxis. In each study, however, a number of the prophylactically treated patients still developed DIP. There have been few studies showing negative results of prophylaxis.

The issue of whether and when to stop antiparkinson medications has been even more unclear. Studies have offered conflicting results: some showed the discontinuation of antiparkinson drugs to be well tolerated in most patients [12, 32, 152, 171–173] while others showed that parkinsonian signs frequently worsened [174–177].

Many patients do not need antiparkinson medications at all and fewer need them for the long term. DIP should be treated *only* when the patient is truly symptomatic, using either anticholinergic medications or amantadine, monitoring both for adverse and beneficial effects. Patients who fail to respond to a trial of one drug should have a second added (anticholinergic plus amantadine). If no benefit ensues, the antiparkinson medication should be stopped. It is recommended that a slow taper of antiparkinson medications be attempted after 3 months and periodically thereafter, whether the patient is parkinsonian or not. Should existing parkinsonism worsen or symptomatic DIP ensue, the medications should be restarted. Studies indicate that if DIP recurs on stopping an antiparkinson drug, restarting it should control the DIP.

Future trends

The first edition of this book looked to the development of "a future class of drugs that do not induce EPS. Hopefully these drugs will be less toxic than clozapine." Since that writing, we have made great progress toward that goal, though its actualization remains elusive. Increasing use of AAs has significantly decreased the incidence of DIP, and these drugs offer patients improved efficacy with less risk of extrapyramidal side effects. Ten years ago we lamented the lack of treatment for the "negative symptoms" of schizophrenia, but we now have drugs that begin to address these problems. However, the development of even safer, more efficacious antipsychotic medications that do not induce prominent side effects clearly remains the next step in psychopharmacology. The development of clozapine reveals that antipsychotics do not need to induce extrapyramidal side effects, and the development of a nontoxic clozapine-like drug remains the goal.

Many research questions of interest remain. For example, an obvious question, not yet answered, is whether DIP from one drug predicts DIP on another, either of the same class or of another class. Does the presence of an active non-basal ganglia brain disease such as Alzheimer's or another dementing illness predispose one to DIP? Is the development of DIP on an AA predictive of the later development of IPD? Do different ethnic groups have a different sensitivity to neuroleptics? Is the presence or absence of DIP predictive of the likelihood of later development of tardive dyskinesia? One interesting observation has been the virtual freedom from acute dystonic reactions of olanzapine despite its ability to induce parkinsonism. This is the first drug known to have this property and suggests new opportunities for further investigation of atypical antipsychotics and their role in DIP and other EPS syndromes.

References

1. Freyhan F. Comments on the biological and psychopathological basis of individual variation in chlorpromazine therapy. Encephale 1957; 45: 913–919.
2. Hornykiewicz O. Parkinsonism induced by dopaminergic antagonists. Adv Neurol 1975 1975; 9: 155–164.
3. Freyhan F. Psychomotility and parkinsonism in treatment with neuroleptic drugs. Arch Neurol Psychiatry 1957; 78: 465–472.
4. Carlsson A. The occurrence, distribution and physiological role of catecholemines in the nervous system. Pharmacol Rev 1959; 11: 490–493.
5. Ehringer H, Hornykiewicz O. Verteilung von noradrenalen und doapmine (3-hydroxytyramine) im gehirn des menschen und ihr berhatten bei erkrankingen des extrapyramidalen systems. Klin Wochenschr 1960; 24: 1236–1239.
6. Cotzias G, Woert MV, Schiffer L. Aromatic amino acids and modification of parkinsonism. N Engl J Med 1967; 276: 374–379.
7. Haase H. Extrapyramidal modification of fine movements: a "condtio sine qua non" of the fundamental therapeutic action of neuroleptic drugs. Rev Can Biol 1961; 20: 425–449.
8. Friedman JH, Max J, Swift R. Idiopathic parkinson's disease in a chronic schizophrenic patient: long-term treatment with clozapine and levodopa. Clin Neuropharmacol 1987; 10: 470–475.
9. Marti-Masso J, Poza J. Cinnarizine-induced parkinsonism: ten years later. Mov Disord 1998; 13(3): 453–456.
10. Micheli F, Pardal M, Giannaula R, et al. Movement disorders and depression due to flunarizine and cinnarizine. Mov Disord 1989; 4(2): 139–146.
11. Belforte J, Magarinos-Azcone C, Armando I, Buno W, JH P. Pharmacological involvement of the calcium channel blocker flunarizine in dopamine transmission at the striatum. Parkinsonism Relat Disord 2001; 8(1): 33–40.
12. Hardie R, Lees A. Neuroleptic-induced Parkinson's syndrome: clinical features and results of treatment with levodopa. J Neurol Neurosurg Psychiatry 1988; 51: 850–854.
13. Akbostanci M, Atbasoglu E, Balaban H. Tardive dyskinesia, mild drug-induced dyskenisia, and drug-induced parkinsonism: risk factors and topographic distribution. Acta Neurol Belg 1999; 99: 176–181.
14. Group NIoMHPSCCS. Phenothiazine treatment in acute schizophrenia. Arch Gen Psychiatry 1964; 10: 246–261.
15. Lohr J, Lohr M, Wasli E, et al. Self perception of tardive dyskinesia and neuroleptic induced parkinsonism: a study of clinical correlates. Psychopharmacol Bull 1987; 23: 211–214.
16. Friedman JH. Personal observation.
17. Villeneuve A. The rabbit syndrome: a peculiar extrapyramidal reaction. Can Psychiatr Assoc J 1972;(suppl 2): S69–S72.

18. Hoy J, Alexander B. Rabbit syndrome secondary to risperidone. Pharmacotherapy 2002; 22(4): 513–515.

19. Duvoisin R. Problems in the treatment of parkinsonism. Adv Exp Med Biol 1977; 99: 131–155.

20. Chabolla D, Maraganore D, Ahlskog J, O'Brien P, Rocca W. Drug-induced parkinsonism as a risk factor for Parkinson's disease: a historical cohort study in Olmsted County, Minnesota. Mayo Clin Proc 1998; 73: 724–727.

21. Ayd F. A survey of drug-induced extrapyramidal reactions. JAMA 1961; 175: 1054–1060.

22. Klawans H, Bergen D, Bruyn G. Prolonged drug-induced parkinsonism. Confin Neurol 1973; 35: 368–377.

23. Friedman J, Jennings D, Seibyl J, Marek K. B-CIT SPECT imaging to distinguish drug-induced parkinsonism from idiopathic Parkinson's disease exacerbated by drugs: pilot data, Part I. In 16th Annual Symposia: Movement Disorders, 2002.

24. Hymas N, Lees AJ, Bolton D, et al. The neurology of obsessional slowness. Brain 1991; 114: 2203–2233.

25. Freyhan F. Therapeutic implications of differential effects of new phenothiazine compounds. Am J Psychiatry 1959; 115: 577–585.

26. Medinar C, Kramer M, Kurland A. Biperiden in the treatment of phenothiazine-induced extra-pyramidal reactions. JAMA 1962; 182: 1127–1128.

27. Levinson D, Simpson G, Singh H, et al. Fluphenazine dose, clinical response and extrapyramidal symptoms during acute treatment. Am J Psychiatry 1990; 47: 761–769.

28. Bradley P. Psychopharmacology of antipsychotic drugs. In Bradley P, ed. Psychopharmacology and Treatment of Schizophrenia. Oxford, Oxford University Press, 1986, pp. 27–70.

29. Jenner P, Marsden C. Neuroleptic agents: acute and chronic receptor actions. In Howell D, ed. Drugs in Central Nervous System Disorders. New York, Marcel Dekker, 1985, pp. 149–262.

30. Azima H, Ogle W. Effects of largactil in mental syndromes. Can Med Assoc J 1954; 71: 116–121.

31. Kennedy P, Hershon H, McGuire R. Extrapyramidal disorders after prolonged phenothiazine therapy. Br J Psychiatry 1971; 118: 509–518.

32. DiMascio A, Demirgian E. Antiparkinson drug overuse. Psychosomatics 1970; 11: 596–601.

33. Fernandez HH, Krupp B, Friedman J. The course of tardive dyskinesia and parkinsonism in psychiatric inpatients: 14 year follow-up. Neurology 2001; 56: 805–807.

34. Rocca W, Bower J, McDonnell S, Peterson B, Maraganore D. Time trends in the incidence of parkinsonism in Olmsted County, Minnesota. Neurology 2001; 57: 462–467.

35. Baldereschi M, Di Carlo A, Rocca W, et al. Parkinson's disease and parkinsonism in a longitudinal study: two-fold higher incidence in men. Neurology 2000; 55: 1358–1363.

36. Bower J, Maraganore D, McDonnell S, Rocca W. Incidence and distribution of parkinsonism in Olmsted County, Minnesota, 1976–1990. Neurology 1999; 52: 1214–1220

37. Rajput A, Offord K, Beard C, Kurland L. Epidemiology of Parkinsonism: incidence, classification, and mortality. Ann Neurol 1984; 16: 278–282.

38. de Rijk M, Breteler M, Graveland G, et al. Prevalence of Parkinson's disease in the elderly: the Rotterdam Study. Neurology 1995; 45: 2143–2146.

39. Kessler I. Parkinson's disease in epidemiologic perspective. Adv Neurol 1978; 19: 355–384.

40. Stephen P, Williamson J. Drug-induced parkinsonism in the elderly. Lancet 1984; 2: 1082–1083.

41. Wilson J, MacLennan W. Drug-induced parkinsonism in the elderly. Age Aging 1989; 18: 208–210.

42. Richardson M, Craig T. The coexistence of parkinsonism-like symptoms and tardive dyskinesia. Am J Psychiatry 1982; 139: 341–343.

43. Crane G. Pseudoparkinsonism and tardive dyskinesia. Arch Neurol Psychiatry 1972; 27: 426–430.

44. Kucharski L, Friedman J, Wagner R. An investigation of the co-existence of abnormal involuntary movements, parkinsonism and akathisia in chronic psychiatric patients. Psychopharmacol Bull 1987; 23: 215–217.

45. Inoue F, Vanikowski A. Withdrawal akinesia. J Neurol Neurosurg Psychiatry 1981; 44: 958.

46. Nelli A, Yarden P, Feinberg I. Parkinsonism following neuroleptic withdrawal. Arch Gen Psychiatry 1989; 46: 383–384.

47. Nishimura K, Tsuka M, Horikawa N. Withdrawal-emergent rabbit syndrome during dose reduction of risperidone. Eur Neuropsychopharmacol 2001; 11(4): 323–324.

48. Marsden C, Midham R, Mackay A. Extrapyramidal movement disorders produced by antipsychotic drugs. In: Bradley P (ed) Psychopharmacology and Treatment of Schizophrenia. Oxford, Oxford University Press, 1986, pp. 340–402.

49. Caligiuri M, Lacro J, Jeste D. Incidence and predictors of drug-induced parkinsonism in older psychiatric patients treated with very low doses of neuroleptics. J Clin Psychopharmacol 1999; 19: 322–328.

50. Keepers G, Clappison V, Casey D. Initial anticholinergic prophylaxis for neuroleptic induced extrapyramidal syndromes. Arch Gen Psychiatry 1983; 40: 1113–1117.

51. Chakos M, Mayerhoff D, Loebel A, Alvir J, Lieberman J. Incidence and correlates of acute extrapyramidal symptoms in first episode of schizophrenia. Psychopharmacol Bull 1992; 28(1): 81–86.

52. Myrianthopoulos N, Kurland A, Kurland L. Hereditary predisposition in drug-induced parkinsonism. Arch Neurol 1962; 6: 19–23.

53. Myrianthopoulos N, Waldrop F, Vincent B. A repeat study of hereditary predisposition to drug-induced parkinsonism. Progr Neurogen 1967; 175: 486–491.

54. Metzen W, Newton J, Steele R, al. e. HLA antigens in drug-induced parkinsonism. Mov Disord 1989; 4: 121–128.

55. Knopp W, Fischer R, Kech J, Teitelbaum A. Clinical implications of the relation between taste sensitivity and the appearance of extrapyramidal side effects. Disord Nerv Syst 1966; 27: 729–735.

56. Demars J. Neuromuscular effects of long-term phenothiazine medications, electroconvulsive therapy and parkinsonism. J Nerv Ment Disord 1966; 143: 73–79.

57. Luckins D, Jackman H, Meltzer H. Lateral ventricular size and drug-induced parkinsonism. Psychiatr Res 1983; 9: 9–16.

58. Tune L, Coyle J. Acute extrapyramidal side effects: serum levels of neuroleptics and anticholinergics. Psychopharmacology 1981; 75: 9–15.

59. Hansen L, Larsen N, Vestergard P. Plasma levels of perphenazine related to development of extrapyramidal effects. Psychopharmacology 1981; 74: 306–309.

60. Alpert M, Diamond F, Kesselman M. Correlation between extrapyramidal and therapeutic effects of neuroleptics. Compar Psychiatry 1977; 18: 333–336.

61. Simpson G, Kunz-Bartholini E. Relationship of individual tolerance and behavior in phenothiazine produced extrapyramidal system disturbance. Disord Nerv Syst 1968; 29: 269–274.

62. Baldessarini R, Tarazi F. Drugs and the treatment of psychiatric disorders: psychosis and mania. In Hardman J, Limbird L (eds) Goodman and Gilman's The Pharmacologic Basis of Therapeutics. New York, McGraw Hill, 2002, pp. 485–520.

63. Friedman JH, Factor SA. Atypical antipsychotics in the treatment of drug-induced psychosis in Parkinson's disease. Mov Disord 2000; 15(2): 201–211.
64. Rosebush PI, Mazurek MF. Neurologic side effects in neuroleptic-naive patients treated with haloperidol or risperidone. Neurology 1999; 52: 782–785.
65. Ford B, Lynch T, Greene P. Risperidone in Parkinson's disease. Lancet 1994; 344: 681.
66. Rich SS, Friedman JH, Ott BR. Risperidone versus clozapine in the treatment of psychosis in six patients with Parkinson's disease and other akinetic-rigid syndromes. J Clin Psychiatry 1995; 56(12): 556–559.
67. Kane J, Honigfeld G, Singer J, Meltzer H. Clozapine for the treatment-resistant schizophrenic, a double-blind comparison with chlorpromazine. Arch Gen Psychiatry 1988; 45: 789–796.
68. Friedman J, Fernandez H. Atypical antipsychotics in Parkinson-sensitive populations. J Geriatr Psychiatry Neurol 2002; 15: 156–170.
69. Group TFCPS. Clozapine in drug-induced psychosis n Parkinson's disease. Lancet 1999; 353: 2041–2042.
70. Marder S, Meibach RC. Risperidone in the treatment of schizophrenia. Am J Psychiatry 1994; 151(6): 825–835.
71. Chouinard G. Effects of risperidone in tardive dyskinesia: an analysis of the Canadian multicenter risperidone study. J Clin Psychopharmacol 1995; 15(suppl 1): 36S-44S.
72. Peuskens J. Risperidone in the treatment of patients with chronic schizophrenia: a multinational, multi-centre, double-blind, parallel-group study versus haloperidol. Br J Psychiatry 1996; 166(6): 712–726.
73. Miller CH, Mohr F, Umbricht D, Woerner M, Fleischhacker WW, Lieberman J. The prevalence of acute extrapyramidal signs and symptoms in patients treated with clozapine, risperidone, and conventional antipsychotics. J Clin Psychiatry 1998; 59(2): 69–75.
74. Simpson G, Lindenmayer J-P. Extrapyramidal symptoms in patients treated with risperidone. J Clin Psychopharmacol 1996; 17: 194–201.
75. De Deyn PP, Rabheru K, Rasmussen A, et al. A randomized trial of risperidone, placebo, and haloperidol for behavioral symptoms of dementia. Neurology 1999; 53: 946–955.
76. Steinwachs A, Grohmann R, Pedrosa F, Ruther E, Schwerdtner I. Two cases of olanzapine-induced reversible neutropenia. Pharmocopsychiatry 1999; 32(4): 154–156.
77. Ellis T, Cudkowicz ME, Sexton PM, Growdon JH. Clozapine and risperidone treatment of psychosis in Parkinson's disease. J Neuropsychiatry Clin Neurosci 2000; 12(3): 364–369.
78. Meco G, Alessandri A, Giustini P, Bonifati V. Risperidone in levodopa induced psychosis in advanced Parkinson's disease: an open-label, long-term study. Mov Disord 1997; 12(4): 1241–1254.
79. Leopold N. Risperidone treatment of drug-related psychosis in patients with parkinsonism. Mov Disord 2000; 15(2): 301–304.
80. Mohr E, Mendis T, Hildebrand K, De Deyn PP. Risperidone in the treatment of dopamine-induced psychosis in Parkinson's disease: an open pilot trial. Mov Disord 2000; 15(6): 1230–1237
81. Factor SA, Molho ES, Friedman JH. Risperidone and Parkinson's disease [letter]. Mov Disord 2001; 17(1): 221–225.
82. Beasley CM, Sanger T, Satterlee W, et al. Olanzapine versus placebo: results of a double-blind, fixed-dose olanzapine trial. Psychopharmacology 1996; 124: 159–167.
83. Beasley CM, Tollefson G, Tran P, et al. Olanzapine versus placebo and haloperidol: acute phase results of the North American double-blind olanzapine trial. Neuropsychopharmacology 1996; 14(2): 111–123.

84. Beasley CM, Hamilton S, Crawford AM, Dellva MA, Tollefson G, Tran P, et al. Olanzapine versus haloperidol: acute phase results of the international double-blind olanzapine trial. Eur Neuropsychopharmacol 1997; 7: 125–137.

85. Tollefson G, Beasley CM, Tran P, et al. Olanzapine versus haloperidol in the treatment of schizophrenia and schizophreniform disorders: results of an international collaborative trial. Am J Psychiatry 1997; 154(4): 457–465.

86. Tollefson G, Kuntz AJ. Review of recent clinical studies with olanzapine. Br J Psychiatry 1999; 174(suppl 37): 30–35.

87. Tran P, Hamilton S, Kuntz AJ, et al. Double-blind comparison of olanzapine versus risperidone in the treatment of schizophrenia and other psychotic disorders. J Clin Psychopharmacol 1997; 17(5): 407–418.

88. Wolters EC, Jansen ENH, Tuynman-Qua HG, Bergmans PLM. Olanzapine in the treatment of dopaminomimetic psychosis in patients with Parkinson's disease. Neurology 1996; 47: 1085–1087.

89. Goetz CG, Blasucci LM, Leurgans S, Pappert EJ. Olanzapine and clozapine. Neurology 2000; 55: 789–794.

90. Friedman JH, Goldstein S, Jacques C. Substituting clozapine for olanzapine in psychiatrically stable Parkinson's disease patients: results of an open-label pilot trial. Clin Neuropharmocol 1998; 21: 285–288.

91. Friedman JH, Goldstein S. Olanzapine in the treatment of dopaminomimetic psychosis in patients with Parkinson's disease. Neurology 1998; 50: 1195–1196.

92. Wirshing D, Spellberg B, Erhart S, Marder S, Wirshing W. Novel antipsychotics and new onset diabetes. Biol Psychiatry 1998; 44(8): 778–783.

93. Molho ES, Factor SA. Worsening of motor features of parkinsonism with olanzapine. Mov Disord 1999; 14: 1014–1016.

94. Manson AJ, Schrag A, Lees AJ. Low-dose olanzapine for levodopa induced dyskinesias. Neurology 2000; 55: 795–799.

95. Caroff SN, Mann SC, Campbell EC, Sullivan K. Movement disorders associated with atypical antipsychotic drugs. J Clin Psychiatry 2002; 63(suppl 4): 12–19.

96. Breier A, Sutton V, Feldman P, et al. Olanzapine in the treatment of dopamimetic-induced psychosis in patients with Parkinson's disease. Biol Psychiatry 2002; 52(5): 438.

97. Ondo W, Levy J, Vuong K, Hunter C, Jankovic J. Olanzapine treatment for dopaminergic-induced hallucinations. Mov Disord 2002; 17(5): 1031–1035.

98. Small J, Hirsch S, Arvantis L, et al. Quetiapine in patients with schizophrenia: a high and low dose double blind comparison with placebo. Arch Gen Psychiatry 1997; 54: 549–557.

99. Arvantis L, Miller B, Group tSTS. Multiple fixed doses of "Seroquel" (quetiapine) in patients with acute exacerbations of schizophrenia: a comparison with haloperidol and placebo. Biol Psychiatry 1997; 42: 233–246.

100. Keck PJ, Buffenstien A, Ferguson J, et al. Ziprasidone 40 and 120 mg/day in the acute exacerbation of schizophrenia and schizoaffective disorder: a 4-week placebo-controlled trial. Psychopharmacology 1998; 140: 173–184.

101. Daniel DG, Zimbroff DL, Potkin S, et al. Ziprasidone 80 mg/day and 160 mg/day in the acute exacerbation of schizophrenia and schizoaffective disorder: a 6-week placebo-controlled trial. Neuropsychopharmacology 1999; 20(5): 491–505.

102. Keck PJ, Reeves K, Harrigan EP, Group tZS. Ziprasidone in the short-term treatment of patients with schizoaffective disorder: results from two double-blind, placebo-controlled, multicenter studies. J Clin Psychopharmacol 2001; 21(1): 27–35.

103. Tandon R, Harrigan E, Zorn S. Ziprasidone: A novel antipsychotic with unique pharmacology and therapeutic potential. J Serotonin Res 1997; 4: 159–177.

104. Hirsch SR, Kissling W, Bauml J, Power A, O'Connor R. A 28-week comparison of ziprasidone and haloperidol in outpatients with stable schizophrenia. J Clin Psychiatry 2002; 63(6): 516–523.

105. Weiden PJ, Iqbal N, Mendelowitz AJ, Tandon R, Zibroff DL, Ross R. Best clinical experience with ziprasidone: update after one year experience. J Psychiat Pract 2002; 8(2): 81–97.

106. Davis R, Markham A. Ziprasidone. CNS Drugs 1997; 8(2): 153–162.

107. Shopsin B, Gershon S. Cogwheel rigidity related to lithium maintenance. Am J Psychiatry 1975; 132: 536–538.

108. Ghadirian A, Annable L, Belanger M, Chouinard G. A cross-sectional study of parkinsonism and tardive dyskinesia in lithium-treated affective disordered patients. J Clin Psychiatry 1996; 57(1): 22–28.

109. Armon C, Shin C, Miller P, et al. Reversible parkinsonism and cognitive impairment with chronic valproate use. Neurology 1996; 47: 626–635.

110. Power C, Blume W, Young G. Reversible parkinsonism associated with valproate therapy [abstract]. Neurology 1990; 40(suppl 1): 139.

111. Iijima M. Valproate-induced parkinsonism in a demented elderly patient. J Clin Psychiatry 2002; 63(1): 75

112. Yatham L, Liddle P, Lam R, et al. PET study of the effects of valproate on dopamine D2 receptors in neuroleptic- and mood-stabilizer-naive patients with nonpsychotic mania. Am J Psychiatry 2002; 159: 1718–1723.

113. Negrotti A, Calzetti S. A long-term follow-up study of cinnarizine- and flunarizine-induced parkinsonism. Mov Disord 1997; 12(1): 107–110.

114. Leo R. Movement disorders associated with the serotonin selective reuptake inhibitors. J Clin Psychiatry 1996; 57: 449–454.

115. Schechter D, Nunes E. Reversible parkinsonism in a 90-year-old man taking sertraline. J Clin Psychiatry 1997; 58(6): 275.

116. Gerber P, Lynd L. Selective serotonin-reuptake inhibitor-induced movement disorders. Ann Pharmacother 1998; 32(6): 692–698.

117. Jimenez-Jimenez F, Tejeiro J, Martinez-Junquera G, et al. Parkinsonism exacerbated by paroxetine [Letter]. Neurology 1994; 44: 2406.

118. Jansen ENH. Increase of parkinsonism disability after fluoxetine medication. Neurology 1993; 43: 211–213.

119. Gonul A, Aksu M. SSRI-induced parkinsonism may be an early sign of future Parkinson's disease. J Clin Psychiatry 1999; 60(6): 410.

120. Pina Latorre M, Modrego P, Rodilla F, Catalan C, Calvo M. Parkinsonism and Parkinson's disease associated with long-term administration of sertraline. J Clin Pharmacol Ther 2001; 26(2): 111–112.

121. Dell'Agnello G, Ceravolo R, Nuti A, et al. SSRIs do not worsen Parkinson's disease: evidence from an open-label, prospective study. Clin Neuropharmacol 2001; 24(4): 221–227.

122. Ceravolo R, Nuti A, Piccinni A, et al. Paroxetine in Parkinson's disease: effects on motor and depressive symptoms. Neurology 2000; 55(8): 1216–1218.

123. Tesei S, Antonini A, Canesi M, Zecchinelli A, Mariani C, Pezzoli G. Tolerability of paroxetine in Parkinson's disease: a prospective study. Mov Disord 2000; 15(5): 986–989.

124. Richard IH, Maughn A, Kurlan R. Do serotonin reuptake inhibitor antidepressants worsen parkinson's disease? A retrospective case series. Mov Disord 1999; 14(1): 155.

125. Yamato H, Kannari K, Shen H, Suda T, Matsunaga M. Fluoxetine reduces L-DOPA-derived extracellular DA in the 6-OHDA-lesioned rat striatum. Neuroreport 2001; 12(6): 1123–1126.

126. Leo R, Lichter D, Hershey L. Parkinsonism associated with fluoxetine and cimetidine: a case report. J Geriatr Psychiatry Neurol 1995; 8: 231–233.
127. Reches A, Burke R, Kuker C, et al. Tetrabenazine, an amine-depleting drug, also blocks dopamine receptors. J Pharmacol Exp Ther 1983; 225: 515–521.
128. Snyder S, Banerjee S, Yamaura H, Greenberg D. Drugs, neurotransmitters and schizophrenia. Science 1974; 184: 1243–1253.
129. Mash D. Dopamine receptor diversity. In Factor SA, Weiner WJ (eds) Parkinson's Disease: Diagnosis and Clinical Management. New York, Demos Medical Publishing, 2002, pp. 233–241.
130. Kapur S, Seeman P. Does fast dissociation from the dopamine D2 receptor explain the action of atypical antipsychotics?: a new hypothesis. Am J Psychiatry 2001; 158(3): 360–369.
131. Meltzer H, Matsubara S, Lee J. The ratios of serotonin-2 and dopamine-2 affinities differentiate atypical and typical antipsychotic drugs. Psychopharmacol Bull 1989; 25: 390–392.
132. Ichikawa J, Ishii H, Bonaccorso S, Fowler W, O'Laughlin I, Meltzer H. 5-HT(2A) and D(2) receptor blockade increases cortical DA release via 5-HT(1A) receptor activation: a possible mechanism of atypical antipsychotic-induced cortical dopamine release. J Neurochem 2001; 76: 1521–1531.
133. Meltzer H. Action of atypical antipsychotics [Letter]. Am J Psychiatry 2002; 159(1): 153–154.
134. Rabey J, Burns R. Neurochemistry. In Factor SA, Weiner WJ (eds) Parkinson's Disease: Diagnosis and Clinical Management. New York, Demos Medical Publishing, 2002, pp. 195–209.
135. Fjalland B, Christensen A, Hyttel J. Peripheral and central muscarinic receptor affinity and psychotropic drugs. Naunyn-Schmiedebergs' Arch Pharmacol 1977; 301: 5–12.
136. Richelson E. Neuroleptic affinities for human brain receptors and their use in predicting adverse effects. J Clin Psychiatry 1984; 45: 331–336.
137. Friedman JH. Atypical antipsychotics: mechanism of action. Can J Psychiatry 2003; 48: 62.
138. Mindham R. Assessment of drug-induced extrapyramidal reactions and of drugs given for their control. Br J Clin Pharmacol 1976; 3(suppl): 395–400.
139. Parkinson Study Group. DATATOP: A multicenter controlled clinical trial in early Parkinson's disease. Arch Neurol 1989; 46: 1052–1060.
140. Simpson G, Amuso D, Blair J, Farhas T. Phenothiazine produces extrapyramidal disturbance. Arch Gen Psychiatry 1964; 10: 127–136.
141. DiMascio A, Bernardo D, Greenblatt D, Marder J. A controlled trial of amantadine in drug-induced extrapyramidal disorders. Arch Gen Psychiatry 1976; 33: 599–602.
142. Mindham R, Gaind R, Anstee B, Rimmer L. Comparison of amantadine, orphenadrine and placebo in drug-induced parkinsonism. Psychol Med 1972; 2: 406–443.
143. Simpson G. Controlled studies of antiparkinsonism agents in the treatment of extrapyramidal syndromes. Acta Psychiat Scand 1970; 212: 44–51.
144. Kelly J, Zimmerman R, Abuzzahab F, Schieve B. A double blind study of amantadine HCl versus benztropine mesylate in drug-induced parkinsonism. Pharmacology 1974; 12: 65–73.
145. Adler C. Amantadine and Anticholinergics. In Factor SA, Weiner WJ (eds) Parkinson's Disease: Diagnosis and Clinical Management. New York, Demos Medical Publishing, 2002, pp. 357–364.
146. Greenblatt D, DiMascio A, Harmatz J, et al. Pharamacokinetics and clinical effects of amantadine in drug-induced extrapyramidal syndromes. J Clin Pharmacology 1977; 17: 704–708.

147. Stenson R, Donlon P, Mayer J. Comparison of benztropine and amantadine in neuroleptic-induced extrapyramidal syndromes. Compar Psychiatry 1976; 17: 762–768.
148. Pacific G, Nardini M, Ferrani P, et al. Effect of amantadine on drug-induced parkinsonism: relationship between plasma levels and effect. Br J Clin Pharmacol 1976; 3: 883–889.
149. Carlson A. The occurrence, distribution, and physiologic role of catecholamines in the nervous system. Pharmacol Res 1959; 11: 490–493.
150. Bruno A, Bruno S. Effects of levodopa on pharmacological parkinsonism. Acta Psychiat Scand 1966; 42: 264–271.
151. Angrist B, Sathanathan G, Gershon S. Behavioral effects of levodopa in schizophrenic patients. Psychopharmacologica (Berl) 1973; 31: 1–12.
152. Yaryura-Tobias, Wolpert A, Dana L, Malis S. Action of L-dopa on drug-induced extrapyramidal syndromes. Disord Nerv Syst 1973; 31: 60–63.
153. Inanga K, Inouye K, Tachibana H, et al. Effect of levodopa in schizophrenia. Folia Psychiatr Neurol Jpn 1972; 26: 145–157.
154. Balldin J, Eden S, Granerus A. Electroconvulsive therapy in Parkinson's syndrome with "on-off" phenomenon. J Neur Transm 1980; 47: 11–21.
155. Andersen K, Balldin J, Gottfries C. Double Blind evaluation of electroconvulsive therapy in Parkinson's disease with "on-off" phenomena. Acta Neurol Scand 1987; 76: 191–199.
156. Moellentine C, T R, Ahlskog J, Harmsen W, et al. Effectiveness of ECT in patients with parkinsonism. J Neuropsychiatry Clin Neurosci1998; 10(2): 187–193.
157. Fall P, Granerus A. Maintenance ECT in Parkinson's disease. J Neur Transm 1999; 106 (7–8): 737–741.
158. Wengel S, Burke W, Pfeiffer R, Roccaforte W, Paige S. Maintenance electroconvulsive therapy for intractable Parkinson's disease. Am J Geriatr Psychiatry 1998; 6(3): 263–269.
159. Goswami U, Dutta S, Jurivilla K. Electroconvulsive therapy in neuroleptic-induced parkinsonism. Biol Psychiatry 1989; 26: 234–238.
160. Mukherjee S, Debsikdar V. Absence of neuroleptic-induced parkinsonism in psychotic patients receiving adjunctive electroconvulsive therapy. Convul Ther 1994; 10(1): 53–58.
161. Hanin B, Lerner Y, Srour N. An unusual effect of ECT on drug-induced parkinsonism and tardive dystonia. Convul Ther 1995; 11(4): 271–274.
162. Metzer W, Paige S, Newton J. Inefficacy of propranolol in attenuation of drug-induced parkinsonian tremor. Mov Disord 1993; 8(1): 43–36.
163. Spivak B, Mester R, Abesgaus J, et al. Clozapine treatment for neuroleptic-induced tardive dyskinesia, parkinsonism, and chronic akathisia in schizophrenic patients. J Clin Psychiatry 1997; 58: 318–322.
164. Levine J, Chengappa K. Second thoughts about clozapine as a treatment for neuroleptic-induced akathisia [Letter]. J Clin Psychiatry 1998; 59(4): 195.
165. Fann W, Lake C. On the coexistence of parkinsonism and tardive dyskinesia. Dis Nerv Syst 1974; 35: 324–326.
166. DeFraites E, Davis K, Berger P. Coexisting tardive dykinesia and parkinsonism: a cast report. Biol Psychiatry 1977; 12: 267–272.
167. Fahn S, Mayeux R. Unilateral parkinson's disease and contralateral tardive dyskinesia: a unique case with successful therapy that may explain the pathophysiology of these two disorders. J Neur Transm 1980; 16: 179–185.
168. Jankovic J, Casabona J. Dyskinesia and parkinsonism. Clin Neuropharmacol 1987; 10: 511–521.
169. Honlon T, Shoenrich C, Freinek W. Perphenazine-benztropine mesylate treatment of newly admitted psychiatric patients. Psychopharmacologica (Berl) 1966; 9: 328–329.

170. Chien C, DiMascio A, Cole J. Antiparkinson agents and depot phenothiazine. Am J Psychiatry 1974; 131: 86–90.

171. McGeer P, Bouling J, Gibson W, Foulkes R. Drug-induced extrapyramidal treatment with dyphenhydramine hydrochloride and dihydroxyphenylalanine reactions. JAMA 1961; 177: 166–170.

172. Stratos N, Phillips R, Walker P, Sandifer M. A study of drug-induced parkinsonism. Dis Nerv Syst 1963; 24: 180–181.

173. Cahan R, Parrish D. Reversibility of drug-induced parkinsonism. Am J Psychiatry 1960; 116: 1022–1023.

174. Manos N, Ghiouzepas J, Logothetis J. The need for continuous anti-parkinsonian medication with chronic schizophrenic patients receiving long-term neuroleptic therapy. Am J Psychiatry 1981; 138: 184–188.

175. Grove L, Cramer J. Benzhexol and side effects with long lasting fluphenazine therapy. Br Med J 1972; 1: 276–279.

176. Mandel W, Claffe B, Margolis L. Recurrent thioperazine induced extrapyramidal reaction following placebo substitutions for maintenance antiparkinsonian drugs. Am J Psychiatry 1962; 118: 351–352.

177. St. Jean A, Donald M, Ban T. Interchangeability of antiparkinsonian medication. Am J Psychiatry 1964; 120: 1189–1190.

CHAPTER 7

Acute drug-induced akathisia

Lenard A. Adler, John Rotrosen, and Burt Angrist

Introduction

Akathisia literally means "inability to remain seated." Patients with acute drug-induced akathisia (DIA) have complaints of restlessness, most often referable to the legs, and usually show movements such as constant motion of the legs when seated, inability to remain seated, and rocking from foot to foot or marching in place when standing. This discussion will focus on acute akathisia, the most typical form encountered. Other akathisia variants, such as chronic akathisia and pseudoakathisia, are covered more extensively in Chapter 10. This chapter will review (1) the history of spontaneously occurring syndromes of restlessness and acute DIA, (2) the clinical significance of acute DIA (3) differential diagnosis of DIA, (4) epidemiology of DIA, (5) quantification of DIA, (6) the possible role of iron in DIA, (7) animal models, (8) treatment of DIA, and (9) comments on pathophysiology.

History

Syndromes of spontaneously occurring restlessness were identified long before the introduction of neuroleptic medications. The earliest descriptions were in the 1600s [1], with reports in the 1800s attributing the restlessness to neurasthenia or hysteria [2].

The term akathisia, from Greek derivation (*kathisia* – "the act of sitting" and a – "negative prefix"), was first used by Haskovec in 1902 [3], who also felt that the syndrome derived from psychological causes. Two reports in 1923 were the first to attribute akathisia to extrapyramidal disease. Bing [4] noted the condition in patients with encephalitis lethargica (Von Economo's disease) and recognized that Haskovec's "akathisia" was a symptom of extrapyramidal dysfunction; moreover, he speculated that Haskovec's patients may also have been victims of a prior encephalitis epidemic known as the "Nona" [5]. Sicard also described akathisia in patients with idiopathic and postencephalitic Parkinson's disease [6].

Ekbom described an idiopathic disorder, restless leg syndrome (RLS), which was similar to akathisia with subjective complaints of restlessness in the legs and associated movements [7, 8]. He stressed the disturbing nature of the symptoms with vivid descriptions given by patients, such as "it is something crawling, irritating, unpleasant, deep in the tissues," or "it feels as if ants were running up and down in my bones." RLS, although qualitatively quite similar to akathisia, differs in that patients with RLS have symptoms predominantly in the evening and when at rest [9, 10].

The first report of drug-induced akathisia was by Sigwald in 1947, who reported this syndrome prior to the introduction of neuroleptics in patients treated with promethazine [11]. With the introduction of neuroleptics, there was an increasing number of reports of syndromes of restlessness associated with these agents, which the investigators also termed akathisia [12, 13]. More recently (see below) akathisia has been reported after the administration of both serotonin reuptake-inhibiting antidepressants and atypical antipsychotics. For those interested, a more detailed history of akathisia was published in 1995 [14].

Clinic significance of acute neuroleptic-induced akathisia (NIA)

Signs and symptoms

The akathisia syndrome is composed of both subjective complaints of restlessness and objective movements. Subjective complaints include a sense of inner restlessness, most often referable to the legs, a compulsion to move one's legs, dysphoria, and anxiety [9, 15, 16].

The diagnosis of akathisia may be difficult in patients with the mild form of the syndrome, who exhibit only subjective complaints, without showing movements [15, 17, 18]. Objectively observable movements almost always accompany subjective restlessness in moderate and severe cases. These movements include rocking from foot to foot, "walking on the spot," swinging of the legs, leg shuffling, pacing, or in its most severe form, tasikinesia, an inability to maintain any position [9, 15, 18–20]. The restlessness and accompanying movements are typically bilateral and relatively symmetrical although recently, cases of unilateral akathisia have also been reported [21].

The subjective distress of akathisia is significant in that it can lead to decreased compliance with treatment or a worsening of psychosis. Van Putten [22], in a study of 85 patients on neuroleptics, found that akathisia was significantly more prevalent in patients who refused medication versus those who were compliant with neuroleptics.

The powerful effect akathisia can have in exacerbating psychopathology deserves particular emphasis. Van Putten et al. [23] coined the term *phenothiazine-induced decompensation* to refer to an increase in psychosis associated with akathisia. They found that such decompensations were similar to the original psychosis and that "thought processes became disorganized, secondary symptoms recurred, quality of contact deteriorated, and many complained of an abject fear or terror that was difficult to articulate" [23]. Conversely, when these patients were treated acutely with I.M. biperiden a 35% decrement in psychopathology scores was seen within 2 hours [23]. A similar study by our group showed a greater than 20% decrease in psychopathology 2 hours after treatment with either I.M. benztropine or oral propranolol [24]. In these two studies, the magnitude of symptom improvement that occurred within 2 hours after treatment of akathisia was in the range frequently seen in patients over the course of an entire hospitalization. Finally, the syndrome can be so distressing that it has been associated with aggressive behavior and violence [25–27] or suicide attempts [27–31].

Differential diagnosis

As mentioned above, akathisia was originally felt to be secondary to psychological causes. A variety of psychological diagnoses should still be considered in the differential diagnosis of NIA. Restless leg syndrome and other movement disorders (such as chronic akathisia, pseudoakathisia, and tardive dyskinesia) can also be difficult to distinguish from acute DIA.

Agitation seen with other psychiatric disorders

Agitation associated with major depression, mania, or psychosis may result in significant restlessness or agitated pacing similar to that seen with akathisia. If these patients are receiving neuroleptics, it may not be possible to distinguish these symptoms from akathisia. A pattern of worsening of agitation with increasing neuroleptics may particularly alert the clinician to Van Putten's "phenothiazine-induced decompensation" [23]. In such cases, treatment of suspected akathisia is warranted.

Patients with generalized anxiety disorder may be restless and can pace. Akathisia may be differentiated from generalized anxiety in that in akathisia there is a compulsion to move and the feelings are often described as "driven" or "unnatural" [16, 32]; however, not all patients can articulate such "fine" distinctions. Treatment response may again help differentiate these conditions. Adler et al. [33]. found that in patients with akathisia the benzodiazepine lorazepam improved subjective complaints of restlessness, but not objective movements, while both elements of the syndrome were improved by propranolol. Conversely, one study found that propranolol improved both the subjective restlessness and objective movements of akathisia without significantly affecting Hamilton Anxiety Scale ratings [34].

Drug withdrawal states

Restlessness, painful sensations in the legs, and leg movements are common symptoms of opiate withdrawal which, in fact, led to the expression "kicking the habit" [35]. Similarities between opiate withdrawal and akathisia also extend to agents used to treat these conditions. The α_2 agonist, clonidine, has been found to improve both opiate withdrawal [36] and akathisia [37, 38]. Additionally, low doses of the β-blocker, propranolol, have been reported to improve the restlessness of both conditions [33, 34, 39–43].

Other movement disorders
Restless leg syndrome (RLS)
As mentioned above, patients with RLS complain of uncomfortable sensory phenomena in the legs more consistently than patients with DIA. Myoclonic jerks (a.k.a. "dyskinesia while awake") are also more frequent in RLS. In this disorder, symptoms are more prominent in the evening or at night when attempting to fall asleep and usually lead to insomnia. On the other hand, akathisia does not occur more frequently at any particular time of day. It is not necessarily worsened by lying down and, indeed, many DIA patients find this to be their most comfortable position [44].

Chronic akathisia (see Chapter 10)
Chronic akathisia (or tardive akathisia) occurs late in the course of treatment; this differs from acute akathisia, which is an early side effect. Both forms of the syndrome have subjective complaints of restlessness along with objectively observable movements. Barnes and Braude [45] defined chronic akathisia as occurring more than 6 months after initiation of, or increase in the dose of, neuroleptics.

Chronic akathisia may be more difficult to treat than acute akathisia [46]. The chronic form may also behave like tardive dyskinesia. Jeste and Wyatt [47] noted that in some patients chronic akathisia "has pharmacological characteristics similar to those of other manifestations of tardive dyskinesia." Braude and Barnes [48] reported two patients with chronic akathisia. The akathisia was more pharmacologically similar to tardive dyskinesia than acute akathisia, in that it (1) improved by increasing the dose of neuroleptic, (2) worsened by reduction of the available dose of neuroleptic, and (3) was unresponsive to anticholinergics.

Pseudoakathisia and tardive dyskinesia
Patients with pseudoakathisia have movements seen in akathisia, without subjective complaints of restlessness. The importance of establishing a differential between acute akathisia and pseudoakathisia is that it has been hypothesized that acute akathisia, chronic akathisia, pseudoakathisia, and tardive dyskinesia may be points in a continuum [48–52]. This supposition is based upon several studies finding a relationship between pseudoakathisia and dyskinetic movements. Munetz and Cornes [50] studied 45 patients with tardive dyskinesia; they found that 21 patients had acute akathisia at some prior time and that 11 of these 21 patients had pseudoakathisia at the time of the examination. Barnes and Braude [45] studied 39 patients receiving depot neuroleptics who also had akathisia. They divided the patients according to whether they had acute akathisia, chronic akathisia, or pseudoakathisia. None of the patients with acute akathisia had tardive dyskinesia, while over one-half of the patients with chronic akathisia or pseudoakathisia also had dyskinesias.

Munetz [52] suggested "in distinguishing akathisia from tardive dyskinesia, one tries to determine whether the patient is restless and is therefore moving (akathisia) or moving and therefore restless (tardive dyskinesia)." However, in practice, the differentiation of acute akathisia from some of the movements seen in patients with tardive dyskinesia and the akathisia variants is often difficult, if not at times impossible, especially when the conditions coexist.

Epidemiology of acute DIA

General consideration

Akathisia can develop very rapidly after initiating neuroleptics or increasing their dose and this is true for other dopamine antagonists not primarily used as antipsychotics, SSRIs, or atypical antipsychotics. Barnes et al. [53] have reported akathisia developing within an hour of receiving preoperative medication with droperidol and metoclopramide. The development of akathisia also appears to be dose dependent. Ayd [54] surveyed 3775 patients receiving neuroleptics and found that patients started on higher doses of neuroleptics were more likely to develop akathisia than patients started on lower doses. Braude et al. [19] prospectively studied the development of akathisia in 109 inpatients followed over 23 days and also found a relationship to dosage. Frequently, it can take several weeks for akathisia to develop [15]. Acute akathisia tends to persist, although it fluctuates in intensity, over time [9]. Although extremely infrequent, akathisia has been reported to persist after discontinuation of neuroleptics [55, 56].

Prevalence of acute akathisia after neuroleptics, atypical antipsychotics, and serotonin reuptake inhibitors
Neuroleptics

The reported prevalence of akathisia in patients receiving neuroleptics varies widely. Lower estimates of prevalence, ranging from 3% to 13% [57–59], were found in earlier studies [15]. More recent investigations have found higher prevalences. Gibb and Lees [15] and Van Putten [16] found figures in the 40% to 45% range. More recently, Van Putten et al. [60] studied 32 schizophrenics, who were off neuroleptics and then treated with haloperidol 10 mg per day for 7 days and found a 75% incidence of akathisia. The most common estimate of prevalence is 20% [17, 19, 54]. Several factors may account for this wide variability in prevalence [42]. These include (1) a lack of recognition of akathisia [61], (2) the fact that some investigators exclude patients with only subjective complaints of restlessness, without objective motor movements (as may exist in mild forms of akathisia), and (3) the degree to which high- versus low-potency neuroleptics are used. Although all neuroleptics can cause akathisia, the syndrome occurs more frequently with higher-potency agents [54, 62]. This may, in part, be due to use of nonequivalent doses. Haloperidol, for example was, in the past, frequently raised in 10 mg per day increments. Chlorpromazine, in contrast, is almost never increased at the therapeutically equivalent rate of 500 mg per day because of concerns about causing orthostasis. Thus, the antiadrenergic effects of low-potency agents may, in fact, have forced clinicians to "titrate" these drugs more slowly.

Atypical antipsychotics
With the advent of atypical agents the prevalence of akathisia has clearly diminished, but the symptom has certainly not disappeared. The extrapyramidal symptoms (EPS) caused by risperidone are clearly dose related. In two studies of risperidone for schizophrenia that used doses that are somewhat high by current standards, akathisia was noted in 32% and 24% of patients [63, 64]. On the other hand, two larger studies that explored dose ranges of 2–16 mg per day found that akathisia rates did not differ from those seen after placebo [65, 66]. A study in patients receiving risperidone for at least 3 months (thus avoiding carry-over effects of prior treatment) in which the mean dose used was 4.7 ± 2.1 mg per day found a prevalence of akathisia of 13% [67]. For olanzapine two larger pivotal studies [68, 69] noted low, dose-related rates of akathisia ranging from 0% to 7.2% compared to 15.9% and 14.8%, respectively, in patients randomized to haloperidol. A study in first-episode schizophrenic patients found akathisia in just over 11% of olanzapine-treated patients versus 38% of patients who received haloperidol [70].

A pivotal study [71] of quetiapine found a low prevalence of akathisia of 0–2% across a dose range of 75–750 mg per day versus 8% and 15% for patients randomized to placebo and haloperidol, respectively. A low liability for inducing akathisia for quetiapine is further suggested by a 3.3% prevalence even in patients over 65 years old [72]. In most studies clozapine has been associated with low prevalence rates of akathisia ranging from 5.6% to 7.7% [73–76]. One study, however, noted akathisia in 39% of patients who had taken clozapine for over a month [77].

Serotonin reuptake inhibitors
Fluoxetine was marketed in 1988; however, prior to that, compassionate premarketing use of the drug was permitted at McLean Hospital. In the course of this use Lipinski et al. described five patients who developed akathisia indistinguishable from neuroleptic-induced akathisia [78]. Based on the number of patients who received the drug, the incidence of fluoxetine-induced akathisia was estimated to be between 9.8% and 25%. Reports of akathisia due to sertraline [79–82] and paroxetine [83] were published between 1993 and 1995. The incidence could not be calculated from these reports, since the number of patients who had received these agents was unknown. In 1996, however, Baldasano et al. [84] reported three more cases of paroxetine-induced akathisia among 67 patients treated with the drug, an incidence of 4%. A single case of akathisia induced by nefazodone has also been noted [85]. Thus it is clear that SSRI-induced akathisia occurs, but probably much less frequently than is seen with classical neuroleptics.

In 1990, Teicher et al. described six patients who developed suicidal preoccupation during fluoxetine treatment [86]. Others also noted suicidality in the context of fluoxetine-induced akathisia [87, 88] and a review of this subject appeared in 1992 [89]. This led to an intense controversy. Ayd [90] noted that

> if there is an association between akathisia and suicide, suicidal attempts, and suicidal or homicidal ideation, it must be exceedingly rare. The estimated incidence of akathisia ranges from 20% to 45%, which translates into an estimated 160 to 360 million people who have had akathisia since 1952. Yet, of these only two are suspected to have committed suicide because of akathisia, only two are thought to have made suicidal attempts because of akathisia, and only one may have had akathisia-induced suicidal or homicidal ideation.
>
> In view of the high annual incidence of suicide, suicidal attempts, and suicidal or homicidal ideation, it is far more likely that the five reported cases are a coincidence and not causally linked to akathisia.

In July 1991, in the context of this controversy the American College of Neuropsychopharmacology established a Task Force to study possible relationships between suicidal behavior and psychotropic medications. Fluoxetine was found to decrease the rate of attempted suicide below that which would statistically be expected. Premarketing studies of fluoxetine, sertraline, and paroxetine, in which the index drug was compared to both placebo and an established antidepressant, all showed rates of suicidal ideation or behavior that were equal to or less than that seen with placebo treatment [91].

In Lipinski's initial report [78] the substrate mechanism of SSRI-induced akathisia was, based on clinical and preclinical studies [92, 93], proposed to increase serotonergic inhibition of dopaminergic functioning. This concept has since been confirmed in studies in which endogenous dopamine release was directly quantified with both PET imaging and microdialysis; basal dopamine release was shown to be diminished by citolopram and increased by 5-HT$_2$ receptor antagonists [94].

Quantification of DIA

Rating scales

At least 11 scales have been designed to evaluate akathisia. Lipinski et al. [40, 41] have used the akathisia item from the Chouinard Extrapyramidal Symptom Rating Scale (ESRS) [95]. Subjective complaints are rated 0 to 3 ("none" to "severe"). Objective movements are rated 0 to 6 (O = "none"; 1 = "looks restless, nervous, impatient, uncomfortable"; 2 = "needs to move at least one extremity"; 3 = "often needs to move one extremity or to change position"; 4 = "moves one extremity almost constantly if sitting or stamps feet while standing"; 5 = "unable to sit down for more than a short period of time"; 6 = "moves or walks constantly").

Bartels et al. [96] used a 3-point scale based on subjective and objective measures. Kabes et al. [97] used a global score of "0" (none) to "3" (unable to sit) for a study of piracetam in NIA. Friis et al. [98] devised a 4-point scale of subjective and objective measures to assess effects of biperiden and sodium valproate in neuroleptic-induced EPS.

Adler et al. [33, 34, 42] have measured objective movements with the akathisia item from the Hillside/Long Island Jewish modification of the Simpson-Angus Extrapyramidal Symptom (EPS) Scale. Movements of akathisia are rated 0 to 4 (0 = absent; 1 = mild; occasional restlessness observed during exam; 2 = moderate; continuous restlessness observed; 3 = marked; subject in and out of chair during exam; unable to maintain concentration; and 4 = extreme; heightened activity; panic). Subjective complaints of restlessness were assessed by having the patient mark a 100-mm line with anchor points, relating to the frequency of restlessness and degree of distress (0 = none; 20 = sometimes, a little; 40 = most of the time, a little; 60 = all of the time, sometimes annoying; 80 = all of the time, always very annoying; and 100 = can't stand it anymore).

Braude et al. [19] developed a 23-item rating scale. Subjective complaints were assessed by four items (limb sensations, inner restlessness, inability to remain still, and inability to keep legs still). Objective movements were rated 0 (absent) to 3 (continuous movement) with the patient in three positions (seated, standing, and lying). These authors found that this scale was able to distinguish akathisia from "illness-related movements" (secondary to psychopathology).

These authors have subsequently condensed the critical items from this 23-item scale into a 4-item scale now generally known as the Barnes akathisia scale [20]. Patients are observed for at least 2 minutes in three situations: when they do not know they are being observed and during formal interview, both seated and standing. Objective movements are rated 0 to 3 based upon their frequency (e.g., more or less than one-half the time) and severity. Subjective complaints are divided into awareness and distress subsets, each rated 0 to 3. A global assessment of akathisia is scored 0 ("absent") to 5 ("severe"); the global rating includes assessments of the awareness of, and distress from, subjective complaints and the severity and frequency of objective movements. High interater reliability has been demonstrated for this instrument. Moreover, it is fairly easy to administer. These features have made this the most frequently used instrument for rating akathisia at this time.

The Hillside akathisia scale [99] by Fleischhacker and colleagues rates patients while sitting, standing, and lying down. Subjective complaints are divided into two subsets, the sensation of inner restlessness and the urge to move, each rated 0 ("absent") to 4 ("present and not controllable"). Objective movements are assessed separately in the head and trunk, hands and arms, and feet and legs; they are rated 0 to 4 (0 = "no akathisia"; 1 = "questionable"; 2 = "small amplitude movements, part of the time"; 3 = "small amplitude movements, all of the time or large amplitude movements, part of the time"; 4 = "large amplitude movements, all of the time"). There is also a clinical global impression item, which asks the rater to score the severity of akathisia, based on their experience with patients with akathisia, on a 1 ("normal, not at all akathisic") to 7 ("among the most akathisic of patients") scale.

The Hillside scale's inclusion of ratings of movements in the head/trunk and hands/arms, in addition to those in the lower extremity, constitutes a double-edged sword. Two systematic studies of patients with akathisia have found that movements of the lower extremities (e.g., rocking from foot to foot, pacing, leg waggling, etc.) are more specific for the akathisia syndrome and help differentiate it from other syndromes [15, 19]. Although akathisia may cause movements of other body areas, by including ratings of movements in the head/trunk and upper extremity, the Hillside scale might be more sensitive (by missing fewer cases since it includes movements of these other areas), but less specific than the other scales. Nonetheless, it is one of only three instruments (the other two being the Barnes and the Prince Henry Hospital Scales) for which reliability has been demonstrated.

The Yale Extrapyramidal Symptom Scale [100] was designed to measure parkinsonism and dystonia as well as akathisia. For the latter objective and subjective symptoms are graded from 0 to 5 based on descriptive clinical anchor points. A final instrument, the Prince Henry Hospital Akathisia Rating Scale was developed in 1994. Its development, biometrics, and reliability were reported in detail [101]. It appears to be "user friendly" to administer and may ultimately rival the Barnes scale [20].

Objective measures of akathisia

Objective measures of akathisia via electromechanical devices or the electromyogram (EMG) have been explored since the 1980s. Our group made an early, somewhat crude attempt in this area via the use of a commercially available running shoe with a built-in sensor that measured the number of impacts per unit of time [102]. About half the patients in the study of a β-2 selective antagonist had decreases in the number of impacts that paralleled decreases in akathisia ratings. Ratings did not correlate for those patients who did not actually pace. Therefore, activity monitors are more useful for the study of akathisia than the running shoe, as the latter will only measure restlessness in those patients who pace (and not in those who move their legs continually when seated or rock from foot to foot while standing).

More sophisticated measures include accellerometric devices or direct EMG measures. The first such study by Braude et al. [103] identified large, low-frequency, rhythmic foot movements in patients with akathisia. Similar findings have been reported by two subsequent groups [104, 105]. Moreover, a similar pattern has been noted in four reports using more invasive EMG methods [106–109]. In the last of these reports the presence of akathisia was determined by two clinicians via Barnes Akathisia Scale ratings in 25 patients. The presence of the EMG marker in patients with and without akathisia permitted calculation of the sensitivity and specificity of the EMG pattern as an objective marker for akathisia. Sensitivity was found to be 69% and specificity 70% [109].

The identification of an objective "signature" of akathisia could be valuable in a number of clinical situations. Is anxious dysphoria after starting a neuroleptic an early sign of akathisia? In patients with agitation or known tardive dyskinesia is a component of the activation due to akathisia and should a trial of treatments be undertaken? Finally, since as noted above, akathisia has such a powerful effect on increasing psychopathology, is a patient who shows any restlessness truly at his "baseline"? If akathisia is present we suspect that this is unlikely.

The possible role of iron

An association between Restless Leg Syndrome and low serum iron was noted by Ekbom as early as 1960 [8]. This raised the question of whether this might also be the case in NIA [110, 111]. The first study of iron status in patients with NIA reported decreased iron and percentage saturation and increased iron-binding capacity in patients with akathisia versus a matched group of patients who took neuroleptics without developing NIA. Serum iron levels also correlated inversely with severity of akathisia in the akathisic group [112]. Two subsequent studies [113, 114] showed lower serum iron levels in patients with akathisia than those without the disorder while a third [115] showed no difference in iron levels but lower levels of ferritin in patients with akathisia. Yet another study showed a highly significant negative correlation between transferrin levels and akathisia scores after 2–3 weeks of neuroleptic treatment [116].

However, four studies have found no differences in iron-related indices between patients with and without akathisia [117–120]. Thus the role of iron deficiency as a contributing factor to NIA remains unresolved and controversial.

Finally, after improvement in akathisia was noted during a course of treatment of iron-deficiency anemia in one patient, one group treated two additional patients who were not iron deficient with iron and noted resolution of akathisia over the next 4–10 weeks [121].

A review of the above studies led Gold and Lenox [122] to conclude that "the rationale for iron supplementation in the treatment of akathisia is relatively weak" and to caution that "uncontrolled iron ingestion is not without toxic effects. Prolonged unnecessary dietary iron supplementation can eventually overwhelm regulatory mechanisms and lead to secondary hemochromatosis and hemosiderosis with end organ damage."

Animal models of akathisia

Akathisia clearly has both subjective and objectively observable components. Attempts have been made to model both.

To develop an animal model of a subjective state, which many patients find difficult to describe, is certainly challenging. Sachdev and colleagues noted that, in the rat, increased defecation in a well-habituated environment has been proposed as an index of emotional distress [123]. This easily quantifiable index had been shown to increase with stress and disturbing stimuli including haloperidol administration [124]. Exploring this behavior as a possible index of neuroleptic-induced dysphoria or akathisia Sachdev and colleagues showed [125] that (1) haloperidol-induced defecation was dose dependent, (2) it was centrally mediated, (3) it was probably not secondary to catalepsy, (4) it is not specific to blockade of D_1 versus D_2 receptors, rather the two subtypes have synergistic effects, and (5) haloperidol-induced defecation is antagonized by lipophilic, but not hydrophilic β-blockers, consistent with known effects in human akathisia. The effects of other treatments for akathisia, however, such as anticholinergics and serotonin antagonists, could not be studied because peripheral effects on the gut would confound interpretation of any changes seen [125]. These findings make this behavior the most extensively studied of the animal models of akathisia.

Other attempts to model akathisia have focused on the objectively observable component of restlessness/hyperactivity. The models utilized include:

1. *Ventral tegmental area (VTA) or medial prefrontal cortex lesions in the rat.* Such lesions induce a syndrome of hyperactivity and increased locomotion, which, however, differs from akathisia in that the behavior is associated with difficulty in suppressing previously learned responses, decreased attention span, reduced fear reactions, reduced defecation, and decreased effects of punishment in avoidance conditioning [125]. The neurobiology of this model has been studied in detail and its substrate appears to be selectively decreased dopaminergic function, particularly of the mesocortical system. The increased locomotion correlates with decrease of dopamine levels in the frontal cortex (more closely than the decreases in the nucleus accumbens, which also occur after VTA lesions) and is replicated by a 6-hydroxy-dopamine lesion to the medial prefrontal cortex. Finally, the syndrome is reversed by administration of amphetamine and apomorphine. These features have led some to question whether animals with such lesions may, in fact, model human Attention Deficit Hyperactivity Disorder.

2. *Restlessness induced by fluoxetine in the rat.* Reports of akathisia after the introduction of flouoxetine led Teicher and colleagues [126] to study the motor effects of fluoxetine in fine detail using an infrared motion analysis system. Findings were compared with those after low-dose amphetamine. Amphetamine led to activation (less time spent immobile) and increased locomotion. Fluoxetine led to less time spent immobile, but without increased coordinated locomotion; the animals spent more time in the same vicinity constantly changing position [126]. Large doses of fluoxetine were required to produce this effect but, because of the rapidity of fluoxetine metabolism in the rat, these doses resulted in acute plasma levels similar to those that accumulate in humans during chronic treatment [126]. The effects of drugs used to treat akathisia in patients have not been studied in this model, to date.

3. *Neuroleptic-induced hyperkinesia in dogs.* In a study in which haloperidol and clozapine were administered to dogs on a complex, operant schedule,

the effects of the drugs could be differentiated. Haloperidol produced greater stereotypical scratching, licking, rotating, and persistent walking [127]. The effects of drugs used to treat akathisia have not been studied in this model.

4. *Neuroleptic-induced restlessness in nonhuman primates.* In a study intended to model tardive dyskinesia, monkeys received chronic biweekly injections of depot fluphenazine. Dystonia, parkinsonian symptoms, and restlessness occurred after each injection [128].

In another study of acute and chronic effects of selective dopamine antagonists, motor restlessness and extrapyramidal reactions were noted. These diminished with chronic administration of D1 but not D2 antagonists [129].

This section is a much abbreviated, paraphrased version of a more extensive and thoughtful review of this subject [125] to which the interested reader is enthusiastically referred.

Treatment of DIA

Adjusting the dose of the causative medication or treatment with an alternative agent

In patients on classical neuroleptics the following strategies have been used with some success: (1) reduction of neuroleptic dose [19] (often not feasible in floridly psychotic patients) and (2) switching to a lower potency classical agent [54]. However, since the availability of atypical antipsychotics, most clinicians would choose to use one of those agents as a first response to akathisia in patients treated with typical neuroleptics.

Pharmacological treatment of NIA

The agents that have been used to treat NIA include [42]: (1) antiparkinsonian agents, including anticholinergics and amantadine, (2) benzodiazepines, (3) agents that affect noradrenergic function, such as β-blockers and clonidine and (more recently), (4) serotonergic (5-HT) antagonists.

Antiparkinsonian agents

Antiparkinsonian medications are commonly used to treat akathisia. However, there are few formal prospective studies of these agents in NIA. Many clinicians feel that antiparkinsonian agents are only partially effective; their use is limited by anticholinergic side effects [59, 62] or tolerance to the therapeutic effect of amantadine [130].

Anticholinergics
There are many open-label studies of anticholinergic medications for drug-induced parkinsonism, few of which specifically examined the effects on akathisia. Kruse [131] treated 112 patients with extrapyramidal symptoms for 3 months each with the anticholinergics benztropine and procyclidine; nearly equal numbers of patients had akathisia versus rigidity/tremor as their major symptoms. He found that patients who had akathisia responded less well to

the anticholinergics than those who had rigidity/tremor. (Response rates: (1) benztropine/akathisia group – 21%; (2) rigidity and tremor group – 86%; (3) procyclidine/akathisia group – 57%; (4) rigidity and tremor group – 81%.)

Neu et al. [132] compared the efficacy of single- versus multiple-dose schedules of benztropine (4–6 mg/day) in 71 patients with drug-induced parkinsonism under double-blind conditions. They found that all of the patients with akathisia had substantial improvement after benztropine treatment (regardless of dose schedule).

Van Putten et al. [23] administered double-blind test doses of the anticholinergic agent biperiden (5 mg IM) and placebo to patients in whom the diagnosis of akathisia was uncertain. Patients were considered to have akathisia if their restlessness improved with biperiden, but not with placebo.

Van Putten and coworkers [60] examined the response of akathisia to open treatment with anticholinergic medications (benztropine or trihexyphenidyl) in patients receiving 1 week of treatment with 10 mg per day of thiothixene (n = 37) or haloperidol (n = 32). In the thiothixene group, four patients had a dysphoric reaction to the anticholinergics and were excluded, and 30 of the remaining patients had a complete response of their NIA to anticholinergics. In the haloperidol cohort, 14 patients had a complete remission after anticholinergics. In this study, the investigators were screening for the development of akathisia and therefore rapidly instituted treatment for NIA. Thus, it is not clear what percentage of the patients would have also developed concomitant parkinsonian EPS if anticholinergic treatment had not been initiated.

Friis et al. [98] performed a double-blind, crossover study examining 4 weeks of treatment each with biperiden (6–18 mg/day), the anticonvulsant sodium valproate, and placebo in 15 patients with NIA. Akathisia was rated on a 0 to 3 scale. Seventy-three percent of the patients responded to biperiden (mean akathisia score decreased from 1.4 after placebo to 0.6 after biperiden); no significant effects of sodium valproate or placebo were seen. It is of interest that 11 of the 15 patients had concurrent parkinsonian EPS.

Braude et al. [19] found that only 6 of 20 patients had improvement in NIA after open treatment with anticholinergics. Those patients who improved also had significant parkinsonian EPS. They suggested that there may be two distinct types of akathisia, distinguished by associated parkinsonian EPS and greater response to anticholinergics in this latter form. This may explain the findings by (1) Kruse [131] of a low response rate to anticholinergics in patients who had akathisia alone (vs. those who had parkinsonian EPS alone) and (2) Friis et al. [98] of a high response rate to biperiden in patients with NIA, many of whom had concomitant parkinsonian EPS.

Amantadine
Merrick and Schmitt [133] treated 11 patients with drug-induced parkinsonism in a double-blind, crossover design study that compared 3 weeks of treatment with amantadine (200 mg/day) to benztropine (2–4 mg/day). Substantial and fairly equal improvements in NIA were seen with both medications.

DiMascio et al. [134] compared amantadine (n = 13) and benztropine (n = 11) under double-blind conditions in patients with drug-induced EPS and NIA. Comparable improvement in NIA occurred over 4 weeks of treatment with both agents.

Stenson et al. [135] treated 11 patients with NIA (under parallel group, double-blind conditions) with matching benztropine (4–6 mg/day) (n = 6) or amantadine (200–300 mg/day) (n = 5) for up to 7 days. All of the patients treated with amantadine improved; in the cohort receiving benztropine, four patients improved, one was unchanged, and one had a worsening of akathisia.

Zubenko et al. [130] treated four patients with NIA with amantadine. All four patients initially showed substantial benefit; however, within 1 week, tolerance developed. Transient improvement occurred after raising the dose of amantadine again. One of these four patients had concomitant EPS that responded to amantadine, without the development of tolerance.

Benzodiazepines
Donlon [136] noted improvement in akathisia in 10 of 13 patients who received open treatment with diazepam (15 mg/day). All patients had not improved with prior treatment with diphenhydramine (antihistaminic/anticholinergic; 75 mg/day).

Gagrat et al. [137] performed a double-blind, parallel-group trial of single intravenous (IV) doses of diazepam (5 mg) (n = 9) versus diphenhydramine (50 mg) (n = 11). NIA was rated at baseline and four times up to 2 hours after infusion. Mean postinfusion ratings (at all four times) were significantly lower than baseline for both diazepam- and diphenhydramine-treated groups.

Kutcher et al. [138] reported the results of an open 1-week trial of clonazepam (0.5 mg/day) in 10 adolescents with NIA. Mean akathisia scores (on the ESRS) decreased significantly from 4.1 at baseline to 1.6 at the end of clonazepam treatment. They noted that possible advantages of clonazepam over other benzodiazepines were (1) the low doses required and (2) the long half-life, making once-a-day treatment possible.

These authors then conducted a double-blind, parallel-group study of treatment with clonazepam (1 mg) (n = 7) versus placebo (n = 7) [139]. Substantial improvement was seen in all patients receiving clonazepam; five of the patients receiving placebo were unchanged, while two patients had mild improvement (of one point on the akathisia subscale of the ESRS). Also, all four of the patients in the placebo cohort who received a subsequent open trial of clonazepam responded to this agent. Bartels et al. [96] studied the effects of 2 weeks of open treatment with lorazepam (1.5–5 mg/day) in 16 schizophrenic patients with NIA. Fourteen patients improved with lorazepam (nine had marked response, and five had moderate response), while two patients were unchanged. Improvement occurred after the first week of treatment, with minimal additional amelioration after the second week of treatment.

Beta-blockers

Beta-blockers are currently considered to be the most promising treatments for akathisia. These medications can be classified according to four properties: (1) selectivity, (2) lipophilicity, (3) intrinsic sympathomimetic activity (ISA), and (4) nonspecific properties, such as membrane-stabilizing effects (MSE). Those that predominantly block β_1 receptors (the predominant β-receptor in cardiac tissue) or β_2 receptors (e.g., lung, pancreas) are referred to as "selective" β-blockers. Those that block both β_1 and β_2 receptors are referred to as "nonselective" β-blockers. The more lipophilic β-blockers cross the blood-brain barrier (BBB) during acute administration, while the less lipophilic (relatively hydrophilic) agents have a lower rate of penetrance of the BBB. Beta-blockers with ISA have some partial agonist activity and therefore do not lower the heart rate as much as those agents without this property. Membrane stabilization is a term used to refer to decreased conductivity in isolated preparations of cardiac tissue, which correlates with local anesthetic effects of β-blockers [140–142].

Table 7.1 classifies β-blockers according to these four properties [142]. This table also shows the β_1 blockade potency ratios for each agent [142–144] so that dose comparisons can be made in the treatment studies. Table 7.2 summarizes studies with propranolol; Table 7.3 summarizes studies with other β-blocking agents.

We will divide and discuss the studies of β-blockers in NIA according to these properties. In general: (1) centrally active β-blockers (i.e., relatively lipophilic agents) have proven more efficacious than relatively hydrophilic ones; (2) the data are less clear regarding the relative contributions of β_1 and

Table 7.1 Characteristics of β-blockers

Drugs	Blockade ot β_1 receptors	Blockade of β_2 receptors	MSE	Lipophilicity	β_1 Blockade potency ratio (D/L-propranotol = 1)
D/L-Propranolol	++	++	++	+++	1.0
D-Propranolol	0	0	++	+++	–
Metoprolol*	++	0−+	0−+	++	1.0
Nadolol	++	++	0	0−+	1.0
Atenolol	++	0−+	0	0	1.0
Pindolol**	++	++	+	++	6.0
ICI 118,551	0	++	++	+++	–
Betaxolol***	++	0−+	0	++	3.0–10.0
Sotalol	++	++	0	0	0.3

MSE = Membrane stabilizing effect.
* Metoprolol is selective for β_1 receptors at doses ≤ 100 mg/day.
** Only pindolol has significant ISA.
*** Betaxofot is selective for β_1 receptors at doses ≤ 10 mg/day.

Table 7.2 Studies of propranolol in acute neuroleptic-induced akathisia

Authors	No. of subjects/ design	Drug (mean mg/day)	Response
I. Open Studies			
Lipinski et al. [40]	12 patients	Propranolol: 30	9 patients: complete response 1 patient: 50% response 2 patients 70% response
Kulik and Wilbur [146]	1 patient	Propranolol: 160	response upon initial treatment and rechallenge
Lipinski et al. [41]	14 patients	Propranolol: 42	All improved; 9 patients with complete response
Adler et al. [147]	17 patients; parallel group	Propranolol: 56	9 patients: significant reductions in subjective and objective NIA 8 patients: little change in subjective and objective NIA
II. Controlled Studies			
Adler et al. [33]	6 patients	Propranolol: 25	Significant reduction in subjective and objective NIA
	Single-blind	Lorazopam: 2	Significant reduction only in subjective NIA
	Crossover	No treatment	No significant difference from baseline
Adler et al. [34]	12 patients; double-blind; crossover	Propranolol: 51	Significant reduction in subjective and objective NIA
Kramer et al. [43]	20 patients; double-blind; crossover	Propranolol: 60 placebo	Significant improvement in NIA after 5 days of propranalol
Lipinski et al. [148]	20 patients; double-blind; parallel group	Propranolol placebo	Improvement in NIA greater on propranolol
Adler et al. [149]	11 patients; double-blind; crossover and parallel group	D-propranolol: 80 placebo D/L- propranolol: 80	No difference in subjective and objective NIA after D-propranolol or placebo; Significant improvement in 8 patients after open D/L-propranolol

β_2 receptors as agents selective for either receptor subset have shown efficacy; (3) membrane-stabilizing effects do not seem to contribute significantly to the therapeutic effects, as will be discussed below; (4) intrinsic sympathomimetic activity may diminish efficacy somewhat, but permit use of β-blocker therapy in patients with bradycardia who would not otherwise tolerate these agents.

Table 7.3 Studies of other ß-blockers in acute neuroleptic-induced akathisia

Study	Agent	Characteristics	Results
I. Agents with ISA			
Reiter et al. [153]	Pindolol	Depiphilic	9 patients: 4 showed good
Adler et al. [154]	Pindolol	Nonselective ISA	response; 4 of the remaining 5 improved further after propranolol
II. Hydrophilic Agents			
Lipinski et al. [41]	Nadolol	Hydrophilic Nonselective	Nadolol less effective than propranolol
Ratey et al. [155]	Nadolol	Hydrophilic Nonselective	3 patients; good response after 2 weeks
Adler et al. [156]	Nadolol	Hydrophilic Nonselective	6 patients; good response with at least 9–11 days of treatment; 1 patient with CNS syphilis; rapid response In 1 day
Wells et al. [157]	Nadolol	Hydrophilic Nonselective	Equal improvement after 9 days treatment with both nadolol and placebo
Dupuis et al. [158]	Sotalol	Hydrophilic Nonselective	6 patients with prior response to propranolol were unresponsive to sotalol
III. Selective Agents			
Derom et al. [159]	Atenolol	Hydrophilic β_1 selective	1 patient; no response to atenolol; good response to propranolol
Reiter et al. [160]	Atenolol	Hydrophilic β_1 selective	7 patients; no improvement on atenolol, while propranolol was effective
Zubenko et al. [164]	Metoprolol	β_1 selective $\leq$ 100 mg/day	5 patients; metoprolol as effective as propanolol only at doses $\geq$ 200 mg/day
Kim et al. [166]	Metoprolol	β_1 selective $\leq$ 100 mg/day	9 patients; metoprolol effective in doses <100 mg/day; no additional benefit with subsequent propranolol treatment
Adler et al. [167]	Metoprolol	β_1 selective $\leq$ 100 mg/day	8 patients; equal effects of 1 day treatment with metoprolol (75 mg/day) vs. propranolol
Dupuis et al. [158]	Betaxolol	β_1 selective	4 patients with prior response to propranolol had good response to betaxolol
Adler et al. [169]	Betaxolol	β_1 selective	6 patients; equal response to betaxolol and propranolol
Adler et al. [170]	ICI 118,551	β_2 selective	Improvement with both ICI 118,551 and propranolol (n = 6); no significant effect of placebo (n = 4)

ISA = Intrinsic sympathomimetic activity.

Strang [145] originally described the beneficial effects of propranolol (5–30 mg/day) in parkinsonian patients who had restless leg syndrome. This led Lipinski et al. [40] to undertake the first trial of propranolol in NIA. Twelve patients with NIA were treated (mean dose = 30 mg/day) in an open design. All patients improved, with nine having a complete response. This improvement was rapid with "a considerable clinical response typically [occurring] within an hour of the first dose and the maximum clinical response ... in 24–48 hours." No significant changes in blood pressure or pulse were observed. Concomitant EPS were also unaffected. The rapidity of the response to propranolol and the absence of effects on blood pressure/pulse and parkinsonian symptoms have also been noted consistently in subsequent studies of low-dose propranolol in NIA. In the same year, another case of NIA successfully treated with propranolol was reported by Kulik and Wilbur [145].

There have been several other reports, which are detailed below, of the efficacy of propranolol in NIA. Although the results of these studies have been uniformly positive, these investigations have each studied a relatively small number of patients.

Lipinski et al. [41] also reported an extension of their original open study, which further documented the efficacy of propranolol in NIA.

Adler et al. [33] compared propranolol (20–30 mg/day), lorazepam (2 mg/day), and periods of no treatment in six patients with NIA; this was a crossover study, in which the rater was blind but patients and the treating physician were not. Propranolol significantly decreased subjective and objective measures of NIA, while lorazepam diminished subjective, but not objective akathisia scores. Scores at the end of the no treatment periods did not differ from baseline.

These authors also performed a randomized, double-blind, crossover design study of the efficacy of propranolol (20–60 mg/day, mean dose = 51 mg/day) and matching placebo in treating NIA [34]. Propranolol caused significant overall improvement in both subjective and objective measures of akathisia compared to ratings done both at baseline and on placebo. Placebo caused no significant change in akathisia ratings from baseline. No significant effect of either propranolol or placebo was seen on Hamilton Anxiety scores. Parkinsonian EPS (cogwheeling, rigidity, tremor, akinesia), as measured by the Simpson-Angus EPS Scale were not significantly affected by treatment with propranolol.

Adler et al. [147] treated 17 patients experiencing akathisia with propranolol (n = 9) (40–80 mg/day) or benztropine (n = 8) (1.5–4.0 mg/day). This was a parallel-group design in which nonblinded akathisia ratings were obtained at baseline and at the end of either treatment. Assessments of memory, performed by a rater blind to treatment assignment, were also obtained to examine for possible effects on cognition. As in prior studies, we found approximately 50% decreases in both subjective and objective NIA after treatment with propranolol. No change in objective NIA and a small decrease in subjective NIA occurred after treatment with benztropine. The relative lack of efficacy of benztropine in this study was hypothesized to be possibly due to (1) atypical responses in the small sample and (2) only one of the patients having significant concomitant parkinsonian EPS. Three measures of recent memory (Buschke recall, Buschke consistent retrieval, and superspan digits subtests) and one measure of immediate memory (WAIS digits forward) were impaired in those patients who received benztropine, but not in those treated with propranolol.

Kramer et al. [43] also completed a double-blind placebo-controlled, crossover study of propranolol (60 mg/day) and placebo in 20 patients. Patients were divided into two cohorts, those who received (1) 2 days of placebo, followed by 5 days of propranolol, or (2) 2 days of propranolol followed by 5 days of placebo. There was an overall trend of decrease in subjective and objective akathisia after propranolol treatment. Furthermore, the ratings on two akathisia subscales were significantly lower after 5 days of treatment with propranolol than after 5 days of placebo. Interpretation of the data from this study is compromised by (1) unequal length of treatment in the two groups (i.e., 2 vs. 5 days), and (2) possible carry-over effects of 5 days of propranolol into the 2-day treatment period on placebo.

Lipinski and coworkers [148] have completed a randomized, placebo-controlled parallel-group study of propranolol in 20 patients with NIA. Changes in akathisia scores from baseline were significantly greater with propranolol than with placebo.

We, in collaboration with Lipinski and coworkers at McLean Hospital, studied the effect of d-propranolol on akathisia [149]. Eleven patients (8 at the New York VAMC and 3 at McLean) completed this double-blind, crossover design study of d-propranolol 80 mg per day versus placebo. The clinical formulation of propranolol is a racemate. The d-isomer has a variety of pharmacological actions in common with the racemate, including membrane stabilization; however, the d-isomer does not have clinically significant β-blocking properties (only 1.7% to 6.7% of the racemate, based on clinical and preclinical studies of antagonism of isoproterenol-induced tachycardia) [150–152]. In this study, there were no differences in ratings after placebo versus after d-propranolol. Significant reductions in akathisia were seen in the eight patients who received racemic propranolol (80 mg/day) after the study was completed. This indicates that antagonism of β-receptors and not nonspecific properties, such as MSE, mediates the therapeutic effect of propranolol in NIA.

In all of these studies of racemic propranolol, maximal improvement was noted within 3 days of initiation of treatment (except for Kramer et al. [43] who found significant improvement after 5 days, but not 2 days).

Other nonselective β-blockers
Pindolol (lipophilic, nonselective, with ISA): We have studied pindolol, another nonselective, lipophilic β-blocker, which additionally has the partial agonist

property of intrinsic sympathomimetic activity (ISA), at first in one patient with sinus bradycardia and NIA [153] and then in an additional eight patients [154]. Of these nine patients, four had substantial or complete remissions in their akathisia with 5 mg per day. The five patients who did not respond were then treated with propranolol (mean = 72.0 mg/day) for 2–8 days; four of these five subjects had further improvement. We suggested that the differential response may have been due to pindolol: (1) being less lipophilic than propranolol and (2) having partial agonist activity (ISA) [154].

Nadolol (nonlipophilic, nonselective): Lipinski et al. [41] made the first attempt to treat NIA with other β-blockers besides propranolol, in order to evaluate central versus peripheral and β_1 versus β_2 mechanisms in the therapeutic effect. They found that nadolol (a nonselective, relatively hydrophilic agent) was less effective after acute treatment than propranolol (nonselective, lipophilic) in the treatment of NIA.

In contrast, Ratey et al. [155] described three cases of NIA that improved with nadolol. Interpretation of these data is difficult because (1) the improvement was also coincident with the starting of benzodiazepines, and (2) the clinical effects required approximately 2 weeks with nadolol versus hours to days with propranolol.

Adler et al. [156] treated six patients with NIA with nadolol (60 mg/day) for 12 to 14 days. Akathisia ratings were subdivided into the following epochs: day 0 (baseline), day 1, days 3–4, days 6–7, days 9–11, and days 12–14. Significant improvement in akathisia was not seen until 9–11 days (subjective ratings) and 12–14 days (objective and global ratings) of nadolol treatment. These findings verify both Lipinski's [41] and Ratey's [155] findings of a subacute, but not an acute, onset of action of nadolol, in that the effect was not seen until at least 9–11 days of treatment. During this study, a seventh patient with NIA, a chronic schizophrenic who also had neurosyphilis was treated. He had a complete cessation of akathisia after 1 day of nadolol therapy. The rapid response of this patient suggests a central site of action, as the active CNS syphilis infection presumably led to a more permeable blood-brain barrier and more rapid penetration of nadolol.

It must be noted, however, that the concept of delayed CNS penetration of nadolol has been called into question by a final placebo-controlled study by Wells et al. [157]. In this parallel group comparison of nadolol and placebo improvement of akathisia indeed occurred after day 9 in nadolol-treated patients. However, an equal degree of improvement was seen in the placebo group at that time [157]. This finding suggests that the improvement Adler et al. [156] attributed to delayed CNS penetration of nadolol may have been due to some degree of accommodation to akathisia over 10–14 days' time.

Nonetheless, the overall concept that lipophilicity is required for ß blockers to be effective in akathisia was further reinforced by the finding of Dupuis et al. [158] that patients with proven responsiveness to propranolol failed to respond to the hydrophilic, nonselective agent sotalol.

Studies of selective β-blockers

Atenolol (nonlipophilic, β_1-selective): Derom et al. [159] have reported a patient whose akathisia was improved with propranolol (120 mg/day), but not with atenolol (a nonlipophilic, selective β_1 antagonist; 100 mg/day). Reiter et al. [160] treated seven patients in a parallel group design with atenolol (mean maximum dose = 60.7 mg/day) and propranolol (mean maximum dose = 60.0 mg/day). Propranolol significantly improved both subjective and objective akathisia versus baseline ratings; atenolol did not improve objective akathisia, and in fact worsened subjective complaints of restlessness in several patients. The authors note the following possible reasons for worsening:

1. Differences in these agents in lipophilicity and selectivity (atenolol: hydrophilic, β_1-selective; propranolol: lipophilic, nonselective).

2. An indirect effect of selective peripheral β_1 blockade (with atenolol, but not propranolol) leading to a compensatory increase in central noradrenergic activity. Patterson's [161] report of a syndrome similar to akathisia in a hypertensive patient treated with atenolol (but not receiving neuroleptics) supports this possibility.

3. Pharmacokinetic effects of β-blockers on neuroleptic plasma levels: two studies have shown increased plasma neuroleptic levels in patients treated with propranolol for aggressive behavior. Silver et al. [162] found that high-dose propranolol (up to 800 mg/day) increased thioridazine levels in two patients. Greendyke and Kanter [163] studied 12 patients with organic brain disease who were receiving high doses of propranolol; they found that propranolol increased plasma thioridazine levels, but not haloperidol levels. If atenolol also increases neuroleptic levels, these higher levels plus lack of acute central effects of atenolol could lead to a worsening of akathisia.

Metoprolol (lipophilic, β_1-selective): Zubenko et al. [164] found that metoprolol, which is a lipophilic/β_1-selective (in low doses) blocker, was effective in treating akathisia only in doses (>200 mg/day) where both β_1 and β_2 receptors are nonselectively blocked [165].

Kim and coworkers [166] examined the effect on NIA of increasing doses of metoprolol in nine patients (in the first six, ratings were nonblind; in the last three, the rater was blind to timing of initiation of treatment). All patients were started at 25–50 mg per day of metoprolol, with the dose of metoprolol increased by 25 mg every several days up to a maximum of 100 mg per day or where maximal clinical improvement occurred. Ratings were obtained prior to each dosage increase. All patients were subsequently treated with open propranolol (60 mg/day). The mean dose of metoprolol where maximal improvement occurred was 66.7 mg per day, a dose where selectivity for the β_1 receptor is considered to be maintained [164, 165]. Seven patients had substantial improvements in akathisia after metoprolol. No significant further improvement was seen with subsequent propranolol treatment [166].

We conducted a second study [167] of the effects of metoprolol at β_1-selective doses: (1) because of the conflicting results of studies of this agent at β_1-selective doses and (2) to control for possible carry-over effects that may have been present in our first metoprolol study (as patients were treated with propranolol immediately after their metoprolol trial). This study was a single-blind crossover design study of 1-day trials of metoprolol (75 mg/day) and propranolol (60 mg/day), with an intervening washout period. Eight patients with NIA participated. Both propranolol and metoprolol produced significant decreases in NIA, which were of equal magnitude.

Betaxolol (lipophilic, β_1-selective): Dupuis et al. [158] studied three different β-blockers, propranolol (20–40 mg/day), sotalol (nonlipophilic, nonselective; 40–80 mg/day), and betaxolol (lipophilic, β_1-selective; 10–20 mg/day), with an intervening washout period between each trial. Eight of 16 patients had complete remission of akathisia after propranolol. Six of these eight had recurrences of akathisia after its discontinuation. These patients were then unsuccessfully treated with sotalolol. Four of these remaining, initially propranolol-responsive patients were then treated with betaxolol, with each having complete alleviation of their akathisia [158].

Betaxolol appears to maintain its β_1 selectivity over a larger dose range than metoprolol [168]. When betaxalol became available in the United States, we treated eight patients with NIA with betaxolol (5 mg/day), a dose where β_1 selectivity is quite likely to be maintained [168]. All eight patients improved and there was no further improvement with subsequent treatment with propranolol [169].

ICI 118,551 (Lipophilic, β_2-selective): We have also examined the effects of ICI 118,551 (the only lipophilic β_2-selective agent developed to date) in a double-blind, parallel group study versus placebo in 10 patients (ICI 118,551 = 6; placebo = 4) with NIA. Mean measures of akathisia were lower in the patients who received ICI 118,551 than in those who received placebo. Five of the six patients treated with ICI 118,551 had improvement in their akathisia, while only one of the placebo-treated patients improved ($\chi^2 = 6.53$, df = 2, p ≤ 0.05) [170]. This study, however, was terminated prematurely when ICI 118,551 was withdrawn from clinical evaluation.

Clonidine

Clonidine is an α_2 agonist that decreases central noradrenergic activity [171]. Zubenko et al. [37] conducted an open trial of this agent (0.2–0.8 mg/day) in six patients with NIA. All six patients improved, with four having complete remission. Treatment was limited by hypotension in two cases. These two patients also developed sedation and had only partial responses to clonidine. This lesser response in the patients who developed hypotension/sedation led Zubenko and coworkers to conclude that the therapeutic efficacy of clonidine was not related to its sedative properties.

Adler et al. [38] treated six patients with clonidine (0.15–0.40 mg/day) in a single-blind (rater-blind) design. Both subjective and objective features of akathisia were significantly decreased after treatment compared to baseline. Akathisia ratings were substantially improved in all patients. Hamilton Anxiety Scale scores were also significantly lowered. The use of clonidine was limited by hypotension in five cases and clinically apparent sedation in four patients. Thus the possibility exists that in this study, the efficacy of the clonidine was due to nonspecific sedative effects. Both Adler et al. [38] and Zubenko et al. [37] noted that the sedation encountered with clonidine was not observed with β-blockers. Clonidine also differed from propranolol in that in the Adler et al. study, clonidine decreased Hamilton Anxiety scores, while, in a prior study [34] propranolol did not.

Studies of 5HT$_2$ antagonists

When the previous edition of this book was published this therapeutic approach was still in its infancy. In 1986, Bersani et al. published observations on ritanserin, which were not widely noted [172]. The efficacy of ritanserin as a treatment for NIA was further suggested by Miller et al. [173]. Since then, progress in this area has made this approach a major addition to the treatment for NIA.

In 1992 Miller et al. [174] reported three patients whose akathisia was resistant to anticholinergic, beta blocker, and benzodiazepine treatment, who then showed a rapid and substantial response to ritanserin. This was important both for nonresponders to propranolol and for those unable to be treated with β blockers because of medical contraindications.

This approach to therapy was then explored systematically by an Israeli group. Cyproheptadine, mianserin, and mirtazapine were shown to have efficacy in both open label [175–177] and double blind studies [178–180]. In addition, the critical role of 5HT$_2$ antagonism was shown by demonstrating the lack of efficacy of the 5HT$_1$, partial agonist buspirone [176], and the 5HT$_3$ antagonist granisetron [181] on NIA.

This body of work is both theoretically and clinically important and provides the clinician with an alternative therapy for patients unresponsive to or intolerant of beta blockers or anticholinergics. We would agree with the conclusion of a recent review by Poyurovsky and Weizman [182]: "When the decision is made to initiate an anti akathisia compound the β-adrenergic blocking agent propranolol" (or, we would add, betoxolol) –"or a 5HT$_{2a}$ antagonist" – "are the first choices. In cases of NIA associated with neuroleptic-induced parkinsonism, priority may be given to anticholenergic agents" [182].

Some comments on pathophysiology

In a perfect world, study of etiology and pathogenesis leads to incisive interventions. Neurologists and (particularly) psychiatrists live in a very imperfect world in which much of the pathogenesis is inferred from pharmacological evidence.

Review of the causes and treatment of DIA leads to a certainty that diminished dopaminergic function plays a key role. This statement is about as bold as a politician asserting he strongly supports morality and motherhood. A more precise characterization of the pathophysiology of akathisia, however, is difficult because of gaps in current knowledge. In this context, we will review the main evidence about the pathophysiology of DIA.

The relationship of akathisia to decreased dopaminergic function was originally suggested by its frequent occurrence in idiopathic and postencephalitic parkinsonism [5, 6, 183]. With respect to pharmacologic evidence, the main causative offenders are the classical neuroleptics. Akathisia, reported after administration of known dopamine receptor antagonists used for other medical indications such as metoclopramide and droperidol [9, 53, 184] has, of course, identical implications with respect to pathogenic mechanisms.

That blockade of dopamine receptors per se is not the only way in which dopamine function can be reduced to a threshold at which akathisia occurs is evident from reports of the syndrome due to depletors-like reserpine [9, 54], and tetrabenazine [185] or synthesis inhibitors such as alpha methyl paratyrosine [185].

A heterogeneous group of other agents has also been reported to cause akathisia. These include atypical antipsychotics (see above), serotonin reuptake inhibitors (see above), calcium channel blockers [186–188] – amoxapine, [189, 190] and lithium [191]. Are antidopaminergic effects part of these agents' pharmacologic profiles?

Probably! Atypical antipsychotics all block dopamine receptors although with rather low affinity in some cases. Serotonin reuptake inhibitors are known to diminish dopaminergic function [92] and dopamine release [94]. The calcium channel blockers reported to be associated with akathisia include a single case with diltiazem [186] and particularly flunarizine and cinnarizine [187, 188]. Evidence was cited [188] that the latter two of these agents has direct neuroleptic-like effects [192–194]. Diltiazem is not, to our knowledge, a dopamine receptor blocker but some antidopaminergic properties can, perhaps, be inferred from its effects on tardive dyskinesia [195]. Finally, amoxopine or a metabolite thereof, is known to have antidopaminergic properties and lithium treatment has been shown to inhibit dopamine synthesis in some studies [196].

If agents that cause akathisia reduce basal dopaminergic function via a variety of mechanisms, is the converse true; do drugs that treat akathisia have positive modulatory effects on dopaminergic function [7]? A series of studies from the 1990s give rather direct evidence that this is indeed the case. In these studies positron emission tomography (PET) imaging is used to measure dopamine efflux in basal ganglia. This is done via measuring competitive displacement of a radiolabeled neuroleptic (raclopride) by endogenous dopamine from D_2 receptors. In these studies, it should be noted, decreases in raclopride binding reflect large changes in dopamine efflux. An important methodological paper [197] measured amphetamine-induced dopamine efflux in nonhuman primates *simultaneously* with *both in vivo* microdialysis and C^{11} raclopride displacement. A 44% increase in dopamine efflux (seen during microdialysis) was found to correspond to a 1% decrease in C^{11} raclopride binding [197]. Using this methodology, both benztropine [198] and the $5HT_2$ antagonist altanserin [94] have been shown to increase dopamine release as measured by decrements in raclopride binding.

Propranolol has not been studied with this PET technique but some evidence for prodopaminergic effects has been shown, at least when high doses are used [199]. Amantadine is generally considered to cause increased dopaminergic function [200] (although more recently this has been questioned [201]).

However, benzodiazepines, which have been used extensively and with benefit in akathisia actually diminish basal dopamine efflux (as indicated by increases of C^{11} raclopride binding) [202]. In the context of this apparent paradox we will note that there is still some question as to whether benzodiazepines specifically affect akathisia or whether their effects ameliorate the subjective aspects of akathisia in a nonspecific manner [33].

Thus agents that cause akathisia all probably decrease dopaminergic function, while most therapies have prodopaminergic effects. Further studies will tell whether these comments constitute an oversimplified Procrustian bed.

Acknowledgment

The authors thank Juanita Forde for the extensive work she did in preparing this manuscript. They would also like to thank Jordan Gellis for his assistance in performing clerical work in preparation of this manuscript.

References

1. Willis T. The London Practice of Physick, 1st edition. London, Thomas Bassett and William Crooke, 1685, p. 404.
2. Beard GM. A Practical Treatise on Nervous Exhaustion, 2nd edition. New York, William Wood, 1880, pp. 41–42.
3. Haskovec L. Akathisie. Arch Bohemes Med Clin 1902; 3: 193–200.
4. Bing R. Ueber Einige bemerkenswerte Begleiterscheinunger der exrapyram idalen Rigiditat (Akathesie-Mikrographie-Kinesia paradoxica). Schweiz Med Wochenschr 1923; 53: 167–171.
5. Sachs 0. Awakenings. New York, Vintage Books, 1976, pp. 30.
6. Sicard JA. Akathisie and tasikinesie. Presse Med 1923; 31: 265–266.
7. Ekbom KA. Asthenia crurum paraesthetica ("irritable legs"). Acta Med Scand 1944; 118: 197–209.
8. Ekbom KA. Restless leg syndrome. Neurology 1960; 10: 868–873.
9. Akathisia and antipsychotic drugs [Editorial]. Lancet 1986; ii: 1131–1132.
10. Gibb WR, Lees AJ. The restless leg syndrome. Postgrad Med J 1986; 62: 329–333.
11. Sigwald J, Grossiord A, Duriel P, Dumont G. Le traitement de la maladie de Parkinson et des manifestations extrpyramidales par le diethyl aminoethynthiodiphenylamine (2987 RP): resultats d'une annee d'application. Rev Neurol (Paris) 1947; 79: 683–687.
12. Steck H. Le syndrome extrapyramidal et d'encephalique au cours des traitements au largactil et au serapsil. Ann Med Psychol 1954; 112: 737–743.
13. Freyhan FA. Psychomotility and parkinsonism in treatment with neuroleptic drugs. Arch Neurol Psychiatry 1957; 78: 465–472.
14. Sachdev P. The development of the concept of akathisia: a historical overview. Schizophrenia Res 1995; 16: 33–45.

15. Gibb WR, Lees AJ. The clinical phenomenon of akathisia. J Neurol Neurosurg Psychiatry 1986; 49: 861–866.
16. Van Putten T. The many faces of akathisia. Compr Psychiatry 1975; 16: 43–47.
17. Barnes TRE, Braude WM. Toward a more reliable diagnosis of akathisia [in reply]. Arch Gen Psychiatry 1986; 43: 1016.
18. Van Putten T, Marder SR. Behavioral toxicity of antipsychotic drugs. J Clin Psychiatry 1987; 48(suppl): 13–19.
19. Braude WM, Barnes TRE, Gore SM. Clinical characteristics of akathisia. Br J Psychiatry 1983; 143: 134–150.
20. Barnes TRE. A rating scale for drug-induced akathisia. Br J Psychiatry 1989; 154: 672–676.
21. Hermesh H, Munitz H. Unilateral neuroleptic-induced akathisia. Clin Neuropharmacol 1990; 13: 253–258.
22. Van Putten T. Why do schizophrenic patients refuse to take their drugs? Arch Gen Psychiatry 1974; 31: 67–72.
23. Van Putten T, Mutalipassi LR, Malkin MD. Phenothiazine-induced decompensation. Arch Gen Psychiatry 1974; 30: 102–105.
24. Duncan EJ, Adler LA, Stephanides M, Sanfilipo M, August B. Akathisia and exacerbation of psychopathology: a preliminary report. Clinical Neuropharmacol 2000; 23: 169–173. .
25. Keckich WA. Violence as a manifestation of akathisia. JAMA 1978; 240: 2185.
26. Kumar BB. An unusual case of akathisia. Am J Psychiatry 1979; 136: 1088.
27. Schulte JR. Homicide and suicide associated with akathisia and haloperidol. Am J Forensic Psychiatry 1985; 6: 3- 7.
28. Shear K, Frances A, Weiden P. Suicide associated with akathisia and depot fluphenazine treatment. J Clin Psychopharmacol 1983; 3: 235–236.
29. Weiden P. Akathisia from prochlorperazine. JAMA 1985; 253: 635.
30. Drake RE, Ehrlich J. Suicide attempts associated with akathisia. Am J Psychiatry 1985; 142: 499–501.
31. Shaw ED, Mann JJ, Widen P, Sinsheimer LM, Brunn RD. A case of suicidal and homicidal ideation and akathisia in a double-blind neuroleptic crossover study. J Clin Psychopharmacol 1986; 6: 196–197.
32. Kendler K. A medical student's experience with akathisia. Am J Psychiatry 1976; 133: 454–455
33. Adler LA, Angrist B, Peselow E, Corwin J, Rotrosen J. Efficacy of propranolol in neuroleptic-induced akathisia. J Clin Psychopharmacol 1985; 5: 164–166.
34. Adler LA, Angrist B, Peselow E, Corwin J, Maslansky R, Rotrosen J. A controlled assessment of propranolol in the treatment of neuroleptic-induced akathisia. Br J Psychiatry 1986; 149: 42–45.
35. Film: Clinical manifestations of Drug Abuse. NIDA.
36. Gold MS, Redmond DE, Kleiber HD. Clonidine blocks the acute opiate withdrawal syndrome. Lancet 1978; ii: 403–405.
37. Zubenko GS, Cohen BM, Lipinski JF, Jonas JM. Use of clonidine in the treatment of akathisia. Psychiatry Res 1984; 13: 253–259.
38. Adler LA, Angrist B, Peselow E, Reitano J, Rotrosen J. Clonidine in neuroleptic-induced akathisia. Am J Psychiatry 1987; 144: 235–236.
39. Roehrich H, Gold MS. Propranolol as adjunct to clonidine in opiate detoxification. Am J Psychiatry 1987; 144: 1099–1100.
40. Lipinski JF, Zubenko GS, Barriera P, Cohen BM. Propranolol in the treatment of neuroleptic-induced akathisia. Lancet 1983; ii: 685–686.

41. Lipinski JF, Zubenko GS, Cohen BM, Barriera PJ. Propranolol in the treatment of neuroleptic-induced akathisia. Am J Psychiatry 1984; 141: 412–415.
42. Adler LA, Angrist B, Reiter S, Rotrosen J. Neuroleptic-induced akathisia: a review. Psychopharmacology 1989; 97: 1–11.
43. Kramer SM, Gorkin RA, DiJohnson C, Sheves P. Propranolol in the treatment of neuroleptic-induced akathisia (NIA) in schizophrenics: a double-blind, placebo-controlled study. Biol Psychiatry 1988; 24: 823–827.
44. Sachdev P. The present status of akathisia: J Neur Ment Disord 1991; 179: 381–391.
45. Barnes TRE, Braude WM. Akathisia variants and tardive dyskinesia. Arch Gen Psychiatry 1985; 42: 874–878.
46. Simpson GM. Neurotoxicity of major tranquilizers. In Roizin L, Shiroki H, Grcevic N (eds) Neurotoxicology, New York, Raven Press, 1977, p 3.
47. Jeste DV, Wyatt RJ. Understanding and Treating Tardive Dyskinesia. New York and London, The Guilford Press, 1982, p 64.
48. Braude WM, Barnes TRE. Late onset akathisia: an indicant of covert dyskinesia. Two case reports. Am J Psychiatry 1983; 140: 611–612.
49. Chouinard G, Annable L, Ross-Chouinard A, Nestoros JN. Factors related to tardive dyskinesia. Am J Psychiatry 1979; 136: 79–83.
50. Munetz MR, Cornes CL. Distinguishing akathisia and tardive dyskinesia: a review of the literature. J Clin Psychopharmacol 1982; 3: 343–350.
51. Stahl SM. Akathisia and tardive dyskinesia: changing concepts. Arch Gen Psychiatry 1985; 42: 915–917.
52. Munetz MR. Akathisia variants and tardive dyskinesia. Arch Gen Psychiatry 1986; 43: 1015.
53. Barnes TRE, Braude WM, Hill DJ. Acute akathisia after oral droperidol and metoclopramide preoperative medication. Lancet 1982; ii: 48–49.
54. Ayd FJ. A survey of drug-induced extrapyramidal reactions. JAMA 1961; 175: 1054–1060.
55. Kruse W. Persistent muscular restlessness after phenothiazine treatment: report of three cases. Am J Psychiatry 1960; 11: 152–153.
56. Weiner WJ, Luby ED. Persistent akathisia following neuroleptic withdrawal. Ann Neurol 1983; 13: 466–467.
57. Goldman D. Parkinsonism and related phenomena from administration of drugs: their production and control under clinical conditions and possible relation to therapeutic effect. Rev Can Exp Biol 1961; 20: 549–560.
58. National Institute of Mental Health. Psychopharmacology survey center collaborative study group. Phenothiazine treatment in acute schizophrenia. Arch Gen Psychiatry 1964; 10: 246–261.
59. Freyhan FA. Extrapyramidal Symptoms and Other Side Effects of Trifluoperazine: Clinical and Pharmacological Aspects. Philadelphia, Lea and Febiger, 1958.
60. Van Putten T, May PRA, Marder SR. Akathisia with haloperidol and thiothixene. Arch Gen Psychiatry 1984; 41: 1036–1039.
61. Weiden P, Mann JJ, Haas G, Mattson M, Frances A. Clinical nonrecognition of neuroleptic-induced movement disorders: a cautionary study. Am J Psychiatry 1987; 144: 1148–1153.
62. Ayd FJ. Drug-induced extrapyramidal reactions: their clinical manifestations and treatment with akineton. Psychosomatics 1960; 1: 143–150.
63. Kopala L, Good K, Honer WG. Extrapyramidal signs and clinical symptoms in first episode schizophrenia: response to risperidone. J Clin Psychopharmacol 1997; 17: 308–313.

64. Wirshing DA, Marshall BD, Green FM, Mintz J, Marder SR, Wirshing WC. Risperidone in treatment—refractory schizophrenia. Am J Psychiatry 1999; 156: 1374–1379.
65. Chouinard G, Jones B, Remington G, et al. Canadian multi-centered placebo controlled study of fixed doses of risperidone and haloperidol in the treatment of chronic schizophrenic patients. J Clin Psychopharmacol 1993; 13: 25–40.
66. Marder SR, Meibach RC. Risiperidone in the treatment of schizophrenia. Am J Psychiatry 1994; 151: 825–835.
67. Miller CH, Mohr F, Umbricht D, Woerner M, Fleischacker WW, Lieberman JA. The prevalence of acute extrapyramidal signs and symptoms in patients treated with clozopine, risperidone and conventional neuroleptics. J Clin Psychiatry 1998; 59: 69–75.
68. Beasley CM Jr., Sanger T, Satterlee W, Tollefson G, Tran P, Hamilton S and the olanzapine study group. Olanzapine versus placebo: results of a double-blind fixed dose olanzapine trial. Psychopharmocology (Berl) 1996; 124: 159–167.
69. Beasley CM Jr, Hamilton SH, Crawford AN, et al. Olanzapine versus haloperidol acute phase results of the international double-blind olanzapine trial. Eur Neuropsychopharmacol 1997; 7: 125–137.
70. Sanger TM, Lieberman JA, Tohen M, Grundy S, Beasley C, Tollefson GD. Olanzapine versus haloperidol treatment in first episode psychosis. Am J Psychiatry 1999; 156: 79–87.
71. Arvanitis LA, Miller BG and the "Seroquel" I3 study group. Multiple fixed dose of "Seroquel" in patients with acute exacerbation of schizophrenia: a comparison with haloperidol and placebo. Biol. Psychiatry 1997; 42: 233–245.
72. McManus DG, Arvanitis LA, Kowalcyk BB. Quetiapine, a novel antipsychotic: experience in elderly patients with psychotic disorders. J Clin Psychiatry 1999; 60: 292–298.
73. Claghorn J, Hongfield G, Abuzzahab FS, et al. Risks and benefits of clozapine versus chlorpromazine. J Clin Psychopharmacol 1987; 7: 377–384.
74. Chengappa KN, Shelton MD, Baker RW, Schooler NR, Baird J, Delaney J. The prevalence of akathisia in patients receiving stable doses of clozapine. J Clin Psychiatry 1994; 55: 142–144.
75. Kurz M, Hummer M, Oberbauer H, Fleischacker WW. Extrapyramidal side-effects of clozapine and haloperidol. Psychopharmacology 1995; 118: 52–56.
76. Miller CH, Mohr F, Umbricht D, Woerner M, Fleischacker WW, Lieberman JA. The prevalence of acute extrapyramidal signs and symptoms in patients treated with clozapine, risperidol and conventional antipsychotics. J Clin Psychiatry 1998; 59: 69–75.
77. Cohen BM, Keck PE Satlin A, Cole JO. Prevalence and severity of akathisia in patients on clozapine. Biol. Psychiatry 1991; 29: 1215–1219.
78. Lipinski JFJ, Mallya G, Zimmerman P, Pope HGJ. Fluoexetine-induced akathisia: clinical and theoretical implications. J Clin Psychiatry 1989; 50: 339–342.
79. Settle ECJ. Akathisia and sertraline [letter]. J Clin Psychiatry 1993; 54: 321.
80. Klee B, Kronig MH. Case report of probable sertraline-induced akathisia. Am J Psychiatry 1993; 150: 836–837.
81. LaPorta LD. Setraline-induced akathisia. J Clin Psychopharmacol 1993; 13: 219–220.
82. Shihabuddin L, Rapport D. Sertraline and extrapyramidal side effects. Am J Psychiatry 1994: 151–288.
83. Adler LA, Angrist B. Paroxetine and akathisia. Biol Psychiatry 1995; 37: 336–337.
84. Baldasano CF, Truman CJ, Neurenberg H, Ghoemi SN, Sachs JS. Akathisia: a review and report following paroxetine treatment. Compr Psychiatry 199; 37: 122–124.
85. Eberstein S, Adler LA, Angrist B. Nefazodone and akathisia. Biol. Psychiatry 1996; 40: 798–799.

86. Teicher MH, Glod C, Cole JD. Emergence of intense suicidal preoccupation during flu-oxetine treatment. Am J Psychiatry 1990; 147: 207–210.

87. Opler LA. Fluoxetine and preoccupation with suicide [letter]. Am J Psychiatry 1991; 148: 1259.

88. Wirshing WC, Van Putten T, Rosenberg J, et al. Fluoxetine, akathisia, and suicidality: is there causal connection? [letter with comment] Arch Gen Psychiatry 1992; 49: 580–581.

89. Hamilton MS, Opler LA. Akathisia, suicidality and fluoxetine. J Clin Psychiatry 1992; 53: 401–406.

90. Ayd, FJ Jr. The present status of akathisia [letter]. J Nerv Ment Disord 1991; 179: 208–210.

91. ACNP Task Force. Suicidal behavior and psychotropic medication. Neuropschophar-macology 1993; 8: 177–183.

92. Meltzer HY, Young M, Metz J, et al. Extrapyramidal side effects and increases of serum prolactin following fluoxetine, a new antidepressant. J Neur Transm 1979; 45: 165–175.

93. Goldstein JM, Litwin LC, Malick JB. Ritanserin increases spontaneous activity of A9 and A10 dopamine neurons [abstract]. 1987; Fed Proc 46: 966.

94. Dewey SL, Smith GS, Logan J, et al. Serotonergic modulation of striatal dopamine mea-sured with positron emission tomography (PET) and in vivo microdialysis. J Neurosci 1995; 15: 821–829.

95. Chouinard G, Ross-Chouinard A, Annable L, Jones BD. Extrapyramidal rating scale. Can J Neurol Sci 1980; 7: 233.

96. Bartels M, Gaertner HJ, Golfinopoulis G. Akathisia syndrome: involvement of noradren-ergic mechanisms. J. Neural Trans 1981; 52: 33–39.

97. Kabes J, Sikora J, Pisvejc J, Hanzlicek L, Skondia V. Effect of piracetam on extrapyramidal side effects induced by neuroleptic drugs. Int Pharmacopsychiatry 1982; 17: 185–192.

98. Friis T, Christensen TR, Gerlach J. Sodium valproate and biperiden in neuroleptic-induced akathisia, parkinsonism and hyperkinesia: a double-blind cross-over study with placebo. Acta Psychiatr Scand 1982; 67: 178–187.

99. Fleischacker WW, Bergmann KJ, Perovich R, et al. The Hillside Akathisia Scale: a new rating instrument for neuroleptic-induced akathisia. Psychopharmacol Bull 1989; 25: 222–226.

100. Mazure CM, Cellar JS, Bowers MB, Nelson JC, Takeshita J, Zigun B. Assessment of extrapyramidal symptoms during acute neuroleptic treatment. J Clin Psychiatry 1995; 56: 94–100.

101. Sachdev P. A rating scale for acute drug induced akathisia: development, reliability and validity. Biol Psychiatry 1994; 35: 263–271.

102. Adler L, Duncan E, Kim A, Hemdal P, Rotrosen J, Angrist B. Akathisia: selective beta blockers and rating instruments. Psychopharmcol Bull 1989; 25: 451–456.

103. Braude WM, Charles IP, Barnes TRE. Coarse jerky foot tremorographic investigation of an objective sign of acute akathisia. Psychopharmocology 1984; 82: 95–101.

104. Rapoport A, Stein D, Grinshpoon A, Elizur A. Akathisia and pseudoakathisia: clinical observations and accelerometric ratings. J Clin Psychiatry 1994; 55: 493–497.

105. Tuisku K, Lauevma A, Holi M, Markula J, Rimon R. Measuring neuroleptic induced akathisia by 3 channel actometry. Schizophr Res 1999; 40: 105–110.

106. Cunningham SL, Richardson GA, Dorsey CM. Polysomographic features of akathisia syndrome in two patients. Sleep Res 1991; 20: 62.

107. Walters AS, Hening W, Rubinstein M, Chokroverty S. A clinical and polysominographic comparison of neuroleptic induced akathisia and the ideopathic restless leg syndrome. Sleep 1991; 14: 339–345.

108. Lipinski JF, Hudson JI, Cunningham SL, et al. Polysominographic characteristics of neuroleptic-induced akathisia. Clin Neuropharmacol 1991; 14: 413–419.
109. Cunningham SL, Winkelman JW, Dorsey CM, et al. An electromyographic marker for neuroleptic induced akathisia: preliminary measures of sensitivity and specificity. Clin Neuropharmacol 1996; 19: 321–332.
110. Blake DR, Williams AC, Pall WS, Fonsero A, Beswick T. Iron and akathisia. Br Med J 1986; 292: 1393.
111. Pall WS, Williams AC, Blake DR. Iron, akathisia and antipsychotic drugs. Lancet 1986 II. 1469.
112. Brown KW, Glen SE, White T. Low serum iron status and akathisia. Lancet 1987 I: 1234–1236.
113. Horiguchi J. Low serum iron in patients with neuroleptic-induced akathisia and dystonia under antipsychotic drug treatment. Acta Psychiatr Scand 1991; 84: 301–303.
114. Valles V, Guillamat R, Vilaplana C, Duno R, Almenar C, Almenar C. Serum iron and akathisia. Biol Psychiatry 1992; 31: 1174–1175.
115. Barton A, Bowie J, Ebmeier Y. Low plasma iron status and akathisia. J Neurol Neurosurg Psychiatry 1990; 53: 671–674.
116. O'Loughlin V, Dickie AC, Ebmeier K. Serum iron and transferrin in acute neuroleptic induced akathisia. J Neurol Neurosurg Psychiatry 1991; 54: 363–364.
117. Nemes ZC, Rotrosen J, Angrist B, Peselow E, Schoentag R. Serum iron levels and akathisia. Biol Psychiatry 1991; 29: 411–413.
118. Sachdev P, Loneragan C. Acute drug-induced akathisia is not associated with low serum iron status. Psychopharmacology 1991; 103: 138–139.
119. Barnes TRE, Halstead SM, Little PW. Relationship between iron status and chronic akathisia in an inpatient population with chronic schizophrenia. Br J Psychiatry 1992; 161: 791–796.
120. Soni SD, Tench D, Routledge RC. Serum iron abnormalities in neuroleptic induced akathisia in schizophrenic patients. Br J Psychiatry 1993; 163: 669–672.
121. Chengappa KNR, Baker RW, Baird J. Iron for chronic and persistent akathisia? J Clin Psychiatry 1993; 54: 320–321.
122. Gold R, Lenox RH. Is there a rationale for iron supplementation in the treatment of akathisia? A review of the evidence. J Clin Psychiatry 1995; 56: 476–483.
123. Broadhurst PL. Determinants of emotionality in the rat. 1. Situational factors. Br J Psychol 1957. 48: 7–12.
124. Russell KH, Hagenmeyer-Hauser SH, Sanberg PR. Haloperidol-induced emotional defecation: a possible model for neuroleptic anxiety syndrome. Psychopharmacology 1987; 91: 45–49.
125. Sachdev P, Brüne M. Animal models of acute drug-induced akathisia—a review. Neurosci Behav Rev 2000; 24: 269–277.
126. Teicher MH, Klein DA, Andersen SL, Wallace P. Development of an animal model of fluoxetine akathisia. Progr Neuropsychopharmacol Biol Psychiatry 1995; 19: 1305–1319.
127. Bruwyler J, Chleide E. Hobeau G, Waegeneer N, Mercier M. Differentiation of haloperidol and clozopine using a complex operant schedule in the dog. Pharmacol Biochem Behav 1993; 44: 181–189.
128. Kovacis B, Domino EF. A monkey model of tardive dyskinesia (TD): evidence that reversible TD may turn into irreversible TD. J Clin Psychopharmacol 1982; 2: 305–307.
129. Christensen AV. Long term effects of D1 and D2 antagonists in vervet monkeys. Behav Neurol 1990; 3: 49–60.

130. Zubenko GS, Barreira P, Lipinski JF. Development of tolerance to the therapeutic effect of amantadine on akathisia. J Clin Psychopharmacol 1984; 4: 218–219.

131. Kruse W. Treatment of drug-induced extrapyramidal symptoms. Dis Nerv Syst 1960; 21: 79–81.

132. Neu C, DiMascio A, Demirgian E. Antiparkinsonian medication in the treatment of extrapyramidal side-effects: single or multiple doses? Curr Ther Res 1972; 4: 246–251.

133. Merrick EM, Schmitt PP. A controlled study of the clinical effects of amantadine hydrochloride [symmetrel]. Curr Ther Res 1973; 15: 552–558.

134. DiMascio A, Bernardo DL, Greenblatt D, Marder JE. A controlled trial of amantadine in drug-induced extrapyramidal disorders. Arch Gen Psychiatry 1976; 33: 559–602.

135. Stenson RL, Donlon PT, Meyer JE. Comparison of benztropine meslyate and amantadine HCl in neuroleptic-induced extrapyramidal symptoms. Compr Psychiatry 1976; 17: 763–768.

136. Donlon P. The therapeutic use of diazepam for akathisia. Psychosomatics 1973; 14: 222–225.

137. Gagrat D, Hamilton J, Belmatier R. Intravenous diazepam in the treatment of neuroleptic-induced dystonia or akathisia. Am J Psychiatry 1978; 135: 1232–1233.

138. Kutcher SP, Mackenzie S, Galerraga W, Szalia S. Clonozepam treatment of adolescents with neurocephalic induced akathisia. Am J Psychiatry 1987; 144: 823–824.

139. Kutcher SP, Willaman P, Mackenzie S, Marton P, Church M. Successful clonazepam treatment of neuroleptic induced akathisia in older adolescents and young adults: a double-blind study. J Clin Psychopharmacol 1989; 9: 403–406.

140. Cruickshank DM. The clinical importance of cardioselectivity and lipophilicity in beta blockers. Am Heart J 1980; 100: 160–178.

141. Shanks RG. The properties of β-adrenoceptor antagonists. Postgrad Med J 1976; 52(suppl 4): 14–20.

142. Frishman WM, Sonnenblick EH. Beta-adrenergic blocking drugs. In Hurst JW, Logue RB, Rackley CE, Sonnenblick EH, Wallace AG, Wenger NK (eds) The Heart, 6th edition. New York, McGraw Hill, 1986, pp 1606–1621.

143. Guidicelli JF, Richer C, Ganansia J, Warrington S, Abriol C, Rulliere R. Betaxolol: β-adrenoceptor blocking effects and pharmacokinetics in man. In Morselli PL, Kilborn JR, Cavero I, Harrison DC, Langer SZ (eds) Betaxolol and Other Beta-Adrenoceptor Antagonists. New York, Raven Press, 1983, p. 89.

144. Shanks RG. Clinical pharmacology of β-adrenoceptor drugs. In Morselli PL, Kilborn JR, Cavero I, Harrison DC, Langer SZ (eds) Betaxolol and Other Beta-Adrenoceptor Antagonists. New York, Raven Press, 1983, pp 73–78.

145. Strang RR. The symptom of restless legs. Med J Australia 1967; 24: 1211–1213.

146. Kulik AV, Wilbur R. Case report of propranolol (Inderal) pharmacotherapy for neuroleptic-induced akathisia and tremor. Progr Neuropsychopharmacol Biol Psychiatry 1983; 7: 223–225.

147. Adler LA, Reiter S, Corwin J, Hemdal P, Angrist B, Rotrosen J. Differential effects of benztropine and propranolol in akathisia. Psychopharmacol Bull 1987; 23: 519–521.

148. Lipinski JF, Mallya G, Cohen B, Waternaux CW. A double-blind, placebo controlled study of propranolol in neuroleptic-induced akathisia. In preparation. (Personal communication.)

149. Adler LA, Angrist B, Fritz P, Rotrosen J, Mallya G, Lipinski JF. Lack of efficacy of d-propranolol in neuroleptic-induced akathisia. Neuropsychopharmacology 1991; 4: 109–115.

150. Howe R, Shanks RG. Optical isomers of propranolol. Nature 1966; 210: 1336–1338.

151. Fitzgerald JD. Perspectives in adrenergic β-receptor blockade. Clin Pharmacol Ther 1969; 10: 292–306.

152. Rahn KH. Relationship between adrenergic blocking and antihypertensive effects of beta receptor antagonists. Adv Clin Pharmacol 1976; 11: 14–18.

153. Reiter S, Adler L, Erle S, Duncan E. Neuroleptic-induced akathisia treated with pindolol. Am J Psychiatry 1987; 144: 383–384.

154. Adler LA, Reiter S, Angrist B, Rotrosen J. Pindolol and propranolol in neuroleptic-induced akathisia. Am J Psychiatry 1987; 144: 1241–1242.

155. Ratey JJ, Sorgi P, Polakoff S. Nadolol as a treatment for akathisia. Am J Psychiatry 1985; 142: 640–642.

156. Adler LA, Angrist B, Weinreb H, Rotrosen J. Studies on the time course and efficacy of β-blockers in neuroleptic-induced akathisia and the akathisia of idiopathic Parkinson's disease. Psychopharmacol Bull 1991; 27: 107–111.

157. Wells BG, Cold JA, Marken DA, et al. A placebo-controlled trial of nadolol in the treatment of neuroleptic-induced akathisia. J Clin Psychiatry 1991; 52: 255–260.

158. Dupuis B, Catteau J, Dumon J-P, Libert C, Petit H. Comparison of propranolol, sotalol, and betaxolol in the treatment of neuroleptic-induced akathisia. Am J Psychiatry 1987; 144: 802–805.

159. Derom E, Elinck W, Buylaert W, Van Der Straeten M. Which β-blocker for the restless leg? Lancet 1984; i: 857.

160. Reiter S, Adler L, Angrist B, Corwin J, Rotrosen J. Atenolol and propranolol in neuroleptic-induced akathisia. J Clin Psychopharmacol 1987; 7: 279–280.

161. Patterson JF. Pseudoakathisia associated with atenolol. J Clin Psychopharmacol 1986; 6: 390.

162. Silver JM, Yudofsky SC, Kogan M, Katz BI. Elevation of thioridazine plasma levels by propranolol. Am J Psychiatry 1986; 143: 1290–1292.

163. Greendyke RM, Kanter DR. Plasma propranolol levels and their effect on thioridazine and haloperidol concentrations. J Clin Psychopharmacol 1987; 7: 178–182.

164. Zubenko GS, Lipinski JF, Cohen BM, Barriera PJ. Comparison of metoprolol and propranolol in the treatment of akathisia. Psychiatry Res 1984; 11: 143.

165. Koch-Weser J. Metoprolol. N Engl J Med 1979; 301: 698–703.

166. Kim A, Adler L, Angrist B, Rotrosen J. Efficacy of low-dose metoprolol in neuroleptic-induced akathisia. J Clin Psychopharmacol 1989; 9: 294–296.

167. Adler LA, Angrist B, Rotrosen J. Metoprolol versus propranolol. Biol Psychiatry 1990; 27: 673–675.

168. Barrett AM. Therapeutic applications of β-adrenoceptor antagonists. In Morselli PL, Kilborn JR, Cavero I, Harrison DC, Langer SZ (eds) Betaxolol and Other Beta-Adrenoceptor Antagonists. New York, Raven Press, 1983, pp. 65–72.

169. Adler LA, Angrist B, Rotrosen J. Efficacy of betaxolol in neuroleptic-induced akathisia. Psychiatry Res 1991; 39: 193–198.

170. Adler L, Duncan E, Angrist B, Hemdal P, Rotrosen J, Slotnick V. Effects of a specific β_2 receptor blocker in neuroleptic-induced akathisia. Psychiatry Res 1989; 27: 1–4.

171. Langer SZ. Presynaptic receptors and their role in the regulation of transmitter release. Br J Pharmacol 1977; 60: 481–497.

172. Bersani G, Grispini A, Marinia S, Pasini A, Valducci M, Ciani N. Neuroleptic-induced extrapyramidal side effects: clinical perspectives with ritanserin (R 55667), a new selective 5-HT2 receptor blocking agent. Curr Ther Res 1986; 40: 492–499.

173. Miller C, Fleischhacker WW, Ehrmann H, Kane JM. Treatment of neuroleptic induced akathisia with the 5HT2 antagonist ritanserin. 1990; Psychopharmacol Bull 1990; 26: 373–376.

174. Miller CH, Hummer M, Pycha R, Fleischhacker WW. The effect of ritanserin on treatment-resistant neuroleptic-induced akathisia: case reports. Progr Neuropsychopharmacol Biol Psychiatry 1992; 16: 247–251.

175. Weiss D, Aizenberg D, Hermesh H, et al. Cyproheptadine treatment in neuroleptic-induced akathisia. Br J Psychiatry 1995; 167: 483–486.

176. Poyurovsky M, Weizman A. Serotonergic agents in the treatment of acute neuroleptic-induced akathisia: open-label study of buspirone and mainserin. Int Clin Psychopharmacol 1997; 12: 263–268.

177. Poyurovsky M, Fuchs C, Weizman A. Low-dose mianserin in the treatment of acute neuroleptic-induced akathisia. J Clin Psychopharmacol 1998; 18: 253–254.

178. Poyurovsky M, Weizman A, Mirtazapine for neuroleptic-induced akathisia. Am J Psychiatry 2001; 158: 819.

179. Poyurovsky M, Shardorodsky M, Fuchs C, Schneidman M, Weitzman A. Treatment of neuroleptic-induced akathisia with the 5-HT$_2$ antagonist mainserin: double-blind, placebo-controlled study. Br J Psychiatry 1999; 174: 238–242.

180. Fischel T, Hermesh H, Aizenberg D, et al. Cyproheptidine versus propranolol for the treatment of acute neuroleptic-induced akathisia: a comparative double-blind study. J Clin Psychopharmocol 2001; 1: 612–615.

181. Poyurovsky M, Weizman A. Lack of efficacy of the 5-HT$_2$ receptor antagonist granisetron in the treatment of acute neuroleptic-induced akathisia. Int Clin Psychopharmacol 1999; 14: 357–360.

182. Poyurovsky M, Weizman A. Serotonin-based pharmacotherapy for acute neuroleptic-induced akathisia: a new approach to an old problem. Br J Psychiatry 2001; 179: 4–8.

183. Lang AE, Johnson K. Akathisia in idiopathic Parkinson's disease. Neurology 1987; 37: 477–481.

184. Kris I, Tyson LB, Grolla RF. Extrapyramidal reaction with high dose metoclopramide. N Engl J Med 1983; 309: 433.

185. Lang AE. Akathisia and the restless leg syndrome. In Janovic J, Tolosa E (eds) Parkinson's Disease and Movement Disorders, 2nd edition. Baltimore, MD, Lippincott, Williams and Wilkins, 1993, pp. 399–418.

186. Jacobs MB. Diltiazem and akathisia. Ann Intern Med 1983; 99: 794–795.

187. Chouza C, Chamano JL, Aljanati R, Scaramelli A, DeMedina O, Romero S. Parkinsonism, tardive dyskathisia, akathisia and depression induced by flunarizine. Lancet 1986; 1: 1303–1304.

188. Mecheli F, Pardal MF, Gotto M, et al. Flunarizine and cinnarizine-induced extrapyramidal reactions. Neurology 1987; 37: 881–884.

189. Ross DR, Walker J, Peterson J. Akathisia induced by amoxapine. Am J Psychiatry 1983; 140: 115–116.

190. Hullett FJ, Levy AB. Amoxapine-induced akathisia [Letter]. Am J Psychiatry 1983; 140: 820.

191. Channalbasavanna SM, Goswami V. Akathisia during lithium prophylaxis [Letter]. Br J Psychiatry 1984; 144: 555–556.

192. Godfraind T, Towse G, Vanrueter JM, Cinnarizine: a selective calcium entry blocker. Drugs Today 1982; 18: 27–42.

193. Holmes B, Bragden RN, Heel RC, Speight TM, Avery GS. Flunarizine: a review of the pharmacodynamic and pharmacokinetic properties and therapeutic use. Drugs 1984; 27: 6–44.

194. Leysen JE, Gonmerin W. Receptor-binding profile of flunarizine: preclinical research report. Janssen Pharmaceutical Research Laboratories R 14950/24, March 1983.

195. Adler L, Duncan EJ, Reiter S, Angrist B, Peselow E, Rotrosen J. Effects of calcium channel antagonists on tardive dyskinesia and psychosis. Psychopharmacol Bull 1988; 24: 421–425.
196. Friedman E, Gershon S. Effect of lithium on brain dopamine. Nature 1973; 243: 520–521.
197. Breier A, Su TP, Saunders R, et al. Schizophrenia is associated with elevated amphetamine-induced synapic dopamine concentrations: evidence from a novel positron emission tomography method. Proc Natl Acad Sci USA 1997; 94: 2569–2574.
198. Dewey S, Brodie JD, Fowler JS, et al. Positron emission tomography (PET) studies of dopaminergic/cholinergic interactions in baboon brain. Synapse 1990; 6: 321–327.
199. Wiesel FA. Effects of high dose propranolol treatment on dopamine and norepinephrine metabolism in regions of mouse brain. Neurosci Lett 1976; 2–35–38.
200. Bailey EV, Stone TW. The mechanism of action of amantadine in parkinsonism: a review. Arch Int Pharmacodyn 1975; 216: 246–262.
201. Jackisch R, Link T, Neufang B, Koch R. Studies on the mechanism of action of the antiparkinson drugs memantine and amantadine: no evidence for direct dopaminergic or antimuscarinic properties. Arc Int Pharmacodyn 1992; 320: 21–42.
202. Dewey SL, Smith GS, Logan J, et al. GABAergc inhibition of endogenous dopamine release measured in vivo with C^{11} raclopride and positron emission tomography. J Neurosci 1992; 12: 3773–3780.

CHAPTER 8

Neuroleptic malignant syndrome

Stewart A. Factor

History

Neuroleptic malignant syndrome (NMS) is a potentially fatal drug-induced movement disorder that was first described by Delay and associates in 1960 during the proceedings of the Societé Medico-Psychologique [1]. This presentation was a communication on the efficacy and safety of haloperidol. Initially referred to as the "syndrome malin," in their chapter in the *Handbook of Clinical Neurology* [2], the term neuroleptic "malignant" syndrome was introduced. This was the first English report on the subject and they described it as the "most serious but also the rarest and least known of complications of neuroleptic chemotherapy." Three main groups of signs were discussed. Changes in the "general condition" included hyperthermia and pallor. Psychomotor signs included "akinesis with a greater or lesser degree of stupor, or hypertonicity and varying dyskinesias." It was initially thought that these signs were seen exclusively in "brain-damaged" individuals. Finally, "signs in the lungs" included congestion and infarction with resultant dyspnea and asphyxia. The poor prognosis was clear "... death in hyperthermia supervenes unless appropriate measures are instituted in time." These measures included discontinuation of antipsychotic medications, rehydration, and correction of electrolyte abnormalities. They suggested antipyrexic medication, including chlorpromazine (a drug now known to cause neuroleptic malignant syndrome) and antiparkinsonian medications in the later stages, if necessary.

After the original description the syndrome remained relatively unknown, as it was underdiagnosed, underrecognized, and rarely reported. Approximately 60 cases were published over two decades before 1980 when Caroff [3] reviewed them. Most were from the French literature, and few were from the United States. In addition, NMS received little or no attention in psychiatric and psychopharmacological textbooks. At that time, it was believed that NMS was related only to treatment with high-potency neuroleptics. Caroff's landmark review stimulated increased interest and recognition and has been followed by numerous reports, studies, and reviews. All neuroleptics have now been implicated in the development of the disorder including atypical agents (see Chapter 11). In addition, it is now clear that NMS is not just related to neuroleptic use. In 1981, Burke and associates [4] reported NMS in a patient with Huntington's disease treated with the dopamine-depleting agent, tetrabenazine, with several other reports following, and in the same year NMS was reported in patients with Parkinson's disease after sudden withdrawal of their dopaminergic medications [5]. These situations strongly suggest that NMS is related to an alteration in dopaminergic transmission in the CNS [6]. Based on this hypothesis, it was in 1983 that treatment with the dopamine agonist, bromocriptine, was recommended [7]. Over the last two decades there is a better understanding of the clinical features and pathophysiology, which has resulted in a rational treatment regimen and improved outcomes.

Clinical aspects

Signs and symptoms (Table 8.1)

The principal clinical features of NMS are hyperthermia, muscle rigidity, autonomic dysfunction, and mental status changes. The presence and severity of each of these can be quite varied from case to case. Hyperthermia is present in nearly all cases of NMS [8–10]. Rare afebrile patients have been reported [11] but these cases may not actually represent NMS cases [12]. Patients may have low-grade temperature or one as high as 42.2°C [13]. Addonizio et al. [14] reported temperatures above 38°C (100.4°F) in 92% of patients, temperatures equal to or higher than 40°C (104°F) in 40% of patients, and temperatures equal to or higher than 41°C (105.8°F) in 13%. The elevation in temperature usually occurs either at the same time or after the onset of motor signs [15]. It usually reaches a peak within 48 hours [9].

Muscle rigidity is typically described as being "lead pipe" or "plastic" in nature [3, 8, 13, 16]. Cogwheel rigidity, as seen in parkinsonism, has also been described but less frequently [17]. Rigidity is reported in over 90% of patients [8–10, 14, 18]; however, a small portion of them may not be rigid [12, 19, 20] although it has been questioned as to whether these nonrigid cases actually had NMS [12]. When present, the rigidity may be severe enough to result in a decrease in chest wall compliance resulting in tachypenic hypoventilation

Table 8.1 Clinical signs of neuroleptic malignant syndrome

Hyperthermia
Muscle rigidity:
  Lead pipe, plastic, cogwheel
Autonomic dysfunction:
  Respiratory – tachypena, dyspnea
  Cardiovascular – arrhythmia, tachycardia, lability of blood pressure, hypotension, hypertension
  Other – diaphoresis, pallor, flushing of the skin, urinary incontinence, dysuria
Mental status change:
  Agitation, lethargy, muteness, confusion, delirium, catatonia, stupor, coma
Movement disorders:
  Akinesia, bradykinesia, tremor, dystonia, chorea, myoclonus
Other neurological signs:
  Seizures, ataxia, nystagmus, gaze paresis, ocular fluttering, reflex changes, Babinski signs

requiring respiratory support [16, 21]. The presence of rigidity has led some investigators to conclude that NMS is simply a severe form of drug-induced parkinsonism [22]; however, the obvious differences between these two disorders makes this unlikely [23]. Musculoskeletal complications resulting from muscle rigidity include joint dislocations, muscle loss with secondary avulsions, and orthopedic deformities of the hands and feet if the disorder is prolonged [24, 25]. Rigidity of the muscles of the pharynx and esophagus may also result in dysphagia, dysarthria, and sialorrhea [10, 13, 24]. Other parkinsonian features may accompany the rigidity. Akinesia (the loss of voluntary movements) and/or bradykinesia (slowness of movement) have frequently been described as features of NMS [3, 8, 13, 16, 21] occurring in nearly 40% in one study [8]. Tremor has also been well described with NMS [9, 10, 13, 16, 26–28]. Resting tremor, similar to that seen in Parkinson's disease [10] and a coarse tremulousness of the trunk and extremities has been described [9]. Tremor occurs in approximately half of the patients with this syndrome [8, 10, 14]. In addition, parkinsonian gait disorder has been occasionally described; however, the frequency is difficult to assess since most patients are unable to walk [9].

Varying dyskinesias were mostly reported in early papers on NMS [1–3]. Dystonia is probably the most frequent, occurring in approximately one third of patients [8, 10, 14, 27, 29]. Blepharospasm [10], opisthotonos [10, 21, 30], oculogyric crises [10, 16, 21, 30], and trismus [10, 21, 30] may all represent manifestations of this movement disorder. Chorea, including orobuccolingual dyskinesia, has also been well described [10, 13, 21, 30] and is probably less frequent than dystonia [10]. Myoclonus has occasionally been seen [26]. Other less common neurological features include seizures, Babinski signs, reflex changes, ataxia, nystagmus, gaze paresis, and ocular fluttering [10, 11, 15, 21, 30–35].

Autonomic abnormalities other than hyperthermia are also frequently present. Cardiovascular autonomic changes include tachycardia, cardiac arrhythmias, and instability of blood pressure. Hypertension, hypotension, and lability of blood pressure have all been described [3, 9, 10, 13–16, 21, 24, 30, 36]. Diastolic hypertension has been found to be common and perhaps a specific early feature of NMS [14, 24]. This may allow early detection when monitoring patients at risk. Autonomic changes affecting the respiratory system result in tachypnea, dyspnea, and pulmonary edema [3, 9, 10, 16, 20, 30]. Other dysautonomic features include diaphoresis, pallor, flushing of the skin, urinary incontinence, and dysuria [3, 9–16, 21, 24, 30, 36].

Alterations in mental status are a hallmark of NMS. In the early stages, there may be various degrees of fluctuating alertness. Patients may go from being alert, responsive, and perhaps even agitated to being more lethargic and mute. During this period, emotional distress, confusion, and delirium may predominate [9, 24]. Some suggest that the variations in behavior associated with muteness, immobility, and lack of response may be the result of catatonic behavior [36]. Although mutism is a common manifestation of catatonia, it is not specific. Various combinations of the "classic" features should be present if a diagnosis of catatonia is to be considered. These features include catalepsy, waxy flexibility, automatic obedience, stereotypic mannerisms, and echophenomenon often associated with extremes of hyper- and hypoactivity [37].

At least three of these features should be present. These symptoms are not typically exhibited in NMS [37]. In general, catatonics frequently become withdrawn and lack any desire to cooperate or communicate. However, NMS patients have been described as attempting to communicate but being unable to because of their muteness. In such cases, they are not actually withdrawn [38]. In addition, patients have been described as having "a striking, frightened facial expression." These patients apparently have an inability to speak because of an impending sense of doom and a high level of anxiety [9]. These findings would suggest that true catatonia does not occur very often in NMS but catatonic signs may be seen [39]. In the later stages, the fluctuating mental status may lead to depressed consciousness, stupor, and coma [3, 13, 16, 21, 36]. Some variation in consciousness occurs in 75% of patients [10]. There have been occasional cases where the initial feature is psychosis with delusions, inattention, hallucinations, and disorganized thinking followed by the more typical symptoms [40]. This may lead to delayed diagnosis.

Laboratory features (Table 8.2)

Laboratory findings in NMS are nonspecific but supportive of the diagnosis. There are two abnormalities, in particular, which are consistently found. The first is an elevation of creatine kinase (CK) [3, 9–11, 13, 18, 21, 30, 36]. In reviews of previously reported cases, elevated CK was found in 44% [10], 71% [18], 92% [8], and 97% [14]. In a prospective evaluation of 24 consecutive patients with NMS, CK was elevated in all cases in which it was measured [9]. Elevations vary widely from >200 to hundreds of thousands. In one study [9], 86% had elevations above 1000 IU/L and 33% had elevations higher than 10,000 IU/L. The mechanism of CK elevation probably relates to myonecrosis developing during intense sustained muscle rigidity. Monitoring the CK levels can be a useful way of tracking the course of the syndrome. Polymorphonuclear leukocytosis is the other commonly reported abnormality [3, 8–11, 13, 14, 18, 21, 30]. The elevation can be anywhere from 10,000 to 30,000 cells per mm [3, 21]. It

Table 8.2 Laboratory features of neuroleptic malignant syndrome

Elevated creatine kinase
Polymorphonuclear leukocytosis
Elevated aldolase, alkaline phosphatase, LDH, SGOT, SGPT
Hypocalcemia
Hypomagnesemia
Hypoferremia
Proteinuria
Myoglobinuria

occurs in half to three-quarters of patients with NMS [9, 10, 18]. It may or may not be associated with a left shift. Other enzyme abnormalities include elevated aldolase, alkaline phosphatase, lactate dehydrogenase, SGOT, and SGPT [9, 10, 21, 30]. Although many of these enzyme abnormalities were originally thought to be hepatic in origin, Rosebush et al. [9] have discussed the more likely possibility that these changes originate from muscle. All enzymes are elevated to a much lesser extent than CK. Only 14% of cases had an elevation in LDH above 1000 IU/L. SGOT, which is elevated in about 80% of patients, rarely goes above 700 IU/L, and SGPT, elevated in 64%, is rarely greater than 500 IU/L. Alkaline phosphatase has been elevated in a small number of patients and bilirubin is always normal [9]. Other features include hypocalcemia, which may be due to rhabdomyolysis. This was found to be present in about half of those with NMS and in all patients with CK elevated above 10,000 IU/L. Hypomagnesemia was also observed in over 60% of patients [9] and hyponatremiais was also occasionally seen [20]. Serum iron levels have been found to be diminished in 95% of patients within a week. The etiology of this hypoferremia is thought to be related to muscle injury and may turn out to be an important marker for this illness [9]. The total iron-binding capacity and ferritin levels are normal. Finally, thrombocytopenia has rarely been associated with NMS but this relationship remains unclear [41]. At least one fatality occurred because of disseminated intravascular coagulation. Abnormalities seen on urinalysis include proteinuria and myoglobinuria [9, 21].

Computerized tomography scans, radionuclide brain scans, and cerebrospinal fluid evaluation are typically normal in NMS [8–10, 14, 21, 30, 36, 38]. Electroencephalogram may be normal or shows signs of diffuse slowing without focal changes. These findings are usually suggestive of a metabolic encephalopathy [3, 8–11, 13, 14, 18, 21, 30, 32, 36, 38].

Diagnosis

There is no stereotyped manner in which NMS presents making diagnosis difficult. The DSM-IV criteria include rigidity and fever accompanied by two of the following: diaphoresis, dysphagia, tremor, incontinence, altered mentation, mutism, tachycardia, labile blood pressure, elevated white count, and elevated creatine kinase for diagnosis [42]. However, any of the above features can herald the disorder and varied combinations may be seen. Levenson [11] also developed a set of criteria for diagnosis. They consider major criteria to be fever, rigidity, and elevated CK; minor manifestations were tachycardia, blood pressure instability, tachypnea, altered consciousness, diaphoresis, and leukocytosis. Criteria for diagnosis were met if the patient had all three major or two major and four minor manifestations in the absence of other disorders. Although these criteria are not universally accepted [15], they are helpful in making a diagnosis. One other study indicated that 80% of patients have either mental status change or rigidity [43] suggesting that both should be major features. Nevertheless, each symptom taken by itself is nonspecific and

Table 8.3 Complications of neuroleptic malignant syndrome

Respiratory
  Tachypneic hypoventilation from decreased chest wall compliance
  Aspiration pneumonia
  Pulmonary embolism
  Pulmonary edema
Cardiovascula:
  Arrhythmia
  Myocardial infarction
  Cardiovascular collapse
  Cardiac arrest
Renal
  Prerenal azotemia from dehydration
  Renal failure secondary to rhabdomyolysis and myoglobinuria
Neurological (long-term sequelae)
  Parkinsonism
  Tardive dyskinesia
  Dystonia
  Cerebellar degeneration (secondary to hyperpyrexia)
  Peripheral neuropathy
  Dementia progression
  Anoxic complications
Orthopedic
  Contractures
  Compartment syndrome

heterogeneity makes the diagnosis difficult. It is the combination of features in particular situations that should lead to a high index of suspicion.

Course and complications (Table 8.3)

Once NMS develops, it usually progresses at a rapid rate. The syndrome typically reaches peak intensity within 72 hours of onset [2, 3, 10–16, 21, 36]. However, this may vary from 45 minutes to as long as 65 days [8, 14, 26]. Features of NMS may vary in severity and combination. Some of the less severe forms may represent aborted episodes due to rapid diagnosis and intervention; however, NMS may take on a mild self-limited course that clears quickly with little or no intervention and causes very few complications or sequelae [44]. Such cases are sometimes associated with or preceded by a mild viral illness. On the other hand, a very malignant course may occur that ultimately will result in death despite rigorous treatment. The overall duration of illness has varied from 8 hours to as long as 40 days [10, 11, 13, 14, 21, 24]. This varies depending on whether oral or depot neuroleptics are the causative agents. With oral medications, NMS typically lasts about 7–14 days after discontinuing the drug; however, depot drugs increase the duration by two to three times [13–16, 21, 45].

Approximately 40% of patients with NMS suffer from medical complications, many of which are life threatening. The presence and severity of these complications depend primarily on the severity and duration of NMS. Respiratory complications are the most common cause of death in patients [13, 36]. These include tachypneic hypoventilation from decreased chest wall compliance, aspiration pneumonia probably resulting from dysphagia, pulmonary embolism secondary to thrombophlebitis, and immobility, DIC, and pulmonary edema [10, 11, 13, 16, 18, 21, 36]. Approximately 20% of patients require endotracheal intubation and respiratory support [9, 11]. Cardiovascular complications include arrhythmia, myocardial infarction, cardiac arrest, cardiovascular collapse, and phlebitis [3, 10, 11, 13, 18, 21]. Renal complications include prerenal azotemia and renal failure [3, 9, 10, 13, 18, 21]. Renal failure is generally the result of myoglobinuria from rhabdomyolysis and hemodynamic factors [8, 11]. If death occurs, it is within 30 days [3, 21, 26]. Early reviews reported a mortality rate between 11% and 30% in NMS [3, 8, 10, 11, 14, 26]. This seems to be changing as the result of increased recognition of the syndrome and early, more aggressive therapy.

Long-term sequelae have been reported in a number of patients recovering from NMS and are of significant concern. Of those abnormalities described, parkinsonism is the most frequent. It was observed in three patients followed for 5 months [9] and in four others after 10 months [46]. In one study parkinsonism was only part of the residual syndrome but lasted up to 6 months [45]. Other sequelae include permanent dystonia [8], tardive dyskinesia (oral-buccal-lingual dyskinesia) lasting up to 6 months [46, 47], peripheral neuropathy [48], and cerebellar degeneration due to hyperpyrexia [35, 49]. Several patients have had anomia that lasted several weeks. In some it cleared [9] while in others it did not [35]. One patient had a worsening of dementia that lasted 3 months before the patient returned to baseline [9]. In two others, the worsened dementia was still present after 10 months [46]. Caroff et al. [45] reported five patients who had, as residual effects, catatonic signs lasting 1–6 months including stupor, coma, mutism, and rigidity. Two of three responded to ECT. Should anoxia occur during an episode, complications such as memory deficits and alterations in level of consciousness may be observed [8].

Several sequelae from orthopedic complications have also been reported. One paper described a man who developed bilateral forearm compartment syndromes as a result of the rhabdomyolysis that occurred with NMS [50]. After surgical intervention it took 2 years before full recovery was achieved. Flexion contractures of upper or lower extremities may occur due to a bed-ridden state and severe dystonia. Physical therapy and botulinum toxin injections have been utilized to treat these problems that may persist for months or longer [51, 52].

Situations resulting in NMS (Table 8.4)

NMS was originally described in psychiatric patients treated with neuroleptics [1–3] It is now clear that this syndrome is not confined to psychiatric patients only but can occur in any patient treated with neuroleptics [6, 53]. All

Table 8.4 Situations resulting in NMS

Psychiatric patients (any diagnosis)
   Treated with neuroleptic for the first time
   Treated with a neuroleptic after a drug free period
   Increase in neuroleptic dose or potency
   Stable dose of neuroleptics accompanied by dehydration or metabolic disturbance
   Sudden withdrawal of parkinsonian drugs (i.e., amantadine)
Nonpsychiatric, non-neurological patients
   Treatment with neuroleptics for sedation, anxiety or sleep disturbance
   Treatment with antiemetics (metoclopramide, prochlorperazine)
   Cocaine abuse
Neurological disease
   AIDS dementia treated with neuroleptics
   Use of tetrabenazine in neurological disease
   Parkinson's disease
      Sudden withdrawal of medications for
         Drug holiday
         Hospitalized patients
         Patient decision due to side effects
         Surgical patients
         DBS patients
      Medication adjustments
      Treatment with neuroleptics – typical and atypical, or lithium
      Off periods
      Premenstrual

groups of neuroleptics have been associated with NMS, including phenothiazines, butyrophenones, thioxanthenes, and atypical agents. The drugs most commonly associated with this disorder are haloperidol and fluphenazine alone or in combination with other neuroleptics [3, 9, 10, 13, 16, 18, 21, 36]. Levenson [11] has suggested that the high association with haloperidol may be related to its frequent use. In most cases, serum levels are therapeutic and not toxic, suggesting that this is not related to drug toxicity [13, 38, 54]. Despite these findings, other studies have indicated that it still may be dose related [9]. Allan and White [28] revealed a clear relationship between drug concentrations and NMS. In their case, signs improved as concentrations of urinary fluphenazine metabolites decreased. In addition, duration of therapy does not appear to be important. Neuroleptic potency may also play an important role given the more frequent occurrence of NMS with more potent agents and depot agents. Despite this, several cases have occurred in apparently susceptible individuals with low doses or from low potency agents [50, 55].

Sixty percent of patients have a history of earlier uncomplicated neuroleptic exposure before the onset of NMS [9]. The disorder usually occurs either when patients are treated for the first time, when neuroleptics are reintroduced after a drug-free interval, or if the dose is increased within a short time [3, 8, 9, 14]. The onset of NMS occurs within 24 hours of initiating the drug in more than 20% patients, within the first week in about 60% and within a month in nearly all patients in whom it occurs [56]. In a small number of cases, NMS may develop while the patient receives a stable dose of neuroleptics [57]. In these patients, it is possible that other risk factors such as agitation and dehydration may play an important role in the onset of the syndrome [9]. Psychiatric patients are frequently given amantadine to treat or prevent extrapyramidal side effects. In two reports, NMS occurred with cessation of this drug [58, 59]. An unusual picture is the apparent occurrence of NMS in psychiatric patients who had their neuroleptics reduced abruptly or stopped [60, 61]. In these patients, the syndrome probably began before the drug doses were diminished and continued to progress to a clearly recognizable stage after the drugs were stopped [60].

Patients with any psychiatric diagnosis who are prescribed a neuroleptic are at risk for NMS. Evaluation of psychiatric diagnoses preceding the onset of NMS indicates that approximately 50% of patients have schizophrenia [8, 10, 11, 14]. Affective disorders have been reported less commonly in some studies [14–18]; however, in a 6-year prospective study, two-thirds of the patients diagnosed had an underlying affective disorder [9]. Other psychiatric diagnoses have included acute psychosis, atypical psychosis, brief reactive psychosis, schizophreniform psychosis, paranoia, character disorder, and postpartum psychosis [3, 8–11, 14, 62].

Finally, treatment with a combination of a neuroleptic and lithium may result in a more severe course of NMS [16, 46]. Lithium by itself does not cause NMS. In the acute manic state of manic-depressive psychosis, neuroleptics are frequently utilized in combination with lithium. Since lithium requires 5 to 10 days to become effective, neuroleptics are given for immediate amelioration of symptoms [46, 47]. In 1974, Cohen and Cohen [46] described a rare "severe encephalopathic syndrome" in four patients treated with lithium and haloperidol. Each patient experienced hyperpyrexia, mental status change, and parkinsonian signs and symptoms. The syndrome described by Delay and associates [1, 2] was not mentioned in the paper but the descriptions were typical of NMS. In two cases, symptoms did not clear until lithium was discontinued. All patients suffered from long-term sequelae, most notably oral-buccal-lingual dyskinesia. It was concluded that a "summative or synergistic effect" between the two drugs caused the syndrome. Interestingly, Baastrup et al. [63] reviewed the hospital records of 425 patients who had been treated with that combination and found that none had developed a syndrome resembling what Cohen and Cohen had described. Others have also argued against such an interaction [16, 21, 64]. In fact, Donaldson et al. [65] indicate that all the cases described by Cohen and Cohen were simply cases of severe lithium intoxication with persistent neurologic sequelae. My own interpretation of these cases was that at least two of them experienced NMS and all four cases had sequelae of lithium-induced toxicity so that in at least two of them the syndrome represented a combination of side effects of both drugs. Spring and Frankel [47] reported a similar case caused by the same drug combination. They noted that the syndrome was identical to NMS except for the residual dyskinesia. These residual findings suggested that lithium may have enhanced the NMS. Since lithium can worsen drug-induced parkinsonism, cause a recurrence of tardive dyskinesia, and decrease central dopaminergic transmission [66], it was felt that lithium must be playing some enhancing role in NMS [47]. In particular, it was felt that patients in the acute manic state were susceptible to NMS when treated with this drug combination [47]. Since haloperidol alone can cause NMS and tardive dyskinesia and since the lithium/haloperidol combination is commonly utilized without adverse effects, it is not surprising that this role for lithium has met with some resistance [16, 21, 47]. Currently, it is difficult to prove whether or not any relationship between lithium and NMS actually exists. Sachdev, in a case control study, did not find lithium to be a risk factor for the development of NMS [67].

NMS can occur in anyone treated with neuroleptics. Several otherwise normal individuals receiving dopamine-blocking agents have developed this syndrome. Several examples follow. A patient treated with haloperidol presurgically to induce sedation experienced NMS after a single dose [68]. A single dose of trimeprazine, a phenothiazine, utilized for sedation and pruritus, resulted in fatal NMS in a normal child [69]. Metoclopramide, an antiemetic drug, has also been reported to cause NMS [70, 71]. One patient seen personally was given a low dose of phenothiazines for hiccups and developed NMS with significant long term sequelae. Two patients developed NMS after autologous peripheral blood stem cell transplantation for neoplastic conditions [53]. These patients are frequently treated with neuroleptics in the peritransplant period.

NMS can occur in patients with various neurological diseases. Burke et al. [4] first reported NMS in a patient with Huntington's disease (HD) treated with tetrabenazine, a dopamine-depleting agent, and alpha-methyl-tyrosine in 1981. Since then two other HD patients have been reported to develop NMS with tetrabenazine [72, 73]. The doses utilized ranged from 100 to 350 mg per day and had been increased within weeks of the occurrence. Two of the cases were rechallenged without incident. In all three patients the chorea from HD disappeared when NMS occurred. Tetrabenazine causes NMS not only in HD patients but in others as well. A patient given tetrabenazine to treat tardive dystonia (history of psychosis and depression treated with thiothixene) developed NMS as well [40]. This patient was on a stable dose for years before the syndrome began. Interestingly, the dystonia improved not just during the time of NMS but for 8 months before returning to baseline. This syndrome has not been reported with reserpine, another dopamine-depleting agent. However, tetrabenazine has dopamine receptor-blocking properties as well, and this may be the cause of NMS when it occurs. This drug is not available in the United States yet. That may explain the low frequency of occurrence of NMS. When available, the treating physicians will need to be vigilant.

HIV-infected individuals represent a particularly high-risk group for NMS. Several patients have been reported [74, 75] and they usually are diagnosed with AIDS dementia. The NMS is frequently secondary to low-dose neuroleptic therapy. These patients are either treated with neuroleptics because of disease-related psychosis or other dopamine-blocking agents for nausea. The risk factors typical for NMS in psychiatric patients are similar in the HIV setting but the prognosis seems to be worse, perhaps because of lack of recognition [75]. Patients with AIDS dementia appear to be more susceptible to extrapyramidal syndromes from neuroleptics than non-HIV patients. This was confirmed by Hriso et al. [76] who retrospectively reviewed the medical records of 31 AIDS patients and 32 non-AIDS psychiatric patients, all of whom were treated with neuroleptics. The AIDS patients had an estimated 2.4 times higher likelihood of experiencing parkinsonism or dystonia. When only haloperidol therapy was taken into account the number rose to 3.4 times. This occurred despite the use of lower neuroleptic doses in the AIDS group. Current evidence supports the notion that this increased susceptibility is due to selective vulnerability of the basal ganglia and, in particular, the dopaminergic system to HIV infection [77–80]. This is demonstrated by the occurrence *de novo* of parkinsonism in AIDS patients and neuropsychological testing abnormalities similar to basal ganglia disorders such as Huntington's disease. Neuroimaging studies also demonstrate abnormalities in the basal ganglia such as reduction of the basal ganglia volume out of proportion to generalized atrophy on MRI, hypometabolism in the basal ganglia by FDG PET, and abnormalities on proton MRI spectroscopy such as decreased NAA/choline ratio in the lenticular nucleus [78, 80]. Pathological studies provide further evidence for this phenomenon. Basal ganglia bear the brunt of infection with the findings of multinucleated giant cells, microglial nodules, and HIV-infected microglia and macrophages being most prominent in the caudate nucleus and putamen [78–80]. Other pathological findings include a greater neuronal loss in the globus pallidus [81] and substantia nigra [78], high concentrations of structural envelop proteins gp41 and gp120, core protein p24 and regulatory protein Tat of the HIV in the globus pallidus, striatum, midbrain, thalamus, and dentate nucleus of the cerebellum [78–80]. Finally, it has been shown that HIV RNA is not distributed uniformly in the brain in patients with AIDS dementia. The basal ganglia represent one region that is selectively infected by the HIV virus [82]. Thus, the increased susceptibility to neuroleptics likely relates to neuronal dysfunction and loss in the basal ganglia, including substantia nigra, which, in turn, causes an increased reaction to the dopamine receptor blockade caused by the neuroleptics and increased risk of extrapyramidal syndromes including NMS.

Parkinson's disease (PD) is a neurodegenerative disorder associated with CNS dopamine depletion. Therefore, based on the hypothesis that NMS relates to decreased dopaminergic activity, it is not surprising that we see this disorder in PD patients. The syndrome seen in PD has been referred to by several names. While it is often referred to as NMS, since it is usually not related to neuroleptic therapy, others have used the terms neuroleptic malignant-like syndrome (NMLS) [83–85], parkinsonism hyperpyrexia syndrome [86], levodopa withdrawal hyperthermia, and lethal hyperthermia [87]. This disorder in PD has the same features of typical NMS, both clinical and laboratory. In the cases reported, the course has lasted 5 to 22 days. The situation that most commonly leads to NMS in PD is withdrawal of anti-PD medications as in a "drug holiday" [5, 30, 33, 83, 85, 88–90]. Drug holidays were utilized in the past to treat psychosis and severe motor complications of PD. However, because of the potentially severe consequences of this treatment strategy it is no longer (and should not be) practiced. This phenomenon has not only been seen with complete withdrawal of dopaminergic drugs but partial withdrawal as well. For instance, one patient developed NMS when immediate release levodopa was switched to controlled release and bromocriptine was tapered off from 40 mg per day to zero in a few days [91] and another developed NMS when tolcapone was stopped but levodopa was initially continued [90]. That patient worsened when the levodopa was stopped as well. NMS has also been described in patients with schizophrenia and PD who were treated with neuroleptics without adverse events but then discontinued antiparkinsonian medications, including levodopa and amantadine [30, 92]. Although drug holidays are no longer practiced there are still situations where anti-PD medications may be stopped and thus there is increased risk for NMS. One situation involves hospitalization for medical illness. It is not uncommon for medications to be held. Also, patients who have surgical procedures will often have their medications held. Since there is no injectable form of dopaminergic medication widely available at present, many patients go days without treatment. Sometimes patients take matters into their own hands and stop medications abruptly because of side effects. Patients need to be warned of the dangers of this practice. Some patients with PD and hallucinations are treated with atypical antipsychotics [93], all of which can cause NMS (see Chapter 11). Finally, subthalamic nucleus deep brain stimulation is a new surgical treatment for fluctuating PD patients. Its use has allowed for the decrease in daily levodopa dose. Some have suggested being quite aggressive with this strategy [94]. This may represent an important risk for NMS. NMS has also occurred in several patients who have not stopped medications. NMS may occur during an "off" period in patients with the "on/off" phenomenon [87]. An "off" period is pharmacologically similar to medication withdrawal. In this particular patient mild episodes were occurring over several years. On one occasion the episode was fatal in a period of 10 hours. One report described two premenstrual episodes in a patient with unchanged medications [95] and there have been patients with episodes associated with hypernatremia and hyponatremia [96]. One patient had three episodes associated with small increases in sodium (149 to 152). An NMS-like syndrome was also described in parkinsonian patients treated with lithium for "on/off" phenomenon [27], a treatment no longer utilized. There have been several deaths associated with this disorder in PD [85, 87, 88] so care must be taken when altering medications in PD patients. Fortunately, NMS is rare in PD. It is important to keep in mind that NMS can occur under the same situations in other parkinsonian syndromes such as multiple system atrophy [97].

Recently, NMS has been reported in association with cocaine abuse [98, 99]. Kosten et al. [98] reported seven people who experienced a syndrome that resulted in rapid death after cessation of acute intense cocaine abuse. Clinical features included hyperthermia, delirium, and agitation followed by akinesia and various degrees of rigidity. In each case, respiratory failure and death ensued within hours. While cocaine bingeing is known to cause an agitation syndrome with hyperthermia, delirium, respiratory arrest, and death the rigidity that characterizes NMS is usually absent with a few exceptions. However, this syndrome most likely represents a form of NMS. It has been demonstrated with ligand binding and autoradiographic methods that the dopamine system is significantly affected. In these patients there is a decreased ability to clear excess dopamine from the synapses and a reduction in the number of D2 receptors is found, particularly in the hypothalamus [99]. A similar syndrome has been described with the 3,4-methylenedioxymethamphetamine (MDMA), also known as ecstasy [100].

Differential diagnosis (Table 8.5)

There are a number of illnesses and syndromes that are characterized by features similar to NMS. In the fully developed syndrome, these disorders can be differentiated; however, in the early and very late stages, this may not be easy

Table 8.5 Differential diagnosis

Medical disorders
  Infection (encephalitis, meningitis)
  Post-infectious encephalomyelitis
  Metabolic encephalopathy
  Myocardial infarction
  Drug allergy
  Tetanus
  Strychnine poisoning
Malignant hyperthermia
Heat stroke
Lethal catatonia
Other drug reactions
  Central anticholinergic syndrome
  Monoamine oxidase inhibitor intoxication and interactions with
    Meperidine
    Dextromethorphan
    Tricyclic antidepressants
    Selective serotonin reuptake inhibitors
  Serotonin syndrome
  Other neuroleptic induced movement disorders:
    Parkinsonism
    Acute dystonia
    Tardive syndromes
  Baclofen withdrawal
  Methylphenidate intoxication
  Benzodiazepine intoxication
Polymyositis
Brainstem stroke (locked in syndrome)
Wilson's disease (acute dystonic form)

[101]. Since NMS is potentially fatal, any situation in which this diagnosis is considered warrants immediate attention.

Infection and other medical illnesses

A diagnosis of NMS is assured if other causes of febrile illness are ruled out. Most important in the differential diagnosis is *infection*. While any infection can result in elevation of temperature, central nervous system infection such as encephalitis, meningitis, or meningoencephalitis can result in elevated temperature, mental status changes, increases in muscle tone and autonomic features [9, 10, 21, 24]. Infection may be viral, bacterial, or fungal in origin. Lumbar puncture and CT scan are warranted in these patients. In many cases, antibiotic therapy is instituted concomitantly with treatment for NMS. It is important to keep in mind that NMS and infection may coexist. NMS predisposes patients to infection because of dysphagia, respiratory complications, and immobility. Infection may increase the risk of NMS [9]. Other considerations related to infection include *postinfectious encephalomyelitis* and *tetanus* [10]. When NMS arises after starting a new neuroleptic, another possibility to consider is *drug allergy* [4, 9, 30]. In one study, 7 of 20 patients had a skin rash during development of NMS [9]. Absence of eosinophilia and lack of a consistent relationship between initiation of neuroleptics and the onset of the rash make it unlikely that NMS is an allergic reaction [9, 30]. In either case, withdrawal of the offending agent is necessary. Other medical illnesses to consider include *diabetic ketoacidosis, tetany, thyrotoxicosis, metabolic encephalopathies* (renal or hepatic), *myocardial infarction* (because of elevated CK), and *strychnine poisoning* [12, 102].

Malignant hyperthermia

Malignant hyperthermia (MH) is a myopathic disorder with varied inheritance (autosomal dominant and recessive forms are reported) [4, 9, 10, 21, 30]. It generally occurs immediately after exposure to halogenated inhalation anesthesics and depolarizing muscle relaxants, such as succinylcholine. Within minutes of exposure, symptoms of hyperpyrexia, muscle rigidity, and changes in mentation occur. There is an associated elevation in CK and myoglobinurea. The disorder is felt to be a peripheral nervous system disease resulting from an abnormality of muscle membranes. In particular, there appears to be defective regulation of the transport of calcium in the sacroplasmic reticulum in the presence of general anesthetic agents. MH occurs frequently in patients who have other myopathic disorders such as muscular dystrophy, myotonic dystrophy, and congenital myopathies. In addition, there is often a family history of anesthesia-associated MH and possibly death. In those at risk for MH, there usually is an elevation in resting CK. In addition, relatives may also have a high resting level of CK. MH is treated with dantrolene sodium, a muscle relaxant that may inhibit the release of calcium ions from the sacroplasmic reticulum [10]. Because of similarities in clinical features of MH and NMS, a similar pathophysiological mechanism has been proposed. These disorders are easily differentiated by the inciting situation.

Heat stroke

Phenothiazines impair heat dissipation mechanisms by interrupting tempera-ture regulation and inhibiting sweating, especially on hot humid days and in association with exercise or agitation. This effect may relate to anticholinergic and anti-alpha adrenergic effects [35]. The resulting syndrome is *heat stroke*. This disorder manifests with hyperpyrexia, dry skin, a depressed level of con-sciousness, seizures, and pallor associated with multiple organ dysfunction. Muscle rigidity, profuse diaphoresis, and dyskinesias do not occur. The use of anticholinergic drugs in combination with neuroleptics may increase the risk of heat stroke, particularly in the elderly. This diagnosis should be considered in the differential diagnosis of NMS since the etiologic agents may be the same [4, 9, 10, 21, 30]. In either case, neuroleptics should be stopped and dehydration addressed.

Lethal catatonia

NMS resembles the psychiatric disorder *lethal catatonia* (LC), which is also re-ferred to as malignant catatonia, a rare catatonia variant. This disorder was described in the 19th century (long before neuroleptics became available) and has gone by many other names in the literature including Bell's mania, mortal catatonia, acute delirious mania, manic depressive exhaustion death, psychotic exhaustion syndrome, delirium acutum, Scheid's cyanotic syndrome, and per-nicious catatonia [103, 104]. In 1934, Stauder [105] coined the term "lethal cata-tonia" when describing 27 cases. In 1987, Kalinowsky felt a better term would be "pernicious catatonia" because it was not uniformly fatal [106]. LC repre-sents a syndrome that may occur in varying circumstances. It is most frequently seen in association with psychiatric disorders such as depression, mania, and psychosis (schizophrenia). In a small percentage (10–15%), it occurs in relation to organic illness including infection, cerebrovascular disorders, tumors, head injury, seizure disorders, and toxic-metabolic disorders [103].

Clinical features of LC occur in three phases [9, 10, 21, 30, 37, 103]. The prodromal phase, which lasts approximately 2 weeks, is characterized by a labile mood, insomnia, and anorexia. The second, hyperactive, phase is most prominent. Intense motor excitement is characterized by violent destructive behavior, unprovoked assaultiveness, and suicide attempts. There is usually disorganization of thought, incoherent speech, hallucinations (visual and au-ditory), and bizarre delusions. Patients also demonstrate the classic features of catatonia including mutism, negativism, and rigidity and refuse nutrients. Autonomic features have been reported in this phase. These include tachy-cardia, diaphoresis, labile blood pressure, and cyanosis of extremities. Fever up to 43.3°C also emerges in this phase that lasts an average of 8 days but may continue for weeks. The patients may also have laboratory abnormalities such as elevated CK, elevated WBC, and in some cases reduced serum iron. In the final phase, excitement gives way to exhaustion, electrolyte imbalance, ex-treme hyperthermia, stupor, coma, and cardiovascular collapse. In this phase, Stauder [105] described rigidity with bizarre posturing. This is not a common feature, and if rigidity is present, it is usually intermittent and alternates with flaccidity. The final phase lasts 36 hours to 4 days before death, which occurs in over 60% of the patients.

In the contemporary literature, this classic presentation is observed in approximately 70% of patients [103]. The other 30% present with a catatonic stupor without intense hyperactivity. In many of these patients, fever and rigidity occur after initiation of neuroleptics, suggesting that these may be cases of NMS in catatonic patients. Autopsy results in patients with LC have been unrevealing [103]. The pathophysiology of LC is hypothesized to be similar to NMS with abnormal dopaminergic transmission in mesolimbic/mesocortical pathways, resulting in catatonia and in the hypothalamus causing fever. This alteration occurs spontaneously and is not related to medications. The other possibility is that there is a reduction in GABAergic activity [107]. Treatment of choice in LC is electroconvulsive therapy (ECT) and benzodiazepines. Controversy surrounds the use or withdrawal of neuroleptics. Mann and associates [103] suggest that withdrawal of these medications is the best route to take. Finally, corticosteroids and ACTH have been utilized with some success.

Controversy surrounds whether LC and NMS are different entities. Some authors claim that NMS and LC may have very similar clinical features but are actually different disorders [9, 10, 21, 56], while others feel they may actually be the same disorder [107–111]. Mann and associates [103, 112] suggest that NMS might be viewed as a "neuroleptic-induced toxic or iatrogenic form of organic lethal catatonia." Similarities include fever, stupor, coma, rigidity, response to ECT, and laboratory abnormalities including low-serum iron levels. These similarities have suggested to some authors that the pathophysiology is the same and therefore the disease is the same [107, 110]. If these two entities were both forms of catatonia then one might consider that NMS actually does not exist. Similar arguments have surrounded tardive dyskinesia and have yet to be proven. It would seem that the enormous literature on NMS suggests otherwise. Furthermore, it is very possible that the recognition of NMS as a specific disorder related to neuroleptic therapy may have been delayed because of consideration that it was simply another form of catatonia associated with the subjects' psychiatric disease. For other investigators the differences are more conspicuous and can allow for differentiation on a clinical basis [56, 104]. LC does not occur in relation to neuroleptic therapy. And catatonia is not considered an essential feature of NMS and is not seen in all cases. In particular, it is not seen in nonpsychiatric patients who develop the syndrome. While mutism and akinesia are thought to be catatonic features in NMS the more distinctive features are not usually seen [56]. The extrapyramidal features of NMS are not usually seen in LC. When seen in the early stages, LC is easily distinguished from NMS since it is a syndrome of hyperactivity and resulting exhaustion and not a drug reaction. Although hyperactivity may be a risk factor in NMS, it is not as constant a feature and does not reach the extremes of that seen in LC. Some investigators [56, 112] suggest using the time of onset of hyperpyrexia to differentiate "classic" LC from NMS. In NMS, fever does not occur during excitement but afterward when the typical features emerge after neuroleptic therapy is initiated. In LC, hyperthermia starts in the excitement phase and progresses relentlessly. Treatment of the two syndromes is different indicating that the primary pathophysiological mechanisms are different. Although ECT may be useful in treating NMS, it is not the treatment of choice. NMS does not respond uniformly to benzodiazepines and LC has rarely been reported to respond to dopamine agonists or dantrolene. Finally, death rates are substantially higher in LC than NMS. It is when LC is seen in its final stage, resembling any "near-death acute confusional state," without clear history, and in the presence of neuroleptic therapy, that differentiation from NMS is difficult [104]. It may be that the similarities relate to the fact that LC and NMS overlap because LC is a risk factor for the development of NMS when neuroleptics are utilized (see risk factors) [110].

Other drug reactions

Adverse reactions to nonneuroleptic psychotropic medications may be similar to NMS, some of which have been termed "neuroleptic-like malignant" syndrome or "nonneuroleptic malignant" syndrome. The differential of these syndromes may be impossible since patients are frequently treated with multiple drugs. Patients may also have combined syndromes when treated with multiple medications [46, 113]. A *central anticholinergic syndrome* often results in confusion, mild temperature elevation, dry flushed skin, dry mouth, dilated pupils, decreased bowel sounds, and urinary retention. Superficially, this may appear similar to NMS; however, in NMS, there is diaphoresis and no change in pupillary function or dry mouth. In addition, anticholinergic toxicity does not result in rigidity or CK elevation [9, 21]. *Monoamine oxidase (MAO) inhibitors* by themselves or in combination with other monaminergic medications may result in a toxic syndrome of agitation, delirium, hyperpyrexia, convulsions, and hypertension [21, 102]. These symptoms may take up to 12 hours to develop. The concurrent administration of meperidine, dextromethorphan, or tricyclic antidepressants and monoamine oxidase inhibitors results in agitation, delirium, hypotension, hyperpyrexia, and even death. In none of these cases have patients been rigid nor have they had elevation of CK. Additional cases have been reported with zopiclone, a benzodiazepine [114], methylphenidate [115], and abrupt withdrawal of baclofen [116].

The serotonin syndrome closely resembles NMS but is caused by SSRIs or other drugs that increase brain serotonin levels. Its similarity to NMS may not be a surprise since serotonin acts to decrease dopamine levels in the brain. It generally occurs with a variety of combinations of medications but most commonly with antidepressants (tricyclics or SSRIs) in combination with nonselective MAO inhibitors. The syndrome may have onset hours to days after initiation of the combined therapy or after an increase in dose of either agent. The clinical features include motor symptoms, mental status change, and autonomic dysfunction. The motor symptoms are movement disorders, particularly myoclonus and tremor, muscle rigidity, hyperreflexia. The mental status changes include agitation, confusion, disorientation, and restlessness. Finally, autonomic instability manifests itself as low-grade fever, nausea, diarrhea, headache, shivering, flushing, diaphoresis, tachycardia, tachypnea, blood pressure change, and pupillary dilatation [117]. Laboratory changes are usually nonspecific but can involve small increases in creatine kinase and white blood cell count. Rarely, the syndrome can be associated with high fevers, seizures, oculogyric crisis, opisthotonus, and Babinski signs. Death may ensue because of DIC, myoglobinuria with renal failure, and cardiac arrhythmias. Diagnostic criteria for this syndrome have been recommended [118]. They include (1) recent increase or addition of known serotonergic agent to an established regimen; (2) at least three of the following: mental status change, agitation, myoclonus, hyperreflexia, diaphoresis, shivering, tremor, diarrhea, incoordination, fever; (3) no other possible etiologies are found; and (4) no addition or change in neuroleptics.

The cause of the serotonin syndrome is related to an excess of serotonin at 5HT1A and 5HT2 receptors and this has been demonstrated in animal models [117, 118]. The treatment involves withdrawal of the causative agents and usually the syndrome will resolve over hours to days. Patients should be closely observed until resolution and supportive measures may be given if needed including antipyretics, and IV fluids. On rare occasions patients will require treatment for myoclonus with clonazepam, lorazepam, or anticholinergics. Antiserotonergic medications such as cyproheptadine, methylsergide, or propranolol are helpful.

There has been some question about the association of the serotonin syndrome with the use of antidepressants combined with selegiline in PD patients. The package insert for selegiline contains a warning. This issue has been studied in some detail [119] and it has been found that 0.24% of PD patients treated with this combination have symptoms possibly consistent with this syndrome and 0.04% of patients had a serious disorder. There have been no deaths in PD patients. None of the PD patients treated with this combination experienced myoclonus, a key feature of the disorder. Fluoxetine may inhibit the metabolism of selegiline therefore leading to accumulation of the drug and loss of MAO-B selectivity. Since serotonin is mainly metabolized by MAO-A it is this scenario that probably leads to symptoms in those patients experiencing the adverse event. Thus, because the syndrome is so rare in PD, in some patients the benefit might outweigh the risks in utilizing this combination of medications.

Other syndromes

Other syndromes inducing increased muscle tone, akinesia, dyskinesia, and elevations in CK can be differentiated from NMS on the basis of the history and physical findings. These include *neuroleptic-induced parkinsonism, acute dystonic reactions, tardive dyskinesia/dystonia,* and *combined drug-induced extrapyramidal syndromes* [11, 120, 121] *Polymyositis* and *brain stem infarction* resulting in a "locked in" syndrome might also be considered. Finally, the rare *acute dystonic form of Wilson's disease,* which occurs preterminally and is characterized by dystonia, rigidity, fever, and rapid emaciation should be considered. One case has been reported with elevated serum CK. This disorder may be difficult to differentiate from NMS, particularly if the diagnosis of Wilson's disease is not known [122].

Epidemiology

The incidence of NMS is not known but it is rare. A number of publications (reviews, retrospective and prospective studies) have reported that the incidence ranges from 0.01% to greater than 2% in those treated with neuroleptics [3, 8, 12, 21, 57, 123–125]. However, the three separate prospective evaluations since 1987 have reported frequencies below 1% [57, 123, 125]. Keck et al. [123] diagnosed six cases in an acute care hospital setting from 679 patients treated with neuroleptics over an 18-month period. This suggests an incidence of 0.9% (±0.3%). Friedman and associates [57] diagnosed one case of NMS from 495 patients treated with neuroleptics in a state hospital over a 6-month period. This finding indicates a frequency of 0.2%. Finally, Gelenberg and associates [125] examined the incidence of NMS in a short-term psychiatric hospital over 1 year. Of 1470 patients treated with neuroleptics, NMS was diagnosed in one patient. This indicates an incidence of 0.07% (95% confidence interval 0.007–0.4%). Reasons for a lower incidence in this hospital were thought to be related to the short stay of patients, use of modest doses of neuroleptics, and fewer false-positive diagnoses of NMS. Since prospective analyses lack the methodological flaws of retrospective studies, it is likely that an incidence of <1% is accurate for the hospital setting and the figure is probably much lower in those treated as outpatients. In all studies, only psychiatric patients treated with neuroleptics were evaluated. The frequency of NMS in other at-risk groups has not been examined. It is expected that, with increased use of atypical agents, the frequency will drop further.

A number of reviews of case reports indicate that there may be a male predominance in this disorder, with a ratio of approximately 2:1 (male:female) [3, 8, 11, 14, 18]. It is unclear whether these findings suggest a true increased susceptibility in males. Alternatively, there may be a predominance of male subjects in populations treated with neuroleptics, or males may require treatment with higher doses of more potent neuroleptics more often than females. In one prospective study of 20 consecutive patients with this disorder seen over 6 years, the male-to-female ratio was the opposite, 1:2 [9]. Although Caroff [3] initially reported a higher incidence in young patients, age of onset has been shown to vary from 1 to 92 years [8, 9, 14, 57].

Pathogenesis and pathology

The pathogenesis of NMS is not completely understood. It is generally accepted that alterations in dopaminergic transmission in the central nervous system associated with drug therapy are the most important mechanism. Abnormalities in muscle membrane function, changes in peripheral and central sympathetic outflow, and alterations in central serotonin metabolism have also been implicated. It is possible that all mechanisms simultaneously play a role in the development of this disorder.

Central dopaminergic systems

That central dopaminergic mechanisms are important in the pathogenesis of NMS is strongly suggested by a number of clinical observations. These include the situations in which the disorder arises [6], signs and symptoms [54], and the response to dopamine replacement or dopamine agonist therapy. The treatment situations that result in NMS all have one feature in common: a decrease in central dopaminergic transmission. Neuroleptics, clozapine, metoclopramide, and tetrabenazine all act by blocking central dopamine receptors [126]. Those agents with the strongest ability to block dopamine receptors are most commonly associated with NMS, further emphasizing that this feature is important [21]. Tetrabenazine and alpha methyltyrosine are central dopamine depletors that can cause NMS [4, 40, 72, 73]. Withdrawal of dopaminergic agents in PD and sudden "off" periods also result in a decrease in dopaminergic activity [5, 85, 87, 88]. Cocaine blocks dopamine reuptake in the synapse. As a result, there is an initial increase in dopaminergic activity in the synapse; however, continuous use ultimately leads to depletion of dopamine in the presynaptic neurons and secondary receptor changes. With a sudden cessation of cocaine use, a relative decrease in postsynaptic dopamine availability occurs [98].

Many of the clinical features of NMS can be readily explained by central dopaminergic blockade [36]. Rigidity, akinesia, and dyskinesias are most probably the result of nigrostriatal dopamine pathway interruption [13, 16, 30, 33]. Many of these features are seen in PD, which is a disease with known central dopamine deficiency. The role of dopamine in thermal regulation is well known [127, 128]. These dopamine pathways are probably within the hypothalamus [4, 13, 16, 28, 30, 33]. The preoptic area and anterior hypothalamus are particularly concerned with thermal detection, and dopamine receptors have been located in this region [98]. Two types of thermosensitive cells are present; warm sensitive (which activate cold effectors to lower body temperature) and cold sensitive (which activate heat effectors to raise body temperature). Activation of one is associated with inhibition of the other under normal circumstances, a coordinated response [128]. The posterior hypothalamus is more involved with the generation of effector signals [30, 33]. The thermosensitive neurons respond to local changes in blood temperature as well as to afferent information from peripheral thermosensors. Dopamine and dopamine agonists modulate hypothalamic temperature regulation while dopamine receptor antagonists block this ability [4, 33]. Hashimoto et al. [54] reported increased levels of prolactin in NMS, which decreased as the serum neuroleptic levels did. Prolactin levels are regulated by hypothalamic-pituitary dopamine systems with a decrease in dopaminergic transmission resulting in increases in prolactin. Ansseau et al. [129] reported that apomorphine failed to elicit an adequate growth hormone response in a patient with NMS. These findings indicate that the hypothalamic dopamine system is altered in NMS. Interruption of other dopamine systems may explain mental status changes and autonomic dysfunction including fever [16]. Gurrera and Chang [128] postulated that the hyperthermia of NMS might occur from two possible sources, central or peripheral. Either the hypothalamus signals the body to raise temperature as a reaction to the dopamine blockade of the neuroleptic, or an excessive heat load is perceived by the hypothalamus emanating from the increased muscle rigidity and metabolism. They retrospectively studied 46 episodes in 36 patients to try and answer which one of the mechanisms is in play based on the associations of cold and warm effector symptoms and hyperthermia. They examined the clinical features that would indicate a cold or heat response and associated them with the febrile response. For instance, pallor, which would be associated with a low temperature state, was common with hyperthermia of NMS. Thus, they found that cold and heat effectors are activated simultaneously in an uncoordinated fashion. Based on these findings it is not possible to decipher which mechanism is the primary cause. However, such unpredicted symptoms as pallor may relate to other pharmacological effects of the drugs such as anticholinergic properties. So the current prevailing hypothesis now is a central effect. Further evidence that NMS is the result of a decrease in central dopaminergic activity derives from its response to dopaminergic agents. Bromocriptine, levodopa, amantadine and others have all been found to be very useful in the treatment of NMS.

Cerebrospinal fluid studies of homovanillic acid (HVA) concentrations (the principal metabolite of dopamine) also support the hypothesis that NMS is related to altered central dopaminergic transmission. Results of studies have varied, but the most common finding has been a decrease in HVA concentrations during NMS. These results suggest a decrease in dopamine metabolism. Nisijima and Ishiguro [130] reported these findings in eight patients who were compared to 10 normal controls. Verhoeven et al. [131] and Nisijima et al. [132] reported similar findings in single cases of NMS. It was suggested that the decreased metabolism was due to abnormal sensitivity of presynaptic autoreceptors. Ansseau et al. [129] reported a slightly elevated HVA concentration in one patient while Granato and associates [133] reported normal HVA concentrations in another. The reasons for these discrepancies are unclear but may be related to the timing of lumbar puncture, number of milliliters of fluid removed, and previous or concurrent therapy. One group [131] noted that HVA levels returned to normal with bromocriptine therapy. Another [130] found that lower levels of HVA continued 14 to 121 days after recovery from NMS. The significance of these findings is not clear. In PD, Ueda et al. [84] compared CSF HVA levels in patients who developed NMS (n = 9) and those who did not (n = 12) when parkinsonian drugs were withdrawn. They looked at levels in the unmedicated and remedicated state. It was found that those who developed NMS had significantly lower levels in both states supporting the notion that dopamine systems played a major role in the development of these symptoms. There was no difference in metabolites of serotonin or norepinephrine. They also found that low-serum HVA levels at baseline were an independent predictor of the occurrence of the NMS, further supporting the dopamine hypothesis [84].

In a single case, Jauss et al. [134] utilized [^{123}I] iodobenzamide SPECT to examine dopamine receptor occupancy in NMS. Serial studies were performed. In the acute phase there was complete absence of binding. With time there was increased ligand binding that correlated with changes in extrapyramidal signs. Thus, this represents additional evidence of the involvement of dopamine systems in NMS. This study also demonstrated that receptor binding could be affected long after the serum drug level reaches zero.

A definite pathological lesion has not been identified in NMS. In two reports, anterior hypothalamic abnormalities were described. Jones et al. [135] described tiny parenchymal hemorrhages and perivascular hemorrhage within the hypothalamus. In addition, tiny foci of acute ischemia were seen in the globus pallidus, internal capsule, and lateral corpus collosum. Horn et al. [136] found bilateral foci of pyknosis and disintegration of neurons and sponginess within the anterior and lateral hypothalamic areas and the tuberal nuclei. Less severe changes were seen in the ventral medial hypothalamic nucleus. Scattered petechial hemorrhages were also present in the periventricular gray matter of the anterior and posterior hypothalamus. The basal ganglia was not involved. The cerebral cortex had widespread small foci of nuclear pyknosis and increased cytoplasmic acidophilia, with vacuolation and disintegration of neurons. The normal brain has also been described [38], and in patients with PD and NMS, autopsy findings have been typical of PD with no additional pathological changes [87, 88].

Muscle

NMS and MH share the clinical features of hyperthermia, muscle rigidity, and elevations in CK. It has been suggested that these two disorders may share pathophysiology as well [135, 137]. The symptoms and signs of MH result from defective membrane regulation of the transport of calcium in the presence of particular general anesthetics. Therefore, MH is considered to be a primary disorder of muscle. Despite overwhelming evidence that NMS is the result of disruption of the central nervous system dopaminergic pathways, muscle abnormalities similar to those seen in MH may exist [13, 135]. In order to explore this possibility, muscle from patients with NMS has been studied by examining halothane- and caffeine-induced contraction of muscle fibers and by pathological evaluation. A screening procedure utilized for MH involves exposing muscle biopsy specimens to various concentrations of halothane and caffeine. Those at risk for MH have strong muscle contractions with small concentrations of these agents. The contractions are the result of changes in permeability and a sudden rise in intracellular calcium. Using muscle strips,

Caroff et al. [137] found muscle from a patient with NMS to be as sensitive to halothane as muscle from MH would be. In single-fiber studies, Araki et al. [138] observed that six of eight NMS patients had increased sensitivity to caffeine. It should be noted that neuroleptics can interfere with sarcoplasmic reticulum function in pharmacological concentrations by causing release of calcium in a manner similar to that of caffeine and halothane. Muscle strips from an NMS patient tested with fluphenazine demonstrated increased contraction and an increase in the release of calcium [137]. Muscle from patients with MH did not respond in the same manner. Muscle from patients with NMS and MH appear to be oversensitive to agents that cause muscle contraction. The role of this feature in muscle rigidity of NMS remains to be clarified.

Pathological studies have also supported the role of direct muscle involvement. In one study, [138] type IIB atrophy was seen in six cases of NMS. Electron microscopy demonstrated glycogen particles accumulated in intermyofibrillar spaces in all examined muscles and mitochondria were either disrupted or were shown to have inner membrane and cristae swelling. In another report [135] increased muscle fiber size, which was "myopathic" in appearance, and acute disseminated segmental necrosis with regeneration and occasional multivacuolated fibers was observed. Finally, Behan et al. [139] described different muscle pathology in three presumed cases of NMS. One of the problems with the paper was inadequate clinical data to confirm the diagnosis. Only their case 1 appeared to demonstrate the typical features of NMS. Nevertheless, they described focal edema of the fibers with vacuolation and, in some instances, necrosis. This was associated with endomysial edema, contraction bands, and ringbinden (one fiber wrapped around another). This pathology affected both fiber types with no inflammation. Lipid and glycogen were normal as was the morphology of mitochondria. Normal muscle biopsy in NMS has also been described in a psychiatric patient [38], one parkinsonian patient [88], and a patient with Huntington's disease [4]. Despite clinical, pathophysiological, and pathological similarities, NMS and MH are distinct disorders. In NMS, many of the features are the result of abnormalities in the central nervous system while all features of MH are the result of peripheral myopathic disturbances. The situations resulting in MH and NMS are distinct. In addition, the clinical course of the two disorders differs. Following a short exposure to anesthetic agents, MH has an explosive onset reaching a plateau in hours. In NMS, onset can occur anywhere from hours to weeks after changes in neuroleptic medication, and may even occur at stable doses. NMS progresses less rapidly, reaching a plateau in about 3 days. The mortality rate of MH is approximately 70% while in NMS, early estimates were 20% [3]. In NMS, diazepam, curare, and pancurium result in muscle flaccidity while this does not occur in MH [13, 21, 36, 38]. MH does not seem to occur in patients with a history of NMS or in their families [4, 64, 140, 141]. It seems that some abnormality of muscle may be present in NMS. Whether or not this abnormality causes some features of NMS or is the result of NMS or neuroleptic therapy is unclear.

Peripheral and central sympathetic systems

Some features of NMS may be the result of interruption of the sympathoadrenomedullary system [142]. In one case, urinary and plasma catecholamines were increased during an episode of NMS. After the patient recovered, the catecholamine levels returned to normal. This abnormality may play an important role in autonomic dysfunction in this disorder. The reason for this increase in turnover of catecholamine in the adrenal medulla is unclear; however, dopamine receptors are present in the adrenal gland [143] and blockade of these receptors may be important. There is also evidence suggesting that central sympathetic function is affected. In one report [130], noradrenalin concentrations in CSF were increased during an episode of NMS and returned to normal with recovery. In addition, a clonidine challenge test, which assesses central alpha noradrenergic receptor sensitivity, failed to generate an adequate response [129]. Gurrera [144] hypothesized that there was disruption of inhibitory effects on the sympathetic nervous system and that this hyperactivity led to uncoordinated sympathetic activity. This, in turn, led to increased muscle tone and metabolism, unregulated vasomotor activity, labile blood pressure, flushing, and pallor. The significance of these abnormalities in the pathophysiology of NMS remains to be proven.

Central serotonergic system

The concentration of 5-HIAA (the principal serotonin metabolite) was diminished in the CSF of eight patients during an NMS episode in one report [130] and one patient in another [132]. While this might suggest alteration in serotonin systems the significance of this finding remains unclear.

Risk factors

Decreased dopaminergic transmission is a necessary condition for the occurrence of NMS. However, there are other factors that may result in an increase in susceptibility. In a number of reports, physical exhaustion and dehydration were frequently present in patients prior to the onset of NMS [9, 21, 36, 92]. Evidence of the importance of dehydration is found in a description of four patients in whom NMS occurred despite stable doses of neuroleptics. Each of these patients became dehydrated just before the onset of the disorder [9]. Hyponatremia [145, 146], hypokalemia, thyrotoxicosis, and hypothyroidism [147] have also been considered as factors that might increase the risk of NMS. In a case-control study of 18 patients, Keck et al. [148] found that psychomotor agitation prior to NMS was important. In addition, those patients with higher total mean and maximal doses of neuroleptics, those with a greater number of IM injections, and those with increasing doses were all at significantly higher risk for NMS. Sachdev et al. [67] reported a similar study of 25 cases, each matched with two cases for age, gender, psychiatric diagnosis, and time and place of admission. Their results were similar. NMS was more likely to occur in patients who were agitated, dehydrated, often needed restraint or seclusion, and received large doses of neuroleptics initially and over several days. Drug potency did not emerge as an important factor. In addition, a history of ECT was found to be a risk factor. The implications of this finding are unclear, especially since ECT has been found to a potentially effective treatment of the syndrome. Finally, a third case-control study by Berardi et al. [149] examined 12 patients during an NMS event and compared them to 24 matched patients. Significant differences were similar to the other studies including psychomotor agitation (usually severe, sometimes violent), confusion, disorganization, neuroleptic dose increase in prior 5 days, and mean and maximum doses. However, there were some additional factors such as catatonia, parkinsonism, and akathisia prior to the onset of NMS that represented risks for its occurrence. The catatonia varied in its features from acute excitement to stupor with other features including mutism, rigidity, and withdrawal. Parenteral administration of the neuroleptics was a risk. The potency of neuroleptics again was not.

While decreased serum iron levels have been associated with NMS, some authors have indicated that a low serum iron level prior to the onset of NMS may itself represent a risk factor. It has been noted that some patients with an excited form of catatonia have low iron levels and that they are at increased risk of developing NMS if neuroleptics are used as therapy. Lee [110] measured serum iron levels in 39 catatonic episodes and in 17 episodes the level was reduced. Post-resolution it returned to normal in 16 episodes. Sixty percent of those patients with low serum iron had excited catatonia while this was the case in 23% of those with normal iron levels. Seven subjects in the low iron group had symptoms suggestive of LC while this was true in none of those with normal serum iron. Five were treated with neuroleptics and all developed NMS. None of the subjects with normal iron developed NMS with neuroleptic therapy. However, they were responsive to benzodiazepines and thus may not have required the rapidly escalating dose used in benzodiazepine nonresponders. Statistically, those with low iron were more likely to have LC, were less likely to respond to benzodiazepines, and more likely to have excited agitated symptoms. Thus, those patients with excited catatonia or, more specifically, LC and a low serum iron level are probably at greater risk of developing NMS when exposed to neuroleptics [110]. Low serum iron alone is not a risk since those with simple retarded catatonia and low iron did not develop NMS when neuroleptics were given.

Another possible risk factor for the development of NMS is being in the early postpartum period. Alexander et al. [150], in a prospective study of all NMS cases over 30 months, diagnosed 11 patients with NMS, three of whom were in the postpartum period. All had depressive episodes and were treated with low doses of neuroleptics. A confounding finding is that all three had agitation and electrolyte imbalance. An additional study examined 900 women treated with neuroleptics prospectively over a 5-year period [151]. Sixty five had postpartum psychiatric disorders and 6.3% (4 patients) developed NMS. These patients were treated with fairly high doses in the first few days after childbirth. Both studies suggest that a state-dependent vulnerability occurs in the postpartum period and that caution is required when treating such patients with neuroleptics.

The clinical situation that seems most likely to predispose to NMS appears to exist in a patient with significant psychomotor agitation, perhaps catatonic excitement, dehydration, physical exhaustion, mild hyperthermia, and early onset of EPS, who is then treated with large and rapidly escalating doses of IM (or oral) dopamine antagonist drugs. Careful monitoring for the symptoms of NMS is important in these cases. It has been suggested that, in this situation, treatment with lower doses of neuroleptics and the use of diazepam, carbamazepine, verapamil, and electroconvulsive shock therapy might prevent the onset of this potentially fatal disorder [148].

In the original description of NMS [1, 2], it was thought that this disorder would "supervene selectively in brain-damaged subjects. . . ." Some evidence to support this concept has been presented [3, 9]. Rosebush et al. [9] found that 42% of 20 consecutive patients with NMS had another form of brain pathology. Other reviews, however, have not indicated that this is an important risk factor [8, 14, 67]. One other possible risk factor is the presence of acute infectious encephalitis. Caroff et al. [152] reported five patients who developed psychiatric symptoms due to acute viral encephalitis and then developed NMS from the neuroleptics prescribed. They all developed the characteristic extrapyramidal features and mental status changes after neuroleptics were instituted as well as escalating hyperthermia. All had CSF confirmation of viral encephalitis. Acute symptoms resolved within days of stopping the neuroleptics but cognitive sequelae were noted for up to a year. The authors used these cases as examples to support a strong association between encephalitis and NMS. Neuroleptics need to be used with caution in patients with infectious encephalitis.

Genetic risk factors have also been sought. Considering the apparent involvement of dopaminergic and serotonergic systems several groups have pursued associations of NMS and polymorphisms in various receptor types. One study examining 5HT receptor genes found no association between the occurrence of NMS and 5HT1A and 5HT2A polymorphisms [153]. On the other hand, another group of investigators did find an association between NMS and the TaqI A1 polymorphism of the dopamine D2 receptor gene [154]. This polymorphism alters the density and function of D2 receptors and may predispose patients to the development of NMS. Further studies to confirm this are needed. Other negative associations have been with the CYP2D6 [155, 156] and with RYR1 gene that has been associated with malignant hyperthermia [157].

In PD, one study examined potential risk factors for the NMS seen with medication withdrawal [83]. The authors compared PD patients admitted to the hospital who experienced NMS (n = 11) to those who never did (n = 87). They found that those with NMS had more severe disease, were on higher doses of levodopa and significantly lower CSF levels of homovanillic acid. The CSF HVA levels independently increased the risk of NMS by a factor of three. There was no significant difference with regard to CSF norepinephrine or serotonin metabolites. Other possible risk factors in PD are the presence of neuropsychiatric complications, motor fluctuations and dehydration.

Treatment

The diagnosis of NMS requires a high index of suspicion in appropriate situations. Early recognition and intervention are the keys to patient survival [56, 158]. If the diagnosis is suspected, treatment should be initiated immediately and aggressively. In those patients on neuroleptics, initial supportive steps include stopping the offending agent, treatment of dehydration with IV fluids, mechanical cooling for fever, correction of metabolic abnormalities, and support for renal, pulmonary, or cardiovascular complications including preventative measures for thrombophlebitis. The mortality rate of 20% reported in 1980 [3] was probably the result of late recognition and treatment with supportive measures only. When it occurs, mortality is likely due to the prolonged duration of symptoms [133]. Further steps are needed to shorten the duration of the clinical course and improve survival.

Although antiparkinsonian agents were recommended for therapy in the 1960s it was not until 1983 that drug therapy was utilized regularly. There have been no controlled therapeutic trials because of the rare occurrence of the syndrome and potentially lethal outcome. All data are based on case reports. Nevertheless, there are data to support the use of some of these agents. The two most frequently used drugs are bromocriptine [7, 18, 32, 59, 159, 160] and dantrolene sodium [21, 24, 31, 162–165] or a combination of the two [32, 59, 133]. In a review of 67 cases [18], 56 cases were treated with dantrolene, bromocriptine, or a combination and the mortality rate dropped to 5%. Early treatment with these drugs can shorten the course of NMS compared to supportive care alone [18] and improve the outcome. An additional study reviewing reported cases also demonstrated a reduction of mortality by over 50% with bromocriptine and/or dantroline compared to supportive care [164]. Dantrolene sodium, a muscle relaxant, was first utilized in NMS because of therapeutic success in MH and its ability to inhibit muscle contraction and heat production. It has the advantage of being available in a parenteral form. Suggested doses of intravenous dantrolene are 2 to 3 mg per kg three or four times a day for a total of approximately 10 mg per kg per day. Higher doses may result in hepatotoxicity. Oral doses of 50 to 600 mg per day have been recommended [21, 24, 165]. Bromocriptine, a direct dopamine receptor agonist, was utilized because of the apparent central dopaminergic abnormalities in NMS. First used successfully in 1983 [7, 160], it is now considered the treatment of choice in those patients in whom oral medications can be administered. The initial dose should be 2.5 mg t.i.d. with increasing increments of 2.5 mg t.i.d. every 24 hours until a response is seen. A total daily dose as high as 60 mg per day has been administered [133]. Despite the ability of this drug to induce psychosis, in this situation, it appears that it is well tolerated in both psychiatric and nonpsychiatric patients. Return to the original psychiatric state is related to improvement of NMS and not treatment with bromocriptine [161]. It has been recommended that in patients who cannot swallow, intravenous dantrolene should be started and bromocriptine could replace it as the patient improves [24]. Others have suggested using dantrolene and bromocriptine in combination since they address different pathophysiological aspects of the disorder [32, 59, 133]. It is believed that dantrolene would diminish CK levels and fever while bromocriptine would improve the extrapyramidal aspects and mental status changes. Dhib-Jalhut et al. [32]. have pointed out that in those treated with only supportive measures, it may take 14 days for the CK to begin to drop, 4–17 days for fever to decrease, and perhaps weeks for improvement in rigidity, with the entire syndrome lasting several weeks. With bromocriptine or combined bromocriptine and dantrolene, the CK dropped in 48 hours, fever diminished in 24 hours, rigidity diminished in 48 hours to 4 days, and autonomic changes reversed in 24 to 72 hours. The whole episode may resolve in a week. If the syndrome is caused by orally administered neuroleptics, treatment should be continued for at least 10 days since recurrence may develop with early withdrawal from treatment. When depot neuroleptics are utilized, 2–3 weeks of therapy may be warranted since it may take this amount of time for the neuroleptics to be cleared. It may be helpful to follow these patients with serial CK and myoglobin levels, in the urine and blood, and close monitoring of clinical features.

Other therapies have been shown to be beneficial in small numbers of patients. Amantadine (up to 400 mg/day) has been useful possibly because of its dopaminergic effects [166]. One retrospective study found that it may lower mortality of NMS [164]. Since amantadine therapy has failed to improve signs of NMS in some cases [133], starting bromocriptine from the outset would be a more sound strategy. If the patient is on amantadine when the episode begins it should be continued. Levodopa has also been examined as a treatment for NMS with some success [10, 17, 167]. However, only a few cases have been reported and although one would expect it to be as efficacious as bromocriptine, it is not uniformly successful [38]. This may be related to timing and dosage since unsuccessful trials of bromocriptine have also been reported [58]. A single patient responded to treatment with combined levodopa and subcutaneous lisuride, a D_2 receptor agonist. Lisuride was started because the patient could not tolerate bromocriptine or levodopa in higher doses (nausea and vomiting). Parenteral forms of dopaminergic drugs (e.g., lisuride, apomorphine) may be useful in a patient with dysphagia [168]. In one case report subcutaneous apomorphine 2 mg every 3 hours was given for 3 days with no other agents and the patient responded rapidly without recurrence [169].

Benzodiazepines such as diazepam and clonazepam have been utilized in NMS when catatonic symptoms are present. In fact, those suggesting that NMS is a form of catatonia suggest that this be the treatment of choice [39, 107, 111]. However, they have been associated with variable success [27, 32, 45, 56]. An inadequate number of patients have been treated to judge their usefulness. In addition, use of benzodiazepines in the pre-NMS state has not been preventative [56]. When used in high doses respiratory status needs to be monitored carefully. Anticholinergic drugs such as benztropine, trihexyphenidyl, and diphenhydramine have often been the first drugs given to patients when NMS arises because of their effectiveness in other extrapyramidal syndromes such as acute dystonic reactions and parkinsonism. In fact, they are probably given initially because of a misdiagnosis. However, these drugs have not been useful in NMS and should not be administered if NMS with hyperthermia is suspected [3, 31, 160, 163, 165]. No decrease in mortality or duration of NMS has been reported with these drugs. In fact, some report that anticholinergics may actually be harmful in patients with NMS [159]. The symptoms of hyperthermia, autonomic dysfunction, and elevated CK should lead one to suspect NMS and not other extrapyramidal syndromes. If anticholinergic agents have been prescribed at the onset of symptoms they should be slowly tapered off [12]. It should be noted that there have been occasional case reports of carbamazepine effectively treating NMS but this needs to be confirmed [170], especially when reports have been published of carbamazepine inducing NMS in patients on long-term stable neuroleptic doses [171]. The reason for choosing carbamazepine in these cases was not made clear by the authors.

Finally, electroconvulsive therapy (ECT) has been utilized to treat NMS and coexisting psychosis [141, 172]. This has been used because it is considered the second line treatment for catatonia after benzodiazepines. When an acutely psychotic patient develops NMS after administration of neuroleptics, cessation of the drugs could lead to worsening of psychosis and NMS. These patients are difficult to manage and ECT is considered appropriate. ECT, in some instances, has been used to treat PD [173, 174]. It is thought to act by increasing nigrostriatal dopaminergic transmission. This may be true in NMS as well. Of 17 NMS cases treated with ECT reviewed by Addonizio and Susman [141], a rapid therapeutic response was obtained in eight. Four patients experienced cardiac arrhythmias, including ventricular fibrillation and cardiac arrest, indicating that ECT is not without serious adverse effects. Others had no response. In four patients treated with ECT for persistent psychosis shortly after NMS cleared, no recurrences of NMS were seen despite reinstitution of neuroleptic therapy. Similar results were described by Mann et al. [175] where 23 of 27 patients had complete or partial improvement of NMS with ECT. However, four patients experienced cardiac arrhythmias. ECT led to a decrease in mortality of about 50% in NMS patients compared to supportive therapy [176]. Nisijima and Ishiguro [177] demonstrated, in five patients, that complete resolution occurred within 6 days confirming the quick response. The role, if any, of ECT as a treatment modality in NMS remains to be established. Some NMS patients may be at risk for the development of cardiac arrhythmias when given succinyl choline and must be monitored closely or given other muscle relaxants when preparing for ECT [12]. A single case report demonstrated improvement of NMS with plasmapheresis in the patient who failed medical therapy [178].

Caroff et al. [176] have suggested that the treatment of NMS needs to be individualized depending on the severity of the episodes and the primary symptoms. In patients who are diagnosed early with mild symptoms just supportive measures may be all that is needed. Benzodiazepines can be utilized in those who have symptoms of catatonia or severe agitation. Bromocriptine and/or dantrolene are utilized in more fulminant cases. Finally, ECT is the choice when the NMS symptoms appear to be resistant to pharmacotherapy and in those with significant psychosis in the post-NMS period.

In the case of PD, where NMS occurs most commonly from withdrawal of antiparkinsonian medications, the usual supportive measures should be instituted and parkinsonian medications should be reinitiated immediately [89]. This situation has been more prevalent during "drug holidays." Drug holidays should no longer be considered a therapeutic option in PD except in extreme situations [179]. In those cases the patients should be hospitalized and vital signs monitored closely. The decreased usage of this therapeutic measure will most likely decrease the frequency of NMS. However, other situations may arise that increase the risk.

Since NMS occurs most frequently in psychiatric patients treated with neuroleptics, it is likely that a large percentage will require retreatment with antipsychotic agents. Obvious questions include whether these patients can be safely rechallenged with neuroleptics and what factors are important in reducing the risk of recurrence of NMS? It is clear that neuroleptics can eventually be reintroduced successfully in a majority of patients [180, 181]. Recurrences have been described as mild and self-limited in some patients while fatalities have also been reported [180, 181]. While recurrences may be early or late [145], the most important factor that might reduce the risk is the time from resolution of NMS to the reintroduction of antipsychotic agents. Studies have demonstrated that waiting 2 weeks or more (longer with depot drugs) allows for a safer rechallenge [180, 181]. In situations where neuroleptics are started sooner, the occurrence of NMS may actually represent an exacerbation of the original episode. This may also occur with early withdrawal of treatment for NMS. The dopamine-blocking potency of the drug used in the rechallenge of patients is another factor that may alter the risk of recurrence. Since NMS may be related to the degree of dopamine receptor blockade, it seems likely that lower-potency drugs, such as thioridazine or atypical agents, may result in fewer recurrences. This has been substantiated in a number of studies [180, 182]. For the same reason, if patients are restarted on the same drug that originally caused NMS or one of similar potency, use of lower doses would also allow for safer rechallenge [180, 181]. Other factors that may reduce the risk of recurrence include making sure the patient is well hydrated and that no metabolic imbalances exist. After reintroduction of the drug, the patient must be monitored carefully for any signs of recurrent NMS.

Future consideration

Major strides have been made in understanding NMS in the past two decades. More data are being captured in large prospective series. However, a good portion of the information presented continues to be based on case reports, retrospective reviews of case reports, and uncontrolled studies performed on small numbers of patients. As a result, conflicting results and conclusions still exist in the literature and many unanswered questions remain. Future goals include a better understanding of the pathogenesis and risk factors so that NMS can be better recognized and avoided. This would require the development of animal models, which at this point do not exist. In relation to this direction of study it would be important to develop a marker for the disease so that its relationship to catatonia could be better delineated. Rosebush et al. [9] have shown how useful prospective analysis can be in describing clinical features. Similar studies of the situations leading the NMS will be useful. Closer examination of CSF, serum, and urine concentrations of catecholamines and their metabolites may provide more clues to the pathogenesis and risk factors. Pharmacological (and neuroendocrinological) studies, and examination of genetic risk factors will also enhance understanding. Improved treatment for those cases that do occur can only evolve through controlled clinical trials that take advantage of multicenter collaboration. Finally, with the development of atypical antipsychotics the possibility of prevention is a reality.

Acknowledgments

I would like to thank Faith Wood for her assistance in the preparation of the manuscript. This work was supported by the AMC Parkinson's Research Fund and the Riley Family Chair of Parkinson's Disease.

References

1. Delay J, Pichot P, Lemperiere T, et al. Un neuroleptique majeur non-phenothiazinique et non-reserpinique, l'haloperiol, dans le traitment des psychosis. Ann Med Psychol 1960; 118: 145–142.
2. Delay J, Denicker P. Drug induced extrapyramidal syndromes. In Vinken PJ, Bruyun GW (eds) Handbook of Clinical Neurology. Amsterdam, North Holland, 1968, pp. 258–259.
3. Caroff SN. The neuroleptic malignant syndrome. J Clin Psychiatry 1980; 41: 79–82.
4. Burke RE, Fahn S, Mayuex R, et al. Neuroleptic malignant syndrome caused by dopamine-depleting drugs in a patient with Huntington's disease. Neurology 1981; 31: 1022–1026.
5. Toro M, Matsuda O, Mikizuich K, Sugano K. neuroleptic malignant syndrome-like state following withdrawal of antiparkinsonian drugs. J Nerv Ment Disord 1981; 169: 324–327.
6. Genis D. Neuroleptic malignant syndrome: impaired dopaminergic systems? Neurology 1985; 35: 1806.
7. Zubenko G, Pope HG. Management of a case of neuroleptic malignant syndrome with bromocriptine. Am J Psychiatry 1983; 140: 1619–1620.
8. Shalev A, Munitz H. The neuroleptic malignant syndrome: agent and host interaction. Acta Psychiatr Scand 1986; 73: 337–347.
9. Rosebush P, Stewart T. A prospective analysis of 24 episodes of neuroleptic malignant syndrome. Am J Psychiatry 1989; 146: 717–725.
10. Kurlan R, Hamill R, Shoulson I. Neuroleptic malignant syndrome. Clin Neuropharmacol 1984; 7: 109–120.

11. Levenson JL. Neuroleptic malignant syndrome. Am J Psychiatry 1985; 142: 1137–1145.
12. Susman VL. Clinical Management of neuroleptic malignant syndrome. Psychiatr Q 2001; 72: 325–336.
13. Smego RA, Durack DT. The neuroleptic malignant syndrome. Arch Intern Med 1982; 142: 1183–1185.
14. Addonizio G, Sussman VL, Roth SD. Neuroleptic malignant syndrome: review and analysis of 115 cases. Biol Psychiatry 1987; 22: 1004–1020.
15. Scrinvasan AV, Murugappan M, Kristamurty SG, Sayeed ZA. Neuroleptic malignant syndrome. J Neurol Neurosurg Psychiatry 1990; 53: 514–516.
16. Szabadi E. Neuroleptic malignant syndrome. Br Med J 1984; 288: 1399–1400.
17. Clarke CE, Shand D, Yuill GM, Green MHP. Clinical spectrum of neuroleptic malignant syndrome. Lancet 1988; 2: 969–970.
18. Rosenberg MR, Green M. Neuroleptic malignant syndrome: review of response to therapy. Arch Intern Med 1989; 149: 1927–1931.
19. Wong MM. Neuroleptic malignant syndrome: two cases without muscle rigidity. Austr N Z J Psychiatry 1996; 30: 415–418.
20. Patel U, Agrawal M, Krishnan P, Nirajan S. Neuroleptic malignant syndrome presenting as pulmonary edema and severe bronchorrhea. J Natl Med Assoc 2002; 94: 279–282.
21. Guze BH, Baxter LR. Neuroleptic malignant syndrome. N Engl J Med 1985; 313: 163–166.
22. Cohen BM, Baldessarini RJ, Pope HG, Lipinski JF. Neuroleptic malignant syndrome. N Engl J Med 1985; 313: 1293.
23. Adityanjee, Singh S, Singh G, Ong S. Spectrum concept of neuroleptic malignant syndrome. Br J Psychiatry 1988; 153: 107–111.
24. Mueller PS. Diagnosis and treatment of neuroleptic malignant syndrome: a review. Neuroview 1987; 3: 1–5.
25. Cullinane CA, Brumfeld C, Flint LM, Ferrara JJ. Neuroleptic malignant syndrome associated with multiple joint dislocations in a trauma patient. J Trauma Injury Infect Crit Care 1998; 45: 168–171.
26. Weinberg S, Twerksy RS. Neuroleptic malignant syndrome. Anesth Analg 1983; 62: 848–850.
27. Koehler PJ, Mirandolle JF. Neuroleptic malignant-like syndrome and lithium. Lancet 1988; 2: 1499–1500.
28. Allan RN, White HC. Side effects of parenteral long-acting phenothiazines. Br Med J 1972; 1: 221–222.
29. Lew, TY, Tollefson G. Chlorpromazine-induced neuroleptic malignant syndrome and its response to diazepam. Biol Psychiatry 1983; 18: 1441–1445.
30. Henderson VW, Wooten GF. Neuroleptic malignant syndrome: a pathogenetic role for dopamine receptor blockage? Neurology 1981; 31: 132–137.
31. Coons DJ, Hillman FJ, Marshall RW. Treatment of neuroleptic malignant syndrome with dantrolene sodium: a case report. Am J Psychiatry 1982; 139: 944–945.
32. Dhib-Jalbut, Hesselbrock R, Brott T, Silbergeld D. Treatment of neuroleptic malignant syndrome with bromocriptine. JAMA 1983; 250: 484–485.
33. Figa'-Talamanca L, Gualandi C, DiMeo L, et al. Hyperthermia after discontinuance of levodopa and bromocriptine therapy: impaired dopamine receptors a possible cause. Neurology 1985; 35: 258–261.
34. Yoshino A, Yoshimasu H, Tatsuzawa Y, Asakura T, Hara T. Nonconvulsive status epilepticus in two patients with neuroleptic malignant syndrome. J Clin Psychopharmacol 1998; 18: 347–349.

35. Lal V, Sardana V, Thussu A, Sawhney IMS, Prabhakar S. Cerebellar degeneration following neuroleptic malignant syndrome. Postgrad Med J 1997; 73: 735–736.
36. Editorial. Neuroleptic malignant syndrome. Lancet 1984; 1: 545–546.
37. Taylor MA. Catatonia: a review of a behavioral neurologic syndrome. Neuropsychiatry Neuropsychol Behav Neurol 1990; 3: 48–72.
38. Morris, HH, McCormick WF, Reinarz JA. Neuroleptic malignant syndrome. Arch Neurol 1980; 37: 462–463.
39. Koch M, Chandragiri S, Rizvi S, Peterides G, Francis A. Catatonic signs in neuroleptic malignant syndrome. Compr Psychiatry 2000; 41: 73–75.
40. Petzinger GM, Bressman SB. A case of tetrabenazine-induced neuroleptic malignant syndrome after prolonged treatment. Mov Disord 1997; 12: 246–248.
41. Ghani SO, Ahmed W, Marco LA. Neuroleptic malignant syndrome and severe thrombocytopenia: case report and literature review. J Clin Psychiatry 2000; 12: 51–54.
42. American Psychiatric Association. Diagnostic and Statistical Manual of Mental Disorders, 4th edition. Washington DC, American Psychiatric Association, 1994.
43. Velamoor VR, Norman RMG, Caroff SN, et al. Progression of symptoms of neuroleptic malignant syndrome. J Nerv Ment Disord 1994; 182: 168–173.
44. Mezaki T, Ohtani SI, Abe K, et al. Benign type of malignant syndrome. Lancet 1989; 1: 49.
45. Caroff SN, Mann S, Keck PE, Francis A. Residual catatonic state following neuroleptic malignant syndrome. J Clin Psychopharmacol 2000; 20: 257–259.
46. Cohen WJ, Cohen NH. Lithium carbonate, haloperidol and irreversible brain damage. JAMA 1974; 230: 1283–1287.
47. Spring G, Frankel M. New data on lithium and haloperidol incompatability. Am J Psychiatry 1981; 138: 818–821.
48. Anderson Sa, Weinschank K. Peripheral neuropathy is a component of the neurologic malignant syndrome. Am J Med 1987; 82: 169–170.
49. Lee S, Merriam A, Kim TS, Leibling M, Dickson DW, Moore GRW. Cerebellar degeneration in neuroleptic malignant syndrome: neuropathologic findings and review of the literature concerning heat related nervous system injury. J Neurol Neurosurg Psychiatry 1989; 52: 387–391.
50. Scheider JM, Roger DJ, Uhl RL. Bilateral forearm compartment syndromes resulting from neuroleptic malignant syndrome. J Hand Surg 1996; 21A: 287–289.
51. Craddock B, Craddock N. Contractures in neuroleptic malignant syndrome. Am J Psychiatry 1997; 154: 436.
52. Black KJ, Racette B, Perlmutter JS. Preventing contractions in neuroleptic malignant syndrome and dystonia. Am J Psychiatry 1998; 155: 1298–1299.
53. Garrido SM, Chauncey TR. Neuroleptic malignant syndrome following autologous peripheral blood stem cell transplantation. Bone Marrow Transplant 1998; 21: 427–428.
54. Hashimoto F, Sherman CB, Jeffrey WH. Neuroleptic malignant syndrome and dopaminergic blockage. Arch Intern Med 1984; 144: 629–630.
55. Gonner F, Baumgartner R, Schupbach D, Merlo MCG. Neuroleptic malignant syndrome during low dosed neuroleptic medication in first-episode psychosis: a case report. Psychopharmacology 1999; 144: 416–418.
56. Caroff SN, Mann SC, Keck PE. Specific treatment of the neuroleptic malignant syndrome. Biol Psychiatry 1998; 44: 378–381.
57. Friedman JH, Davis R, Wagner RL. Neuroleptic malignant syndrome: the results of a 6 month prospective study of incidence in a state psychiatric hospital. Clin Neuropharmacol 1988; 11: 373–377.

58. Lazarus A. Neuroleptic malignant syndrome and amantadine withdrawal. Am J Psychiatry 1985; 142: 142.
59. Rosse R, Ciolino C. Dopamine agonists and neuroleptic malignant syndrome. Am J Psychiatry 1985; 142: 270–271.
60. Corrigan FM, Coulter F. Neuroleptic malignant syndrome, amitriptyline and thioridazine. Biol Psychiatry 1988; 23: 320–321.
61. Spivak B, Weizman A, Wolovick L, et al. Neuroleptic malignant syndrome during abrupt reduction of neuroleptic treatment. Acta Psychiatr Scand 1990; 81: 168–169.
62. Price DK, Turnbull GJ, Gregory RP, Stevens DG. Neuroleptic malignant syndrome in a case of post-partum psychosis. Br J Psychiatry 1989; 155: 849–852.
63. Baastrup PC, Holinagel P, Sorensen R, Shou M. Adverse reactions in treatment with lithium carbonate and haloperidol. JAMA 1976; 236: 2645–2646.
64. Levenson JL, Fisher JG. Long term outcome after neuroleptic malignant syndrome. J Clin Psychiatry 1988; 49: 154–156.
65. Donaldson IM, Cunningham J. Persisting neurologic sequelae of lithium carbonate therapy. Arch Neurol 1983; 40: 747–751.
66. Friedman E, Gershon S. Effect of lithium on brain dopamine. Nature 1973; 243: 520–521.
67. Sachdev P, Mason C, Hadzi-Pavlovic D. Case control study of neuroleptic malignant syndrome. Am J Psychiatry 1997; 154: 1156–1158.
68. Konikoff F, Kuritzky A, Jerushalmi Y, Theodor E. Neuroleptic malignant syndrome by a single injection of haloperidol. Br Med J 1984; 289: 1228–1229.
69. Moyes DG. Malignant hyperpyrexia caused by trimeprazine. Br J Anaesth 1973; 45: 1163–1164.
70. Robinson MB, Kennett RP, Harding AE, Legg NJ, Clarke B. Neuroleptic malignant syndrome associated with metoclopramide. J. Neurol Neurosurg Psychiatry 1985; 40: 1304.
71. Samie MR. Neuroleptic malignant-like syndrome induced by metoclopramide. Mov Disord 1987; 2: 57–60.
72. Mateo D, Munoz-Blanco JL, Gimenez-Roldan S. Neuroleptic malignant syndrome related to tetrabenazine introduction and haloperidol discontinuation in Huntington's disease. Clin Neuropharmacol 1992; 15: 63–68.
73. Osseman M, Sindic CJM, Laterre C. Tetrabenazine as a cause of neuroleptic malignant syndrome. Mov Disord 1996; 11: 95.
74. Breitbart W, Marotta RF, Call P. AIDS and Neuroleptic malignant syndrome. Lancet 1988; 2: 1488–1489.
75. Hernandez JL, Palacios-Araus L, Echevarria S, Herran A, Campo JF, Riancho JA. Neuroleptic malignant syndrome in the acquired immunodeficiency syndrome. Postgrad Med J 1997; 73: 779–784.
76. Hriso E, Kuhn T, Masdeu JC, Grundman M. Extrapyramidal symptoms due to dopamine blocking agents in patients with AIDS encephalopathy. Am J Psychiatry 1991; 148: 1558–1561.
77. Kieburtz KD, Epstein LG, Gelbard HA, Greenamyre T. Excitotoxicity and dopaminergic dysfunction in the acquired immunodeficiency syndrome dementia complex: therapeutic implications. Arch Neurol 1991; 48: 1281–1284.
78. Berger JR, Nath A. HIV dementia and the basal ganglia. Intervirology 1997; 40: 122–131.
79. Nath A, Anderson C, Jones M, et al. Neurotoxicity and dysfunction of dopamine systems associated with AIDS dementia. J Psychopharmacol 2000; 14: 222–227.

80. Lopez OL, Smith G, Meltzer CC, Becker JT. Dopamine systems in human immunodeficiency virus-associated dementia. Neuropsychiatry Neuropsychol Behav Neurol 1999; 12: 184–192.

81. Factor SA, Podskalny GD, Barron KD. Persistent neuroleptic induced rigidity and dystonia in AIDS dementia complex: a clinico-pathological case report. J Neurol Sci 1994; 127: 114–120.

82. Wiley CA, Soontornniyomkij V, Radhakrishnan L, et al. Distribution of brain HIV load in AIDS. Brain Pathol 1998; 8: 277–284.

83. Ueda M, Hamamoto M, Nagayama H, et al. Susceptibility to neuroleptic malignant syndrome in Parkinson's disease. Neurology 1999; 52: 777–781.

84. Ueda M, Hamamoto M, Nagayama H, Okubo S, Amemiya S, Katayama Y. Biochemical alterations during medication withdrawal in Parkinson's disease with and without neuroleptic malignant-like syndrome. J Neurol Neurosurg Psychiatry 2001; 71: 111–113.

85. Friedman JH, Feinberg SS, Feldman RG. A neuroleptic malignant like syndrome due to levodopa therapy withdrawal. JAMA 1985; 254: 2792–2795.

86. Gordon PH, Frucht SJ. Neuroleptic malignant syndrome in advanced Parkinson's disease. Mov Disord 2001; 16: 960–961.

87. Pfeiffer RF, Sucha EL. "On-off"-induced lethal hyperthermia. Mov Disord 1989; 4: 338–341.

88. Sechi GP, Tanda F, Mutani R. Fatal hyperpyrexia after withdrawal of levodopa. Neurology 1984; 34: 249–251.

89. Hirschorn KA, Greenberg HS. Successful treatment of levodopa induced myoclonus and levodopa withdrawal-induced neuroleptic malignant syndrome: a case report. Clin Neuropharmacol 1988; 11: 278–281.

90. Iwuagwa CU, Riley D, Bonomo RA. Neuroleptic malignant-like syndrome in an elderly patient caused by abrupt withdrawal of tolcapone, a catechol-o-methyltransferase inhibitor. Am J Med 2000; 108: 517–518.

91. Cunningham MA, Darby DG, Donnan GA. Controlled-release delivery of L-dopa associated with nonfatal hyperthermia, rigidity and autonomic dysfunction. Neurology 1991; 41: 942–943.

92. Simpson DM, David GC. Case report of neuroleptic malignant syndrome associated with withdrawal from amantadine. Am J Psychiatry 1984; 141: 796–797.

93. Friedman JH, Factor SA. Atypical antipsychotics in the treatment of drug-induced psychosis in Parkinson's disease. Mov Disord 2000; 15: 201–211.

94. Vingerhoets FJG, Villemure JG, Temperli P, Pollo C, Pralong E, Ghika J. Subthalamic DBS replaces levodopa in Parkinson's disease: two-year follow-up. Neurology 2002; 58: 396–401.

95. Mizuta E, Yamasaki S, Nakatake M, Kuno S. Neuroleptic malignant syndrome in a Parkinsonian woman during the premenstrual period. Neurology 1993; 43: 1048–1049.

96. Cao L, Katz RH. Acute hypernatremia and neuroleptic malignant syndrome in Parkinson disease. Am J Med Sci 1999; 318: 67–68.

97. Konishi T, Konagaya Y. Neuroleptic malignant syndrome – like condition in multiple system atrophy. J Neurol Neurosurg Psychiatry 1997; 63: 120–121.

98. Kosten TR, Kleber HD. Rapid death during cocaine abuse: a variant of neuroleptic malignant syndrome. Am J Drug Alcohol Abuse 1988; 14: 335–346.

99. Wetli CV, Mash D, Karch SB. Cocaine associated agitated delirium and the neuroleptic malignant syndrome. Am J Emerg Med 1996; 14: 425–428.

100. Demirkiran M, Jankovic J, Dean JM. Ecstasy intoxication: an overlap between serotonin syndrome and neuroleptic malignant syndrome. Clin Neuropharmacol 1996; 19: 157–164.

101. Friedman JH. Recognition and treatment of neuroleptic malignant syndrome. Curr Opin Neurol Neurosurg 1988; 1: 310–311.

102. Lazarus A. Neuroleptic malignant syndrome: detection and management. Psychiatr Ann 1985; 15: 706–712.

103. Mann SC, Caroff SN, Bleier Hr, et al. Lethal catatonia. Am J Psychiatry 1986; 143: 1374–1381.

104. Castillo E, Robin RT, Holsboer-Trachler E. Clinical differentiation between lethal catatonia and neuroleptic malignant syndrome. Am J Psychiatry 1989; 146: 324–328.

105. Stauder KH. Die toldliche katatonie. Arch Psychiatry Nervenkr 1934; 102: 614–634.

106. Kalinowsky LB. Lethal catatonia and neuroleptic malignant syndrome. Am J Psychiatry 1987; 144: 1106.

107. Fink M. Neuroleptic malignant syndrome and catatonia: one entity or two? Biol Psychiatry 1996; 39: 1–4.

108. Kellam AMP. The neuroleptic malignant syndrome, so-called: a survey of the world literature. Br J Psychiatry 1987; 150: 752–759.

109. Carroll BT, Goforth HW. Serum iron in catatonia. Biol Psychiatry 1995; 38: 776–777.

110. Lee JWY. Serum iron in catatonia and neuroleptic malignant syndrome. Biol Psychiatry 1998; 44: 499–507.

111. Carroll BT, Taylor RE. The nondichotomy between lethal catatonia and neuroleptic malignant syndrome. J Clin Psychopharmacol 1997; 17: 235–236.

112. Mann SC, Caroff SN. Lethal catatonia and neuroleptic malignant syndrome. Am J Psychiatry 1987; 144: 1106–1107.

113. Bennett DA. Combined neuroleptic malignant syndrome and central cholinergic syndrome. J Neurol Neuorsurg Psychiatry 1990; 53: 711.

114. Larner AJ, Smith SC, Farmer SF. "Non-neuroleptic malignant" syndrome. J Neurol Neurosurg Psychiatry 1998; 65: 613.

115. Ehara H, Maegaki Y, Takeshita K. Neuroleptic malignant syndrome and methylphenidate. Pediatr Neurol 1998; 19: 299–301.

116. Turner MR, Gainsborough N. Neuroleptic malignant-like syndrome after abrupt withdrawal of baclofen. J Psychopharmacol 2001; 15: 61–63.

117. Bodner RA, Lynch T, Lewis L, Kahn D. Serotonin syndrome. Neurology l995; 45: 219–223.

118. Sternbach H. The serotonin syndrome. Am J Psychiatry 1991; 148: 705–713.

119. Richard IH, Kurlan R, Tanner C, Factor S, Hubble J, Suchowersky O, Waters C and the Parkinson study group. Serotonin syndrome and the combined used of deprenyl and an anti-depressant in Parkinson's disease. Neurology l997; 48: 1070–1077.

120. Weiner WJ, Lang AE. Movement Disorders: A Comprehensive Survey, Mount Kisco, NY, Futura Publishing, 1989.

121. Factor SA, Matthews MK. Persistent dystonic-rigid syndrome caused by combined metoclopramide and prochlorperazine therapy. South Med J 1991; 84(5): 626–628.

122. Denning TR, Berrios GE. Potential confusion of neuroleptic malignant syndrome and Wilson's disease. Lancet 1989; 2: 43.

123. Keck PE, Pope HG, McElroy SL. Frequency and presentation of neuroleptic malignant syndrome: a prospective study. Am J Psychiatry 1987; 144: 1344–1346.

124. Pope HG, Keck PE, McElroy SL. Frequency and presentation of neuroleptic malignant syndrome in a large psychiatric hospital. Am J Psychiatry 1986; 143: 1227–1233.

125. Gelenberg AJ, Bellingham B, Wojcik JD, et al. A prospective survey of neuroleptic malignant syndrome in short-term psychiatric hospital. Am J Psychiatry 1988; 145: 517–518.

126. Peringer E, Jenner P, Donaldson IM, Marsden CD, Miller R. Metoclopramide and dopamine receptor blockade. Neuropharmacology 1976; 15: 463–469.

127. Cox B. Dopamine. In Lomax P, Schonbaum E (eds) Body Temperature, Regulation, Drug Effects ad Therapeutic Implications, New York, Marcel Dekker, 1979, pp. 234–255.

128. Gurrera RJ, Chang SS. Thermoregulatory dysfunction in neuroleptic malignant syndrome. Biol Psychiatry 1996; 39: 207–212.

129. Ansseau M, Reynolds CF, Kupfer DJ, et al. Central dopaminergic and noradrenergic receptor blockade in a patient with neuroleptic malignant syndrome. J Clin Psychiatry 1986; 47: 320–321.

130. Nisijima K, Ishiguro T. Neuroleptic malignant syndrome: a study of CSF monoamine metabolism. Biol Psychiatry 1990; 27: 280–288.

131. Verhoeven WMA, Elderson A, Westenberg HGM. Neuroleptic malignant syndrome: successful treatment with bromocriptine. Biol Psychiatry 1985; 20: 680–684.

132. Nisijima K, Oyafuso K, Shimada T, Hosino H, Ishiguro T. Cerebrospinal fluid monoamine metabolism in a case of neuroleptic malignant syndrome improved by electroconvulsive therapy. Biol Psychiatry 1996; 39: 383–384.

133. Granato JE, Stern BJ, Ringel A, et al. Neuroleptic malignant syndrome: successful treatment with dantrolene and bromocriptine. Ann Neurol 1983; 14: 89–90.

134. Jauss M, Krack P, Franz M, et al. Imaging of dopamine receptors with [^{123}I]Iodobenzamide Single-Photon Emission-Computed Tomography in neuroleptic malignant syndrome. Mov Disord 1996; 11: 726–728.

135. Jones EM, Dawson A. Neuroleptic malignant syndrome: a case report with post mortem brain and muscle pathology. J Neurol Neurosurg Psychiatry 1989; 52: 1006–1009.

136. Horn E, Lach B, Lapierre Y, Hrdina P. Hypothalamic pathology in the neuroleptic malignant syndrome. Am J Psychiatry 1988; 145: 617–620.

137. Caroff S, Rosenberg H, Gerber J. Neuroleptic malignant syndrome and malignant hyperthermia. Lancet 1983; 1: 244.

138. Araki M, Takagi A, Higuchi I, Sugita H. Neuroleptic malignant syndrome: caffeine contracture of single muscle fibers and muscle pathology. Neurology 1988; 38: 297–301.

139. Behan WMH, Madigan M, Clark BJ, Goldberg J, McLellan DR. Muscle changes in the neuroleptic malignant syndrome. J Clin Pathol 2000; 53: 223–227.

140. Hermesh H, Aizenberg D, Lapidot M, Munitz H. Neuroleptic malignans. Neurology 1989; 39: 1273.

141. Addonizio G, Susman VL. ECT as a treatment alternative for patients with symptoms of neuroleptic malignant syndrome. J Clin Psychiatry 1987; 48: 102–105.

142. Feibel JH, Schiffer RB. Sympathoadenomedullary hyperactivity in neuroleptic malignant syndrome: a case report. Am J Psychiatry 1981; 138: 1115–1116.

143. Bigornia L, Suozzo M, Ryan KA, Napp D, Schneider AS. Dopamine receptors on adrenal chromaffin cells modulate calcium uptake and catecholamine release. J Neurochem 1988; 51: 999–1006.

144. Gurrera RJ. Sympathoadrenal hyperactivity and the etiology of neuroleptic malignant syndrome. Am J Psychiatry 1999; 156: 169–180.

145. Gibb WRG, Wedzicha JA, Hoffbrand BI. Recurrent neuroleptic malignant syndrome and hyponatremia. J Neurol Neurosurg Psychiatry 1986; 49: 960–961.

146. Tomson CRV. Neuroleptic malignant syndrome associated with inappropriate antidiuresis and psychogenic polydipsia. Br Med J 1986; 292; 171.

147. Moore AP, Macfarlane FA, Blumhardt LD. Neuroleptic malignant syndrome and hypothyroidism. J Neurol Neurosurg Psychiatry 1990; 53: 517–518.

148. Keck PE, Pope HG, Cohen BM, et al. Risk factors for neuroleptic malignant syndrome: a case controlled study. Arch Gen Psychiatry 1989; 46: 914–918.
149. Berardi D, Amore M, Keck PE, Troia M, Dell'Atti M. Clinical and pharmacologic risk factors for neuroleptic malignant syndrome: a case control study. Biol Psychiatry 1998; 44: 748–754.
150. Alexander PJ, Thomas RM, Das A. Is risk for neuroleptic malignant syndrome increased in the postpartum period? J Clin Psychiatry 1998; 59: 254–255.
151. Fido AA. Postpartum period: a risk factor for neuroleptic malignant syndrome. Ann Clin Psychiatry 1999; 11: 13–15.
152. Caroff SN, Mann SC, McCarthy M, Naser J, Rynn M, Morrison M. Acute infectious encephalitis complicated by neuroleptic malignant syndrome. J Clin Psychopharmacol 1998; 18: 349–351.
153. Kawanishi C, Hanihara T, Shimoda Y, et al. Lack of association between neuroleptic malignant syndrome and polymorphisms in the 5HT1A and 5HT2A receptor genes. Am J Psychiatry 1998; 155: 1275–1277.
154. Suzuki A, Kondo T, Otani K, et al. Association of the TaqI A polymorphism of the dopamine D(2) receptor gene with predisposition of neuroleptic malignant syndrome. Am J Psychiatry 2001; 158: 1714–1716.
155. Kawanishi C, Hanihara T, Maruyama Y, et al. Neuroleptic malignant syndrome and hydroxylase gene mutations: no association with CYP2D6A or CYP2D6B. Psychiatr Genet 1997; 7: 127–129.
156. Iwahashi K, Yoshihara E, Nakamura K, et al. CYP2D6 HhaI genotype and neuroleptic malignant syndrome. Neuropsychobiology 1999; 39: 33–37.
157. Miyatake R, Iwahashi K, Matsushita M, Nakamura K, Suwaki H. No association between neuroleptic malignant syndrome and mutations in the RYR1 gene associated with malignant hyperthermia. J Neurol Sci 1996; 143: 161–165.
158. Velamoor VR, Fernando MLD, Williamson P. Incipient neuroleptic malignant syndrome? Br J Psychiatry 1990; 156: 581–584.
159. Dhib-Jalbut S, Hesselbrock R, Mouradian MM, Means ED. Bromocriptine treatment of neuroleptic malignant syndrome. J Clin Psychiatry 1987; 48: 69–73.
160. Mueller PS, Vester JW, Fermaglich J. Neuroleptic malignant syndrome: successful treatment with bromocriptine. JAMA 1983; 249: 386–388.
161. Adityanjee, Das P, Chawle HM. Neuroleptic malignant syndrome and psychotic illness. Br J Psychiatry 1989; 155: 852–854.
162. May DC, Morris SW, Stewart RM, et al. Neuroleptic malignant syndrome: response to dantrolene sodium. Ann Intern Med 1983; 98: 183–184.
163. Goekoop JG, Carbaat PA Th. Treatment of neuroleptic malignant syndrome with dantrolene. Lancet 1982; 2: 49–50.
164. Sakkas P, Davis JM, Hua J, Wang Z. Pharmacotherapy of neuroleptic malignant syndrome. Psychiatr Ann 1991; 21: 157–164.
165. Goulon M, de Rohan-Chabot P, Elkharrat D, et al. Beneficial effects of dantrolene in the treatment of neuroleptic malignant syndrome: a report of two cases. Neurology 1983; 33: 516–518.
166. McCarron MM, Boettger ML, Peck JJ. A case of neuroleptic malignant syndrome successfully treated with amantadine. J Clin Psychiatry 1982; 43: 381–382.
167. Harris M, Nora L, Tanner CM. Neuroleptic malignant syndrome responsive to carbidopa/levodopa: support for a dopaminergic pathogenesis. Clin Neuropharmacol 1987; 10: 186–189.
168. Rodriguez ME, Luquin MR, Lera G, et al. Neuroleptic malignant syndrome treated with subcutaneous lisuride infusion. Mov Disord 1990; 5: 170–172.

169. Wang H-C, Hseih Y. Treatment of neuroleptic malignant syndrome with subcutaneous apomorphine monotherapy. Mov Disord 2001; 16: 765–767.
170. Thomas P, Maron M, Rascle C, et al. Carbamazepine in the treatment of neuroleptic malignant syndrome. Biol Psychiatry 1998; 43: 303–305.
171. Nisijima K, Kusakabe Y, Ohtuka K, Ishiguro T. Addition of carbamazepine to long-term treatment with neuroleptics may induce neuroleptic malignant syndrome. Biol Psychiatry 1998; 44: 930–931.
172. Jessee SS, Anderson GF. ECT in the neuroleptic malignant syndrome: case report. J Clin Psychiatry 1983; 44: 186–188.
173. Fochtmann L. A mechanism for efficacy of ECT in Parkinson's disease. Convulsive Ther 1988; 4: 321–327.
174. Douyon R, Serby M, Klutchko, B, Rotrosen J. ECT and Parkinson's disease revisited: a "naturalistic" study. Am J Psychiatry 1989; 146: 1451–1455.
175. Mann SC, Caroff SN, Bleier HR, Antelo RE, Un H. Electroconvulsive therapy of the lethal catatonia syndrome: case report and review. Convulsive Ther 1990; 6: 239–247.
176. Caroff SN, Mann SC. Neuroleptic malignant syndrome. Psychopharmacol Bull 1988; 24: 25–29.
177. Nisijima K, Ishiguro T. Electroconvulsive therapy for the treatment of neuroleptic malignant syndrome with psychotic symptoms: a report of five cases. J ECT 1999; 15: 158–163.
178. Gaitini L, Fradis M, Vaida S, Krimerman S, Beny A. Plasmapheresis in neuroleptic malignant syndrome. Anaesthesia 1997; 52: 165–168.
179. Mayeux R, Stern Y, Mulvey K, Cote L. Reappraisal of temporary levodopa withdrawal ("drug holiday") in Parkinson's disease. N Engl J Med 1985; 313: 724–728.
180. Rosebush PI, Stewart TD, Gelenberg AJ. Twenty neuroleptic rechallenges after neuroleptic malignant syndrome in 15 patients. J Clin Psychiatry 1989; 50: 295–298.
181. Susman VL, Addonizio G. Recurrences of neuroleptic malignant syndrome. J Nerv Ment Disord 1988; 176: 234–241.
182. Shalev A, Hermesh H, Aisenberg D, Munitz H. Neuroleptic malignant syndrome. N Eng J Med 1985; 313: 1292–1294.

CHAPTER 9

Tardive dyskinesia

Thomas M. Hyde, Jose A. Apud, Whitney C. Fisher, and Michael F. Egan

Introduction

The introduction of neuroleptics in 1954 for the treatment of psychotic disorders was a major landmark in medicine, and psychiatry in particular. While the clinical efficacy of these agents was quickly established, the subsequent discovery of a sometimes-persistent involuntary movement disorder tardive dyskinesia (TD) associated with long-term administration led to more cautious use. The recent introduction of clozapine and other atypical antipsychotics may have reduced the frequency of TD (see Chapter 12). Nevertheless, some patients continue to require typical neuroleptics and TD remains a clinical problem. In this chapter, we will discuss the clinical issues related to TD, including minimizing the risk of TD, whether to continue neuroleptics in patients with TD, and what medications may be useful for suppressing TD.

History of TD

In 1957, five years after the introduction of chlorpromazine Delay and Deniker [1], and Schonecker [2] described what were probably the first reported cases of TD. Following 2 to 8 weeks of exposure to chlorpromazine, three elderly women developed lip-smacking dyskinetic movements. TD was first described in the American literature in 1960 [3]. Several years later, Hunter and associates [4] described dyskinesias in 13 female inpatients with chronic psychiatric illness, all of whom had been treated with phenothiazines. The notion that TD was uncommon persisted until large studies in the late 1960s began to reveal relatively high prevalence rates. General acceptance of the association of TD with long-term neuroleptic treatment occurred in the early 1970s. The first therapeutic trials for TD followed shortly thereafter [5–7]. In the 1970s, reports of TD in children and severe, disabling TD in adults [8–10] began to appear [11].

Epidemiology

Although epidemiological data point to neuroleptic exposure as being the most significant etiologic factor in the development of TD, some authors have continued to question this relationship [12, 13]. For example, in a study comparing chronic schizophrenic inpatients treated with neuroleptics with a neuroleptic-naïve group, Owens and associates [12] did not find a significant difference between prevalence rates of spontaneous dyskinesia (53.2%) and TD (67%). When the data were reanalyzed adjusting for a difference in the age of the two groups, a slightly higher prevalence in the neuroleptic-treated patients was found [14]. Fenton et al. [15] found that the prevalence of spontaneous orofacial dyskinesias was 15% when reviewing detailed records of neuroleptic-naïve patients with schizophrenia. This study highlights the difficulty of distinguishing spontaneous from tardive dyskinesia in any given patient. Despite the presence of spontaneous dyskinesias in patients with schizophrenia, epidemiological studies [16] strongly suggest that neuroleptics produce dyskinesias in patients with a wide variety of psychiatric diagnoses.

Estimates of the prevalence of TD have ranged from 0.5 to 62% [16, 17]. Several factors may complicate these estimates and explain such widely divergent results. These include differences in diagnostic criteria, assessment methods, patient age, gender and psychiatric diagnoses, possible comorbid medical and neurological illnesses, and duration and type of neuroleptic exposure. The most recent and well-controlled studies (1980–1988) have estimated the average prevalence to be about 30% with typical neuroleptic therapy [18–21].

Data on incidence provide a more accurate estimate of risk per year with exposure to typical neuroleptics. These data have been generated from several, rigorous, large-scale, prospective studies. Results indicate that the average yearly rate of developing TD is about 5% per year for the first several years. The cumulative 5-year incidence rate appears to be 20–26% [22, 23]. It is unclear whether the risk levels off after 5 years or continues to increase linearly. Glazer et al. [24] have suggested that the risk may indeed be linear for 10 years or more, with the 10-year risk estimated at 49% and the 25-year risk estimated at 68%.

Epidemiological studies have uncovered a variety of risk factors that increase the chance of developing TD (e.g., [16, 25, 22]). Demographic risk factors include increased age, psychiatric diagnosis (mood disorders have increased risk), and gender. Regarding the latter, initial studies suggested that females had increased rates, but these findings were confounded by differences in age or treatment variables between groups. More recent, controlled studies only find higher rates in women over 65 years, while gender effects are not apparent in younger cohorts. In fact, some studies have found greater severity in young men, compared to young women [17]. The presence of diabetes, organic brain damage, and negative symptoms (in patients with schizophrenia) also may significantly increase risk, perhaps through their effects on the corticostriatal input or striatal function itself. Studies focused on patients with organic brain damage, patients with diabetes, or the elderly suggest these factors may increase 1-year incidence rates up to 20% or more. Treatment variables associated with increased risk include higher dose of neuroleptics, number of medication-free periods, and a history of acute extrapyramidal side effects. The association with increased dose has not been found in many studies, but has intuitive appeal [22, 23]. How medication-free periods and acute extrapyramidal side effects increase TD incidence is unclear but could theoretically be mediated through their impact on the D1-mediated striato-nigral pathway (e.g., [26]).

In the United States, clozapine, a highly effective novel atypical antipsychotic, is rarely associated with TD, if at all [23, 27]. This observation indicates that it is possible for a medication to be a highly potent antipsychotic while not causing TD. Unfortunately, the use of clozapine has been severely limited by a variety of other potential side effects, such as agranulocytosis and seizures. As a consequence, new medications have been designed to mimic clozapine's therapeutic profile but with fewer potential serious side effects. A number of atypical agents are now in common use. These new "atypical" agents, which include risperidone, olanzapine, quetiapine, sertindole, ziprasidone, and aripiprizole, appear to cause fewer acute extrapyramidal side effects than older, "typical" agents. Moreover, with long-term use they appear to be associated with a lower incidence of TD (see Chapter 11). However, these agents are not a panacea, as they have other serious side effects including weight gain, diabetes, and sedation.

Data supporting the notion that atypical antipsychotics have a markedly lower propensity to cause TD is only gradually emerging. Initial reports on this issue suggested that atypical agents did produce some cases of TD, but these reports were problematic. First, many were single case reports rather than systematic prospective studies. Second, most of the patients who develop TD while on atypical agents had previous long-term exposure to high-potency typical drugs. It can take up to several months for the elimination of high-potency typical neuroleptics from the brain after years of treatment. The dyskinesias might have been masked, only to appear several months after a change from typical to atypical agents. Later case reports, however, appeared more convincing, with dyskinesias developing after prolonged administration of these atypical agents and without prior typical agent exposure (28, 29]).

One of the first well-executed studies demonstrating the markedly lower propensity of TD with atypical agents was a double-blind randomized trial of olanzapine versus haloperidol over 2.6 years. This study revealed a dramatically lower incidence of TD in olanzapine-treated subjects (0.52% vs. 7.45%) [30]. Glazer [31] reported similar findings. Kane and colleagues [27] concluded that if clozapine does cause TD, it does so at an extremely low rate. They were unable to demonstrate that clozapine definitively induced TD with long-term treatment in 28 patients. The relatively abrupt cessation of clozapine has been associated with the transient appearance of dyskinesias [32]. However, these may have been dyskinesias suppressed by clozapine rather than induced by this medication. A reduction in clozapine dose also has been associated with the reemergence of TD suppressed by a higher dose of this medication [33]. Risperidone has been associated with the production of TD in a few case reports [34, 35]. In a more systematic study, Jeste [36] found a much lower rate of TD with risperidone treatment in comparison to haloperidol, in agreement with an earlier report from Chouinard [37]. A meta-analysis of risperidone clinical trials noted an extremely low incidence of TD among risperidone-treated subjects [0.23%] [38]. This analysis is limited by the comparatively short duration of risperidone treatment (12 months maximum). For quetiapine, a somewhat convincing case report also was published in 1999 [39]. However, this patient had been treated with high-potency typical neuroleptics for many years prior to receiving quetiapine. Therefore, the appearance of TD on quetiapine could just as easily have resulted from an unmasking of latent dyskinesias suppressed by typical neuroleptic therapy. These studies provide strong support for the notion that atypical agents dramatically lower the incidence of TD.

Despite the promise of atypical agents, many patients, for various reasons, continue to require older typical neuroleptic agents, and continue to develop and suffer from TD. Thus, although the pool of patients developing this disorder is undoubtedly shrinking, TD remains a therapeutic issue. The challenges facing clinicians include how to minimize the risk of TD, and what to do with patients once they develop TD. Awareness of the alternatives will hopefully facilitate treating patients chronically with neuroleptics.

Prevention of TD

The mainstay of TD prevention has been to limit exposure to typical neuroleptic agents whenever possible. For patients who require neuroleptics, most experts recommend that one use the smallest effective dose and atypical agents as first-line pharmacological therapy. The idea that increased dose of typical agents has a significant impact on the incidence or severity of TD has intuitive appeal but limited empirical support [23, 40]. Most studies have actually failed to find such a relationship. Those that have are often criticized for methodological confounds that cloud their interpretation [23, 41–43]. A recently published study that addressed some of the typical methodological pitfalls suggests that each 100 mg chlorpromazine equivalent increase in dose is associated with a 5% increase in the chance of developing TD [44]. On the other hand, very low-dose neuroleptic therapy carries a higher risk of psychiatric relapse [42, 45, 46]. The rate of relapse must be balanced against the risk of acute nondyskinetic side effects (e.g., sedation), which are frequently dose-related and often lead to medication noncompliance. For long-term treatment, intermediate doses (e.g., 400–900 mg chlorpromazine equivalents) may be as effective as the higher doses often used in acute settings [40, 47, 48].

Intermittent treatment or use of "drug holidays" has been examined as a way to reduce cumulative neuroleptic exposure. While one study suggested that this strategy might benefit some patients [49], it is often an impractical and possibly dangerous strategy. In fact, well-controlled studies suggest that intermittent neuroleptic treatment is less effective at preventing psychotic relapse [50], does not prevent the development of TD [51–53], and may even *increase* the likelihood of developing TD [54]. "Drug holidays" should be used with great caution, and the prevention of TD is an inadequate rationale for their use.

Depot neuroleptics are often used to improve medication compliance and reduce relapse rates. Currently, these preparations are limited to the high-potency typical agents, haloperidol and fluphenazine (although depot forms of atypical agents are in development). One report found that depot neuroleptics have a higher tendency to cause TD [55], but this requires additional study. Such an association could be due to poor compliance and the subsequent intermittent treatment of patients who are treated with depot preparations.

Long-term use of neuroleptics is indicated primarily for a subset of psychiatric patients. These include patients with chronic psychotic disorders, especially schizophrenia and schizoaffective disorder, who demonstrate a clear therapeutic response. A variety of other patient groups are often administered neuroleptics, including those with treatment-resistant bipolar disorder, unipolar depression, obsessive-compulsive disorder, and borderline personality disorder. Many of these patients can be maintained on other agents that are much less likely to produce TD. These include lithium, anticonvulsants (e.g., carbamazepine and valproic acid), tricyclics, serotonin reuptake inhibitors, mixed norepinephrine and serotonin reuptake inhibitors, and benzodiazepines. The preferred strategy to minimize the risk of TD is to use atypical neuroleptics. However, some patients will not respond as well to clozapine as they do to other neuroleptics. Unfortunately, clozapine's expense, and the need for regular blood monitoring, have been other major factors limiting its use.

Risperidone was the first of the new generation of putative atypical neuroleptics modeled after clozapine. Clinical and preclinical studies indicate that risperidone has a reduced liability to produce acute extrapyramidal side effects (EPS) [56]. Because lower acute EPS liability has been hypothesized to be associated with a lower risk of producing TD, such results are encouraging [57]. Recent case reports, however, indicate that risperidone can induce TD [58–60]. In one case, a schizophrenic patient had been medication-free for 6 months before risperidone was started; abnormal movements developed after 1 year on risperidone [60]. More recent prospective studies have confirmed that risperidone has lower propensity to induce TD compared to typical agents [36, 38]. Based largely on its clinical efficacy and reduced liability for acute EPS and TD, risperidone has become a drug of choice at many centers in consideration for the prevention of TD.

The development of additional "atypical" neuroleptics has proceeded rapidly. For olanzapine and sertindole, phase II and III studies convincingly demonstrated that both medications are very effective in treating psychosis and have a low incidence of EPS [61–63]. Additional "atypical" agents, including quetiapine, ziprasidone, and aripiprazole also are available. In preclinical studies, sertindole produced dose-related EPS in Cebus monkeys. It was also effective in suppressing spontaneous dyskinesias in monkeys [64], suggesting that it might also be effective in suppressing TD. Of course, antipsychotics that induce EPS and suppress dyskinesias also have the potential to produce TD. Nevertheless, the introduction of "atypical" neuroleptics, without the onerous blood testing regimen required with clozapine, is perhaps the most exciting development related to TD prevention in decades. Their use has largely supplanted the use of high-potency typical agents.

Another untested strategy is the prophylactic use of protective agents to reduce the incidence of TD during chronic neuroleptic treatment. Data using animal models indicate that antioxidants, such as vitamin E [65] and GM1 ganglioside [66] reduce dyskinesia scores in animals treated with long-term haloperidol decanoate. Vitamin E has also been shown to attenuate the development of D_2 supersensitivity [67], a likely important step in the genesis of TD. Clinical studies in humans have typically found that Vitamin E reduces severity of preexisting TD (see the discussion under TD suppression: medication trails). These observations suggest that prophylactic treatment (e.g., 1,200–2,000 IU/day) with vitamin E could reduce the risk of developing TD. While no human studies are available to support this strategy, long-term use of vitamin E has little risk. Lithium has also been suggested to reduce the incidence of TD [68], although recent data are conflicting [43, 69]. Routine use of lithium for TD prevention is uncommon.

Finally, two other interventions may help patients avoid developing TD. First, medication compliance should be emphasized, as this will limit drug-free periods and reduce any risk for TD that this entails. Secondly, vigorous treatment of comorbid substance abuse disorders is important. Anecdotal reports suggest that patients who abuse stimulants such as cocaine may develop more severe symptoms. Thus, the physician has a number of tools, such as the use of atypical agents, encouraging medication compliance, the administration of antioxidants, and treatment of comorbid substance abuse that can reduce a patient's chance of developing TD.

Management of patients with TD

When symptoms of TD first appear, a thorough medical evaluation should be considered. Briefly, this includes physical and neurological examination, laboratory testing, and a review of the differential diagnosis [70]. Fortunately, the incidence of organic disorders masquerading as TD appears to be very low [71]. The next issue is the continuation of neuroleptic therapy. Most published recommendations suggest that drug withdrawal or marked dose reduction, when possible, are indicated; the likelihood of psychotic relapse, however, is fairly high and is a major risk of this approach. Conversion to a high-potency "atypical" agent is often a safer option. A third issue is whether additional medications are needed to suppress TD. Often, mild-to-moderate symptoms are either unnoticed or have little functional impact. For those whom suppressive therapy is needed, the treating physician can choose from a number of mildly-to-moderately successful interventions.

It is imperative to involve both the patient and their family from the outset, so that informed decisions can be made and documented. Patients educated with printed information sheets [72] appear better informed than those educated verbally [73]. Routine monitoring of TD is essential to quantitatively track symptomatic changes and treatment response. The most popular rating procedure is the AIMS examination [74]. Ratings should be performed every

4 to 6 months on patients with TD and perhaps more often when medication changes are made. Moreover, an examination should also be performed at least semiannually on patients at risk for developing TD.

Clinical course of TD

Data on the natural course of TD is critical for assessing treatment options. Of greatest concern is the possibility that continued treatment could lead to relentless progression. Fortunately, this does not seem to be the case for the large majority of patients. Data from several long-term studies indicate that progression to severe TD, if it does occur, happens only in a small percentage of cases [75–80]. This is supported by epidemiological studies indicating that the prevalence of moderately severe TD is roughly 6% to 10% of patients with TD or about 4% of patients treated with neuroleptics [81, 82]. The prevalence of very severe TD is probably lower than this, but estimates are difficult to come by [83]. By far, the most common course for TD is a waxing and waning of mild-to-moderate symptoms over many years [23, 75, 84–86]. Approximately 50% of patients will show recurrent symptoms with neither marked progression nor extended remission. While estimates between studies vary, many suggest that 10% to 30% will have a reduction in movements or full remission, while 10% to 30% will show some degree of worsening. These data suggest that for many patients, continued treatment with neuroleptics after the development of TD is a reasonable option.

   Risk factors have been examined in attempts to identify those patients that are most likely to show progression and/or persistence of TD with continued treatment. In general, these factors are similar to risk factors for developing TD (although see [23]). They include age [87], gender, and exposure to anticholinergic agents. Increasing age has been associated with fewer spontaneous remissions while on medication and less improvement after medications are withdrawn. Regarding gender, the literature is divided. Many suggest that female gender is associated with increased risk and persistence, although the opposite has also been found [17, 86, 88]. Worse prognosis has been associated less commonly with duration of exposure to neuroleptics, diagnosis (worse with organic brain syndromes and affective disorders), duration of TD [79, 88–90] and frequent on/off manipulations [23]. Overall, these data suggest that efforts to reduce or discontinue neuroleptics might be directed toward those at greater risk.

Neuroleptic discontinuation

Although continued neuroleptic treatment may be a psychiatric necessity for many patients with TD, this must be weighed against the potential benefits of withdrawal and discontinuation. Indeed, many experts [40] recommend neuroleptic withdrawal, with the critical caveat that it should only be done in patients who can tolerate it. Unfortunately, predicting who can or cannot tolerate this is fraught with uncertainty. A recent rigorous review of the literature concluded that there is a lack of evidence to support the efficacy of neuroleptic cessation as a treatment for TD, although dose reduction may be beneficial [91]. In the first several weeks following withdrawal, TD often gets worse [92, 93]. For example, Gardos et al. withdrew neuroleptics from 33 patients and noted significant increases in dyskinesia severity and dysphoria in 33%, resulting in early removal from the study. Glazer et al. [94] withdrew neuroleptics for 3 weeks in 19 patients and noted a relapse of psychosis in 26% and TD worsening in 53% of the patients. The magnitude of TD exacerbation in this study is unclear.

Despite the initial exacerbation that may result from neuroleptic withdrawal, TD does appear to improve over the long term. In a comprehensive review of 20 studies, Jeste and Wyatt [95] reported that 36% of patients withdrawn from neuroleptics showed improvement. Since then, additional studies tend to support their conclusion. Jus and colleagues [96] found improvement in 49 of 62 patients by slowly tapering neuroleptics over 4 years. Improvement has been seen up to 5 years after cessation of treatment [97]. In a mostly nonpsychotic patient group, Fahn [98] reported improvement in 13 out of 22 patients over a 2-to-4-year period. These patients had concurrent treatment with reserpine or tetrabenazine. In contrast, Glazer and colleagues [99] followed 49 patients for an average of 40 weeks after discontinuation of neuroleptics. Complete remission was rare (2%), dyskinesia severity improved in only 20%, and relapse of psychosis for patients with schizophrenia approached 50% [99, 100]. One difficulty with drawing conclusions from these studies is that many were unblinded or poorly controlled. Nevertheless, they suggest that neuroleptic withdrawal is risky but can result in long-term remission of TD in some patients [78].

Degree of improvement following withdrawal may be related to the same risk factors associated with the development of TD and improvement during continued treatment. Poor outcome related to age, over 65 years [87] showing little improvement, organic brain damage, number of extended medication-free periods, and length of neuroleptic treatment [95]. If drug withdrawal is attempted, very gradual tapers appear to be less likely to lead to worsening of psychosis. A variation of this strategy is to initially increase neuroleptic dose to suppress TD followed by very gradual withdrawal (e.g., 10% per month). This has worked in at least several cases of moderate-to-severe TD with dystonic features (Kleinman J, personal communication), but has not been studied in controlled trials.

While withdrawal should be considered, many patients will not be able to tolerate this approach. The risks associated with neuroleptic withdrawal include psychotic decompensation [101] and increased likelihood of injury to self or others. Furthermore, untreated patients with schizophrenia may have a worse long-term prognosis than patients treated with neuroleptics [102]. Over the long term, some patients initially withdrawn from neuroleptics have actually ended up receiving higher total doses of neuroleptics to cope with symptom exacerbation [103]. Many factors may be important in predicting the success of neuroleptic withdrawal, such as psychiatric diagnosis, past history of dangerous behavior, current stressors, living and working environment, and family relationships.

Switching to "atypical" antipsychotics

In lieu of typical neuroleptics, alternate therapeutic agents must be considered. In patients requiring continued neuroleptic therapy, the first choice is to switch patients to an "atypical" drug. These medications offer the advantage of potent antipsychotic efficacy and the possibility of reduction of the risk for TD. Extrapolating, one might conclude that patients with TD will have a greater likelihood of TD remission on atypical neuroleptics. A small retrospective study of the effects of clozapine on TD revealed an 85% reduction in involuntary movements over a 10-month trial [104]. A small open prospective trial found a 52% reduction in the severity of TD with clozapine [105]. Another trial purportedly found no benefit from clozapine. However, this study did not assess the longitudinal course of TD in patients on clozapine, and easily might have missed a reduction in severity over time [106]. Another small short-term trial with clozapine did not demonstrate any effect on the severity of TD [107]. Several case reports have reported a marked improvement in TD when patients were switched from typical neuroleptics to olanzapine [108] and quetiapine [109]. On the other hand, weight gain and an increased risk of diabetes can complicate treatment with clozapine and other atypical agents. As a result, one must clearly delineate the benefits and risks to patients for each treatment option. In particular, with atypical agents, the possible benefits of TD reduction must be balanced against the risk of side effects such as sedation, weight gain, seizures, diabetes, and/or agranulocytosis.

Suppressive therapy for TD

The next important therapeutic decision is whether to attempt suppression of TD. In our experience, suppressive therapy should be considered if TD poses health risks, impairs function, or is otherwise significantly bothersome to the patient (e.g., problems with breathing, eating, walking, or sleeping). Many patients with moderate-to-severe TD will not meet these requirements and may not even be aware of their symptoms. Furthermore, a moderate or severe rating on an item of the AIMS scale does not necessarily mean a patient is functionally impaired or disfigured. Suppression in these cases may not be necessary. Assessment by an occupational or physical therapist can sometimes give insight into functional impairment and may suggest nonpharmacological strategies to cope with the functional disabilities imposed by TD.

Patients with moderate-to-severe TD are the most likely candidates for suppressive treatments. Severe TD is most common in younger men (under 40 years) and older women (over 65 years), and often has a component of dystonia. Several large studies have found that up to 4% of patients who take chronic neuroleptics develop severe TD. Severe TD can produce a variety of functional problems, depending on the area of the body that is affected. For example, truncal TD can interfere with walking, sitting, and even sleeping (although TD disappears, for the most part, once a patient is able to fall asleep). Orofacial dyskinesia can be particularly disfiguring, sometimes interfering with eating and adequate nutrition, and has been linked to reduced life expectancy [110]. Respiratory dyskinesia is often overlooked and can produce a variety of respiratory signs and symptoms, including irregular respiratory rate, tachypnea, and grunting [111, 112]. Patients with severe TD are at risk for aspiration and its attendant consequences, including pneumonia, cardiopulmonary arrest, and death. A variety of risk factors have been examined, such as number of medication-free periods [82] (although see Gardos et al. [83]), but it is difficult to predict who will develop severe TD. Anecdotal reports suggest that severe TD comes on quickly, developing over the course of several months, rather than being the result of a relentlessly progressive process that develops over a long period of time in the face of continued neuroleptic exposure. Several authors have noted that increased blinking or blepharospasm may be a prodromal symptom [83, 113]. Certainly, many patients have increased blinking and do not go on to develop severe TD. Treatment of severe TD, as with less pronounced forms, often requires continued neuroleptic treatment concomitantly with serial trials of suppressive agents.

Several comprehensive reviews [7, 54, 114–118] have surveyed most of the published data on treatment of TD from the 1970s through the 1990s. In general, the goal of most studies was to demonstrate short-term reduction, or suppression, of dyskinetic symptoms. There are no empirically validated guidelines to follow when choosing a suppressive agent. For patients in need of suppression, carefully trying a number of different agents can sometimes be rewarding. In general, therapeutic trials have attempted to manipulate one of the following neurotransmitter systems: dopamine, GABA, acetylcholine, norepinephrine, and serotonin. These systems have received the most attention in part due to theories about the pathophysiology of TD.

Pathophysiology of TD
Dopamine supersensitivity

The dopamine supersensitivity hypothesis of TD was first proposed in 1970 by Klawans. Based on the similarity between levodopa-induced dyskinesias and TD, he suggested that chronic neuroleptic treatment produced supersensitive striatal dopamine receptors, similar to denervation-induced cholinergic supersensitivity found in peripheral muscles. Since then, dopamine supersensitivity has been an important theoretical construct guiding TD research. Several inconsistencies, however, suggest that it cannot explain entirely the pathogenesis of TD. First, supersensitivity occurs within 2 to 4 weeks of initiating neuroleptic treatment, whereas TD develops after long-term use. Second, in animal studies, most subjects develop supersensitivity, in contrast to the minority of patients that develop TD. Finally, supersensitivity disappears within weeks after neuroleptics are withdrawn, while TD can persist for months and years. The original version of this idea has been supplanted with the notion that D_2 supersensitivity may be a necessary first step in a path that ultimately leads to the development of TD. Interestingly, clozapine does not induce D_2 supersensitivity at standard doses.

Consistent with this are data suggesting that subjects with parkinsonian symptoms are at higher risk for developing TD. A second variation on this theme is the idea that parkinsonian symptoms and subsequent TD are due to sustained high levels of D_2 receptor occupancy with typical agents [119, 120]. In contrast, antipsychotic efficacy may be achieved with lower levels of D_2 occupancy for relatively shorter periods as seen with atypical antipsychotics [121].

A related idea implicates the "balance" between acetylcholine and dopamine. This is supported, for example, by the observations that parkinsonian symptoms are alleviated by dopamine agonists or cholinergic antagonists. Higher doses of dopamine agonists can also induce dyskinesias. If dopamine and acetylcholine work in the opposite direction, this implies that cholinergic agonists could alleviate dyskinesias. While this idea has been heuristically useful, initial attempts at cholinergic potentiation as a treatment for TD were largely unsuccessful. Relatively few data are available regarding the efficacy of newer cholinesterase inhibitors available for the treatment of Alzheimer's disease.

GABA depletion

Considerable attention has been focused on the GABA (gamma amino butyric acid) system, which is a major inhibitory component of basal ganglia pathways [122–124]. A number of studies point to decreased GABA turnover or increased GABA binding sites in one or more areas of the basal ganglia in rodents and primates following chronic neuroleptic treatment. This reduction in turnover is most prominent in animals that have dyskinesias [125]. Furthermore, changes in GABA activity (e.g. GAD 67 mRNA expression levels) are produced by typical but not atypical neuroleptics [126]. Anderson and colleagues [127], in a very small human postmortem study found a significant decrease in subthalamic glutamic acid decarboxylase (GAD) activity (the rate-limiting enzyme in the metabolic pathway for GABA) in patients with TD compared with patients without TD. Other attempts to assess GABAergic neurotransmission in living patients have also suggested that individuals with TD have particular abnormalities [128, 129]. Traditional clinical-neuropathological studies strongly implicate the basal ganglia in involuntary movement disorders. GABAergic neurons play a central role in the subcortical regions that generate abnormal movements. Further study of this system has led to more detailed notions of those components that may be abnormal. GABA agonists have some therapeutic efficacy in either suppressing or ameliorating TD, such as the anticonvulsant gabapentin [130].

Neurotoxicity

The possibility that long-term neuroleptic treatment may have a toxic effect on the brain has led to many studies that look for evidence of neuronal injury. The neurotoxicity hypothesis is particularly engaging given the persistence of TD, in some cases, and the similarity between TD and degenerative diseases of the basal ganglia, such as Huntington's disease. Unfortunately, most postmortem studies in animals and patients exposed to long-term neuroleptic treatment have been inconsistent or have suffered from methodological problems [131–138]. Neuroleptics could produce more subtle damage, however, through mechanisms other than simple neuronal degeneration. Dopamine is metabolized by MAO to DOPAC (and then HVA). A byproduct of this reaction is hydrogen peroxide, a potent oxidant. It has been hypothesized that hydrogen peroxide could generate a cascade of free radicals that react with proteins, lipids, and other cellular constituents, ultimately leading to significant neuronal dysfunction. Indeed, several groups have found evidence suggesting that free radical formation may occur both in rodents and humans treated with neuroleptics [139]. Neuroleptics may also alter striatal glutaminergic neurotransmission, perhaps impacting excitotoxic mechanisms, as some data from animal models suggest [140]. Melatonin is a lipid-soluble free-radical scavenger that is highly active as an antioxidant. Interestingly, a small double-blind, placebo-controlled study using 10 mg per day for 6 weeks found that melatonin was effective in ameliorating TD [141]. On the other hand, vitamin E, another antioxidant, has been tried in a number of small studies but its efficacy remains uncertain (as reviewed [115, 116, 142, 143]). While stronger evidence is clearly required, this hypothesis has led to trials of antioxidants as a treatment for TD.

Striatal dysfunction

Studies on the basal ganglia and movement disorders suggest that the final common pathway for dyskinesias is increased activation of the D_1-mediated striatonigral/striatopallidal (or "direct") pathway [144–146]. These medium spiny striatal neurons are primarily GABAergic, but also use several neuropeptides as cotransmitters, including substance P, and dynorphin. The direct pathway inhibits neurons in the substantia nigra, pars reticulata, and its associated nucleus, the internal segment of the globus pallidus. These areas, in turn, project to the thalamus, which is thought to act as a filter for cortical input. The theory is that increased inhibition of the inhibitory GABAergic nigral/pallidal outflow produces a net increase (or loss of inhibition) in the activity of thalamocortical projections. The other major outflow tract from the striatum [144–146], the D_2-mediated striatopallidal (or "indirect") loop (projective to the external segment of the globus pallidus), may also play a role. The medium spiny neurons of this pathway are also GABAergic and use the neuropeptide enkephalin as a cotransmitter. Increased activity of this pathway that results from blockade of the inhibitory D_2 receptors, may facilitate the expression of D_1 overactivation [26]. Indeed, animal studies suggest that haloperidol increases D_1 agonist-induced dyskinetic mouth movements in rodents. The specific molecular changes underlying persistent motor abnormalities are unclear but could be related to subtle cytoarchitectural changes in enkephalinergic [147] or glutamatergic terminals [148].

While the hypothesis that TD is a result of such alterations in basal ganglia physiology remains unproven, it suggests that a variety of neurotransmitters and receptors could play a role. Examples include D_1 and D_2 receptors, CCK, neurotensin, GABA, NMDA receptors, and opiate receptors (mu, kappa, and possibly delta). Drugs targeting these transmitter systems may possibly affect TD symptoms. Unfortunately, animal studies using such agents have been inconclusive, and human studies are limited. Moreover, while an imbalance between the direct and indirect basal ganglia pathways may explain the involuntary movements themselves, the etiology and nature of the basal ganglia pathology that underlies these movements remains obscure.

TD suppression: medication trials

The competing theories on TD have led to clinical trials of a wide variety of medications. Many of these trials have serious deficiencies, and none has been successful in the majority of patients. As a result, one may have to try several medications before finding one with some utility. Selection is guided by the underlying psychiatric diagnosis, risk/benefit analysis, success in prior studies, potential side effects of the suppressing agent, and interactions with other medications.

Suppression with typical antipsychotics

Typical neuroleptics themselves may be effective to some degree in suppressing TD. A 1979 review of 50 studies, totaling 501 patients, found that 67% of the patients showed clinical improvement with neuroleptic suppression, the highest improvement rate of any suppressive strategy [95]. However, a subsequent review [114] suggested a lower rate of response. Suppressive effects are most pronounced in short-term studies [7, 40, 149, 150], although some well-controlled studies have found that suppression is often minimal [151, 152]. The therapeutic efficacy of long-term (more than 8 weeks) suppression is unclear, in part due to problems with study design. Most studies have first withdrawn patients from neuroleptics and then compared changes between neuroleptic and placebo treatment [5, 153–156]. This may be a better measure of ability to suppress withdrawal dyskinesias than persistent TD. For example, haloperidol was able to dramatically reduce TD in a small cohort of patients withdrawn from neuroleptics for 80 days, and then reassessed after 21 days of haloperidol treatment [107]. Other studies are either unblinded or lacked appropriate control groups [96, 154, 157, 158]. Of three particularly well-controlled studies, two found significant long-term suppression [159, 160], while the third did not [161]. A fourth study using depot neuroleptics showed brief improvement (i.e, 1–2 days) along with increased blood levels immediately following drug injection in four of six patients [162]. While potentially useful, the safety and efficacy of increased neuroleptic dose for long-term suppression remains questionable.

A primary concern with using higher neuroleptic doses for suppression is the potential that TD could become worse. Nevertheless, in severe cases with life-threatening complications, increasing dose or a switch to a high-potency typical neuroleptic may be the only maneuver that will provide immediate help. Higher-potency neuroleptics such as haloperidol may be more effective at suppressing movements than those of lower potency such as molindone. Glazer and colleagues [163] were able to suppress 66% of patients with withdrawal TD using haloperidol, but only 39% with molindone. If withdrawal dyskinesias are similar pharmacologically to persistent dyskinesias, they may also be suppressed more effectively by high-potency neuroleptics. Giving medications in smaller divided doses throughout the day has also been helpful in masking symptoms of TD. In a variation of this, we have seen improvement in several patients after stopping neuroleptic treatment for several weeks and then restarting at a lower dose. This has not been studied under controlled conditions.

Suppression with atypical antipsychotics

Beyond their use as drugs with less TD liability, atypical antipsychotics, particularly clozapine, have also been tried as suppressive agents. Early experience with clozapine was generally disappointing [164–166], or mixed [167]. A description of published reports is provided in Table 9.1. Briefly, of 16 publications, seven are case reports, four open trials, one single-blind, and four double-blind or controlled crossover studies. All seven case reports found improvement. Two described rapid TD suppression [168, 169] while four observed dramatic responses only after months or years [170–172]. Four open uncontrolled trials [167, 173–175] also found beneficial effects with clozapine. The most significant results were observed after at least 4 weeks of treatment and in patients with severe TD and tardive dystonia [167–169]. In most cases, TD symptoms returned to baseline after discontinuation of clozapine [167, 173–175]. This suggests that TD was suppressed.

Of the four double-blind, controlled, or crossover studies, two found significant improvement with clozapine [176, 177]. In both positive studies, clozapine was administered for 22 to 52 weeks. The negative studies lasted only 3 to 5 weeks. The study by Tamminga and colleagues was particularly lengthy, and included a control group of 32 patients treated with haloperidol during a 12-month blind treatment period. Comparison of the different studies is complicated by the use of different doses of clozapine, lack of appropriate controls, and inconsistent patient follow-up. Two noteworthy trends are that a long duration of treatment is needed and that dystonic features may be more responsive than dyskinetic [178]. The mixed results in controlled studies suggest that further investigations of clozapine's suppressive properties are warranted.

If clozapine is shown to have therapeutic effects in TD, several mechanisms could potentially play a role. An early acute response to clozapine suggests a *suppressive effect* similar to classical neuroleptics. Longer-term improvement could be due to a *passive* mechanism in which dyskinetic movements improve with time in the absence of the offending agent. A third possibility would

Table 9.1 Studies on the effect of atypical neuroleptics on tardive dyskinesia

Reference	Drug	Design	Duration	Maximal dose	Outcome
Gerlach et al. [165]	Clozapine	Double-blind, cross-over	3 weeks	225 mg/day	No significant effect
Caine et al. [164]	Clozapine	Double-blind, placebo-controlled	3–5 weeks	425 mg/day	No significant effect
Gerlach and Simmelsgaard [166]	Clozapine	Cross-over	4 weeks	62.5 mg/day	No significant effect
Carroll et al. [168]	Clozapine	Case report	18 days	1000 mg/day	Significant improvement
Simpson et al. [176]	Clozapine	Single-blind, placebo-controlled, double cross-over	22 weeks	523–775 mg/day	Significant improvement
Cole et al. [173]	Clozapine	Open, uncontrolled	Up to 12 weeks or more	100–500 mg/day	Significant improvement, mainly after >12 weeks
Gerbino et al. [174]	Clozapine	Open	4 weeks and 12 months	4 weeks: 650 mg/day; 12 months: down to 50% of the initial dose	Significant improvement at both times
Meltzer and Luchins [169]	Clozapine	Case report	2 weeks	900 mg/day	Significant improvement
Small et al. [175]	Clozapine	Open, uncontrolled	7 weeks	340 mg/day	Significant improvement in only 7/19 patients
Van Putten et al. [326]	Clozapine	Case report	14 weeks	250 mg/day	Significant improvement
Lamberti and Bellnier [171]	Clozapine	Case report	11 months	300 mg/day	Significant improvement
Lieberman et al. [167]	Clozapine	Open, uncontrolled	36 months	486 mg/day (average daily dose at end-point)	At least 50% improvement in 43% of patients
Friedman [170]	Clozapine	Case report	>3 years	350–500 mg/day	Significant improvement
Trugman et al. [172]	Clozapine	Case report	4 years	625 mg/day	Significant improvement

(*continued*)

Table 9.1 (*continued*)

Reference	Drug	Design	Duration	Maximal dose	Outcome
Tamminga et al. [177]	Clozapine	Double-blind, controlled, random-ized, non-cross-over	12 months	293.8 mg/day	Significant improvement
Levkovitch et al. [327]	Clozapine	Case report	48 months	450–550 mg/day	Significant improvement
Meco et al. [182]	Risperidone	Cross-over, placebo controlled	4 weeks	6 mg/day	No significant effect
Kopala and Honer [183]	Risperidone	Case report	4 weeks	4 mg/day	Significant improvement
Chouinard [37]	Risperidone	Double-blind, parallel	8 weeks	6–16 mg/day	Significant improvement
Bassitt et al. [179]	clozapine	Open trial	6 months	390 mg/day	52% improvement
Dalack et al. [104]	clozapine	Retrospective chart review	10 months	358 mg/day	85% improvement
Spivak et al. [180]	clozapine	Open trial	18 weeks		74% improvement

be that clozapine has an *active* (not simply suppressive) therapeutic effect on dyskinetic movements. Teasing these differences out could have an impact on the design of future neuroleptics. From a molecular standpoint, clozapine displays affinity for a variety of neurotransmitter receptors. Its higher affinity for the D_1 and 5-HT_2 compared to D_2 receptors and its overall very low affinity for striatal D_2 receptor may be consistent with the low EPS profile of clozapine. The relatively early suppression of dyskinetic movements could be mediated by D_1 receptors. On the other hand, the potent anticholinergic properties of clozapine may explain its efficacy in treating tardive dystonia [181].

Little is known about the efficacy of risperidone in suppressing symptoms of TD. Surprisingly, an early short-term, controlled study found no evidence of suppression, [182]. One case report found suppression of severe TD with risperidone [183]. More convincingly, the Canadian Multicenter Risperidone study showed an antidyskinetic effect in a double-blind, placebo-controlled trial [37]. Thus, risperidone may be useful as suppressive medication.

Other new atypical antipsychotics also may provide alternatives for the treatment of TD. Olanzapine, sertindole, quetiapine, and ziprasidone have been shown to be efficacious for the treatment of psychosis and produce fewer EPS than traditional neuroleptics [61–63, 184, 185]. Similar to clozapine, these drugs are more effective in blocking the 5-HT_2 than the D_2 receptor site, and also have lower D_2 receptor occupancy *in vivo*, particularly quetiapine [121]. On the other hand, in contrast to clozapine, most are relatively potent D_2 antagonists. The finding that clozapine is associated with a lower incidence of TD [57] and may suppress TD suggests that there are important advantages to using clozapine-like medications with selectivity for the 5-HT$_2$ receptor. It is unclear how effectively the new atypical neuroleptics will be in suppressing TD.

Dopamine-depleting agents

Medications that work primarily by reducing or depleting presynaptic stores of dopamine have sometimes been helpful in reducing TD severity. Dopamine-depleting medications, including reserpine, tetrabenazine, α-methyldopa, and AMPT (alpha methyl-p-tyrosine), work by several different mechanisms. Reserpine and tetrabenazine (not available in the United States) disrupt storage of dopamine in presynaptic vesicles. Alpha-methyldopa reduces dopamine synthesis by competitive inhibition of dopa decarboxylase and the formation of a false neurotransmitter. AMPT also reduces dopamine (and norepinephrine) synthesis via its actions on tyrosine hydroxylase, the rate-limiting enzyme in dopamine synthesis.

Studies of dopamine-depleting medications suggest that they may alleviate symptoms in up to 50% of patients with TD. For example, using reserpine, Huang et al. [186] found at least 50% improvement in 5 out of 10 patients, while Fahn [98] showed improvement in 8 of 17 patients (who were no longer taking neuroleptics). Nasrallah et al. [187] found improvement in 5 of 10 patients in a 4-week, double-blind study using AMPT. Only patients who remained on neuroleptics in addition to AMPT improved. While not all studies have found this degree of success [188], previous reviews of both uncontrolled case reports and controlled studies support the 50% estimate [95, 114]. For example, a review of five studies performed from 1961 to 1977 found that tetrabenazine improved TD in 29 of 42 patients. In the same review, 17 out of 38 patients from another five reports improved on reserpine, and 18 of 32 patients improved on AMPT [95]. While larger, well-controlled studies are needed to validate these findings, the limited available data supports the use of dopamine-depleting medications for TD suppression. Unfortunately, major side effects, including hypotension (reserpine, α-methyldopa), impotence, and depression, as well as parkinsonism and akathisia, often limit their use. Depression, a relatively frequent side effect, has been successfully treated with concurrent antidepressant administration.

Dopamine agonists

Dopamine agonists, in animal studies, downregulate dopamine receptors and theoretically could be useful in TD. A major drawback is that they can initially exacerbate both TD and psychotic symptoms. Direct (apomorphine, bromocriptine and pergolide) and indirect (amantadine and levodopa) dopamine agonists have been tried in patients. Some positive case reports or single-blind studies have been published, but most double-blind studies show limited efficacy [114, 189]. One exception is a recent report of 35 inpatients with severe orofacial TD who showed marked improvement with levodopa after 3 months. Symptoms returned when levodopa was discontinued, and again responded when treatment was restarted [190]. Despite several methodological shortcomings, this study is encouraging but needs to be replicated.

Dopamine autoreceptor agonists (e.g., 3-PPP) decrease the release of dopamine and present another possible mechanism to treat TD. 3-PPP has been shown to improve a model of TD in monkeys [191], but it has not been tried in humans. In low doses, apomorphine is an autoreceptor agonist, while in high doses it is a postsynaptic receptor agonist. Theoretically, low doses should decrease dopamine release and improve symptoms of TD, while high doses should do the opposite. Paradoxically, one study showed that high doses, up to 6.0 mg, reduced TD [192]. The usefulness of apomorphine may be limited by side effects such as nausea and vomiting at therapeutic doses and its short duration of action. Pergolide, which activates both pre- and postsynaptic dopamine receptors, has been suggested as a potential treatment for TD but controlled trials have not been reported [193].

Noradrenergic antagonists

Although noradrenergic innervation of basal ganglia structures is sparse and limited primarily to the thalamus, noradrenergic agents have been used with some success to treat TD. The beta-adrenergic antagonist, propranolol, has been reported in open studies to partially suppress TD in 11 of 15 patients [54]. In a double-blind study of four patients, two improved with long-term treatment [194]. Unfortunately, no larger or more recent studies are available, and it is unclear whether propranolol's suppressive effect is due to increased neuroleptic blood levels. In contrast, pindolol, another beta-blocker, was unsuccessful in suppressing TD in a small, placebo-controlled study [195]. Clonidine, an α_2 agonist, decreases release of norepinephrine by autoreceptor stimulation, and has been reported to have antidyskinetic properties in a majority of patients [196–198]. However, in a rigorous meta-analysis of treatment studies for TD, Soares and McGrath [199] concluded that clonidine offered little if any treatment value. Clonidine may also have antipsychotic properties [196] and has relatively few side effects (hypotension, sedation). Other noradrenergic antagonists with possible suppressive effects include disulfiram [200] and fusaric acid, both of which are dopamine beta-hydroxylase inhibitors. Oxypertine depletes norepinephrine (and dopamine) and may also improve dyskinesias [201]. Unfortunately, this line of treatment has not been pursued with large, well-controlled studies. At the present time, noradrenergic antagonists, particularly clonidine, appear to be relatively safe and possibly effective as suppressive agents.

Anticholinergics

Dopamine and acetylcholine appear to have opposite effects on striatally mediated motor activity. One would predict that anticholinergics should make TD worse. While this has been found in some reports [202], others have found either no change [203] or even improvement. For example, in an acute challenge study using intravenous administration, Lieberman and colleagues [151, 152] showed that benztropine tended to improve movements while physostigmine made them worse (see also Moore and Bowers [204]). This suggests that dopamine and acetylcholine are not simply functional antagonists in the basal ganglia. In general, however, most data indicate that long-term treatment with anticholinergics either does not help or may actually worsen TD [7, 54, 205], and their discontinuation may be helpful in up to 60% of patients [114, 206]. An important exception is tardive dystonia, which may markedly improve with moderate-to-high doses (20 mg/day and higher) of anticholinergics such as trihexyphenidyl [207, 208].

Anticholinergics have also been hypothesized to predispose patients to develop TD [209], although this has been disputed [206]. The issue may be that patients exhibiting acute EPS, who are more likely to be treated with anticholinergics, are more susceptible to TD than patients who do not exhibit acute EPS [210]. In spite of such theoretical considerations, anticholinergics remain useful for acute EPS for many patients.

Cholinergics
Just as anticholinergics might worsen TD, cholinergic agonists might improve it. However, numerous studies conducted primarily in the 1970s with several acetylcholine precursors generally yielded disappointing results [7, 54, 95]. These agents included deanol, choline, and lecithin (a naturally occurring precursor of choline). One difficulty with interpreting these negative findings is the issue of how much drugs like deanol actually raise central cholinergic neurotransmission. Physostigmine, a centrally acting acetylcholinesterase inhibitor, has been used to investigate the pharmacology of TD, with mixed results [151, 152, 211]. An encouraging preliminary study using cholinergic-releasing agent, meclofenoxate, found improvement in 5 out 11 patients [212]. A systematic review of the literature regarding these older cholinomimetic agents was unable to demonstrate any clear-cut value in ameliorating TD [213]. Surprisingly, the new generation of centrally acting cholinomimetics, the acetylcholinesterase inhibitors used for the treatment of Alzheimer's disease, have not been examined with respect to TD with one notable exception. In an open-label study of donepezil, the authors reported that 9 of 10 patients showed improved TD scores after 6 weeks on 5–10 mg per day [214]. While a more careful evaluation of acetylcholinesterase inhibitors is warranted, it remains unclear whether cholinergic agents are useful in suppressing moderately severe TD symptoms.

GABA agonists
A variety of experimental and commercially available GABA agonists have been used to treat TD, some with significant success. Jeste and Wyatt's [7, 54] review describes 19 studies totaling 204 patients, with 54% having greater than 50% improvement, the most effective nonneuroleptic class of drugs reviewed. In a 1988 review of nine additional studies, the efficacy of GABA agonists fell to about 30% [114]. On the other hand, in a selective review of the effects of benzodiazepines, Thaker and colleagues [215] found that, in 15 reports involving a total of 158 patients, 83% of patients improved to some degree. In contrast, another recent review indicated that, of all the studies published, only two met the strict criteria for careful analysis [216]. From these two studies the

authors could not confidently assert that benzodiazepines offered demonstrable clinical benefit in the treatment of TD. While side effects (e.g., sedation, ataxia, addiction) may limit the use of many GABA agonists, they have a role, at least as second-line agents, for the suppression of TD.

Experimental GABA agonists have produced mixed results in clinical studies. For example, THIP, a GABA$_A$ agonist [128], and gamma-vinyl-GABA (GVG), a GABA-transaminase inhibitor [217], improved TD but to a minor degree. Muscimol, another GABA$_A$ agonist, produced a 45% reduction in seven patients [218]. Several reports suggest that progabide, a mixed GABA$_A$ and GABA$_B$ agonist, may have significant therapeutic effects, but more studies are needed. While the efficacy of these experimental agents supports a role for GABA in the pathophysiology of TD, they have limited clinical utility.

The most extensively studied commercially available GABA agonists include valproate, diazepam, clonazepam, and baclofen. Regarding valproate, a 1979 review described three studies using valproate that had mixed results [95]. Since then, three additional reports were not encouraging. In one, three of six patients improved [205], while in a second, none of 10 improved [187]. In a third, well-controlled, double-blind study, 33 patients treated for 6 weeks with valproate were not significantly different than 29 patients treated with placebo [219]. Diazepam, in contrast, has been more effective. Four studies prior to 1979 reported improvement in 26 of 29 patients on diazepam [95]. More recently, in a single-blind study, diazepam was again effective in 11 of 20 patients [220]. One drawback is that diazepam can be habit forming or can cause sedation, depression or, less commonly, impulsiveness and belligerence. Clonazepam is an effective alternative. Two open studies found markedly different results with 42 of 42 patients benefiting in one [221], but only 2 of 18 improving in another [222]. In a more recent, well-controlled, double-blind study by Thaker and colleagues [215], suppression was observed in 26.5% of patients with choreoathetosis and 41.5% of patients with dystonia. Tolerance can develop to clonazepam's therapeutic effects, but this may be overcome by a brief withdrawal period [215]. In eight studies with baclofen, only two showed significant results [223]. In one of these, 3 out of 13 patients improved [223], while in the second, 9 of 13 patients improved [224]. Baclofen appears to act primarily on GABA$_B$ receptors, which may not be as important in TD. A recent review of a variety of GABA agonists studied in randomized trials concluded that there is no convincing evidence that these agents reduce the severity of TD [225]. Many studies purporting clinical efficacy of GABA agonists were eliminated from consideration in this review due to a lack of randomization, the use of unstable doses of neuroleptics, a lack of placebo control, or other major methodological flaws.

In summary, of GABA agonists, benzodiazepines have the most promise in clinical studies for suppressing TD. On average, 58% of patients in open studies have improved, while in double-blind studies, 43% have improved [226]. Thus, clonazepam or diazepam is potential therapeutic options in treating TD. Valproate and baclofen are probably less effective, and cannot be strongly endorsed. Newer agents, such as gabapentin, have not been employed in controlled studies.

Antioxidants
One of the more interesting treatments for TD is vitamin E (α-tocopherol), an antioxidant and free radical scavenger. The original use of this compound was motivated by the notion that neuroleptics produce toxic-free radicals that can cause neural dysfunction via cell damage and/or death. Differences in the production and handling of free radicals among patients may underlie TD [227]. There is a recent report that a polymorphism of the manganese superoxide dismutase gene confers increased risk toward the development of TD [228]. Eleven double-blind, placebo-controlled studies have examined the effects of vitamin E (Table 9.2) [229]. Of these, three reported no evidence of a therapeutic effect [230–232]. These negative studies were either brief (2 weeks), included older patients, or studied patients with a relatively long duration of TD. In contrast, nine other studies found some evidence of reduced TD severity with doses ranging from 1200 to 1600 IU per day for 4 to 12 weeks. Vitamin E's effects have been most pronounced in patients with relatively recent onset (e.g., within 5 years) [229, 233, 234]. Overall, improvement in positive studies has ranged form 18.5 to 43%. In addition, several open trials or case reports have also found evidence for therapeutic effects in TD or tardive dystonia [235–237]. On the other hand, a recent large, multicenter study funded by the Veteran's Administration of 107 subjects with TD treated either with a daily dose of 1600 IU of vitamin E or placebo for 1 year found no difference between the two groups [238]. Similarly, several other drugs with antioxidant properties have not been effective in TD (e.g., selegiline and coenzyme Q). These results raise significant doubts about the efficacy of vitamin E and other antioxidants in the treatment of TD.

Calcium channel blockers
Observations that calcium channel blockers may help TD symptoms came initially from case reports in the late 1980s [239–242] (see Table 9.3). Unfortunately, despite the plethora of anecdotes, only three double-blind, placebo-controlled, or crossover studies have been published. Suppressive efficacy is most convincing for nifedipine. Two open, one single-blind, and one double-blind study all found significant improvement with nifedipine (Table 9.3). Data on verapamil are more limited; three case reports [239, 240, 244] and one single-blind, placebo-controlled study of nine patients found that verapamil suppressed moderate-to-severe TD [245]. Case reports suggest diltiazem may also have at least a temporary suppressive effect [241, 242]. Similarly, an acute, single-dose, double-blind challenge study concluded that diltiazem suppressed TD [246]. In contrast, in a 3-week double-blind crossover study, diltiazem was no different than placebo [247]. One recent review of calcium channel blockers was inconclusive. The authors felt that all of the studies exhibited significant methodological flaws and larger randomized crossover studies were needed [115, 116].

Table 9.2 Studies of vitamin E in tardive dyskinesia

Reference	Maximum dose	Design	Duration of TD (yrs)	Number of patients	Outcome
Lohr et al. [243]	1200 IU	Double-blind, cross-over	2.6 ± 1.9 yrs	15	43% improvement
Elkashef et al. [328]	1200 IU × 4 wks	Double-blind, cross over	3.8 ± 2.8 yrs	8	27% improvement
Schmidt et al. [230]	1200 mg × 2 wks	Double-blind, cross over	10 pts > 1yr 9 pts < 1yr	19	No overall effect
Egan et al. [233]	1600 IU × 6 wks	Double-blind, cross over	5.9 ± 4.8 yrs	18	No overall effect. 9 pts with TD for 5 yrs or less showed 18.5% improvement
Shriqui et al. [231]	1200 IU × 6 wks	Double-blind, cross over	"long duration"	27	No effect
Junker et al. [329]	1200 mg	Double-blind, cross over	n.s.	16	Significant improvement in patients over age 40
Adler et al. [234]	1600 IU 8 to 12 weeks	Double-blind, parallel	9 patients >5 yrs 4 patients <5 yrs	28	32% improvement on vitamin E. Patients w/TD <5 yrs did better (52% vs. 27%)
Akhtar et al. 1993	1200 mg 4 weeks	Double-blind, parallel	6.5 yrs	32	Greater improvement in patients on vitamin E (20%) vs. placebo (8%)
Lam et al. [232]	1200 IU 4 weeks	Double-blind, cross over	Not available	12	No difference. Older patients (61.8 years). Long duration of illness(over 20 years)
Dabiri et al. [330]	1200 IU 12 weeks	Double-blind, parallel	14 weeks	11	36% improvement
Lohr and Caliguri [229]	1600 IU 2 months	Double-blind, parallel	11 months	35	24% improvement
Adler et al. [238]	1600 IU 36 weeks	Double-blind, parallel	4 yrs	40	30% improvement, greater in patients with shorter duration of TD
Adler et al. [238]	1600 IU 12 months	Double-blind, parallel	4 yrs	107	No difference

Table 9.3 Studies on the effect of calcium channel blockers on tardive dyskinesia

Reference	Drug	Design	Duration	Maximal dose	Outcome
Kushnir and Ratner [248]	Nifedipine	Open	1–8 months	20–80 mg/day	Significant improvement
Duncan et al. [249]	Nifedipine	Single blind	7–14 days	60 mg/day	Significant improvement
Steadman et al. [250]	Nifedipine	Open	6 weeks	60 mg/day	Significant improvement
Suddath et al. [331]	Nifedipine	Double-blind, cross-over	8 weeks	90 mg/day	Significant improvement
Barrow and Childs [239]	Verapamil	Case report	Unspecified	320 mg/day	Significant improvement
Buck and Havey [240]	Verapamil	Case report	6 months	320 mg/day	Significant improvement
Reiter et al. [245]	Verapamil	Single-blind	2–5 days	160–320 mg/day	Significant improvement
Abad and Ovsiew [244]	Verapamil	Case report	1 week and >1 month	1 week: 240 mg/day; >1 month: 360 mg/day	Significant improvement
Ross et al. [241]	Diltiazem	Case report	Few hours to 3 weeks	120–240 mg/day	Significant improvement
Falk et al. [242]	Diltiazem	Case report	25 weeks	240 mg/day	Temporary improvement
Leys et al. [246]	Diltiazem	Single dose, double-blind, placebo controlled	180 minutes	60 mg	Temporary improvement up to 90 minutes
Adler et al. [251]	Diltiazem	Single blind	2–12 days	240 mg/day	No significant effect
Loonen et al. [247]	Diltiazem	Randomized, double-blind, cross-over	3 weeks	240 mg/day	No significant effect

While the paucity of controlled, double-blind studies for calcium channel blockers limit conclusions, several trends emerge from prior reports: (a) of the three, nifedipine may be the most effective [248–250]; (b) regardless of the calcium channel blocker used, there seems to be a dose-related response [245, 248–251]; (c) older rather than younger patients may respond better to nifedipine [240, 248].

Several mechanisms could be involved in the action of calcium channel blockers. The effects may be due to unanticipated pharmacokinetic effects, as nifedipine has been shown to produce increased plasma neuroleptic levels [250]. Alternatively, these drugs may exert therapeutic effects by their actions on dopamine neurotransmission. In animals, calcium channel antagonists have been reported to block postsynaptic D-2 receptors and inhibit presynaptic dopaminergic activity [252]. SPECT studies show that calcium channel blockers reduce [127]iodobenzamide binding (a D_2 ligand) to D-2 receptors in the striatum, suggesting a weak antidopaminergic effect [253]. Finally, calcium channel blockers exert a number of indirect effects [254], such as reducing noradrenergic activity that could be related to the apparent decrease in TD severity. While more data on the neurochemical effects and well-controlled clinical studies are needed, the data to date suggest that these agents may be useful for patients requiring TD suppression.

Serotoninergic modulation

The observation that most atypical antipsychotic medications block $5HT_{2A}$ receptors suggests that serotonin plays a role in the biology of TD. Could serotonergic drugs play a role in TD suppression? Preclinical studies have shown that serotonin modulates striatal dopamine release [255]. Limited clinical data suggests that serotonergic agents may impact TD in humans. Buspirone, for example, a serotonin $5HT_{1A}$ partial agonist, has been observed to suppress TD [256] and levodopa-induced dyskinesias [257]. Subsequent reports, however, raise doubts about the utility of buspirone as a robust suppressive agent. In two open trials, one found that TD improved in eight patients [258], while a second found that, if anything, buspirone worsened TD in seven patients [259]. In a third open trial of 19 patients treated for 6 weeks, a nonsignificant 25% reduction in TD severity was observed; haloperidol levels, however, were significantly increased by 26% in these patients [260]. Paradoxically, buspirone has also been reported to induce akathisia [261], dystonia [262], and oral dyskinesia [263]. Buspirone's disparate effects could be attributed to neurotransmitter systems other than serotonin; it is weakly antidopaminergic with mixed D_2 agonist/antagonist properties, and reverses neuroleptic-induced D_2 supersensitivity in rats [264]; it is also a sigma receptor antagonist. Based on these few reports, its routine use for TD suppression cannot be recommended. In patients who have failed other modalities, however, it could be considered.

Serotonin reuptake inhibitors (SRIs) are a second class of serotonergic medications that sometimes appear to affect hyperkinetic disorders. Preclinical studies show that SRIs reduce dopamine synthesis in a variety of brain areas, including the striatum [265]. In monkeys, SRIs inhibit amphetamine-induced repetitive movements and worsen neuroleptic-induced parkinsonism [161]. Furthermore, in patients, SRIs have been noted to exacerbate parkinsonian symptoms [266]. Theoretically, one might expect that SRIs might improve symptoms of TD. Surprisingly, these medications appear to induce "oral hyperkinesias" in monkeys [161], although it is difficult to know the relationship between these movements and TD. Case reports have suggested that SRIs occasionally produce dyskinesia in humans phenotypically similar to TD, but usually subsiding when the SRI is withdrawn [267–271]. These limited observations, while supporting the role of serotonin in the suppression and enhancement of movement disorders, do not indicate a prominent role for SRIs as suppressive medications.

If SRIs fail to improve TD, one might try the opposite strategy by using a serotonin antagonist. Two such studies have noted some improvement with the 5-HT$_2$ and antihistamine agent cyproheptadine [272, 273], while a third found no effect [274]. A second 5-HT$_{2a}$ receptor antagonist, nefazadone, which also is a weak SRI, has been tried in patients and improves parkinsonian symptoms but has little effect on TD [275]. Another recent open-label study of 20 patients with schizophrenia reported improvement in both psychosis and TD using 12 mg per day of the 5-HT$_3$ receptor antagonist, ondansetron [276]. TD ratings performed blindly from videotapes improved by almost 50%, a remarkable change certainly meriting replication. Thus, while many interventions manipulating the serotonin system have not been rewarding, both the possible role of 5-HT$_{2a}$ receptors in mediating the atypicality of new antipsychotics and the idea that ondansetron could suppress TD symptoms continue to suggest a role for serotonin in TD.

Botulinum toxin

Advances in treating other movement disorders are often put to use to treat TD. This strategy has been particularly successful with the recent introduction of botulinum toxin to treat tardive dystonia, especially torticollis [277]. Botulinum toxin (type A) blocks acetylcholine release at the neuromuscular junction, producing a chemical denervation. The resulting focal muscle paresis persists for up to 3 to 6 months [278]. Botulinum toxin injections have been used to treat blepharospasm, laryngeal and limb dystonias, hemifacial spasm, tremor, tics, and torticollis [279, 280]. Patients responsive to botulinum injections may also do well with a newly described surgical procedure involving selective peripheral denervation of the involved musculature, although such a radical irreversible approach must be used with caution [281].

Miscellaneous therapeutic agents

A variety of other drugs and neurotransmitter systems have been implicated in the pathophysiology of dyskinetic movements and could theoretically play a role in the suppression of TD. Many potential therapeutic agents are described only in case reports, small series, animal studies, or unblinded trials, making conclusions problematic. One particularly interesting approach has been to use ceruletide, a CCK analogue. CCK is a neuropeptide coexpressed in dopaminergic neurons and appears to function as a neuromodulator in the striatum. CCK purportedly exhibits neuroleptic-like effects on dopamine receptors, metabolism, and behavior. Ceruletide itself appears to inhibit some of the behavioral effects of amphetamine, reduces striatal dopamine metabolism [282], and blocks dyskinetic mouth movements in an animal model of TD [283]. Ceruletide has been found to be beneficial in one study of seven patients [284], which included several with severe TD. In a much larger (N = 77), well-controlled, parallel study, long-lasting moderate-to-marked improvement was seen in 42.5% of patients receiving the active drug, compared with 9.1% improvement in the placebo group [285]. While seemingly promising, one difficulty with interpreting these data is that ceruletide is a peptide, which, administered peripherally, may not get into the brain in appreciable amounts [286]. On the other hand, peripherally administered ceruletide has been shown to have central effects on dopamine neuronal activity [287] and metabolism in rats [282].

Lithium is frequently mentioned in conjunction with TD, although few data on its effects are available. Lithium appears to prevent dopamine supersensitivity in rats when used with neuroleptics [288]. In humans, epidemiological data suggest that when lithium is added to neuroleptic treatment, the incidence of TD is reduced [23]. In contrast, lithium has not been successful as a suppressive agent [226].

Anecdotes of successful treatments with a pharmacopoeia of other, often unusual interventions abound. A very low dose of prednisolone, for example, surprisingly produced a complete remission in two patients with severe TD [289]. Estrogen replacement produced marginal improvement in postmenopausal women [223]. An experimental neurotensin receptor antagonist inhibits dyskinesias in a rodent model of TD [290]. Another unusual and perhaps unorthodox approach is the use of branched chain amino acids [291]. This group has reported a significant improvement in TD symptoms in 18 patients treated for 3 weeks with 222 mg per kg of branched chain amino acids, compared to 18 placebo-treated patients. Remarkably, the authors noted a positive correlation between decreases in TD ratings and aromatic amino acid plasma concentrations [292]. The use of dentures and correction of other dental problems has been observed to markedly reduce oral TD. Canes, braces, or biofeedback may offer limited benefit in severe cases. ECT has had variable effects with a few patients reportedly having dramatic improvements [293]. Once again with ECT, as with so many reported treatments for TD, controlled trials are lacking. These experimental interventions may merit some consideration in severe cases of TD when all other therapeutic options have failed.

Neurosurgical interventions
Neurosurgical interventions for movement disorders have gained a new currency with improved functional outcomes and decreased mortality and morbidity [294]. Stereotactic guidance utilizing CT or MRI scanning in conjunction with intraoperative electrophysiological monitoring has greatly advanced the field [295]. There is at least one case report of dramatic improvement in TD following pallidotomy [296]. Another case of severe TD with dystonic components has been effectively treated with a ventral thalamotomy [297]. Serious potential side effects, including damage to the optic tract and other nearby vital structures, probably will limit this form of treatment as "the treatment of last resort."

Future research strategies
Theoretically, attempts to reduce stimulation from the D_1-mediated striatonigral pathway should reduce hyperkinetic movements by increasing GABAergic activity in projections from the substantia nigra and globus pallidus interna to the thalamus. This, in turn, would decrease thalamocortical activity, and, ultimately, motor activity. What is not clear, however, is how one might reduce striatonigral activity. One strategy, from animal behavioral work, is to

use D_1 antagonists. A number of investigators have looked at the role of D_1 antagonists in movement disorders and dyskinesia (e.g., [298]). While no D_1 antagonist is currently available for clinical use in the United States, and controlled studies are few, at least one trial of a mixed D_1 and D_2 antagonist was no better than a more pure D_2 antagonist in suppressing TD [299]. Furthermore, in spite of preclinical data from rats and primate studies ([298], see discussion in [300]) suggesting a role for D_1 receptors in levedopa-induced dyskinesias, at least one study in humans did not support this notion [301].

A second approach might be to alter neurotransmission by the colocalized basal ganglia neuropeptides, including dynorphin, enkephalin, and substance P. In humans, several case reports suggest that intravenous naloxone, a relatively nonspecific opioid receptor antagonist, reduces levodopa-induced dyskinesias [302] and tardive dyskinesia [303, 304]. Paradoxically, morphine, an opioid receptor agonist, may improve dystonic posturing in patients with tardive dyskinesia [305] and levodopa dyskinesias in parkinsonian patients [306]. In an additional complication, naltrexone failed to improve levedopa-induced dyskinesias in parkinsonian patients [307]. While such case reports are suggestive, more data are needed before the clinical utility or feasibility of modulating basal ganglia pathways through agents directly acting on neuropeptides is considered. Indeed, a greater understanding of the neurobiological meaning of this concept is a goal of current research. Nevertheless, for the intractable patient who has exhausted other options, this approach may offer some hope.

New laboratory techniques hold the promise of increasing our understanding of the molecular mechanisms underlying TD, and all hyperkinetic movement disorders. Perhaps the most exiting is high throughput molecular profiling with cDNA microarrays [308]. Microarrays simultaneously assay the relative levels of mRNA expression of thousands of genes from a single tissue sample. The interrogation of the transcriptome of basal ganglia structures holds great promise. Microarray studies can either be performed on tissue from animal models of TD or postmortem human specimens comparing individuals with and without TD. Such studies hold the promise of defining the molecular mechanisms underlying this disorder. Equally importantly, microarrays might also help identify new therapeutic strategies.

Another emerging molecular genetic research strategy involves looking for alleles that either increase the risk of or protect individuals from the development of TD. Functional genomic studies have begun to clarify the impact of normal genetic variation on complex behaviors, susceptibility to neuropsychiatric illness, information processing, and patterns of neural activation on functional imaging studies. Normal variation in several genes has been associated with differential biological function and several neuropsychiatric illnesses. One of the first reports suggesting a link between genotype and the susceptibility to TD involved the CYP2D6 gene, a cytochrome p450 enzyme important in the metabolism of neuroleptics and other drugs [309]. This was confirmed independently by several groups [310, 311]. Subsequent studies have suggested a link between TD and polymorphisms in the dopamine D-2 receptor [312, 313], dopamine D-3 receptor [314, 315], μ opioid receptor [316], serotonin 2-A receptor [317, 318], serotonin 2-C receptor [319], and manganese superoxide dismutase genes [228]. Many of these reports are underpowered with respect to the size of the patient cohorts, and several have been disputed [320–324]. The association with a polymorphism in the dopamine D-3 receptor gene seems to be the best established [325]. This strategy holds the promise of identifying those individuals at risk for the development of TD, and modifying their treatment accordingly. Moreover, pharmacogenomics may yield important clues into the pathophysiology of TD, and help devise novel and more effective treatments for those individuals already suffering from this disorder.

Summary

Despite the promise of a new generation of "atypical" antipsychotic neuroleptics with reduced EPS, TD remains a vexing albeit diminishing clinical issue. Prevention is still an important approach; clinicians must consider whether other treatments are more effective than neuroleptics. This is particularly true for high-risk groups, such as the elderly and patients with brain damage or diabetes. For many patients, neuroleptics are unavoidable for the treatment of chronic psychosis. In such patients, initiation of therapy with an atypical agent may lower the risk for the subsequent development of TD. If TD develops, a thorough neurological evaluation should be considered. Switching from a typical to an atypical agent is a common first step although the efficacy of this approach is unclear (see Table 9.1). If typical agents are needed, the dose should be tapered to the lowest possible effective level. Adding vitamin E to typical agents may also be worthwhile albeit still unproven. Targeted dosing has generally not been better than continuous treatment for the majority of patients. Neuroleptic discontinuation is frequently recommended and has limited success, but is fraught with risks of its own.

Fortunately, the incidence of severe TD is relatively low. When TD does cause distress, disfigurement, or adversely affects health or function, suppressive agents may be needed. Some studies suggest that atypical antipsychotics may be useful in such cases, although more data are needed. At present, many consider them to be a first-line treatment for suppression. Clozapine is often considered a second-line agent due to complications associated with its use. Suppression can be tried with drugs that are fairly safe and have at least some moderate record of success. These third-line agents include vitamin E, calcium channel blockers, and adrenergic antagonists, such as clonidine. Medications that have more side effects or risks, but that are probably more effective in the short term, include benzodiazepines and dopamine-depleting agents. These fourth-line agents are sometimes used first by movement disorder specialists when a rapid response is needed. A fifth approach is to increase the dose of typical neuroleptics in an attempt to achieve temporary suppression, followed by a gradual reduction. This does not always produce suppression and runs the theoretical risk of long term-worsening. More experimental agents can be tried when other attempts fail. These include cholinergic agonists (e.g., tacrine), melatonin, dopamine agonists (e.g, amantadine), buspirone, GABA agonists (e.g., gabapentin), cyproheptadine, ondansetron, opioid agonists or antagonists, estrogen, steroids, or even ECT. When dystonia is a prominent feature, specific therapeutic agents include anticholinergics and, if sufficiently localized, botulinum toxin injections.

The use of suppressive agents is typically a highly individualized process. The steps outlined here should be considered only a proposal based on our experience. It has not been prospectively evaluated, and other experts may have differing approaches. Furthermore, this approach may not be the best one in all circumstances. Many patients will have special needs indicating that third- or fourth-line agents should be tried first. Often, a trial of at least several drugs is needed before an effective one is found. In our experience, success can sometimes be achieved by patiently trying a number of agents one after another. This requires not only familiarity with the many strategies described above, but a strong, working alliance with the patient.

Tardive dyskinesia will remain a major public health issue in psychiatry at least for the near future. With advances in the understanding of the mechanisms of action of atypical antipsychotics and the physiology of the basal ganglia, continued improvements can be anticipated. With the discovery of susceptibility genes for TD, individuals at high risk might be identified prior to the initiation of neuroleptic therapy, and the application of alternative pharmacological approaches might reduce this risk. While the treatment of TD remains a formidable problem, prevention through the use of atypical agents, alternative psychotherapeutic agents, and pharmacogenomics promise to make TD an increasingly rare clinical entity for future generations of clinicians and patients.

References

1. Delay J, Deniker P. Trente-huit cas de psychoses traites par la cure prolongee et continue de 4568 R. Ann Med Psychol 1952; 110: 364.
2. Schonecker M. Ein eigentumliches syndrom im oralen bereich bei megaphen applikation. Nervenartz 1957; 28: 35.
3. Kruse W. Persistent muscular restlessness after phenothiazine treatment: report of 3 cases. Am J Psychiatry 1960; 117: 152–153.
4. Hunter R, Earl JC, Thornicroff S. An apparently irreversible syndrome of abnormal movements following phenothiazine medication. Proc R Soc Med 1964; 57: 758–762.
5. Kazamatsuri H, Chien C-P, Cole JO. Treatment of tardive dyskinesia II. Short-term efficacy of dopamine-blocking agents haloperidol and thiopropazate. Arch Gen Psychiatry 1972; 27: 100–103.
6. Kazamatsuri H, Chien C, Cole JO. Treatment of tardive dyskinesia: clinical efficacy of a dopamine-depleting agent, tetrabenazine I. Arch Gen Psychiatry 1972; 27: 95–99.
7. Jeste DV, Wyatt RJ. Therapeutic strategies against tardive dyskinesia: two decades of experience. Arch Gen Psychiatry 1982; 39: 803–816.
8. Keegan DL, Rajput AH. Drug-induced dystonia tarda: treatment with L-dopa. Dis Nerv Sys 1973; 38: 167–169.
9. Tarsy D, Granacher R, Bralower M. Tardive dyskinesia in young adults. Am J Psychiatry 1977; 134: 1032–1034.

10. Casey DE, Rabins P. Tardive dyskinesia as a life-threatening illness. Am J Psychiatry 1978; 135: 486–488.
11. Tarsy D. History and definition of tardive dyskinesia. Clin Neuropharmacol 1983; 6: 9199.
12. Owens DG, Johnstone EC, Frith CD. Spontaneous involuntary disorders of movement. Arch Gen Psychiatry 1982; 39: 452–461.
13. Waddington JL. Abnormal involuntary movements and psychosis in the preneuroleptic era and in unmedicated patients: implications for the concept of tardive dyskinesia. In The Neurobiology of Dopamine Systems. Manchester, UK, Manchester University Press 1986, pp. 51–66.
14. Owens DG. Involuntary disorders of movement in chronic schizophrenia: the role of the illness and its treatment. In Casey DE, Chase TN, Christensen AV, et al. (eds) Research and Treatment. Berlin, Springer-Verlag, 1985, pp. 79–87.
15. Fenton WS, Wyatt RJ, McGlashan TH. Risk factors for spontaneous dyskinesia in schizophrenia. Arch Gen Psychiatry 1994; 51(8): 643–650.
16. Kane JM. Tardive dyskinesia. In Jeste DV, Wyatt RJ (eds) Neuropsychiatric Movements Disorders. Washington, DC, American Psychiatric Press, 1984, pp. 68–95.
17. Yassa R, Jeste DV. Gender differences in tardive dyskinesia: a critical review of the literature. Schizophr Bull 1992; 18: 701–715.
18. Chouinard G, Annable L, Rose-Chouinard A, et al. A 5-year prospective longitudinal study of tardive dyskinesia: factors predicting appearance of new cases. J Clin Psychopharmacol 1988; 8(suppl): 21–26.
19. Baldessarini RJ, Cole JO, Davis JM. Tardive Dyskinesia: A Task Force Report. Washington DC, American Psychiatric Association, 1980.
20. Casey DE, Hansen TE. Spontaneous dyskinesia. In Jeste DV, Wyatt RJ (eds) Neuropsychiatric Movement Disorders. Washington DC, American Psychiatric Press, 1984, pp. 68–95.
21. Kane JM, Woerner M, Lieberman J. Tardive dyskinesia: Prevalence, incidence, and risk factors. In Casey DE, Chase T, Christensen AV, Gerlach J (eds) Dyskinesia Research and Treatment (Psychopharmacology suppl 2). Berlin, Springer, 1985, pp. 72–78.
22. Morgenstern H, Glazer WM. Identifying risk-factors for tardive dyskinesia among long-term outpatients maintained with neuroleptic medications. Arch Gen Psychiatry 1993; 50: 723–733.
23. Kane JM. Tardive dyskinesia: epidemiological and clinical presentation. In Bloom FE, Kupfer DJ (eds) Psychopharmacology: The Fourth Generation of Progress. New York, Raven Press, 1995.
24. Glazer, WM, Morgenstern, H., Doucette, JT. Predicting the long-term risk of tardive dyskinesia in out patients maintained on neuroleptic medications. J Clin Psychiatry 1993; 54: 133–139.
25. Waddington JL. Tardive dyskinesia in schizophrenia and other disorders: association with aging, cognitive dysfunction, and structural brain pathology in relation to neuroleptic exposure. Hum Psychopharmacol 1987; 2: 11–22.
26. Egan MF, Hurd Y, Hyde TM, et al. Alterations in mRNA levels of D2 receptors and neuropetides in striatonigral and striatopallidal neurons of rats with neuroleptic-induced dyskinesias. Synapse 1994; 18: 178–189.
27. Kane JM, Woerner M, Pollack S, et al. Does clozapine cause tardive dyskinesia? J Clin Psychiatry 1993; 54: 327–330.
28. Ananth J, Kenan J. Tardive dyskinesia associated with Olanzapine monotherapy. J Clin Psychiatry 1999; 60: 870.
29. Herran A, Vazquez-Barquero JL. Tardive dyskinesia associated with olanzapine. Ann Intern Med 1999; 131: 72.

30. Beasley CM, Dellva MA, Tamura RN, et al. Randomised double-blind comparison of the incidence of tardive dyskinesia in patients with schizophrenia during long-term treatment with olanzapine or haloperidol. Br J Psychiatry 1999; 174: 23–30.

31. Glazer WM. Expected incidence of tardive dyskinesia associated with atypical antipsychotics. J Clin Psychiatry 2000; 61: 21–26.

32. Ahmed S, Chengappa KNR, Naidu VR, et al. Clozapine withdrawal-emergent dystonias and dyskinesias: a case series. J Clin Psychiatry 1998; 59: 472–477.

33. Uzun O, Cansever A, Ozsahin A. A case of relapsed tardive dyskinesia due to clozapine dose reduction. Int Clin Psychopharmacol 2001; 16: 369–371.

34. Chandler M. Risperidone-induced tardive dyskinesia in first-episode psychotic patients. J Clin Psychopharmacol 1999; 19: 276–277.

35. Hong KS, Cheong SS, Woo J-M, et al. Risperidone-induced tardive dyskinesia. Am J Psychiatry 1999; 156: 1290.

36. Jeste DV. Tardive dyskinesia in older patients. J Clin Psychiatry 2000; 61: 27–32.

37. Chouinard G. Effects of risperidone in tardive dyskinesia: an analysis of the Canadian Multicenter Risperidone Study. J Clin Psychopharmacol 1995; 15(1)(suppl): 36s–44s.

38. Lemmens P, Brecher M, Van Baelen B. A combined analysis of double-blind studies with risperidone versus placebo and other antipsychotic agents: factors associated with extrapyramidal symptoms. Acta Psychiatr Scand 1999; 99: 160–170.

39. Gehlber D, Belmaker RH. Tardive dyskinesia with quetiapine. Am J Psychiatry 1999; 156: 796–797.

40. APA Task Force on Tardive Dyskinesia: Tardive Dyskinesia – A Task Force Report of the American Psychiatric Association. APA Press, Washington, DC, 1992.

41. Kane JM, Smith JM. Tardive dyskinesia: prevalence and risk factors, 1959–1979. Arch Gen Psychiatry 1982; 39: 473–481.

42. Kane JM, Rifkin A, Woerner M, et al. Low dose neuroleptic treatment of outpatient schizophrenics. Arch Gen Psychiatry 1983; 40: 893–896.

43. Kane JM, Woerner M, Sarantakos S. Depot neuroleptics: a comparative review of standard, intermediate, and low dose regimens. J Clin Psychiatry 1986; 47(5)(suppl): 30–33.

44. Chakos MH, Alvir JM, Woerner MG, et al. Incidence and correlates of tardive dyskinesia in first episode of schizophrenia. Arch Gen Psychiatry 1996; 53(4): 313–319.

45. Johnson, DA, Ludlow, JM, Street, K, Talor, RD. Double-blind comparison of half-dose and standard-dose flupenthixol decanoate in the maintenance treatment of stabilised out-patients with schizophrenia. Br J Psychiatry 1987; 151: 634–638.

46. Marder SR, Van Putten T, Mintz J. Low- and conventional-dose maintenance therapy with fluphenazine decanoate: two year outcome. Arch Gen Psychiatry 1987; 44: 518–521.

47. Baldessarini RJ, Davis JM. What is the best maintenance dose of neuroleptics in schizophrenia? Psychiatry Res 1980; 3: 115–122.

48. Van Putten T, Marder SR. Low dose treatment strategies. J Clin Psychiatry 1986; 47(5)(suppl): 12–16.

49. Jolley AG, Hirsch SR, McRink A, et al. Trial of brief intermittent neuroleptic prophylaxis for selected schizophrenic outpatients: clinical outcome at one year. Br Med J 1989; 298: 985–990.

50. Carpenter WT, Hanlon TE, Heinrichs DW, et al. Continuous versus targeted medication in schizophrenic outpatients: outcome results. Am J Psychiatry 1990; 147: 11138–11148.

51. Jeste, DV, Potkin, SG, Sinha, S, Feder, S, Wyatt, RJ. Tardive dyskinesia-reversible and persistent. Arch Gen Psychiatry 1979; 36: 585–590.

52. Newton JEO, Cannon DJ, Couch L, et al. Effects of repeated drug holidays on serum haloperidol concentration, psychiatric symptoms, and movement disorders in schizophrenic patients. J Clin Psychiatry 1989; 50: 132–135.

53. Kane JM Marder SR. Pharmacologic treatment of schizophrenia. Schizophr Bull 1993; 19: 287–302.

54. Jeste DV, Wyatt RJ. Understanding and Treating Tardive Dyskinesia. New York, Guilford Press, 1982, pp. 72–170.

55. Gibson A. Depot injections and tardive dyskinesia. Br J Psychiatry 1978; 132: 361–365.

56. Klieser E, Lehman E, Kinzler E, et al. Randomized, double-blind, controlled trial of risperidone versus clozapine in patients with chronic schizophrenia. J Clin Psychopharmacology 1995; 15: 455–515.

57. Casey DE. Serotonergic aspects of acute extrapyramidal syndromes in non-human primates. Psychopharmacol Bull 1989; 25: 457–459.

58. Buzan RD. Risperidone-induced tardive dyskinesia. Am J Psychiatry 1996; 153: 734–735.

59. Daniel DG.. Smith K, Hyde T, et al. Neuroleptic-induced tardive dyskinesia. Am J Psychiatry 1996; 153: 734.

60. Woerner MG, Sheitman BS, Lieberman JA, et al. Tardive dyskinesia induced by risperidone? Am J Psychiatry 1996; 153: 843.

61. Tollefson GD, Beasley CM, Tran PV. Olanzapine versus haloperidol: results of the multicenter, international trial. Schizophr Res 1996; 18: 131.

62. Beasley CM, Tollefson G, Tran P, et al. Olanzapine versus placebo and haloperidol: acute phase results of the North American double-blind olanzapine trial. Neuropsychopharmacology 1996; 14: 111–123.

63. Schulz SC, Mack R, Zborowski J, et al. Efficacy, safety and dose-response of three doses of sertindole and three doses of Haldol in schizophrenia patients. Schizophr Res 1996; 18: 133.

64. Casey DE. Behavioral effects of sertindole, risperidone, clozapine and haloperidol in cebus monkeys. Psychopharmacology 1996; 124: 134–140.

65. Klugewicz DA, Tracy K, Lafargue T, et al. Effects of antioxidant treatment on the VCM syndrome. Soc Neurosci Abstr, 1996.

66. Andreassen OA, Jorgensen HA. GM1 ganglioside attenuates the development of vacuous chewing movements induced by long-term haloperidol treatment of rats. Psychopharmacology (Berl) 1994; 116(4): 517–522.

67. Gattaz WF, Emrich A, Behrens S. Vitamin E attenuates the development of haloperidol-induced dopaminergic hypersensitivity in rats: possible implications for tardive dyskinesia. J Neural Transm 1993; 92: 197–201.

68. Cole JO, Gardos G, Rapkin RM. Lithium carbonate in tardive dyskinesia and schizophrenia. In Gardos G, Casey DE (eds) Dyskinesia and Affective Disorder. Washington DC, American Psychiatric Press, 1984, pp. 49–73.

69. Ghadirian AM, Annable L, Belanger MC, et al. A cross sectional study of parkinsonism and tardive dyskinesia in lithium treated affective disordered patients. J Clin Psychiatry 1996; 57(1): 22–28.

70. Hyde T, Hotson JR, Kleinman JE. Differential diagnosis of choreiform tardive dyskinesia. J Neuropsychiatry 1991; 3: 255–268.

71. Woerner M, Kane JM. Leiberman JA, et al. The prevalence of tardive dyskinesia. J Clin Psychopharmacology 1991; 11: 34–42.

72. Wyatt RJ. Practical Psychiatric Practice: Clinical Interview Forms, Rating Scales and Patient Handouts. Washington DC, American Psychiatric Press, 1995.

73. Kleinman I, Schacter D, Kouter E. Informed consent and tardive dyskinesia. Am J Psychiatry 1989; 28: 117–118.

74. Guy W. (ed) ECDEU Assessment Manual for Psychopharmacology: Publication ADM 76–358. Washington DC, U.S. Department of Health, Education, and Welfare, 1976, pp. 534–537.

75. Gardos G, Perenyi A, Cole JO, et al. Seven year follow up of tardive dyskinesia in Hungarian outpatients. Neuropsychopharmacology 1988; 1: 169–172.

76. Gardos G, Casey D, Cole JO, et al. Ten year outcome of tardive dyskinesia. Am J Psychiatry 1994; 151: 836–841.

77. Gerlach J, Casey DE. Tardive dyskinesia. Acta Psychiatr Scand 1988; 77: 369–378.

78. Casey DE, Gerlach J. Tardive Dyskinesia: what is the long-term outcome. In Casey DE, Gardos G (eds) Tardive Dyskinesia and Neuroleptics: From Dogma to Reason. Washington DC, American Psychiatric Press, 1986, pp. 75–97.

79. Gardos G, Cole J. The prognosis of tardive dyskinesia. J Clin Psychiatry 1983; 44: 177–179.

80. Bergen JA, Eyland EA, Campbell JA, et al. The course of tardive dyskinesia in patients on long term neuroleptics. Br J Psychiatry 1989; 154: 523–528.

81. Kane JM, Woerner M, Lieberman J. Tardive dyskinesia: prevalence, incidence, and risk factors. J Clin Psychopharmacology 1988; 8: 52S–56S.

82. Yassa R, Nair NPV, Iskandar H, et al. Factors in the development of severe forms of tardive dyskinesia. Am J Psychiatry 1990; 147: 1156–1163.

83. Gardos G, Cole JO, Salomon M, et al. Clinical forms of severe tardive dyskinesia. Am J Psychiatry 1987; 144: 895–902.

84. Barnes TRE, Kidger T, Gore SM. Tardive dyskinesia: a 3 year follow up study. Psychol Med 1983; 13: 71–81.

85. Robinson ADT, McCreadie RG. The Nithsdale schizophrenia survey. V. Follow up of tardive dyskinesia at 31/2 years. B J Psychiatry 1986; 149: 621–623.

86. Bergen J, Kitchin R, Berry G. Predictors of the course of tardive dyskinesia in patients receiving neuroleptics. Biol Psychiatry 1992; 32: 580–594.

87. Smith JM, Baldessarini RJ. Changes in prevalence, severity and recovery in tardive dyskinesia with age. Arch Gen Psychiatry 1980; 37: 1368–1373.

88. Yassa R, Nair NPV. A 10-year follow-up study of tardive dyskinesia. Acta Psychiatr Scand 1992; 86: 262–266.

89. Glazer WM, Morgenstern H, Doucette JT. The prediction of chronic persistent versus intermittent tardive dyskinesia. A retrospective follow-up study. Br J Psychiatry 1991; 158: 822–828.

90. Bergen, J, Kitchin, R., Berry, G. Predictors of the course of tardive dyskinesia in patients receiving neuroleptics. Biol Psychiatry 1992; 32: 580–594.

91. McGrath JJ, Soares-Weiser KVS. Neuroleptic-reduction and/or cessation and neuroleptics as specific treatments for tardive dyskinesia. The Cochrane Database System Reviews. 3. Oxford, Update Software, 2002.

92. Gardos G, Cole JO, Rapkin RM, et al. Anticholinergic challenge and neuroleptic withdrawal. Arch Gen Psychiatry 1984; 41: 1030–1035.

93. Dixon L, Thaker G, Conley R, et al. Changes in psychopathology and dyskinesia after neuroleptic withdrawal in a double blind design. Schizophr Res 1993; 10: 267–271.

94. Glazer WM, Bowers MB, Charney DS, et al. The effect of neuroleptic discontinuation on psychopathology, involuntary movements, and biochemical measures in patients with persistent tardive dyskinesia. Biol Psychiatry 1989; 26: 224–233.

95. Jeste DV, Wyatt RJ. In search of treatment for tardive dyskinesia: review of the literature. Schizophr Bull 1979; 5: 253–293.

96. Jus A, Jus K, Fontaine P. Long-term treatment of tardive dyskinesia. J Clin Psychiatry 1979; 40: 72–77.

97. Klawans HL, Tanner CM, Barr A. The reversibility of "permanent" tardive dyskinesia. Clin Neuropsychopharmacol 1984; 7: 153–159.

98. Fahn S. A therapeutic approach to tardive dyskinesia. J Clin Psychiatry 1985; 464: 19–24.

99. Glazer WM, Moore DC, Schooler NR, et al. Predictors of improvement in tardive dyskinesia following discontinuation of neuroleptic medication. Br J Psychiatry 1990; 157: 585–592.

100. Glazer WM, Moore DC, Schooler NR, et al. Tardive dyskinesia: a discontinuation study. Arch Gen Psychiatry 1984; 41: 623–627.

101. Gilbert PL, Harris J, McAdam LA, et al. Neuroleptic withdrawal in schizophrenic patients. Arch Gen Psychiatry 1995; 52: 173–188.

102. Wyatt RJ. Neuroleptics and the natural course of schizophrenia. Schizophr Bull 1991; 17: 235–280.

103. Johnson DAW, Pasterski G, Ludlow JM, et al. The discontinuation of maintenance neuroleptic therapy in chronic schizophrenic patients: drug and social consequences. Acta Psychiatr Scand 1983; 67: 339–352.

104. Dalack GW, Becks L, Meador-Woodruff JH. Tardive dyskinesia, clozapine, and treatment response. Progr Neuropsychopharmacol Biol Psychiatry 1998; 22: 567–573.

105. Bassitt DP, Neto MRL. Clozapine efficacy in tardive dyskinesia in schizophrenic patients. Eur Arch Psychiatry Clin Neurosc 248: 209–211.

106. Modestin J, Stephan PK, Erni T, et al. Prevalence of extrapyramidal syndromes in psychiatric inpatients and the relationship of clozapine treatment to tardive dyskinesia. Schizophr Res 2000; 42: 223–230.

107. Andia I, Zumarraga M, Zabalo MJ, et al. Differential effect of haloperidol and clozapine on plasma homovanillic acid in elderly schizophrenic patients with or without tardive dyskinesia. Biol Psychiatry 1998; 43: 20–23.

108. Soutullo CA, Keck PE, McElroy SL. Olanzapine in the treatment of tardive dyskinesia: a report of two cases. J Clin Psychopharmacology 1999; 19: 100–101.

109. Veseley C, Kufferle B, Brucke T, et al. Remission of severe tardive dyskinesia in a schizophrenic patient treated with the atypical antipsychotic substance quetiapine. Int Clin Psychopharmacology 2000; 15: 57–60.

110. McClelland HA, Dutta D, Metcalf A, et al. Mortality and facial dyskinesia. Br J Psychiatry 1986; 148: 310–316.

111. Chui HFK, Lee S, Chan CHS. Misdiagnosis of respiratory dyskinesia. Acta Psychiatr Scand 1991; 83: 494–495.

112. Nishikawa T, Kanaeda W, Uegaki A, et al. Respiratory dyskinesia: a variety of forms differentially diagnosed by using a spirophraph. Clin Neuropharmacol 1992; 15: 315–321.

113. Wojcik JD, Falk WE, Fink JS, et al. A review of 32 cases of tardive dystonia. Am J Psychiatry 1991; 148: 1055–1059.

114. Jeste DV, Lohr JB, Clark K, et al. Pharmacological treatments of tardive dyskinesia in the 1980s. J Clin Psychopharmacology 1988; 8(suppl): 38–48.

115. Soares KVS, McGrath JJ. Calcium channel blockers for neuroleptic-induced tardive dyskinesia (Cochrane Review). Cochrane Database System Review 3. Oxford, Update Software, 2001.

116. Soares KVS, McGrath JJ. Vitamin E for neuroleptic-induced tardive dyskinesia. (Cochrane Review). Cochrane Database System Review 4. Oxford, Update Software, 2001.

117. Soares KVS, McGrath JJ, Deeks JJ. Gamma-aminobutyric acid agonists for neuroleptic-induced tardive dyskinesia. Cochrane Database System Review 3. Oxford, Update Software, 2001.

118. Soares-Weiser KV, Joy C. Miscellaneous treatments for neuroleptic-induced tardive dyskinesia. Cochrane Database System Review. 2. Oxford, Update Software, 2003.

119. Turrone P, Remington G, Kapur S, et al. Differential effects of within-day continuous versus transient dopamine D_2 receptor occupancy in the development of vacuous chewing movements in rats. Neuropsychopharmacology 2003; 28: 1433–1439.

120. Turrone P, Remington G, Kapur S, et al. The relationship between dopamine D_2 receptor occupancy and the vacuous chewing movement syndrome in rats. Psychopharmacology (Berl) 2003; 165: 166–171.

121. Kapur S, Seeman P. Does fast dissociation from the dopamine D_2 receptor explain the action of atypical antipsychotics? A new hypothesis. Am J Psychiatry 2001; 158: 360–369.

122. Mao CC, Cheney DC, Marco E, et al. Turnover times of gamma aminobutyric acid and acetylcholine in nucleus caudatus, nucleus accumbens, globus pallidus, and substantia nigra: effects of repeated administration of haloperidol. Brain Res 1977; 132: 375–399.

123. Gale K. Chronic blockade of dopamine receptors by antischizophrenic drug enhances GABA binding in substantia nigra. Nature 1980; 283: 569–570.

124. Fibiger HC, Lloyd KG. Neurobiological substrates of tardive dyskinesia: the GABA hypothesis. Trends Neurosci 1989; 12: 462–464.

125. Gunne LM, Haggstrom JE, Sjokvist B. Association with persistent neuroleptic-induced dyskinesia of regional changes in the brain GABA synthesis. Nature 1984; 309: 347–349.

126. Sakai K, Gao XM, Hashimoto T, et al. Traditional and new antipsychotic drugs differentially alter neurotransmission markers in basal ganglia-thalamocortical neural pathways. Synapse 2001; 39: 152–160.

127. Anderson U, Haggstrom JE, Levi ED, et al. Reduced glutamate decarboxylase activity in the subthalamic nucleus in patients with tardive dyskinesia. Mov Disord 1989; 4: 37–46.

128. Thaker GK, Tamminga CA, Alphs LD, et al. Brain gamma-aminobutyric acid abnormality in tardive dyskinesia. Arch Gen Psychiatry 1987; 44: 522–529.

129. Thaker GK, Nguyen JA, Tamminga CA. Increased saccadic distractability in tardive dyskinesia: functional evidence for subcortical GABA dysfunction. Biol Psychiatry 1988 1: 49–59.

130. Hardoy MC, Hardoy MJ, Barta MG, et al. Gabapentin as a promising treatment for antipsychotic-induced movement disorders in schizoaffective and bipolar patients. J Affective Disord 1999; 54: 315–317.

131. Christensen E, Moller JE, Faurbye A. Neuropathological investigation of 28 brains from patients with dyskinesias. Acta Psychiatr Scand 1970; 46: 14–23.

132. Jellinger K. Neuropathological findings after neuroleptic long-term therapy. In Roizin L, Shnaki H, Grcevic N (eds) Neurotoxicology. New York, Raven Press, 1977, pp. 25–42.

133. Colon RJ. Long-lasting changes in cerebral neurons induced by drugs. Biol Psychiatry 1975; 10: 227.

134. Gerlach J. Long-term effects of perphenazine on the substantia nigra in rats. Psychopharmacologia 1975; 45: 51.

135. Pakkenberg H, Fog R, Nikkantan B. The long-term effect of perphenazine enanthate on the rat brain: some metabolic and anatomic observations. Psychopharmacologia 1973; 29: 329–336.

136. Pakkenberg H, Fog R. Short-term effect of perphenazine evantoate on the rat brain. Psychopharmacologia 1974; 40: 165–169.

137. Fog R, Pakkenberg H, Jaul P, et al. High dose treatment of rats with perphenazine enanthate. Psychopharmacology 1976; 50: 3305–3307.

138. Nielsen EB, Lyon M. Evidence for cell loss in corpus striatum after long-term treatment with a neuroleptic drug (fluphenthixol) in rats. Psychopharmacology 1978; 59: 85–89.

139. Pai B, Nagesh JN, Gangadhar BN, et al. Depletion of glutathione and enhanced lipid peroxidation in the CSF of acute psychotics following haloperidol administration. Biol Psychiatry 1994; 36: 489–491.

140. Andreassen OA, Jorgensen HA. Neurotoxicity associated with neuroleptic-induced oral dyskinesias in rats. Implications for tardive dyskinesia? Progr Neurobiol 2000; 61: 525–541.

141. Shamir E, Barak Y, Shalman I, et al. Melatonin treatment for tardive dyskinesia: a double-blind, placebo-controlled, crossover study. Arch Gen Psychiatry 2001; 58: 1049.

142. Gupta S, Mosnik D, Black DW, et al. Tardive dyskinesia: review of treatment past, present, and future. Ann Clin Psychiatry 1999; 11: 257–266.

143. Lohr JB. Kuczenski R, Niculescu AB. Oxidative mechanisms and tardive dyskinesia. CNS Drugs 2003; 17: 47–62.

144. Albin RL, Young AB, Penney JB. The functional neuroanatomy of the basal ganglia disorders. Trends Neurosci 1989; 12: 366–375.

145. Crossman AE. A hypothesis on the pathophysiological mechanisms that underlie levodopa- or dopamine agonist-induced dyskinesia in Parkinson's disease: implications for future strategies in treatment. Mov Disord 1990; 5: 100–108.

146. DeLong MR. Primate models of movement disorders of basal ganglia origin. Trends Neurosci 1990; 13: 281–289.

147. Meredith GE, De Souza IE, Hyde TM, et al. Persistent alterations in dendrites, spines, and dynorphinergic synapses in the nucleus accumbens shell of rats with neuroleptic-induced dyskinesias. J Neurosci 2000; 20: 7798–7806.

148. Andreassen OA, Meshul CK, Moore C, et al. Oral dyskinesias and morphological changes in rat striatum during long-term haloperidol administration. Psychopharmacology (Berl) 2001; 157: 11–19.

149. Doongaji DR, Jeste DV, Jape NM, et al. Effects of intravenous metoclopramide in 81 patients with tardive dyskinesia. J Clin Psychopharmacology 1982; 2: 376–379.

150. Perenyi A, Arato M, Bagdy G, et al. Tiapride in the treatment of tardive dyskinesia: a clinical and biochemical study. J Clin Psychiatry 1985; 46: 229–231.

151. Lieberman JA, Lesser M, Johns C, et al. Pharmacological studies of tardive dyskinesia. J Clin Psychopharmacology 1988; 8: 57S–63S.

152. Lieberman JA, Pollack S, Lesser MS, et al. Pharmacological characterization of tardive dyskinesia. J Clin Psychopharmacology 1988; 8: 254–260.

153. Singer K, Cheng MN. Thiopropazate hydrochloride in persistent dyskinesia. Br Med J 1971; 4: 22–25.

154. Roxburgh PA. Treatment of persistent phenothiazine-induced oral dyskinesia. Br J Psychiatry 1970; 116: 277–280.

155. Kazamatsuri H, Chien C-P, Cole JO. Long-term treatment of tardive dyskinesia with haloperidol and tetrabenazine. Am J Psychiatry 1973; 130: 479–483.

156. Glazer WM, Hafez H. A comparison of masking effects of haloperidol versus molindone in tardive dyskinesia. Schizophr Res 1990; 3: 315–320.

157. Curran JP. Management of tardive dyskinesia with thiopropazate. Am J Psychiatry 1973; 130: 925–927.

158. Smith JS, Kiloh LG. Six month evaluation of thiopropazate hydrochloride in tardive dyskinesia. J Neurol, Neurosurg Psychiatry 1979; 42: 576–579.

159. Frangos E, Christodoulides H. Clinical observations on the treatment of tardive dyskinesia with haloperidol. Acta Psychiatr Belg 1975; 75: 19–32.

160. Gerlach J, Casey DE. Sulpiride in tardive dyskinesia. Acta Psychiatr Scand 1983; 311(69)(suppl): 93–101.

161. Korsgaard S, Noring U, Gerlack J. Fluperlapine in tardive dyskinesia and parkinsonism. Psychopharmacology 1984; 39: 803–816.
162. Barnes TRE, Wiles DH. Variation in oro-facial tardive dyskinesia during depot antipsychotic drug treatment. Psychopharmacology 1983; 81: 359–362.
163. Glazer WM, Hafez HM, Benarroche LL. Molindone and haloperidol in tardive dyskinesia. J Clin Psychiatry 1985; 46: 4–7.
164. Caine ED, Polinsky RJ, Kartzinel R, et al. The trial use of clozapine for abnormal involuntary movement disorders. Am J Psychiatry 1979; 136: 317–320.
165. Gerlach J, Koppelhaus P, Helweg E. Clozapine and haloperidol in a single-blind crossover trial: therapeutic and biochemical aspects in the treatment of schizophrenia. Acta Psychiatr Scand 1974; 50: 410–424.
166. Gerlach J, Simmelsgaard H. Tardive dyskinesia during and following treatment with haloperidol, haloperidol + biperiden, thioridazine, and clozapine. Psychopharmacology 1978; 59: 105–112.
167. Lieberman JA, Saltz BL, Johns CA, et al. The effects of clozapine on tardive dyskinesia. Br J Psychiatry 1991; 158: 503–510.
168. Carroll BJ, Curtiss CG, Kokmen E. Paradoxical response to dopamine agonists in tardive dyskinesia. Am J Psychiatry 1977; 134: 785–790.
169. Meltzer HY, Luchins DJ. Effect of clozapine in severe tardive dyskinesia: a case report. J Clin Psychopharmacology 1984; 4: 286–287.
170. Friedman JH. Clozapine treatment of psychosis in patients with tardive dystonia: report of three cases. Mov Disord 1994; 9: 321–324.
171. Lamberti JS, Bellnier T. Clozapine and tardive dystonia. J Nerv Ment Disord 1993; 181: 137–138.
172. Trugman JM. Leadbetter R, Zalis ME, et al. Treatment of severe axial tardive dystonia with clozapine: case report and hypothesis. Mov Disord 1994; 9: 441–446.
173. Cole JO, Gardos G, Tarsy D. Drug trials in persistent dyskinesia. In Fann WE, Smith RC, Davis JM (eds) Tardive Dyskinesia, Research and Treatment. New York, SP Medical and Scientific Books, 1980, pp. 419–427.
174. Gerbino L, Shopsin B, Collora M. Clozapine in the treatment of tardive dyskinesia: an interim report. In Fann WE, Smith RC, Davis JM (eds) Tardive Dyskinesia, Research and Treatment. New York, SP Medical and Scientific Books, 1980, pp. 475–489.
175. Small JG, Milstein V, Marhenke JD, et al. Treatment outcome with clozapine in tardive dyskinesia, neuroleptic sensitivity and treatment-resistant psychosis. J Clin Psychiatry 1987; 48: 263–267.
176. Simpson G, Lee JH, Shrivastava RK. Clozapine in tardive dyskinesia. Psychopharmacology 1978; 56: 75–80.
177. Tamminga CA, Thaker GK, Moran M, et al. Clozapine in tardive dyskinesia: observations from human and animal model studies. J Clin Psychiatry 1994; 55 (9)(suppl B): 102–106.
178. Lieberman, JA, Saltz, BL, Johns, CA, Pollack, S, Borenstein, M, Kane, J. The effects of clozapine on tardive dyskinesia. Br J Psychiatry 1991; 158: 503–510.
179. Bassitt, DP and Louza Noto, MR Clozapiine efficacy in tardive dyskinesia in schizophrenic patients. Eur Arch Psychiatry Clin Neurosci 1998; 248: 209–211.
180. Spivak, B, Mester, R, Abegaus, J, Wittenberg, N, Adlersberg, S, Gonen, N, Weizman, A. Clozapine treatment for neuroleptic-induced tardive dyskinesia, parkinsonism, and chronic akathisia in schizophrenic patients. J Clin Psychiatry 1997; 58: 318–322.
181. Lieberman JA, Saltz BL, Johns CA, et al. Clozapine effects on tardive dyskinesia. Psychopharmacol Bull 1989; 25: 57–62.

182. Meco G, Bedini L, Bonifanti V, et al. Risperidone in the treatment of chronic schizophrenia with tardive dyskinesia: a single-blind crossover study versus placebo. Curr Therap Res 1989; 46: 876–883.

183. Kopala LC, Honer WG. Schizophrenia and severe tardive dyskinesia responsive to risperidone. J Clin Psychopharmacology 1994; 14: 430–431.

184. Seeger TF, Seymour PA, Schmidt AW. (CP-88,059): a new antipsychotic with combined dopamine and serotonin receptor antagonist activity. J Pharmacol Exp Therap 1995; 275: 101–113.

185. Borison RL, Arvantis LA, Miller BG. A comparison of five-fixed doses of "Seroquel" (ICI-204,636) with haloperidol and placebo in patients with schizophrenia. Schizophr Res 1996; 18(132): Abst. V.D.2.

186. Huang CC, Wang RH, Hasegawa A, et al. Reserpine and alpha methyl dopa in the treatment of tardive dyskinesia. Psychopharmacology 1981; 73: 359–362.

187. Nasrallah HA, Dunner FJ, McCalley-Whitters M, et al. Pharmacological probes of neurotransmitter systems in tardive dyskinesia: implications for clinical management. J Clin Psychiatry 1986; 47: 56–59.

188. Lang AE, Marsden CD. Alpha-methyl-paratyrosine and tetrabenazine in movement disorders. Clin Neuropharmacol 1982; 5: 375–387.

189. Lieberman JA, Alvin J, Mukherjee SJM. Treatment of tardive dyskinesia with bromocriptine. A test of the receptor modification strategy. Arch Gen Psychiatry 1989; 46: 908–913.

190. Ludatscher JI. Stable remission of tardive dyskinesia by L-dopa. J Clin Psychopharmacology 1989; 9: 39–41.

191. Kovacic B, LeWitt P, Clark D. Suppression of neuroleptic-induced persistent abnormal movement in Cebus apella monkeys by enantiomers of 3-PPP. J Neural Transm 1989; 74: 97–107.

192. Smith RC, Tamminga CA, Harasgti J, et al. Effects of dopamine agonists in tardive dyskinesia. Am J Psychiatry 1977; 134: 763–768.

193. Fuller RW, Clemens JA, Hynes MD. Degree of selectivity of pergolide as an agonist at presynaptic versus postsynaptic dopamine receptors: implications for prevention or treatment of tardive dyskinesia. J Clin Psychopharmacology 1982; 2: 371–375.

194. Schrodt GR, Wright JH, Simpson R, et al. Treatment of tardive dyskinesia with propranolol. J Clin Psychiatry 1982; 43: 328–331.

195. Greendyke RM, Webster JC, Kim J, et al. Lack of efficacy of pindolol in tardive dyskinesia. Am J Psychiatry 1988; 145: 1328–1319.

196. Freedman R, Kirch D, Bell J, et al. Clonidine treatment of schizophrenia. Double-blind comparison to placebo and neuroleptic drugs. Acta Psychiatr Scand 1982; 65: 35–45.

197. Nishikawa T, Tanaka M, Tsuda A, et al. Clonidine therapy for tardive dyskinesia and related syndromes. Clin Neuropharmacol 1984; 7(3): 239–245.

198. Browne J, Silver H, Martin R, et al. The use of clonidine in the treatment of neuroleptic-induced tardive dyskinesia. J Clin Psychopharmacology 1986; 6: 88–92.

199. Soares KVS, McGrath JJ. The treatment of tardive dyskinesia-a systematic review and meta-analysis. Schizophr Res 1999; 39: 1–16.

200. Jeste DV, Lohr JB, Kaufman CA, et al. Pathophysiology of tardive dyskinesia: evaluation of supersensitivity theory and alternative hypotheses. In Casey D, Gardos G (eds) Tardive Dyskinesia: From Dogma to Reason. Washington DC, American Psychiatric Press, 1986, pp. 15–32.

201. Soni SD, Freeman HL, Hussein EM. Oxypertine in tardive dyskinesia: and 8-week controlled study. Br J Psychiatry 1984; 144: 48–52.

202. Klawans HL. The pharmacology of tardive dyskinesia. Am J Psychiatry 1973; 130: 82–86.

203. Wirshing WC, Freidenberg DL, Cummings JL, et al. Effects of anticholinergic agents on patients with tardive dyskinesia and concomitant drug-induced Parkinsonism. J Clin Psychiatry 1989; 9: 407–411.

204. Moore DC, Bowers MB. Identification of a subgroup of tardive dyskinesia patients by pharmacological probes. Am J Psychiatry 1980; 137: 1202–1205.

205. Friis T, Christensen TR, Gerlach J. Sodium valproate and biperiden in neuroleptic-induced akathisia, parkinsonism, and hyperkinesia. Acta Psychiatr Scand 1983; 67: 178–187.

206. Yassa R. Tardive dyskinesia and anticholinergic drugs: a critical review of the literature. Encephale 1988; 14: 233–239.

207. Burke RE, Fahn S, Jankovic J, et al. Tardive dystonia: late onset and persistent dystonia caused by antipsychotic drugs. Neurology 1982; 32: 1335–1346.

208. Fahn S. High dose anticholinergic therapy in dystonia. Neurology 1983; 33: 1255–1261.

209. Klawans HL. Therapeutic approaches to neuroleptic-induced tardive dyskinesia. In Yahr MD (ed) The Basal Ganglia. New York, Raven Press, 1976, pp. 447–457.

210. Keepers GA, Casey DE. Use of neuroleptic-induced extrapyramidal symptoms to predict future vulnerability to side effects. Am J Psychiatry 1991; 148: 1.

211. Yagi G; Takamuja M; Kauba S, et al. Mortality rates of schizophrenic patients with tardive dyskinesia during 10 years: a controlled study. Keio J Med 1989; 38: 70—72.

212. Izume K, Tominaga H, Koja T, et al. Meclofenozate therapy in tardive dyskinesia: a preliminary report. Biological Psychiatry 1986; 21: 151–160.

213. Tammenmaa IA, McGrath JJ, Sailas E, et al. Cholinergic medication for neuroleptic-induced tardive dyskinesia. The Cochrane Library. 3. Oxford, Update Software, 2002.

214. Caroff SN, Campbell EC, Havey J, et al. Treatment of tardive dyskinesia with donepezil: a pilot study. J Clin Psychiatry 2001; 62: 772–775.

215. Thaker GK, Nguyen JA, Strauss ME, et al: Clonazepam treatment of tardive dyskinesia: a practical GABA-mimetic strategy. Am J Psychiatry 1990; 147: 445–451.

216. McGrath JJ, Soares, KVS. Benzodiazepines for neuroleptic-induced tardive dyskinesia. The Cochrane Database System Review. 3. Oxford, Update Software, 2002.

217. Stahl SW, Thornton JE, Simpson ML, et al. Gamma-vinyl-GABA treatment of tardive dyskinesia and other movement disorders. Biol Psychiatry 1985; 20: 888–983.

218. Tamminga CA, Crayton J, Chase T. Improvement in tardive dyskinesia after muscimol therapy. Arch Gen Psychiatry 1979; 36: 595–598.

219. Fisk GG, York SM. The effect of sodium valproate on tardive dyskinesia-revisited. Br J Psychiatry 1987; 150: 542–456.

220. Singh MM, Becker RE, Pitman RK, et al. Sustained improvement in tardive dyskinesia with diazepam: indirect evidence for corticolimbic involvement. Brain Res Bull 1983; 11: 179–185.

221. O'Flannagan PM. Clonazepam in the treatment of drug-induced dyskinesia. Br Med J 1975; 1: 269–270.

222. Sedman G. Clonazepam in the treatment of tardive oral dyskinesia. Br Med J 1976; 2: 583.

223. Glazer WM, Naftolin F, Morgenstern J, et al. Estrogen replacement and tardive dyskinesia. Psychoneuroendocrinology 1985; 10: 345–350.

224. Stewart RM, Robbin J, Beckham B. Baclofen in tardive dyskinesia patients maintained on neuroleptics. Clin Neuropharmacol 1982; 5: 365–373.

225. Soares, KV, McGrath, JJ, Deeks, JJ Gamma-aminobutyric acid agonists for neuroleptic-induced tardive dyskinesia. Cochrane Database Syst Rev 2001; CD000203. Review.

226. Gardos G, Cole JO. The treatment of tardive dyskinesia. In Bloom FE, Kupfur DJ (ed) Psychopharmacology: The Fourth Generation of Progress. New York, Raven Press, 1995, pp. 1503–1511.

227. Matsumoto T, Uchimura H, Hirano M, et al. Differential effects of acute and chronic administration of haloperidol on homovanillic acid levels in discrete dopaminergic areas of rat brain. Eur J Pharmacology 1983; 89: 27–33.
228. Hori H, Ohmori O, Shinkai T, et al. Manganese supraoxide dismutase gene polymorphism and schizophrenia: relation to tardive dyskinesia. Neuropsychopharmacology 2000; 23: 170–177.
229. Lohr JB. Caliguri MP. A double blind placebo-controlled study of vitamin E treatment of tardive dyskinesia. J Clin Psychiatry 1996; 57: 167–173.
230. Schmidt M, Meister P, Baumann P. Treatment of tardive dyskinesia with vitamin E. Eur Psychiatry 1991; 6: 201–207.
231. Shriqui CL, Bradwejn J, Annable L, et al. Vitamin E in the treatment of tardive dyskinesia: a double-blind placebo-controlled study. Am J Psychiatry 1992; 149: 391–393.
232. Lam LCW, Chiu HFK, Hun SF. Vitamin E in the treatment of tardive dyskinesia: a replication study. J Nerv Ment Disord 1994; 182: 113–114.
233. Egan MF, Hyde TH, Albers GW, et al. Treatment of tardive dyskinesia with vitamin E. Am J Psychiatry 1992; 149: 773–777.
234. Adler L, Peselow E, Rotrosen J, et al. Vitamin E treatment of tardive dyskinesia. Am J Psychiatry 1993; 150: 1405–1407.
235. Spivak B, Schwartz B, Radwan M, et al. Alpha-tocopherol treatment for tardive dyskinesia. J Nerv Ment Disord 1992; 180: 400–401.
236. Peet M, Laugharne J, Rangarajan N, et al. Tardive dyskinesia, lipid peroxidation and sustained amelioration with vitamin E treatment. Int J Clin Psychopharmacol 1993; 8: 151–153.
237. Coupland N, Nutt D. Successful treatment of tardive oculogyric spasms with vitamin E. [letter]. J Clin Psychopharmacol 15: 285–286.
238. Lohr, JB, Cadet Jl, Lohr, MA, Jeste, DV, Wyatt, RJ. Alpha-tocopherol in tardive dyskinesia. Lancet 1987; 1: 913–914.
239. Adler LA, Rotrosen J, Edson R, et al. Vitamin E treatment for tardive dyskinesia. Veterans Affairs Cooperative Study 394 Study Group. Arch Gen Psychiatry 1999; 56: 836–841.
240. Barrow N, Childs A. An anti-tardive-dyskinesia effect of verapamil. Am J Psychiatry 1986; 143: 1485.
241. Buck OD, Havey P. Treatment of tardive dyskinesia with verapamil. J Clin Psychopharmacol 1988; 8: 303–304.
242. Ross JL, Mackenzie TB, Hanson DR, et al. Diltiazem for tardive dyskinesia. Lancet 1987; 1: 824–825.
243. Casey, DE Extrapyramidal syndromes and new antipsychotic drugs: findings in patients and non-human primate models. Br J Psychiatry Suppl. 1996; 29: 32–39.
244. Falk WE, Wojcik JD, Gelenberg AJ. Diltiazem for tardive dyskinesia and tardive dystonia. Lancet 1988; 1: 824–825.
245. Abad V, Ovsiew F. Treatment of persistent myoclonic tardive dystonia with verapamil. Br J Psychiatry 1993; 162: 554–556.
246. Reiter S, Adler L, Angrist B, et al. Effects of verapamil on tardive dyskinesia and psychosis in schizophrenic patients. J Clin Psychiatry 1989; 50: 26–27.
247. Leys D, Vermersch P, Comayras S, et al. Diltiazem for tardive dyskinesia. Lancet 1988; 1: 250–251.
248. Loonen AJM, Verwey AH, Roels PR, et al. Is diltiazem effective in treating the symptoms of (tardive) dyskinesia in chronic psychiatric inpatients? A negative, double-blind, placebo-controlled trial. J Clin Psychopharmacol 1992; 12: 39–42.
249. Kushnir SL, Ratner JT. Calcium channel blockers for tardive dyskinesia in geriatric patients. Am J Psychiatry 1989; 146: 1218–1219.

250. Duncan E, Adler L, Angrist B, et al. Nifedipine in the treatment of tardive dyskinesia. J Clin Psychopharmacol 1990; 10: 414–416.

251. Steadman TJ, Whiteford HA, Eyles D, et al. Effects of nifedipine on psychosis and tardive dyskinesia in schizophrenic patients. J Clin Psychopharmacol 1991; 11: 43–47.

252. Adler L, Duncan E, Reiter S, et al. Effect of calcium channel antagonists on tardive dyskinesia and psychosis. Psychopharmacol Bull 1988; 24: 421–425.

253. Mena MA, Garcia MJ, Tabernero C, et al. Effects of calcium antagonists on the dopamine system. Clin Neuropharmacol 1995; 18: 410–426.

254. Brucke T, Wober C, Podreka I, et al. D2 receptor blockade by flunarizine and cinnarizine explains EPS side effects. A SPECT study. J Cerebral Blood Flow Metab 1995; 15: 513–518.

255. Sabria J, Pastor C, Clos MV, et al. Involvement of different types of voltage-sensitive calcium channels in the presynaptic regulation of noradrenaline release in rat brain cortex and hippocampus. J Neurochem 1995; 64: 2567–2571.

256. Seibyl JP, Glazer WM, Innis RB. Serotonin function in tardive dyskinesia. Psychiatr Ann 1989; 19: 310–314.

257. Neppe VM. High dose buspirone in case of tardive dyskinesia [letter] Lancet 1989; 2: 1458.

258. Kleedorfer B, Lees AJ, Stern GM. Buspirone in the treatment of levodopa induced dyskinesias. J Neurol, Neurosurg Psychiatry 1991; 54(4):376–377.

259. Moss LE, Neppe VM, Drevets WC. Buspirone in the treatment of tardive dyskinesia. J Clin Psychopharmacol 1993; 13: 204–209.

260. Brody D, Adler KA, Kime T, et al. Effects of buspirone in seven schizophrenic subjects. J Clin Psychopharmacol 1990; 10: 68–69.

261. Goff DC, Midha KK, Brotman AW, et al. An open trial of buspirone added to neuroleptics in schizophrenic patients. J Clin Psychopharmacol 1991; 11: 193–197.

262. Newton RE, Maranycz JD, Alderice MT, et al. Review of the side effect profile of buspirone. Am J Med 1986; 80(3)(suppl B): 17–21.

263. Boylan K. Persistent dystonia associated with buspirone. Neurology 1990; 40: 1904.

264. Strauss A. Oral dyskinesia associated with buspirone use in an elderly woman. J Clin Psychiatry 1988; 49: 322–323.

265. McMillan BA. Comparative chronic effects of buspirone or neuroleptics on rat brain dopaminergic neurotransmission. J Neural Transm 1985; 64: 1–12.

266. Baldessarini RJ, Marsh E. Fluoxetine and side effects [letter]. Am J Psychiatry 1990; 147: 191–192.

267. Bouchard RH, Pourcher E, Vincent P. Fluoxetine and extrapyramidal side effects [letter]. Am J Psychiatry 1989; 146: 1352–1353.

268. Budman CL, Bruun RD. Persistent dyskinesia in a patient receiving fluoxetine. Am J Psychiatry 1991; 148: 1403.

269. Stein MH. Tardive dyskinesia in a patient taking haloperidol and fluoxetine. Am J Psychiatry 1991; 148: 683.

270. Arya DK, Szabadi E. Dyskinesia associated with fluvoxamine [letter]. J Clin Psychopharmacology 1993; 13(5): 365–366.

271. Dubovsky SL, Thomas M. Tardive dyskinesia associated with fluoxetine. Psychiatr Serv 1996; 47: 991–993.

272. Leo RJ. Movement disorders associated with the serotonin selective reuptake inhibitors. J Clin Psychiatry 1996; 57: 449–454.

273. Kurata K, Hosokawa K, Koshino Y. Treatment of neuroleptic induced tardive dyskinesia. J Neurol 1977; 215: 295–298.

274. Goldman D. Treatment of phenothiazine-induced dyskinesia. Psychopharmacology 1976; 47: 271–272.

275. Gardos G, Cole J. Pilot study of cyproheptadine (Periactin) in tardive dyskinesia. Psychopharmacol Bull 1978; 14: 18–20.

276. Wynchank D, Berk M. Efficacy of nefazadone in the treatment of neuroleptic induced extrapyramidal side effects: a double-blind randomized parallel group placebo-controlled trial. Hum Psychopharmacol 2003; 18: 271–275.

277. Sirota P, Mosheva T, Shabtay H, et al. Use of the selective serotonin 3 receptor antagonist ondansetron in the treatment of neuroleptic-induced tardive dyskinesia. Am J Psychiatry 2000; 157: 287–289.

278. Tarsy D, Kavfman D, Sethi KD, et al. An open label Study of botulinum toxin type A for treatment of tardive dystonia. Clin Neuropharmacol 1997; 20: 90–93.

279. Hughs AJ. Botulinum toxin in clinical practice. Drugs 1994; 48: 888–893.

280. Goetz CG, Horn SS. Treatment of tremor and dystonia. Neurol Clin 2001; 19: 129–144.

281. Hsiung GY, Das SK, Ranawaya R, et al. Long-term efficacy of botulinum toxin A in treatment of various movement disorders over a 10-year period. Mov Disord 2002; 17: 1288–1293.

282. Braun V, Richter HP. Selective peripheral denervation for the treatment of spasmodic torticollis. Neurosurgery 1994; 35: 58–62.

283. Matsumoto T, Nakahara T, Uchimura H, et al. Effect of systemically administered caerulein on doapmine metabolism in rat brain. Brain Res 1984; 324: 195–199.

284. Stoessl AJ, Dourish CT, Iversen SD. Chronic neuroleptic-induced mouth movement in the rat: suppression by CCK and selective dopamine D1 and D2 receptor antagonists. Psychopharmacology 1989; 98: 372–379.

285. Nishikawa T, Tanaka M, Tsuda A, et al. Treatment of tardive dyskinesia with ceruletide. Progr Neuropsychopharmacol Biol Psychiatry 1988; 12(5): 803–812.

286. Kojima T, Yamauchi T, Miyasaka M, et al. Treatment of tardive dyskinesia with ceruletide: a double-blind, placebo-controlled study. Psychiatry Res 1992; 43: 129–136.

287. Passaro E, Bebas H, Olendorf W, et al. Rapid appearance of intraventricularly administered neuropeptides in the peripheral circulation. Brain Res 1982; 241: 335–340.

288. Skirboll LR, Grace AA, Hommer DW, et al. Peptide-monoamine coexistence: Studies of actions of cholecystokinin-like peptide on the electrical activity of midbrain dopamine neurons. Neuroscience 1981; 6: 2111–2124.

289. Klawans HL, Weiner WJ, Nausieda PA. The effects of lithium on an animal model of tardive dyskinesia. Progr Neuropsychopharmacol 1977; 1: 53–60.

290. Benechke R, Conrad B, Klingehhofer J. Successful treatment of tardive and spontaneous dyskinesias with corticosteroids. Eur Neurol 1988; 28: 146–149.

291. McCormick SE, Stoessl AJ. Central administration of the neurotensin receptor antagonist SR48692 attenuates vacuous chewing movements in a rodent model of tardive dyskinesia. Neuroscience 2003; 119: 547–555.

292. Richardson MA, Bevans ML, Weber JB, et al. Branched chain amino acids decrease tardive dyskinesia symptoms. Pyschopharmacology 1999; 143: 358–364.

293. Richardson MA, Bevans ML, Read LL, et al. Efficacy of branched-chain amino acids in the treatment of tardive dyskinesia in men. Am J Psychiatry 2003; 160: 1117–1124.

294. Hay DP, Hay L, Blackwell B, et al. ECT and tardive dyskinesia. J Geriatr Psychiatry Neurol 1990; 3: 106–109.

295. Abosch A, Lozano A. Stereotactic neurosurgery for movement disorders. Can J Neurol Sci 2003; 30(suppl 1): S72-S82.

296. Ohye C. Use of selective thalamotomy for various kinds of movement disorder, based on basic studies. Stereotact Funct Neurosurg 2000; 75: 54–65.

297. Wang Y, Turnbull I, Calne S, et al. Pallidotomy for tardive dyskinesia. Lancet 1997; 349: 777–778.

298. Hillier CEM, Wiles CM, Simpson BA. Thalamotomy for severe antipsychotic induced tardive dyskinesia and dystonia. J Neurol Neurosurg Psychiatry 1999; 66: 250–251.

299. Boyce S, Rupniak NMJ, Steventon MJ, et al. Differential effects of D1 and D2 agonists in MPTP-treated primates: functional implications for Parkinson's disease. Neurology 1990; 40: 927–933.

300. Lublin H, Gerlack J, Hagert U, et al. Zuclopenthixol, a combined dopamine D1/D2 antagonist, in tardive dyskinesia. Eur Neuropsychopharmacol 1991; 1: 541–548.

301. Nutt JG. Levodopa-induced dyskinesia: review, observations, and speculations. Neurology 1990; 40: 340–345.

302. Braun A, Fabbrini G, Nouradian MM, et al. Selective D-1 receptor agonist treatment of Parkinson's Disease. J Neural Transm 1987; 68: 41–50.

303. Sandyk R, Snider SR. Naloxone treatment of l-dopa induced dyskinesias in Parkinson's disease. Am J Psychiatry 1986; 143: 118.

304. Blum I, Munitz H, Shalev A, et al. Naloxone may be beneficial in the treatment of tardive dyskinesia. Clin Neuropharmacol 1984 7(3): 265–267.

305. Lindenmayer J-P, Gardner E, Goldberg E, et al. High dose naloxone in tardive dyskinesia. Psychiatry Res 1987; 26: 19–28.

306. Berg D, Becker G, Naumann M, et al. Morphine in tardive and idiopathic dystonia. J Neural Transm 2001; 108: 1035–1041.

307. Berg D, Becker G, Reiners K. Reduction of dyskinesia and induction of akinesia induced by morphine in Parkinsonian patients with severe sciatica. J Neural Transm 1999; 106: 725–728.

308. Rascol O, Fabre N, Blin O, et al. Naltrexone, an opiate antagonist, fails to modify motor symptoms in patients with Parkinson's disease. Mov Disord 1994; 9: 437–440.

309. Bunney WE, Bunney BG, Vawter MP, et al. Microarray technology: a review of new strategies to discover candidate vulnerability genes in psychiatric disorders. Am J Psychiatry 2003; 160: 657–666.

310. Armstrong M, Daly AK, Blennerhassett R, et al. Antipsychotic drug-induced movement disorders in schizophrenics in relation to CYP2D6 genotype. Br J Psychiatry 1997; 170: 23–26.

311. Kapitany T, Meszaros K, Lenzinger E, et al. Genetic polymorphisms for drug metabolism (CYP2D6) and tardive dyskinesia in schizophrenia. Schizophr Res 1998; 32: 101–106.

312. Ohmori O, Shinkai T, Kojima H, et al. Tardive dyskinesia and debrisoquine 4-hydroxylase (CYP2D6) genotype in Japanese schizophrenics. Schizophr Res 1998; 32: 107–113.

313. Chen C-H, Wei F-W, Koong F-J, et al. Association of TaqI A polymorphism of dopamine D2 receptor gene and tardive dyskinesia in schizophrenia. Biol Psychiatry 1997; 41: 827–829.

314. Hori H, Ohmori O, Shinkai T, et al. Association between three functional polymorphisms of dopamine D2 receptor genes and tardive dyskinesia in schizophrenia. Am J Med Gen 2001; 105: 774–778.

315. Steen VM, Lovlie R, MacEwan T, et al. Dopamine D3-receptor gene variant and susceptibility to tardive dyskinesia in schizophrenic patients. Mol Psychiatry 1997; 2: 139–145.

316. Segman RH. Neeman T, Heresco-Levy U, et al. Genotypic association between the dopamine D3 receptor and tardive dyskinesia in chronic schizophrenia. Mol Psychiatry 1999; 4: 247–253.

317. Ohmori O, Suzuki T, Hori H, et al. Polymorphisms of the mu and delta opioid receptor genes and tardive dyskinesia in patients with schizophrenia. Schizophr Res 2001; 52: 137–138.

318. Segman RH, Heresco-Levy U, Finkel B, et al. Association between the serotonin 2A receptor gene and tardive dyskinesia in chronic schizophrenia. Mol Psychiatry 2001; 6: 225–229.
319. Tan EC, Chong SA, Mahendran R, et al. Susceptibility to neuroleptic-induced tardive dyskinesia and the T102C polymorphism in the serotonin type 2A receptor. Biol Psychiatry 2001; 50: 144–147.
320. Segman RH, Heresco-Levy U, Finkel B, et al. Association between the serotonin 2C receptor gene and tardive dyskinesia in chronic schizophrenia. Psychopharmacology 2000; 152: 408–413.
321. Basile VS, Ozdemir V, Masellis M, et al. Lack of association between serotonin-2A receptor gene (HTR2A) polymorphisms and tardive dyskinesia in schizophrenia. Mol Psychiatry 2001; 6: 230–234.
322. Kaiser R, Tremblay PB, Klufmoller F, et al. Relationship between adverse effects of antipsychotic treatment and dopamine D(2) receptor polymorphisms in patients with schizophrenia. Mol Psychiatry 2002; 7: 695–705.
323. Chong SA, Tan EC, Tan CH, et al. Polymorphisms of dopamine receptors and tardive dyskinesia among Chinese patients with schizophrenia. Am J Med Genet 2003; 116B: 51–54.
324. Lohmann PL, Bagli M, Krauss H, et al. CYP2D6 polymorphism and tardive dyskinesia in schizophrenic patients. Pharmacopsychiatry 2003; 36: 73–78.
325. Lerer B, Segman RH, Fangerau H, et al. Pharmacogenetics of tardive dyskinesia: combined analysis of 780 patients supports association with dopamine D3 receptor gene Ser9Gly polymorphism. Neuropsychopharmacology 2002; 27: 105–119.
326. Van Putten T, Wirshing W, Marder S. Tardive Meige's syndrome responsive to clozapine. J Clin Psychopharmacology 1990; 10: 381–382.
327. Levkovitch Y, Kronenberg J, Kayser N, et al. Clozapine for tardive dyskinesia in adolescents. Brain Dev 1995; 17: 213–215.
328. Elkashef AM, Ruskin PE, Bacher N, et al. Vitamin E in the treatment of tardive dyskinesia. Am J Psychiatry 1990; 147: 505–506.
329. Junker D, Steigleider P, Gattaz WF. Alpha-tocopherol in the treatment of tardive dyskinesia. Clin Neuropharmacol 1992; 15(suppl 1, pt b): 639b.
330. Dabiri LM, Pasta D, Darby JK, et al. Effectiveness of vitamin E for treatment of long-term tardive dyskinesia. Am J Psychiatry 1994; 151: 925–926.
331. Suddath RL, Straw GM, Freed WJ, et al. A clinical trial of nifedipine in schizophrenia and tardive dyskinesia. Pharmacol Biochem Behav 1991; 39: 743–745.
332. Akhtar S, Jajor TR, Kumar S. Vitamin E in the treatment of tardive dyskinesia. J Postgrad Med 1993; 39: 124–126.
333. Cole JO, Gardos G. Tardive dyskinesia: outcome at 10 years. Schizophr Res 1990; 3: 11.
334. Fleischhacker WW, Linkz CGG, Hurst BC. ICI-204,636 ('Seroquel')-a putative new atypical antipsychotic; results from phase III trials. Schizophr Res 1996; 18:132, Abst. V.D.1.
335. Glazer WM, Moore DC, Bowers MB, et al. The treatment of tardive dyskinesia with baclofen. Psychopharmacology 1985; 87: 480–483.
336. Khot V, Egan MF, Hyde TM, et al. Neuroleptics and classical tardive dyskinesia. In Lang AE, Weiner WJ (eds) Drug-Induced Movement Disorders. Mount Kisco, NY, Futura, 1992, pp. 121–166.
337. Lohr JB, Cadet JL, Lohr MA, et al. Vitamin E in the treatment of tardive dyskinesia: the possible involvement of free radical mechanisms. Schizophr Bull 1988; 14: 291–296.
338. Umbrich P, Soares KV. Benzodiazepines for neuroleptic-induced tardive dyskinesia. Cochrane Database System Review. 2. Oxford, Update Software, 2003.

CHAPTER 10

Neuroleptic-induced tardive dyskinesia variants

Frank Skidmore, William J Weiner, and Robert Burke

Introduction

Since the earliest reports of tardive dyskinesia (TD), a variety of involuntary movements, in addition to the well-known oral-buccal-lingual masticatory movements, have been described, including dystonia, akathisia, myoclonus tics, and tremor. These variants are now well recognized. It is difficult to know why, historically, these forms took longer to gain wide recognition. One probable reason is that while definitive prevalence studies have not been done, it appears that these forms are less common than oral-buccal-lingual dyskinesia. In addition, some of the clinical features of the two major variants, tardive dystonia and tardive akathisia, are quite variable, and not widely known among neurologists and psychiatrists, although movement disorders specialists have come to recognize certain tardive dystonic postures (e.g., retrocollis) as "classic." In spite of the delayed recognition of these variants, there now seems to be a consensus that they do exist as distinct forms of tardive dyskinesia, and that they also occur in isolation. In addition, although they have a clinical pharmacology similar to that of oral dyskinesia, in that they are caused and suppressed by antidopaminergic drugs, there is some evidence that they have their own unique pharmacology as well. Most importantly, these variants deserve distinct recognition because, unlike oral dykinesia, they are usually quite disabling, particularly tardive dystonia. Therefore, the main emphasis here will be on the clinical recognition, differential diagnosis, and treatment of these disorders.

The term *tardive dyskinesia* is used differently by different authors. In this chapter, the term is used to encompass all forms of persistent dyskinesia due to neuroleptics, and it, therefore, includes not only classic oral dyskinesia, but also the variant forms described here. The reader should be aware that in the early literature the term is used to refer strictly to the oral-lingual form of dyskinesia. Although the term *tardive* was originally intended to emphasize the late appearance of these disorders during neuroleptic treatment, it is now clear that these disorders may appear early in the course of therapy, and there is no fundamental distinction between cases appearing early and those appearing late. The current definition emphasizes what is a more important characteristic shared by these disorders, their *persistence*. It is this characteristic that distinguishes these tardive dykinesias from the other neuroleptic-induced movement disorders, including acute dystonia, acute akathisia, and parkinsonism, which typically remit following cessation of neuroleptics.

Tardive dystonia

The nature of dystonic movements

Dystonic movements are strikingly different from the classically described oral-lingual masticatory movements, and it is this clear distinction in clinical phenomenology, which led investigators to identify persistent dystonia as a distinct subtype of tardive dyskinesia [1], although many earlier reports had also noted this occurrence [2–12]. Dystonia is defined as "a syndrome of sustained muscle contractions, frequently causing twisting and repetitive movements, or abnormal postures" [13]. Dystonic movements take on a variable appearance according to the body region involved. For example, dystonia affecting the muscles about the eyes (blepharospasm) appears as frequent blinking in mild form, and sustained spasms of eye closure in more severe form. Dystonia of lower facial muscles appears as facial grimacing, sustained jaw closure, opening, or deviation. Sustained, forceful protrusion of tongue may also occur. Neck involvement may appear as twisting about the long axis of neck (torticollis), backward pulling (retrocollis), forward pulling (anterocollis), or a mixture of these. Further examples of dystonic movements affecting other body regions in tardive dystonia will be discussed.

Two general features of dystonic movements deserve mention. First, many dystonic movements are action-specific, meaning that they occur with some actions but not with others. For example, some individuals with dystonia affecting the hand will develop involuntary movements only during the act of writing ("writer's cramp"). We have observed an individual who had pronounced tardive dystonia of the arms and trunk with walking, but who showed minimal dystonia during dancing. A similar case has been described where truncal and cervical dystonia present with sitting and walking dissipated with dancing [14]. A videotape of this case has been published. Second, many patients with dystonia note that their movements can be partially controlled by simple tactile maneuvers, such as touching the chin to control torticollis, or the brow to control blepharospasm. These "sensory tricks" are quite characteristic. Both the action-specific nature and partial control by sensory tricks often mislead neurologists and psychiatrists to an erroneous diagnosis of hysteria or malingering in patients with true dystonia. It should be noted that these features are present in idiopathic and tardive dystonia.

The evidence that chronic dystonia is associated with neuroleptic drug use

For the oral-buccal-lingual form of tardive dykinesia, retrospective epidemiologic studies have convincingly demonstrated an association between the

Table 10.1 Selected reports of cases of persistent dystonia associated with dopamine antagonist treatment

Authors	Year	Patients (No.)	Age of onset (Years)
Druckman et al. [2]	1962	1	46
Chateau et al. [3]	1966	1	27
Dabbous and Bergman [4]	1966	1	5
Harenko [5]	1967	6	74–89
Burke et al. [1]	1982	42	13–60
Kang et al. [18]	1986	67	13–72
Yassa et al. [20]	1986	7	21–76
Friedman et al. [21]	1987	5	Not listed
Lang [22]	1990	20	22–50
Miller and Jankovic [23]	1990	30	13–89
Wojcik et al. [24]	1992	32	22–69
Van Harten, et al. [16]	1996	26	Not listed
Kiriakakis [25]	1998	107	13–68

use of neuroleptics and the involuntary movements [15, 16]. These data are important to establish a causal relationship between drug use and the oral movements, because oral, masticatory movements apparently can occur in elderly patients spontaneously [17]. Dystonic movements may also occur spontaneously, and therefore, it is important to consider the evidence to support an association between neuroleptic drug use and persistent dystonia. The Curaco study, a prevalence study of extrapyramidal syndromes among all psychiatric inpatients in the Netherland Antilles, strongly supports a connection between dystonia and neuroleptic use [16]. In this well-defined catchment area with only one psychiatric hospital, the investigators used the Fahn-Marsden scale for evaluating dystonia and found that 13.4% of chronic psychiatric inpatients (all on neuroleptics) had dystonic movements. Little is known of the epidemiology of the dystonias, but these are not common disorders (certainly much lower than a prevalence of 13.4%), and the frequent association between dystonias and neuroleptic use in this study population is highly suggestive. Table 10.1 lists a number of reports of dystonia occurring during neuroleptic drug use. This list is undoubtedly not complete, because some authors do not use the term *dystonia* to characterize the involuntary movements; for example, the term *Pisa syndrome* appears to refer to a truncal dystonia that causes leaning. Furthermore, movement disorder neurologists now consider the association between neuroleptic use and persistent dystonia to be so commonplace that these cases are no longer reported, unless there is some aspect of interest.

In addition to the frequently reported association between neuroleptic use and dystonia, a number of other observations suggest a casual relationship. First, there are close temporal relationships between the use of neuroleptics and the occurrence of dystonia in given individuals. In one report, there was a 12% remission rate of dystonia following withdrawal of neuroleptics [18]. The majority of these individuals had nonfocal dystonias that spontaneously remitted. Second, when dystonia occurs during treatment with neuroleptics, it occurs with oral-lingual dyskinesia in 55% of cases or with tardive akathisia in 31% of cases. Strong evidence indicates that both oral-lingual dyskinesia and tardive akathisia are due to neuroleptic drugs, and their cooccurrence with dystonia strongly suggests that it is also due to the drugs [16]. Idiopathic dystonia and dystonia due to other identifiable etiologies do not cause the simultaneous occurrence of oral dyskinesias or akathisia. Third, it is clear that neuroleptics cause acute dystonia, and in a few instances, these occurrences have continued as persistent dystonia [1]. Fourth, the clinical pharmacology of persistent dystonia, which develops during neuroleptic drug treatment is distinctive; it fairly consistently can be suppressed by dopamine receptor-blocking drugs or dopamine depletors [18]. In this respect, it is like other forms of tardive dykinesia (e.g., oral-lingual dyskinesia) and is unlike other forms of dystonia [19]. These considerations have led many movement disorder neurologists to conclude that neuroleptics are capable of causing persistent dystonia.

Diagnostic criteria

Criteria for a diagnosis of tardive dystonia include the following: (1) The patient must have dystonia. (2) The dystonia must develop either during or within 3 months of a course of neuroleptic treatment. This 3-month cutoff is arbitrary in recognition of the fact that neuroleptics may suppress tardive dyskinesia and often movements do not become apparent until some time after drugs have been stopped. In the absence of direct evidence, it seems difficult to claim that a movement disorder due to neuroleptics could first appear more than 3 months after their use. (3) Wilson's disease must be excluded by a 24-hour urine copper and a slit-lamp examination for Kayser-Fleischer rings. In addition, there must be no other neurological signs to suggest one of the many known causes of secondary dystonia [26]. (4) There must be a negative family history for dystonia, or, in a family with a known genetic cause (e.g., DYT1), the known mutation must be excluded. Otherwise, in the presence of a positive family history, it would not be possible to know whether the affected individual had neuroleptic-induced dystonia or had simply expressed an inherited form coincident with neuroleptic use.

In the diagnosis of tardive dystonia by the above criteria, the presence of dystonia is sufficient. Dystonia need not be the dominant movement disorder, and it is not necessary to force a single unitary diagnosis on a patient; thus, a given patient may have not only tardive dystonia, but also classic oral-lingual dyskinesia or tardive akathisia. If all are present, all may be diagnosed. Patients with tardive movement disorders frequently demonstrate a mixture of abnormal movements, and to attempt to choose one as "predominant" is often subjective and arbitrary.

Epidemiology

Tardive dystonia has not been the subject of prospective case-control studies, but it is clear that it is undoubtedly less common than oral-buccalingual tardive dyskinesia. In a survey of 555 psychiatric in- and outpatients, Yassa and colleagues found a prevalence of 34% for oral tardive dyskinesia, and only 1.4% for tardive dystonia [27]. Similarly, Friedman and coworkers found a prevalence of only 1.5% among 352 psychiatric inpatients [21]. Estimates of the prevalence of dystonia depend on the diagnostic criteria used. Sethi et al. [28] found that 27 of 125 veterans on chronic antipsychotic medication had some form of dystonia. Notably, in the latter group "mild dystonia" was taken into account and only 20% of these cases (or 4% of the total cases) were symptomatic. Using the Fahn-Marsden scale to rate dystonia in a large epidemiologic study, van Harten et al. [16] found the prevalence of dystonia to be 13.4% in a defined catchment of patients in the Netherland Antilles; however, the authors noted that only 2.9% of their study population had "moderate-to-severe" dystonia, as defined by dystonia involving at least two body areas moderately or one severely.

Although patient characteristics for oral dyskinesia and tardive dystonia have rarely been compared within the same patient population, it appears that tardive dystonia usually has an earlier mean age of onset. In Yassa's study [27], 11 patients with severe oral dyskinesia had a mean age of onset of 64 years whereas 8 patients with tardive dystonia had a mean age of onset of 40.5 years. Similarly, other investigators have noted an early mean age of onset, ranging from 34 to 39 years [1, 18, 26]. In a patient population referred for neurological evaluation, Miller and Jankovic [23] reported a mean onset of 45 years among 30 tardive dystonics, and 59 years among 79 patients with predominantly oral dyskinesia. In that series, the majority of patients with oral dyskinesia had onset in the sixth to eighth decades, whereas patients with tardive dystonia had a uniform distribution of age of onset. Similarly, Kang et al. [18] found in a series of neurological referrals that age of onset of tardive dystonia was uniformly distributed across a range spanning from 13 to 72 years. There is a relationship between age of onset and distribution of dystonia. Site of onset, for example, is more likely to be in the lower limbs in younger patients. In older patients, the upper limbs, neck, or face are more likely to be involved [1, 25]. As in the primary dystonias, focal and segmental dystonias, including craniocervical dystonias, are more common in older patients. Tardive dystonia is more likely to generalize in younger patients. Regardless of age of onset, however, few dystonias remain strictly focal at the time of maximum severity [1, 25].

There is evidence that gender, like age, can impact the development of tardive dystonia. The literature has been mixed on the point of whether males are more likely to develop tardive dystonia, with some studies showing a male predominance [1, 21, 24, 25, 26], and others showing approximate equal prevalence in males and females [18, 23, 28]. Many earlier studies, however, were based on referral populations, in which referral bias can influence the results. A more complicated picture has arisen in recent studies, which suggests that age of onset may be the largest factor in the differences seen between males and females in earlier studies. A difference in age of onset between male and female patients has long been noted, and both Kang et al. [18] and Kiriakakis et al. [25] have noted differences in the age of onset between males and females. In Kang's series, the mean age of onset in men was 34 years, compared to 33.5 in Kiriakakis' series. Among women, the mean age of onset was 44 years and 43.8 years, respectively [18, 25]. Notably, in Kiriakakis' series, it was noted that the mean age of onset of neuroleptic use for men among the patients was 27.9 years (5.5 years before mean age of onset of dystonia). This is in contrast to women, in whom the mean age of onset of neuroleptic use was 36.4 years (7.4 years before onset of dystonia). Kiriakakis' data suggest that not only do males develop tardive dystonia at an earlier age than females, they may develop dystonia more rapidly after exposure to dopamine-blocking agents [25]. Kiriakakis' findings are supported by those of van Harten et al. [16] in the Curacao study, an epidemiologic study of tardive syndromes in a defined catchment population. In this study, males under 44 years were more than twice as likely to have dystonic movements than females under the age of 44 years. When the investigators looked at patients older than 65 years, however, women were twice as likely as men to have dystonia. Moreover, 62.5% of women with tardive dystonia in this study were older than 70 years. This is notable, as in one earlier study [21] showing a higher prevalence in men, patients over the age of 70 years were excluded. Despite the later age of onset in women, van Harten et al. [16] noted no specific difference in prevalence between male and female patients in their population.

Virtually all of the dopamine (DA) receptor antagonists that have been reported to cause oral tardive dyskinesia have also been reported to cause tardive dystonia. These include the aliphatic, piperazine, and piperidine classes of phenothiazines; butyrophenones (e.g., haloperidol); thioxanthenes (chlorprothixene, thiothixene); dipenzazepines (loxapine); diphenylbutylpiperidines (pimozide); and an indolone (molindone) [1, 18, 23]. Amoxapine, an antidepressant with DA receptor-blocking properties, has also been implicated in cases of tardive dystonia. Several antiemetics with DA receptor-blocking properties have also been associated with tardive dystonia, including prochlorperazine [18], promethazine [1], and metoclopramide [23, 29]. There is hope that the so-called "atypical neuroleptics" may have a lower propensity to cause tardive dystonia. Tardive dystonia, if it occurs at all [30], appears to be extremely rare with the atypical neuroleptic clozapine, although acute reversible withdrawal emergent dystonia has been reported [31]. The record of other "atypical neuroleptics," however, is mixed. Both quetiapine and olanzepine have been implicated in the development of tardive dyskinesia [32, 33], a condition that has similar risk factors. There is a report of a patient developing tardive dystonia on olanzepine, although this patient had a prior history of exposure to other neuroleptics [34]. There has been no report to date of tardive dystonia in association with quetiapine. The rate of tardive syndromes with both these medications may be lower than that found with the use of typical neuroleptic agents [35, 36]. Risperidone was formerly considered an atypical neuroleptic, but now has a well-recognized association with

Neuroleptic-Induced TD Variants/175

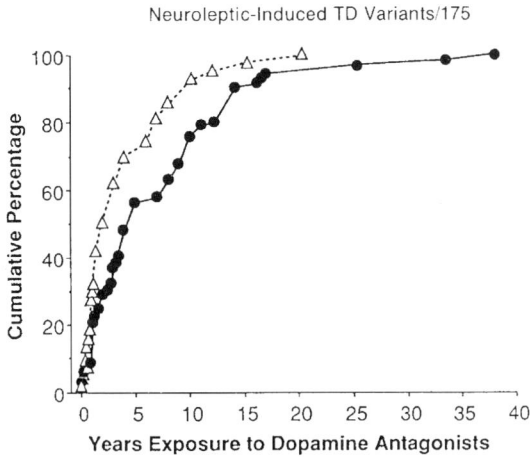

Figure 10.1 Duration of exposure to dopamine antagonists among patients with tardive dystonia (from reference [17]). The cumulative percentage of patients with tardive dystonia is shown in relation to years of exposure to dopamine antagonists, for both the 67 patients in reference [17] (black circles) and 43 patients in the literature as of 1986 (open triangle) (see reference [17] for citations). Instances of tardive dystonia occurred soon after exposure, seen as a rapidly rising cumulative percentage curve arising from the origin. Thus, there was no "safe" minimum exposure less than which this condition was unlikely to occur. (Reproduced with permission [17]).

parkinsonism [37, 38] and tardive syndromes [39–41] including tardive dystonia [42–45].

As there have been no prospective studies, there has been no careful assessment of any possible relationship between duration or dose of antipsychotics and the likelihood of occurrence of tardive dystonia. Retrospective studies have shown that although tardive dystonia usually occurs, on the average, following years of neuroleptic exposure, it can also occur within a few days or weeks [1, 18, 25]. In Burke's original series [1], a patient developed persistent dystonia after just 3 days of exposure. In Kang's series, 20% of patients developed dystonia within the first year of exposure (Fig. 10.1) [18]. The same was true of 43 patients reported in the literature at that time (Fig. 10.1). More recently, Kiriakakis et al. [25] in a series of 107 patients with tardive dystonia found that the onset of dystonia occurred as soon as 4 days after exposure, and as late as 23 years after initial exposure. Anecdotally, one of us (RB) has seen a patient develop persistent, nonreversible dystonia 1 day after initial exposure to a dopamine-blocking agent. There does not appear to be a minimum "safe" period of exposure to neuroleptics during which time tardive dystonia will not occur.

The occurrence of acute dystonia does not appear to be a significant risk factor for the occurrence of tardive dystonia. In Kang's series of 67 patients, only four (6%) had a history of an acute dystonic reaction, which is not much different from the incidence in the general population exposed to neuroleptics [18]. Prior brain injury, however, may impact the development of tardive dystonia. In Burke's original description of 42 cases of tardive dystonia, 7 of 18 patients with onset prior to 30 years had a history of an abnormal birth or development [1]. Subsequently, in a retrospective analysis of neurological referrals, Gimenez-Roldan and coworkers noted mental retardation in 3 of 9 tardive dystonia patients [46]. However, it is difficult to know the significance of these observations made in selected patient groups, referred for neurological evaluation, and in the absence of controls.

The question of genetic predisposition is relevant to the epidemiology of tardive dystonia. The incidence of tardive dystonia in patient populations exposed to dopamine-blocking agents has varied, but even the highest quoted incidence has been less than 22% [26], and most authors quote incidence rates of between 1.4% and 2.7% [20, 21, 25]. The low prevalence of development of tardive dystonia in most studies would suggest some interaction with other factors such as genetic factors. It is, in fact, notable that the one epidemiologic study of tardive dystonia showing a much higher incidence of 13.4% involved a single, well-defined and potentially more genetically homogeneous population [16]. However, to date, there have, been no studies specifically linking DYT1 mutations or other genetic defects to the development of tardive dystonia [47]. In the absence of more knowledge regarding the causes of idiopathic torsional dystonia there is a limit to our current ability to study this issue.

It is unknown, in the absence of adequate epidemiologic data, whether any particular psychiatric diagnosis constitutes a specific risk factor for the development of tardive dystonia. It is clear, however, from multiple retrospective analyses that the full range of possible psychiatric diagnoses is represented among these patients. In Kiriakakis's series [25], only 57% of patients received dopamine-blocking agents for schizophrenia or schizoaffective disorders. Other diagnoses in their patient population included mood disorders, personality disorders, and vertigo or gastrointestinal syndromes. In Kang's series of 67 patients [18], many patients (12 of 67) also had unclear indications of the use of dopamine-blocking agents, indicating that more careful consideration in the use of these drugs may be warranted.

Clinical features

Onset

Tardive dystonia uniformly affects all age groups. In Kang's study of 67 cases the reported ages of onset ranged from 13 to 72 years, with a mean of 39 years [18]. Kiriakakis's later series [25] had a strikingly similar age range and mean age of onset (mean 38.3 years, range 13–68 years). Males develop tardive dystonia earlier than females. In most patients, tardive dystonia begins in the face or neck. This was the case in 67% of patients in Burke's series [1]. Less commonly, the dystonia may begin in one of the arms. In our experience, tardive dystonia never begins as a focal foot dystonia. In this respect, it differs from the primary torsion dystonias, which commonly, in children, begin in a foot.

Clinical course

Since tardive dystonia has never been the subject of a prospective analysis, it is difficult to describe how it typically evolves, either in patients maintained on neuroleptics or in those taken off them. On the basis of retrospective analysis it is known that tardive dystonia usually begins in one location and spreads to other body regions. The clinical presentation of tardive dystonia can be indistinguishable from the presentation of idiopathic torsion dystonia, and patients have been described to clinically resemble cervical dystonia [48, 49], blepharospasm [42, 50, 51], and primary oromandibular dystonia [52]. Tardive dystonia can also present with a unique syndrome of retrocollis, posteriorly arched trunk, internal arm rotation, and elbow extension with wrist flexion [18, 37, 53]. This pattern is almost never described in idiopathic torsion dystonia, and should raise the suspicion of neuroleptic exposure even if the history is not readily available [37]. One clinical finding that can help to differentiate tardive dystonia from idiopathic cervical dystonia is the propensity of tardive dystonia to improve with walking, a finding that is distinctly uncommon in idiopathic torsion dystonia [18, 37]. This is distinctly different from the often-observed improvement in ambulation in primary dystonic gait disorders when patients walk backward. Dystonic ocular deviations, although rare, also diagnostically strongly favor dopamine-blocking agent exposure [54], as this type of dystonic finding is essentially undescribed in idiopathic torsion dystonia. As with idiopathic torsion dystonia, tardive dystonia can sometimes be relieved briefly by "sensory tricks," such as a touch to the chin to relieve torticollis, a touch above the brow to relieve blepharospasm, or a hand lightly resting on the hip to straighten severe axial torsion. In addition, tardive dystonia, like the primary dystonias, can be remarkably action-specific. The action-specific nature of the dystonia can lead to misdiagnosis, especially in a population of patients with a prior psychiatric diagnosis. The clinical diagnosis of tardive dystonia is often aided by the coexistence of other tardive involuntary movements. Classic oral-buccal-lingual tardive dyskinesia occurred sometime during the course in 55% of patients with tardive dystonia Kang's series and in 32% of the patients in Kiriakakis' series. Tardive akathisia, was present in 31% and 22% of these series, respectively [18, 25].

The clinical course and spectrum of tardive dystonia has been described in a number of retrospective reports. In Kang's series [18], only 15% remained focal. Most developed dystonia in multiple regions; an additional 13% developed generalized dystonia. This is in agreement with Kiriakakis' later study of 107 patients [25]. Only 16% of their patients had focal dystonia at maximum severity of symptoms, even though 83% presented with focal dystonia [25]. The craniocervical region was affected in 87% of patients in Kiriakakis' series, and 83% in Kang's series. Retrocollis, anterocollis, and trunk involvement with back arching were more common in patients with tardive dystonia than in those with idiopathic dystonia [18, 25]. Younger patients were more likely to have onset in the lower limbs, while older patients tended to have onset in the upper limbs [25]. In both series, earlier exposure to neuroleptics and younger age were associated with generalized dystonia, while patients with focal or segmental dystonia tended to be older or to have exposure to neuroleptics at a later age. A longer duration of exposure to neuroleptics, however, did not correlate with more severe dystonia. On the contrary, patients who developed generalized dystonia in one study had been treated for shorter periods by the time of dystonia onset (4.9 years) than patients with focal dystonia (13.6 years) [18].

Although significant disability can result from tardive dystonia, the development of a bedridden state is rare, and in Burke's series of 42 patients, only one was bedridden [1]. Case reports of severe disability sufficient to cause a bedridden state are similarly rare [29, 55, 56]. In spite of the rarity of this degree of disability, the bedridden state can occur, and in some instances severe tardive dystonia can lead to life-threatening complications. Severe retrocollis sufficient to cause life-threatening dysphagia has been described [57, 58]. Lazarus and Toglia [59] described a young woman with tardive dystonia who, 3 months after withdrawal of neuroleptics, developed what could be termed a dystonic storm with development of severe dystonic movements that resulted in elevation of serum muscle enzymes, myoglobinuria, renal failure, and death. We have also observed patients with long-standing tardive dystonia who suddenly develop a severe dystonic state with elevation of serum muscle enzymes, either following abrupt neuroleptic withdrawal or in the setting of systemic infection. It can be difficult to differentiate such severe exacerbations of tardive dystonia from neuroleptic malignant syndrome (NMS) (see Chapter 8). A key point of distinction is that a tardive dystonia patient will have a history of chronic dystonic movements, whereas a patient with NMS will develop severe dystonia (and/or rigidity) acutely.

Analysis of patient outcome data in the literature reveals that the chance of remission of tardive dystonia is low, but that chance of remission can be significantly increased by stopping dopamine-blocking treatment at the onset of dystonia [1, 18, 24].

In Kiriakakis's series of 107 patients, only 14% of patients underwent a remission over a mean 8.5-year follow-up period [25]. This is in agreement with Burke et al.' series [1], in which only 12% (5 of 42) underwent remission. Remission in Kiriakakis' series could occur as late as 9 years after stopping dopamine-blocking therapy, but occurred a mean of 2.6 years after discontinuation of dopamine-blocking agents. Length of exposure also affected the likelihood of remission, as patients with ≤ 10 years of exposure to dopamine-blocking agents had a fivefold greater chance of remission than those with >10 years of exposure. Permanently stopping dopamine-blocking therapy in the Kiriakakis study also was associated with remission (12 of 54 patients stopping dopamine-blocking agents had remissions, while only 3 of 52 patients who continued dopamine-blocking agents had remissions) [25]. Other than cessation of dopamine-blocking agents, Kirakakis et al. could find no specific pharmacologic therapy that altered the outcome of tardive dystonia, although a variety of treatment including botulinum toxin have been associated with symptomatic improvement [49, 60, 61].

Differential diagnosis and diagnostic evaluation

In movement disorders, diagnosis is performed in two steps: first the type of involuntary movement is identified (see Chapter 1 for a more detailed discussion of this approach); then, for that particular type of movement, various etiologies are considered. In the diagnosis of tardive dystonia, it is usually possible to readily distinguish the sustained, twisting movements of dystonia from other dyskinesias. Choreic movements are quick, brief, flowing, and random in their timing and location. Myoclonic movements are brief and shock-like. Tremors are regular, oscillatory movements. Some motor tics can resemble dystonic movements, being sustained or twisting. Tics can usually be identified on the basis of their timing. They occur intermittently, sometimes in flurries. Tics are characteristically preceded by a subjective urge to perform the movement and are followed by a sense of relief. Tics can often be entirely suppressed by the patient for prolonged periods, whereas dystonia usually cannot. Finally, patients with tics often have a variety of them, and it is frequently possible to identify a sustained tic (also called a "dystonic tic") by the company it keeps.

One difficulty that many neurologists have in diagnosing dystonia is that they think of it as consisting *exclusively of slow*, sustained movements. While dystonia is always sustained, there can be superimposed rapid, jerking, or even oscillatory movements. These rapid movements are especially likely to be seen when the patient attempts to move against the direction of the sustained, dystonic pull; for example, when some patients attempt to turn their head away from the direction of their torticollis, they develop a rapid, oscillatory movement resembling a tremor. Such rapid movements affecting lower facial muscles can lead to difficulty in distinguishing dystonic tardive dyskinesia. Usually dystonia can be identified as a sustained contraction in association with the rapid movements; there may be sustained facial grimacing or sustained jaw closure. The distinction between tardive dystonia and oral-buccal lingual tardive dyskinesia affecting the face is of more than academic interest; identification of the type of movement has implications for therapy.

Once a diagnosis of dystonia is made, consideration must be given to the possible causes. In a patient on neuroleptics, an acute dystonic reaction must be considered (see Chapter 5). Acute dystonia almost always occurs within the first 5 days of beginning neuroleptics; the only exception is if a substantial increase in dose is made during the course of therapy or concurrent antiparkinson medication (e.g., anticholinergics, amantidine) is discontinued. Acute dystonia is much more likely to be accompanied by oculogyric crisis. Finally, acute dystonia universally responds to administration of diphenhydramine or benztropine. The differential diagnosis includes NMS, which may present with prominent dystonia Generally, the associated alteration in mental status, fever, and serum biochemical evidence of muscle injury makes that diagnosis clear. Only rarely does tardive dystonia become so severe as to cause fever and muscle injury, and in these instances it is typically preceded by a history of chronic dystonia, unlike NMS, which is acute and fulminant in its onset.

After acute causes of dystonia are excluded, Wilson's disease should be ruled out by obtaining a serum cervioplasmin, 24-hour urine copper and a slit-lamp examination. Wilson's disease can present with dystonia (or other movement abnormalities) and any of a number of psychiatric disorders that may encourage the initial inappropriate use of neuroleptic drugs. As it is treatable, it must always be considered. Beyond this evaluation for Wilson's disease, further evaluation depends on the presence or absence of other neurological signs besides dystonia. If there are other neurological signs, the differential diagnosis is lengthy (see Table 5 in Chapter 1). Diagnostic studies to differentiate among these numerous causes may need to be extensive and will not be detailed here. If there are other neurological signs besides dystonia that are *progressive,* then tardive dystonia cannot be the sole diagnosis, as neuroleptics do not induce progressive changes in intellect, sensory function, and so on. If, however, there are other neurological signs that are entirely static (e.g., mental retardation) then once appropriate studies have been performed to rule out metabolic and degenerative conditions listed (see Table 5 in Chapter 1), it is possible to diagnose tardive dystonia associated with a static encephalopathy. As previously noted, in any patient, a diagnosis of tardive dystonia is supported by the presence of other tardive syndromes such as oral-buccal-lingual tardive dyskinesia, or tardive akathisia.

Treatment

When a diagnosis of any form of tardive dyskinesia is made, the first therapeutic step should be to taper and discontinue the causative drugs, if possible. Often, severe psychiatric illness will make it impossible to do so. Nevertheless, it is imperative to carefully reconsider the indications for DA antagonists in a given patient and to consider alternate therapy. Many patients are given these drugs chronically for inappropriate indications (e.g., anxiety and insomnia). Discontinuation of these drugs is an important first therapeutic step because the ideal therapeutic outcome is to have a complete remission of involuntary movements without need for continued drug treatment. The ideal therapeutic response requires discontinuation of the offending drugs as soon as possible, as a shorter duration of exposure is associated with a higher incidence of remission [25]. In patients requiring continued treatment, replacing neuroleptic agents with atypical agents such as clozaril, olanzepine, or quetiapine is an appropriate course of action. These agents have a lower propensity to cause tardive syndromes [31, 32], and in the case of clozapine, may actually suppress the movements [62–66].

After a decision has been made to continue, replace, or discontinue DA antagonists, the degree of disability caused by the involuntary movements must be considered. If DA antagonists cannot be discontinued for psychiatric reasons and they sufficiently suppress the involuntary movements such that they are not disabling, then it is not necessary to treat with additional drugs. If the patient is disabled by the involuntary movements, then additional treatment is indicated.

The most effective pharmacologic treatment of tardive dystonia is antidopaminergic therapy. Tetrabenazine and reserpine, dopamine-depleting agents, improve about 50% of patients, while dopamine receptor-blocking agents are somewhat more effective, improve 77% of patients [18, 37]. The atypical neuroleptic, clozapine, may also be useful [62–66]. With clozapine the improvement may take months to years. A synergistic effect with combined clozapine and clonazepam has been reported [67]. Unlike tardive dyskinesia (but similar to primary idiopathic torsional dystonia), tardive dystonia may also improve with anticholinergic therapy such as trihexphenidyl [18, 37]. Tardive dystonia patients, however, vary in their response to DA-depleting agents and anticholinergics, and unfortunately there is no way of predicting who will respond to which class of drug. Kang et al. [18] compared patients who responded to anticholinergics to those who responded to DA depletors, and found no difference between these patient groups in age at onset of dystonia, sex, distribution of dystonia at onset or at maximum severity, duration of exposure to DA antagonists before dystonia, or presence of classic oral dyskinesia. Without a means of predicting which drug a patient will respond to, the choice is often guided by anticipated side effects. Since older patients are more likely to suffer confusion or memory loss from anticholinergics, DA depletors are chosen. Patients with a history of depression, however, are at risk for recurrence due to DA depletors, favoring the use of anticholinergics.

With all potential pharmacologic treatments of tardive dystonia, it is reasonable to start with a low dose of the drug and gradually increase the dose until either adequate benefit is obtained, or intolerable side effects intervene, or a judicious maximum is reached. Reserpine is started at a dose of 0.25 mg per day and gradually increased. If symptomatic hypotension occurs, the dose is decreased as needed, and mineralocorticoids may be considered. Doses of reserpine of up to 9.0 mg per day may be used, although an average dose of 5.0 mg per day is more typical. Trihexyphenidyl and ethopropazine are started at 5.0 mg per day of the former or 50.0 mg per day of the latter and gradually increased [68]. In treating dystonia, up to 120 mg per day of trihexyphenidyl may be required, but the average dose in treating tardive dystonia is 20 mg per day. One important potential adverse effect of anticholinergics is that the more typical tardive orofacial dyskinesia may be aggravated or even brought out *de novo* in these patients. Benzodiazepines, such as clonzepam or lorazepam, are useful in combination with both anticholinergic and antidopaminergic therapies. Bromocriptine or other dopamine agonists, clonidine, verapamil, amantidine, carbamazepine, valproate, and baclofen have all been reported to be helpful in some patients [37] (see Chapter 9).

There are alternatives to pharmacologic therapy, and in fact, for patients with focal cranial dystonias, botulinum toxin injections into affected muscles are a valuable alternative [61]. Blepharospasm responds well, as does torticollis [50]. There are no common surgical approaches to the management of tardive dystonia; however, there is a single case report in the literature of bilateral globus pallidus internus (GPi) deep brain stimulation being useful in a severe case of medically refractory tardive dystonia [69]. In this 70-year-old patient, who had a 6-year history of medically refractory severe tardive dystonia, bilateral GPi stimulation was associated with rapid improvement of dystonia. Notably, the patient also had bilateral VIM electrode placement, but VIM stimulation had no effect on the dystonia, nor was it observed to augment the effect of bilateral GPi stimulation. Although interesting, given the lack of any additional published data on neurosurgical management of tardive dystonia, at this time such an approach should be considered as experimental and a last resort.

Although it is therapeutically ideal to discontinue DA antagonists in patients with tardive dystonia, there are two situations in which the drugs are used therapeutically for their ability to suppress the dystonic movements. It is appropriate to use DA antagonists when a patient has severe, generalized tardive dystonia that is either painful or causes muscle damage (evidenced by an elevated serum CPK). In this circumstance, tardive dystonia is potentially life-threatening. Parentally administered DA antagonists may suppress the dystonic movements and prevent medical complications. It is also appropriate to use DA antagonists to suppress the movements when DA depletors, anticholinergics, and other drugs have failed, and the patient has either been successfully maintained off DA antagonists for 4 to 5 years without remission or has not tolerated withdrawal.

Tardive akathisia

The nature of akathisia

Many of the early reports of oral-buccal-lingual tardive dyskinesia contain very clear descriptions of motor restlessness associated with the movements [70–73], and yet persistent akathisia as a subtype of the tardive syndromes was not recognized until much later [74]. A possible reason for this delayed recognition is that a consensus on the definition of akathisia does not emerge from the literature. Many authorities have considered the term *akathisia* to refer strictly to an abnormal subjective state, characterized by restlessness [75]. Others, however, consider the characteristic motor phenomena of akathisia (i.e., the movements) as sufficient for a diagnosis of akathisia [72, 76] or at least "pseudoakathisia" [77]. The most satisfactory "gold standard" definition of akathisia for the present must rest on both the subjective and objective features [78]. The degree to which more partial manifestations of the condition may be sufficient to define it remains to be determined by a more complete study of its spectrum. The subjective state of akathisia is reported as an aversion to being still. The patient may or may not use the term "restless." They may instead refer to "nervousness," or "jitteriness," and so on, but they must report discomfort related to being still, which can be relieved by movement. There is a significant mood component in the subjective state of akathisia, and Halstead et al. [79] noted that a significant proportion of patients with the subjective sensation of inner restlessness also reported marked symptoms of dysphoria, namely tension, panic, irritability, and impatience. The motor signs that can be seen in akathisia consist of an increased, abnormal frequency of movements. The movements are often complex and stereotyped, that is, repeated in the same pattern over and over. Unlike other clinical movement syndromes (e.g., chorea, myoclonus, tremor), there are no movements that are abnormal in their patterns or appearance in this syndrome. Instead, the movements are abnormal in frequency, and are constantly repeated by the patient in a stereotyped fashion. Examples of motor behavior seen in akathisia include repetitive crossing/uncrossing or rapidly abducting/adducting the legs while sitting, or marching in place while standing. The combination of these subjective and motor features defines akathisia.

Evidence that chronic akathisia is due to neuroleptic drug use
Like tardive dystonia, tardive akathisia has not been the subject of case-control studies to investigate its relationship to neuroleptic drug use. Unlike dystonia, however, akathisia rarely, if ever, occurs on an idiopathic basis. Today, other than parkinsonism, there are few other causes of akathisia besides treatment with neuroleptic drugs. Thus, there is a broad consensus that persistent akathisia is a complication of treatment with these agents.

The association between neuroleptic drugs and akathisia is further strengthened by a number of other observations. As for tardive dystonia, there are close temporal relationships between the use of these drugs and the occurrence of akathisia. In a number of patients, discontinuation of the drugs has led to remission [78]. In addition, patients who have gone into remission can develop persistent akathisia a second time, during reexposure to a neuroleptic. Tardive akathisia is even more frequently associated with oral-buccal-lingual tardive dyskinesia (90% of cases in one series [78]) than tardive dystonia. Tardive akathisia not infrequently appears to evolve from acute akathisia, which is clearly a complication of neuroleptics. These occurrences have been called "acute persistent" akathisia [74]. Finally, the clinical pharmacology of tardive akathisia is like that of oral-lingual tardive dyskinesia, further indicating a close relationship between these disorders.

Diagnostic criteria
The diagnosis of tardive akathisia is based on the following criteria: (1) akathisia, defined, as above, on the basis of both the subjective and motor features of restlessness, must be present; (2) the akathisia must not have preceded, and must develop during (or within 3 months of cessation of) neuroleptic treatment; and (3) akathisia must be *persistent*, that is, present for at least a 1-month duration. There is no stipulation about the duration of neuroleptic treatment prior to the onset in making diagnosis. Although tardive akathisia

usually develops late in the course of therapy, it can, like tardive dystonia and oral-lingual dyskinesia, develop early. The more important critical feature is its persistence. Individual patients often have difficulty pinpointing when their akathisia began in relation to therapy; therefore, terms such as "acute persistent" and "tardive" akathisia become semantic quagmires. In addition, since there is a smooth continuum for onset in relation to duration of therapy, it seems arbitrary to try to divide between early-onset and late-onset persistent neuroleptic-induced akathisias. Treatment response to DA antagonists is not a necessary diagnostic criterion. It is, however, helpful to attempt to discontinue DA antagonists and observe the response in the particular situation in which a patient develops akathisia early in the course of DA antagonist therapy, and has persistent akathisia (>1 month) while on a constant dose. The patient may have acute akathisia that is persistent due to ongoing therapy, or may have a chronic akathisia, that is, tardive akathisia. The only way to determine which type of akathisia the patient has is to attempt to stop the drugs. If the akathisia promptly abates on drug withdrawal, then the patient had acute akathisia. If, however, the akathisia persists (or worsens) for more than a month following drug withdrawal, then the patient has tardive akathisia. If the patient cannot be taken off neuroleptic drugs, then it is not possible to know for certain which form of akathisia the patient has.

Epidemiology

In his classic monograph, Ayd found acute akathisia to have a prevalence of 21%, making it the most common drug-induced disorder [80]. Multiple studies support that tardive akathisia may also be common. Braude and Barnes examined 82 schizophrenic outpatients to determine the presence of restless movements [81]. Of these 39 patients (48%) had such movements. Of these 39 patients, 6 (7% of the total) apparently had acute akathisia. An additional 10 (12%) had "pseudoakathisia" (i.e., restless movements in the absence of subjective complaints). The remaining 23 (28%) had chronic (tardive) akathisia. The prevalence of 28% found in this outpatient study is similar to an observed prevalence of 20% among 65 schizophrenic outpatients reported by Schilkrut and colleagues [82]. Halstead et al. found the prevalence of chronic akathisia to be 24% in 120 hospitalized chronic schizophrenics. An additional 18% had pseudoakathisia [79]. Van Harten et al. [16] in another study of psychiatric inpatients found a prevalence of 9.4% for akathisia and 12.9% for pseudoakathisia among 194 inpatients in the only psychiatric hospital in the Netherlands Antilles; however, there was also a relatively high level of parkinsonism in their study population (36.1%). Since drug-induced parkinsonism and akathisia have been shown to be negatively correlated [83], the somewhat lower incidence of akathisia may be related to the relatively high prevalence of drug-induced parkinsonism in this study population. Overall, these studies support a relatively high rate of chronic akathisia among patients on long-term neuroleptic or dopamine receptor-blocking therapy.

Neuroleptic-induced tardive dyskinesia variants **273**

Neuroleptic-Induced TD Variants/187

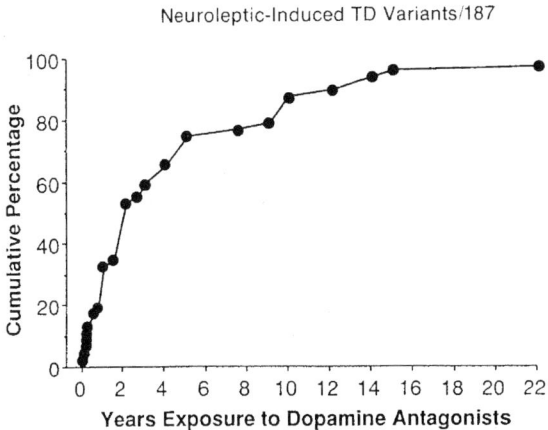

Figure 10.2 This figure demonstrates the relationship between years of treatment with dopamine antagonists and the cumulative onset of tardive akathisia in our group of patients (n = 45; reference [72]). It can be seen that cases begin to occur within the first year of exposure; there is no period of minimum safe exposure to DA antagonists free of risk from inducing tardive akathisia. The first point on the curve is a patient who developed persistent akathisia following 2 weeks of neuroleptic therapy. (Reproduced with permission [72].)

Some epidemiologic data are available on the development of tardive akathisia among various subgroups. In Halstead's study of 120 psychiatric in-patients [79], patients with chronic akathisia tended to be younger than those without akathisia. Affected patients also tended to be on higher doses of neuroleptics, and were more likely to be receiving their neuroleptic dose as a depot injection. Patients with akathisia were more likely to have tardive dyskinesia in the limbs, while patients with pseudoakathisia were more likely to have orofacial dyskinesia. Among the 52 patients with tardive akathisia reported by Burke et al., the ages of those suffering from tardive akathisia ranged from 21 to 82 years [78]. Although women outnumbered men, men tended to have a younger age of onset than women. The average duration of therapy prior to onset was 4.5 years, but as with tardive dystonia, tardive akathisia can occur early in the course of therapy, and Fig. 10.2 shows the time of onset in relation to duration of neuroleptic treatment. It can be seen that many cases developed within the first year of treatment. It can also be seen that onset in relation to duration of therapy is a smooth and continuous function; there is no clear separation between early-onset and late-onset persistent cases. The average age of onset (60.4 years) among early-onset (<1 year of neuroleptic exposure) patients in Burke's series was no different than the others [78].

Like tardive dystonia and tardive dyskinesia, tardive akathisia has been reported following treatment with all classes of dopamine receptor-blocking agents, including metoclopramide [84]. Clozapine is known to cause akathisia as well [84, 85], although the rate of occurrence is much lower. As would be expected, given the wide range of medications that can cause tardive akathisia, patients with tardive akathisia have received dopamine receptor-blocking therapy for a wide variety psychiatric and nonpsychatric indications. In Burke et al.' series [78], 36% of patients were treated for secondary or questionable indications including anxiety, nausea, gastrointestinal distress, and pain.

Clinical features

The subjective state of akathisia

Patients with akathisia frequently complain of an unbearable inner torment and beg repeatedly for relief. There is evidence that akathisia may be associated with suicide [87]. Many patients do not know how to describe what they feel, and they may use a variety of terms other than "restless"; they may complain of "jitteriness," "a tortured sort of feeling," "fidgety," "nervous," "about to jump out of my skin," "all revved up," and so on. Patients who are floridly psychotic or impaired intellectually will be especially unlikely to clearly express their subjective condition. Akathisia may, therefore, be confused with a variety of psychiatric states that lead to agitation, such as mania, agitated depression, or severe anxiety [88, 89]. In addition, the emotions associated with akathisia, including fright or anger, can be associated with a spectrum of abnormal behaviors and "acting out" [90, 91]. Patients with mild akathisia complain of impatience, irritability, or inability to concentrate.

It has been suggested that patients with acute akathisia suffer more severe subjective distress and that the subjective component becomes less severe in the chronic setting. Braude and Barnes have suggested that in the chronic setting, akathisia may evolve to a state of "pseudoakathisia" in which there are motor features of restlessness but no subjective restlessness [74]. Whether this is true, and how often it occurs, will require prospective analysis. In Burke et al.'s retrospective survey [78], there certainly did exist patients who had severe subjective distress that continued for years without abatement. Among these patients, the position most frequently identified as the most uncomfortable was sitting. The most preferred position was lying down. Thus, patients would often complain that they could no longer sit through a meal, or sit for TV or the movies. Inability to stand in one place for a prolonged period also interfered with activities of daily living; many of these patients could not stand in line for shopping or banking.

Motor features

In general, patients with akathisia show an increased frequency of movement, and they make movements that are complex and stereotyped, that is, repeated in the same pattern over and over. Patients can often suppress the movements, if asked to do so, for at least brief periods of time. During the time they suppress the movements, they build a greater inner sense of restlessness or "tension," which is then relieved by performing the movements. The type of movements the patient makes depends on their position; for example, when sitting, they may cross and uncross the legs, whereas on standing, they will march in place.

In Burke et al.'s study [78], analysis of the movements of 52 patients with tardive akathisia demonstrated that the legs were most frequently affected. Marching in place while standing and crossing/uncrossing the legs while sitting occurred in 58% and 48%, respectively. Other common leg movements included pumping the leg up and down or rapidly adducting/abducting while sitting. Truncal movements were also common and included rocking back and forth and frequent shifts of position while sitting. Somewhat less common, but more distinctive, were complex arm and hand movements, including face rubbing, hair rubbing, head or face scratching, folding/unfolding the arms, and picking at clothes. Many of these patients also complain of respiratory irregularities and develop panting or grunting. In addition, some of the most severely affected patients would moan or even shout. Movements of the facial region were less common, but they did occur. Repetitive, lateral tongue movements and repetitive head nodding may also occur [92].

In Burke's 52 patients, tardive akathisia was associated with either oral-buccal-lingual dyskinesia or tardive dystonia in all but one patient. Sixty-three percent had oral dyskinesia, 8% had tardive dystonia, and 27% had both. The few patients with tardive akathisia and tardive dystonia had an earlier age of onset (39 years) than those with akathisia and oral dyskinesia (62.2 years) [78].

Clinical course

In the patients of Burke et al. [78] 67% had persistent akathisia at last follow-up for a mean duration of 4.2 years. Most of these patients had discontinued neuroleptics several years earlier. Among 33% of these patients who did not have akathisia at last follow-up, 6% were in true remission; that is, they had been weaned from therapy without recurrence. The other patients who did not have akathisia at follow-up were receiving ongoing therapy that probably suppressed it. The patients who did not have akathisia at follow-up had an earlier age of onset. Thus, younger patients appear to have a more reversible or treatable condition.

Differential diagnosis

Akathisia can be difficult to differentiate from psychiatric conditions that cause agitation. It is helpful to recall that the subjective distress of akathisia is an aversion to remaining still and is at least partially relieved by movement. Subjective distress due to psychiatric disease does not necessarily show this relationship to movement. In the case of agitation due to psychiatric illness, other aspects of the patient interview will generally reveal other features consistent with exacerbation of the psychiatric condition, such as hallucinations or delusions. An additional differentiating point is the presence of the stereotyped movements that tend to be characteristic of akathisia.

Neuroleptic-induced akathisia must be distinguished from restless legs syndrome. The latter consists of uncomfortable dysesthesias in the legs that occur nocturnally as the patient lies down to go to sleep. The dysesthesias are relieved by pacing about. The sensory complaints, the nocturnal occurrence, the predominant leg involvement, and the worsening rather than improvement in the supine position all help to distinguish restless legs syndrome from akathisia.

One of the few other causes of akathisia today, besides neuroleptic drug treatment, is Parkinson's disease (PD) [93]. In Lang and Johnson's series, 26% of Parkinson patients had true akathisia. In some, it was an early symptom of PD, but in most it developed later, when the diagnosis of parkinsonism was apparent. There have been some scattered reports of akathisia developing in the context of SSRI treatment as well [94, 95], but there have been no descriptions of akathisia persisting after medication was discontinued, and therefore there is no evidence that SSRIs can cause tardive akathisia.

Treatment

The approach to the treatment of tardive akathisia is like that for tardive dystonia and oral dyskinesia. If neuroleptics can be stopped, they should be. A certain percentage of patients will undergo spontaneous remission. Whether or not neuroleptics are stopped, the next step is to assess the degree of disability. If there is only mild akathisia, then the patient can simply be followed. If, however, there is significant disability, then akathisia should be treated whether or not the patient has been taken off neuroleptics. DA-depleting drugs are the most frequently beneficial. Among 30 patients treated at Columbia University, 15 were managed with reserpine; of these, 13 (87%) showed improvement. In 11 of these patients, reserpine gave complete control (n = 3) or marked improvement (n = 8). Tetrabenazine was effective in 7 of 12 (58%) treated patients. Of patients treated with these drugs, about 50% in one study remained on them at follow-up [78]. The approach to using these drugs is similar. One begins with a small dose (0.25 mg/day for reserpine) and very gradually titrates upward. The mean reserpine dose in one study was 5.0 mg per day [78].

It is important to note that tardive akathisia differs dramatically from acute akathisia in its clinical pharmacology. While dopamine antagonists worsen acute akathisia, they have an opposite and antagonistic effect on tardive akathisia. Opiates have been reported to be effective in the management of acute akathisia [96]. However, they are generally ineffective for tardive akathisia [97]. Although a number of investigators have reported that the β-blocker propranolol is effective for the management of acute akathisia [98], this class of medication has not been reported to help in tardive akathisia. It is unclear how the differences in pharmacology relate to the underlying mechanisms of acute and chronic akathisia.

Tardive myoclonus and tardive tics

Myoclonus refers to sudden, brief shock-like jerks. Like dystonia and akathisia, myoclonus was described in early reports of tardive dyskinesia [99]. Several patients have been described with tardive dystonia and myoclonus [1]. Pure myoclonus has also been reported as a complication of neuroleptic treatment [100, 101], and as a complication of treatment with the dopamine-blocking agent, metoclopramide [102]. Tominaga et al. [97], in a brief report, indicated that tardive myoclonic jerks could be suppressed by clonazepam. Burke et al. also observed that clonazepam may be effective among tardive dystonia patients with significant myoclonus.

It has been difficult to ascribe tics to neuroleptic drug treatment with certainty. Transient tics occur quite commonly among children in the general population, and Tourette's syndrome is a common neurological disease of childhood. Tics, unlike oral-buccal-lingual dyskinesia, dystonia, akathisia, and myoclonus, quite characteristically occur and remit spontaneously. Thus, it is more difficult to make meaningful temporal connections between the use of neuroleptics and the occurrence of tics. Finally, a number of reports of "Tourettes" associated with neuroleptic treatment may actually have been cases of tardive akathisia, with repeated complex stereotyped movements and grunting or moaning that resembled motor and vocal tics.

These caveats notwithstanding, there have been a number of reports of tic disorders occurring in patients during or following neuroleptic therapy. Considered together, these cases seem suggestive that, in rare instances, neuroleptics may induce tics [103–112] (Table 10.2). Most of these patients developed their tics in adulthood, long after spontaneously occurring Tourette's syndrome would ordinarily occur. In most of them, the described vocal utterances seem to have been more complex or formed than typically occurs in akathisia; there were barks, clicks, and coprolalia. In Table 10.2, those patients with only nonspecific vocalizations, such as grunting or howling, who may also be observed in tardive akathisia, are noted in the final column to have a possible diagnosis of tardive akathisia.

The average age of onset among the 13 reported cases was 39 ± 5 (SEM) years, ranging from 10 to 71 years. In the majority of these patients (7 of 10 with available information), the tics began after discontinuation of neuroleptics. As in spontaneously occurring Tourette's syndrome, most of the motor tics occurred in the cranial regions (face, head, neck). As in Tourette's syndrome, there was a wide range of vocal utterances: barks, clicks, sniffs, coprolalia, and echolalia. For the ten patients with sufficient information, seven had associated tardive movements, either oral-buccal-lingual dyskinesia or tardive dystonia. These associated movements strengthen the association between the occurrence of the tics and exposure to neuroleptics. Among these 13 patients, adequate information about the clinical course is provided in 11; nine had their tics suppressed by a DA antagonist; two went into spontaneous remission. Occasional reports suggest a relationship between neuroleptic treatment

Table 10.2 Reported cases of Tourette's syndrome associated with dopamine antagonist treatment

Authors	Year	Age of onset	Signs	Other tardive disorders	Comments
Klawans et al. [103]	1978	28	Face/arm tics, barking	Dystonia	
DeVaugh-Geiss [100]	1980	65	Facial tics barking	OBLD	
Stahl [101]	1980	28	Facial tics barking coprolalia	None	
Fog and Pakenberg [102]	1980	20	"Tics of head and body," grunting	NS	? Tardive akathisia
		54	Arm movements, shouting	NS	? Tardive akathisia
		50	Howling (no tics)	OBLD	? Tardive Akathisia
Seeman et al. [107]	1981	25	Blepharospasm, facial grimacing grunting	NS	? Tardive dystonia and akathisia
Mueller and Aminoff [108]	1982	27	Head turning gutteral noises barking	OBLD	
Klawans et al [109]	1982	71	Facial tics	None	
		32	Facial tics	OBLD	
Munetz et al. [110]	1985	60	Head and neck tics, Coprolalia	OBLD	
Karagianis and Nagpurkar [111]	1990	10		OBLD	
Bharucha and Sethi [112]	1995	36	Vocal/motor tics	None	Video documentation of tics presented

and the occurrence of tics, but the new occurrence of tics in adulthood related to neuroleptic treatment appears to be fairly infrequent.

Tardive tremor

Jankovic and Stacy have described a single small series of patients who developed a low frequency (3–5 Hz) postural and kinetic tremor related to chronic neuroleptic treatment [113]. In all patients, the tremor occurred in the presence of other tardive syndromes, including akathisia, chorea, dystonia, myoclonus, and stereotypy. The diagnosis of tardive tremor was made in these patients on the basis of exacerbation of tremor with neuroleptic withdrawal, and improved symptoms after treatment with the dopamine depleting agent tetrabenazine. Only a handful of addition cases of tardive tremor have been reported including one due to metoclopramide [114]. This is clearly one of the least common of tardive syndromes.

Withdrawal emergent phenomena

Although not strictly tardive in nature, it is worthwhile to briefly mention the withdrawal emergent syndromes, which can occur as late complications of dopamine-blocking therapy. Withdrawal emergent chorea is the most commonly recognized of these syndromes. Typically occurring in children, withdrawal emergent chorea occurs when children are suddenly withdrawn from long-standing dopamine antagonist therapy [37, 115]. Phenotypically, withdrawal chorea resembles other causes of chorea (e.g., Sydenham's chorea), from which it must be differentiated. Children display fluid, involuntary, but nonstereotyped movements involving the limbs, trunk, and neck. The oral stereotypies seen in more typical tardive dyskinesia are not commonly seen [37]. The movements typically are suppressed by reinstitution of dopamine blockade, and do not generally recur if agents are tapered slowly [116]. The natural history of withdrawal emergent chorea is for the chorea to disappear gradually over a time course of a few weeks [37].

Withdrawal emergent versions of the other tardive syndromes, including dyskinesia, akathisia, and dystonia have been described [37]. These syndromes differ from tardive versions in their relatively rapid resolution with time. Rapid withdrawal of dopamine-blocking agents can also provoke true tardive syndromes as well; however, slowly tapering of the dose of these agents is the preferred method of stopping therapy.

Conclusion

It is clear that dopamine antagonists cause a broad spectrum of tardive syndromes. Given the frequency with which these medications are used and the protean manifestations of prolonged therapy, it is important for the neurologist to recognize and differentiate these disorders in order to construct appropriate management plans for these patients. It is particularly important to recognize that in many cases the tardive syndromes are fellow travelers, and many patients may have varying degrees of more than one phenomenon. In addition to the motor syndromes described, patients may also complain of unusual sensory symptoms (apart from akathisia). For example, Ford et al. [117] described 11 patients with tardive akathisia, tardive dystonia, or tardive dyskinesias who complained of profoundly distressing chronic oral or genital pain. The long-term social and psychological sequelae of these phenomena require that all physicians develop a healthy respect for agents that have dopamine-blocking activity, and prescribe these medications only when indications for use are appropriate and the benefits of therapy outweigh the risks of the potentially permanent consequences.

References

1. Burke RE, Fahn S, Jankovic J, et al. Tardive dystonia: late onset and persistent dystonia caused by antipsychotic drugs. Neurology (NY) 1982; 32: 1335–1346.

2. Druckman R, Seelinger D, Thulin B. Chronic involuntary movements induced by phenothiazines. J Nerv Ment Disord 1962; 135: 69–76.

3. Chateau R, Fau R, Groslambert R, Perret J. A propos d'un cas de torticollis spasmodique irreversible survenu au cours d'un traitement par neuroleptiques. Ann Med Psychol (Paris) 1966; 122: 110–111.

4. Dabbous IA, Bergman AB. Neurologic damage associated with phenothiazine. Am J Dis Child 1966; 111: 291–296.

5. Harenko A. Retrocollis as an irreversible late complication of neuroleptic medication. Acta Neurol Scand 1967; 43(suppl): 145–146.

6. Angle CR, McIntire MS. Persistent dystonia in a brain-damaged child after ingestion of phenothiazine. J Pediatr 1968; 73: 124–126.

7. Crane GE. Persistent dyskinesia. Br J Psychiatry 1973; 122: 395–405.

8. Keegan DL, Rajput AH. Drug-induced dystonia tarda: treatment with L-Dopa. Dis Nerv Syst 1973; 38: 167–169.

9. Shields WB, Bray PF. A danger of haloperidol therapy in children. J Pediatr 1976; 88: 301–303.

10. Tarsy D, Grancher R, Bralower M. Tardive dyskinesia in young adults. Am J Psychiatry 1977; 134: 1032–1034.

11. McLean P, Casey DE. Tardive dyskinesia in an adolescent. Am Psychiatry 1978; 135: 969–971.

12. Weiner WJ, Nausieda P, Glantz RH. Meige syndrome (blepharospasm-oromandibular dystonia) after long-term neuroleptic therapy. Neurology 1981; 31: 1555–1556.

13. Fahn S. Concept and classification of dystonia. In Fahn S. Marsden CD, Calne DB (eds) Dystonia 2, Advances in Neurology, Volume 50. 1988, pp. 2–8.

14. Molho ES, Factor SA, Podshalny GD, Brown D. The effect of dancing on dystonia. Mov Disord 1996; 11: 225–227.

15. Tardive dykinesia: Report of the American Psychiatric Association Task Force on Late Neurological Effects of Antipsychotic Drugs. Washington, DC, American Psychiatric Association, 1980.

16. van Harten PN, Matroos GE, Hoek HW, Kahn RS. The prevalence of tardive dystonia, tardive dyskinesia, parkinsonism and akathisia The Curacao Extrapyramidal Syndromes Study. Schizophr Res 1996; 19(2–3): 195–203.

17. Weiner WJ, Klawans HL. Lingual-facial-buccal movements in the elderly. J Am Geriatr Soc 1973; 21: 314–317.

18. Kang UJ, Burke RE, Fahn S. Natural history and treatment of tardive dystonia. Mov Disord 1986; 1: 193–208.

19. Greene P, Shale H, Fahn S. Experience with high dosages of anticholinergic and other drugs in treatment of torsion dystonia. In Fahn S, Marsden CD, Caine DB (eds) Dystonia 2, Advances in Neurology, Volume 50. 1988, pp. 547–556.

20. Yassa R, Nair V, Dimitry R. Prevalence of tardive dystonia. Acta Psychiatr Scand 1986; 73: 629–633.

21. Friedman JH, Kucharski LT, Wagner RL. Tardive dystonia in a psychiatric hospital. J Neurol Neurosurg Psychiatry 1987; 50: 801–803.

22. Lang AE. Clinical differences between metoclopramide- and antipsychotic-induced tardive dyskinesias. Can J Neurol Sci 1990; 17: 137–139.

23. Miller LG, Jankovic J. Neurologic approach to drug-induced movement disorders: A study of 125 patients. South Med J 1990; 83: 525–532.

24. Wojcik JD, Falk WE, Fink JS, Cole JO, Gelenberg AJ. A review of 32 cases of tardive dystonia Am J Psychiatry 1991; 148(8): 1055–1059.

25. Kiriakakis V, Bhatia KP, Quinn NP, Marsden CD. The natural history of tardive dystonia. A long-term follow-up study of 107 cases. Brain. 1998; 121(Pt 11): 2053–2066.

26. Calne D, Lang AE. Secondary dystonia. In Fahn S, Marsden CD, Calne DB (eds) Dystonia 2, Advances in Neurology, Volume 50. 1988, pp. 547–556

27. Yassa R, Nair V, Iskandar H. A comparison of severe tardive dystonia and severe tardive akathisia. Acta Psychiatr Scand 1989; 80: 155–159.

28. Sethi KD, Hess DC, Harp RJ. Prevalence of dystonia in veterans on chronic antipsychotic therapy. Mov Disord 1990; 5: 319–321.

29. Factor SA, Matthews MK. Persistent extra pyramidal syndrome with dystonia and rigidity causal by combined. Metoclopramide and prochlorperazine therapy. South Med J 1991; 84; 626–628.

30. Molho ES, Factor SA. Possible tardive dystonia resulting from clozapine therapy. Mov Disord 1999; 14(5): 873–874.

31. Ahmed S, Chengappa KN, et al. Clozapine withdrawal-emergent dystonias and dyskinesias: a case series. J Clin Psychiatry 1998; 59(9): 472—477.

32. Sharma V. Treatment-emergent tardive dyskinesia with quetiapine in mood disorders. J Clin Psychopharm 2003; 23(4): 415–417.

33. Bella VL, Piccoli F. Olanzepine-induced tardive dyskinesia. Br J Psychiatry 2003; 182: 81–82.

34. Dunayevich E, Strakowski S. Olanzapine-induced tardive dystonia. Am J Psychiatry 1999; 156(10): 1662.

35. Beasley CM, Dellva MA, Yamura RN, et al. Randomised double-blind comparison of the incidence of tardive dyskinesia in patients with schizophrenia during long-term treatment with olanzapine or haloperidol. Br J Psychiatry 1999; 174: 23–30.

36. Glazer WM, Morgenstern H, Pultz JA, et al. Incidence of persistent tardive dyskinesia is lower with quetiapine treatment than with typical antipsychotics in patients with schizophrenia and schizoaffective disorder. Schizophr Res 2000; 41(1): B45.

37. Fahn S. The Tardive Syndromes: Phenomenology, Concepts on Pathophysiology & Treatment. A Comprehensive Review of Movement Disorders for the Clinical Practioner 2003; 181–265.

38. Levin T, Heresco-Levy U. Risperidone-induced rabbit syndrome: an unusual movement disorder caused by an atypical antipsychotic. Eur Neuropsychopharmacol 1999; 9(1–2): 137–139.

39. Haberfellner EM. Tardive dyskinesia during treatment with risperidone. Pharmacopsychiatry 1997; 30(6): 271.

40. Silberbauer C. Risperidone-induced tardive dyskinesia. Pharmacopsychiatry 1998; 31(2): 68–69.

41. Hong KS, Cheong SS, Woo JM, Kim E. Risperidone-induced tardive dyskinesia. Am J Psychiatry 1999; 156(8): 1290.

42. Ananth J, Burgoyne K, Aquino S. Meige's syndrome associated with risperidone therapy. Am J Psychiatry 2000; 157(1): 149.

43. Vercueil L, Foucher J. Risperidone-induced tardive dystonia and psychosis [letter]. Lancet 1999; 353: 981.

44. Fdhil H, Krebs MO, Bayle F, Vanelle JM, Olie JP. Risperidone-induced tardive dystonia: a case of torticollis. Encephale 1998; 24: 581–583.

45. Sherr JD, Thaker G. Progression of abnormal involuntary movements during risperidone treatment. J Clin Psychiatry 1998; 59: 478–479.

46. Gimenez-Roldan S, Mateo D, Bartolome P. Tardive dystonia and severe tardive dyskinesia. Acta Psychiatr Scand 1985; 71: 488–494.

47. Molho ES, Feustel PJ, Factor SA. Clinical comparison of tardive and idiopathic cervical dystonia. Mov Disord 1998; 13: 486–489.
48. Brashear A, Ambrosius WT, Eckert GJ, Siemers ER. Comparison of treatment of tardive dystonia and idiopathic cervical dystonia with botulinum toxin type A. Mov Disord 1998; 13: 158–161.
49. Bressman SB, de Leon D, Raymond D, et al. Secondary dystonia and the DYT1 gene. Neurology 1997; 48: 1571–1577.
50. Sachdev P, Tardive blepharospasm. Mov Disord 1998; 13: 947–951.
51. Levin H, Reddy R. Clozapine in the treatment of neuroleptic-induced blepharospasm: a report of 4 cases. J Clin Psychiatry 2000; 61(2): 140–143.
52. Tan EK, Jankovic J. Tardive and idiopathic oromandibular dystonia: a clinical comparison. J Neurol Neurosurg Psychiatry 2000; 68(2): 186–190.
53. Krack P, Schneider S, Deuschl G. Geste device in tardive dystonia with retrocollis and opisthotonic posturing. Mov Disord 1998; 13: 155–157.
54. Fitzgerald PM, Jankovic J. Tardive oculogyric crisis. Neurology 1989; 39: 1434–1437.
55. Gimenez-Roldan S, Mateo D, Bartolome P. Tardive dystonia and severe tardive dyskinesia. Acta Psychiatr Scand 1985; 71: 488–494.
56. Yadalam KG, Korn ML, Simpson GM. Tardive dystonia: four case histories. J Clin Psychiatry 1990; 51.
57. Samie MR, Dannenhoffer MA, Rozek S. Life-threatening tardive dyskinesia caused by metoclopramide. Mov Disord 1987; 2: 125–129.
58. Hayashi T, Nishikawa T, Koga I, Uchida Y, Yamawaki S. Life-threatening dysphagia following prolonged neuroleptic therapy. Clin Neuropharmacol 1997; 20: 77–81.
59. Lazarus AL, Toglia JU. Fatal myoglobinuric renal failure in a patient with tardive dykinesia. Neurology 1985; 35: 1055–1057.
60. Kiriakakis V, Bhatia K, Quinn NP, Marsden CD. Botulinum toxin treatment of tardive syndromes [abstract]. Mov Disord 1997; 12: 27.
61. Tarsy D, Kaufman D, Sethi KD, Rivner MH, Molho E, Factor S. An open-label study of Botolinum toxin A for treatment of tardive dystonia. Clin Neuropharmacol 1997; 20: 90–93.
62. Lieberman J, Johns C, Cooper T, Poolack S, Kane J. Clozapine pharmizology and tardive dyskinesia. Psychopharmacology 1989; 99(S): S54–S59.
63. Lieberman JA, Saltz BL, Johns CA, et al. The effects of clozapine on tardive dyskinesia. Br J Psychiatry 1991; 158: 285–294.
64. Friedman JH. Clozapine treatment of psychosis in patients with tardive dystonia: report of three cases. Mov Disord 1994; 9: 321–324.
65. Wolf ME, Mosnaim AD. Improvement of axial dystonia with the administration of clozapine. Int J Clin Pharm Therap 1994; 32: 282–283.
66. Trugman JM, Leadbetter R, Zalis ME, Burgdorf RO, Wooten GF. Treatment of severe axial tardive dystonia with clozapine: case report and hypothesis. Mov Disord 1994; 9: 441–446.
67. Shapleske J, McKay AP, McKenna PJ. Successful treatment of tardive dystonia with clozapine and clonazepam. Br J Psychiatry 1996; 168: 516–518.
68. Fahn S. High dosage anticholinergic therapy in dystonia. Neurology (Cleveland) 1983; 33: 1255–1261.
69. Trottenburg T, Paul G, et al. Pallidal and thalamic neurostimulation in severe tardive dystonia. J Neurol Neurosurg Psychiatry 2001; 70: 557–559.
70. Uhrbrand L, Faurybe A. Reversible and irreversible dyskinesia after treatment with perphenazine, chlorpromazine, reserpine and electroconvulsive therapy. Psychopharmacologia 1960; 1: 408–418.

71. Druckman R, Seelinger D, Thulin B. Chronic involuntary movements induced by phenothiazines. J Nerv Ment Disord 1962; 135: 69–76.
72. Hunter R, Earl CJ, Thornicroft S. An apparently irreversible syndrome of abnormal movements following phenothiazine medication. Proc R Soc Med 1964; 57: 758–762.
73. Kruse W. Persistent muscular restlessness after phenothiazine treatment: report of three cases. Am J Psychiatry 1960; 117: 152–153.
74. Braude WM, Barnes TRE. Late-onset akathisia – an indicant of covert dyskinesia: two case reports. Am J Psychiatry 1983; 140: 611–612.
75. Duvoisin R. Neurological reactions to psychotropic drugs. In Efron DH (ed) Psychopharmacology: A Review of Progress 1957–1967. Washington, DC, U.S. Government Printing Office, 1968, pp. 561–573.
76. Gibb WRG, Lees AJ. The clinical phenomenon of akathisia. J Neurol Neurosurg Psychiatry 1986; 49: 861–866.
77. Munetz MR, Cornes CL. Akathisia, pseudoakathisia and tardive dyskinesia: clinical examples. Compr Psychiatry 1982; 23: 345–352.
78. Burke RE, Kang UK, Jankovic J, Miller LG, Fahn S. Tardive akathisia: an analysis of clinical features and response to open therapeutic trials. Mov Disord 1989; 4: 157–175.
79. Halstead SM, Barnes TR, Speller JC. Akathisia: prevalence and associated dysphoria in an in-patient population with chronic schizophrenia. Br J Psychiatry 1994; 164(2): 177–183.
80. Ayd F. A survey of drug-induced extrapyramidal reactions. JAMA 1961; 175: 1054–1060.
81. Braude WM, Barnes TRE. Late-onset akathisia- an indicant of covert dyskinesia: two case reports. Am J Psychiatry 1983; 140: 611–612.
82. Schilkrut VR, Duran E, Haverbeck C, Katz I, Vidal P. Verlauf von psychopathologischen und extrapyramidalmotorischen symptomen unter einer Langzeit-Neuroleptika behandlung schizophrener Patienten. Drug Res 1978; 28: 1494–1495.
83. van Harten PN, Hoek HW, Matroos GE, Koeter M, Kahn RS. The inter-relationships of tardive dyskinesia, parkinsonism, akathisia and tardive dystonia: the Curacao Extrapyramidal Syndromes Study II. Schizophr Res 1997; 26(2–3): 235–242.
84. Shearer RM, Bownes IT, Curran P. Tardive akathisia and agitated depression during metoclopramide therapy. Acta Psychiatr Scand 1984; 70: 428–431.
85. Gerlach J, Peacock L. Motor and mental side effects of clozapine. J Clin Psychiatry 1994; 55(suppl B): 107–109.
86. Peacock L, Solgaard T, Lublin H, Gerlach J. Clozapine versus typical antipsychotics. A retro- and prospective study of extrapyramidal side effects. Psychopharmacology (Berl) 1996; 124(1–2): 188–196.
87. Drake RE, Ehrlich J. Suicide attempts associated with akathisia. Am J Psychiatry 1985; 142: 499–501.
88. Kumar B. An unusual case of akathisia. Am J Psychol 1979; 136: 8.
89. Raskin DE. Akathisia: A side effect to be remembered. Am J Psychiatry 1972; 129: 345–347.
90. Van Putten T. The many faces of akathisia. Compr Psychiatry 1975; 16: 43–47.
91. Siris S. Three cases of akathisia and "acting out." Clin Psychiatry 1985; 46: 395–397.
92. Burke RE, Kang UJ, Fahn S, Jankovic J, Miller LG. Tardive akathisia [letter]. Mov Disord 1990; 181–182.
93. Lang AE, Johnson K. Akathisia in idiopathic Parkinson's disease. Neurology 1987; 37: 477–480.
94. Olivera, A. Sertraline and akathisia: spontaneous resolution. Biol Psychiatry 1997; 41: 241–242.
95. Olivera A. A case of paroxetine-induced akathisia. Biol Psychiatry 1996; 39: 909–910.

96. Walters A, Hening W, Chokroverty S., Fahn S. Opiod responsiveness in patients with neuroleptic-induced akathisia. Mov Disord 1986; 1: 119–128.

97. Walters S, Hening W, Chokroverty S. Tardive akathisia [letter]. Mov Disord 1990; 5: 89–90.

98. Adler LA, Angrist B, Peselow E, et al. Noradrenergic mechanisms in akathisia: treatment with propranolol and clonidine. Psychopharmacol Bull 1987; 23: 21–25.

99. Degwitz R. Extrapyramidal motor disorders following long-term treatment with neuroleptic drugs. In Crane GE, Gardner R (eds) Psychotropic Drugs and Dysfunctions of the Basal Ganglia, Public Health Service Publication No. 1938, 1969, pp. 22–33.

100. Tominaga H, Fukuzako H, Izumi K, et al. Tardive myoclonus [letter]. Lancet 1987; 1: 322.

101. Little JT, Jankovic J. Tardive myoclonus. Mov Disord 1987; 2: 307–312.

102. Hyser CL, Drake ME Jr. Myoclonus induced by metoclopramide therapy. Arch Intern Med 1983; 143(11): 2201–2202.

103. Klawans HL, Falk DK, Nausieda PA, Weiner WJ. Gilles de la Tourette's syndrome after long-term chlorpromazine therapy. Neurology 1978; 28: 1064–1068.

104. DeVaugh-Geiss J. Tardive Tourette's syndrome. Neurology 1980; 30: 562–563.

105. Stahl S. Tardive Tourette's syndrome in an autistic patient after long-term neuroleptic administration. Am J Psychiatry 1980; 137: 1267–1269.

106. Fog R, Pakenberg H. Theoretical and clinical aspects of the Tourette syndrome (chronic multiple tic). J Neur Transm 1980;16(suppl): 211–215.

107. Seeman MV, Patel J, Pyke J. Tardive dyskinesia with Tourette-like syndrome. J Clin Psychiatry 1981; 42: 357–358.

108. Mueller J, Aminoff MJ. Tourette-like syndrome after long-term neuroleptic drug treatment. Br J Psychiatry 1982; 141: 191–193.

109. Klawans HL, Nausieda PA, Goetz CC, et al. Tourette-like symptoms following chronic neuroleptic therapy. In Friedhoff AJ, Chase TN (eds) Gilles de la Tourette Syndrome. New York, Raven Press, 1982; pp. 415–418.

110. Munetz MR, Slawsky RC, Neil JF. Tardive Tourette's syndrome treated with clonidine and mesoridazine. Psychosomatics 1985; 26: 254–257.

111. Karagianis JL, Nagpurkar R. A case of Tourette syndrome developing during haloperidol treatment. Can J Psychiatry 1990; 35: 228–232.

112. Bharucha KJ, Sethi KD. Tardive Tourettism after exposure to neuroleptic therapy. Mov Disord 1995; 10(6): 791–793.

113. Stacy M, Jankovic J. Tardive tremor. Mov Disord. 1992; 7(1): 53–57.

114. Tarsy D, Indorf G. Tardive tremor due to metoclopramide. Mov Disord 2002; 17(3): 620–621.

115. Polizos P, Engelhardt DM, Hoffman SP, Waiser J. Neurological consequences of psychotropic drug withdrawal in schizophrenic children. J Autism Child Schizophr 1973; 3: 247–253.

116. Fahn S. The tardive dyskinesias. In Matthews WB, Glaser GH (eds) Recent Advances in Clinical Neurology, volume 4, Edinburgh, Churchill Livingstone, 1984, pp. 229–260.

117. Ford B, Greene, P, Fahn S. Oral and genital tardive pain syndromes. Neurology 1994; 44: 2115–2119.

CHAPTER 11

Movement disorders due to atypical antipsychotics

Karen E. Anderson

Introduction

Standard or typical antipsychotics were first used in the early 1950s, starting with the introduction of chlorpromazine, for the treatment of psychosis. Their use represented a major advance in the treatment of severe, chronic, mental illness. However, the risks of iatrogenic movement disorders associated with the use of these medications quickly became apparent. Development of abnormal movements, termed extrapyramidal symptoms (EPS), was linked to dopamine receptor blockade, which also provided the antipsychotic efficacy of these medications. Atypical antipsychotics were developed with the hope of not only increasing efficacy of treatment for psychiatric symptoms, but also reducing the debilitating and sometimes life-threatening EPS. Since drug-related EPS are thought to be due to the blockade of postsynaptic dopaminergic receptors in the nigrostriatal pathways, it has been suggested that an increase in striatal dopamine activity (which may result from atypical antipsychotic administration) could also counteract EPS (see [1] for a review). Concomitant hyperactivity of the cholinergic system [2] explains why anticholinergic medications are sometimes beneficial for the treatment of EPS. Tardive dyskinesia (TD) is different from other EPS as it may be caused by supersensitivity of the dopaminergic system from chronic blockade and proliferation of postsynaptic nigrostriatal dopamine receptors [3]. However, few data are available to directly support this hypothesis [4].

Given their preclinical profile, atypical antipsychotics were expected to be associated with a reduced incidence of EPS and tardive syndromes. Their unique clinical effects are thought to be due, at least in part, to their greater propensity to block the serotonergic system relative to the dopaminergic system, thus normalizing the imbalances between these systems that may exist in pathological conditions [5]. While there is variation between individual agents, all atypicals share this high serotonin-to-dopamine blockade ratio. When serotonergic activity is inhibited, dopamine release increases and helps to correct the blockade effect at postsynaptic dopaminergic receptors. Thus, a relatively low D2 affinity coupled with higher affinity for serotonin 2A (5-HT2A) receptors is generally accepted to be one possible hallmark of an atypical antipsychotic [6–8]. Other factors seen in preclinical data, which may suggest mechanisms for the reduction of EPS with these agents, include selective inactivation of A10 mesolimbic dopaminergic neurons without this effect on A9 nigrostriatal neurons, and a reduction in antagonism of apomorphine- and amphetamine-related stereotypies [9]. (For further details on the pharmacology of typical agents see Chapter 4.)

Atypical antipsychotics have come into wide clinical use, replacing typical agents as the first line of treatment for psychosis and often for agitation, especially in patients with dementia [10]. They are additionally used as mood stabilizers [11], and as part of augmentation strategies for the treatment of refractory depression [12], and a host other conditions. As use of these agents has increased, especially with off-label prescribing, it has become apparent that although they are associated with an apparently lower incidence of EPS, they are not free of these side effects. Clinicians must continue to judiciously weigh whether treatment with these agents warrants the possibility of exposing patients to the risk of EPS.

This chapter will review the controlled clinical trial data, when available, on EPS with use of the five atypicals currently available in the United States: clozapine, risperidone, olanzapine, quetiapine, and ziprasidone. Many of these studies examine the reduction of EPS in patients treated previously with typical antipsychotics compared with atypicals, although this does not give an index of new onset movement disorders associated with these agents. Direct comparisons with typical antipsychotics, where available, will be discussed. In reviewing these data, it should be noted that most studies and reports are from work with patients with schizophrenia; applicability of these data to other populations may be questionable. The development of tardive dyskinesia (TD) may have a relationship to acute EPS. TD has been thought to be a supersensitivity response to chronic blockade of dopaminergic pathways [3], which would suggest that patients who develop acute EPS are at increased risk for TD. Support has been found for this hypothesis in some [13, 14] but not all [15, 16] studies. Both, the occurrence of TD associated with use of atypicals and the treatment of TD with atypicals, will be reviewed as it provides another measure of these agents' causal relationship to abnormal involuntary movements. In reviewing the data on TD, it should be remembered that outside factors may influence the occurrence of TD in any patient. Spontaneous dyskinesias have been estimated to occur in neuroleptic-naïve schizophrenic populations, the most-studied group, at 1–11%, depending on the abnormal involuntary movement rating used [15, 17], Fenton found differing rates of spontaneous dyskinesias based on age and duration of illness at 4% in first-episode patients, 12% for whom have been ill for a number of years but are under 30 years of age, 25% for those between the ages of 30 and 50 years, and up to 40% for patients over 60 years [18]. These spontaneous abnormal movements may make assessment of drug-related TD problematic, especially in older patient populations (see Chapter 3). Other possible risk factors for development of TD include female gender, length of exposure to neuroleptics, and cumulative neuroleptic dose (see Chapter 9).

The presence of these characteristics in a study population may complicate assessment of a medication's TD liability. In addition, in reports where TD improves with atypical agents it is difficult to decipher if the improvement is due to a "passive" effect from the removal of typical neuroleptics and replacement with agents with fewer dopamine-blocking effects, a "suppression" of symptoms as seen with typical neuroleptics, or some other "active" therapeutic effect. The risk of neuroleptic malignant syndrome associated with the use of atypicals will also be reviewed as potential predictors of susceptibility to EPS. The association between atypical antipsychotic use and abnormal movements in elderly patients in general, and in particular in patients with Parkinson's disease (PD), will also be considered, since sensitivity to EPS is common in these patients and provides important insights into a medication's propensity to cause EPS. Recommendations for use of atypicals to treat psychiatric symptoms in patients with PD are included.

Clozapine

Clozapine, which is a dibenzodiazepine derivative, was the first atypical antipsychotic medication approved for use in the United States (1990). It was developed in the 1950s, but received widespread clinical attention after a study of its use in the treatment of refractory patients in 1988 [19]. The authors reported a significant reduction in acute EPS in those patients treated with clozapine compared to those receiving chlorpromazine with benztropine mesylate. In the many trials comparing clozapine to typical antipsychotics, treatment with clozapine has been shown to reduce incidence of acute EPS and to reduce patient dropout rates. Clozapine treatment has also been found to decrease the need for anticholinergic medications or other treatments for EPS used concomitantly with typicals [20–28]. Clozapine also has not been found to have a dose-dependent increase in EPS [29]. Despite this overall favorable profile for clozapine, with regard to EPS, its use is limited by the necessity of frequent blood draws to monitor for medication-induced leukopenia, which can be fatal. Patients require weekly blood draws for 6 months and then every 2 weeks thereafter for as long as they are on the drug.

Some groups have reported high rates of akathisia with clozapine use (39%) [30]. However, the akathisia seen in that study was mild and doses of clozapine were higher, relative to typical antipsychotics, than was used in other similar studies (e.g., [19, 24]). The incidence of moderate or severe akathisia associated with clozapine use is comparable to that seen with typical neuroleptics. The rate of akathisia related to clozapine treatment averages between 7% and 9% ([19, 20, 31], among others). Based on clinical reports, some groups have recommended the use of clozapine for the treatment of refractory akathisia [32].

Tardive dyskinesia

In several long-term studies, no cases of TD have been found with clozapine) use ([20–23, 31]. Other groups have reported new onset or worsening of TD; however. these were in patient populations that had prior treatment with typical agents, making attribution of side effects purely due to clozapine problematic [26, 27, 33]. Work by Kane et al. is the largest study of clozapine and TD to date; they followed 28 patients who were treated with clozapine for at least 1 year, with average treatment of 7.7 years. Clozapine-treated patients were compared with patients treated with a standard neuroleptic for at least 1 year. Two patients in the clozapine group developed movements meeting criteria for TD at study conclusion, but both had questionable TD during baseline assessment, providing inconclusive results. Survival analysis demonstrated a lower risk of TD development in the clozapine-treated group.

Clozapine has generally been found to be more effective than typical neuroleptics in suppression of TD [20, 26, 28]. A study by Tamminga et al. [34], comparing clozapine with haloperidol, followed 32 schizophrenic patients with TD for a year. Those treated with clozapine showed significantly greater reduction in dyskinesia on standardized ratings compared with those receiving haloperidol. The clozapine treatment group also did not show a drug discontinuation-induced worsening of dyskinesias. However, other groups have found withdrawal dyskinesias following clozapine treatment [35]. Clozapine has been found to be especially efficacious for the suppression of tardive dystonia; the mechanism for this particular effect is unclear but the reversal of dystonia is slow and may take months [36–38].

Neuroleptic malignant syndrome

Surveys have stated the risk of NMS from clozapine to be approximately 0.2%, which does not differ greatly from rates seen with typicals [39] (see Chapter 8). Patients who develop NMS following clozapine treatment display classic signs of NMS, but may show fewer tremors, less rigidity, and have lower temperatures than those who develop the syndrome following treatment with typical agents [40]. Rechallenge rates of NMS with clozapine are not significantly different from those with typical neuroleptics, with recurrence rates of up to 30% reported [40].

Parkinson's disease

Hallucinations and psychosis are common in PD, and can be disabling. Their prevalence has increased substantially with the use of levodopa and dopamine agonists for motor symptoms. Newer studies suggest that between 20% and 45% of PD patients will experience these symptoms [41, 42]. Treatment of psychosis can be extremely challenging, since patients with PD have been found to be very sensitive to neuroleptics with regard to the occurrence of EPS, and tend to experience worsening of their motor symptoms when treated with these agents. Clozapine is the most widely studied atypical antipsychotic in PD patients with hallucinations and delusions [43]. In a 60-subject randomized, double-blind, placebo-controlled trial of low dose (mean dose approximately 25 mg/day) clozapine for hallucinations and psychosis in PD, clozapine significantly improved psychotic symptoms and was additionally found to actually improve tremor without worsening of other parkinsonian symptoms [44]. This study confirmed the results of numerous open-label trials [45] and was followed by a second, equally successful, double-blind study [46]. It remains the only agent proven to be useful in PD patients with psychosis with double-blind trials.

Risperidone

Risperidone, a benzisoxazole, was the next atypical to be introduced in 1994. It was initially hoped that risperidone would provide the favorable EPS profile seen with clozapine without the liabilities of leukopenia risk and the concomitant need for frequent blood monitoring. Although it is an effective and widely used antipsychotic agent, risperidone has not lived up to the expectation that it would provide an alternative to clozapine with respect to low rates of EPS.

Initial studies with risperidone were quite promising, with lower rates of acute EPS and reduction of EPS on objective ratings, decreased dropout rates, and reduction in concomitant anticholinergic use compared with haloperidol treatment [35, 47–56]. These benefits were soon, however, found to be highly dose dependent. When the above studies were reviewed, the advantages of risperidone were greatly diminished at doses greater than 6 mg per day [35, 47–52]. This dose dependency was also seen in drug-naïve patients [57], not only with respect to the occurrence to EPS but also with respect to the use of anticholinergic medications [58]. When lower doses of haloperidol or lower-potency typicals were compared to risperidone, the EPS liability of risperidone was similar [48, 53–55, 59]. In one other study, the authors did a comparison of the frequency of EPS from risperidone and haloperidol in neuroleptic-naïve patients admitted for the first time to an acute case facility with psychosis. It was a prospective analysis of 350 patients, 34 of whom received risperidone. The mean doses were 3.7 mg per day risperidone and 3.7 mg per day for haloperidol. Measures for akathisia, parkinsonism acute dystonia, and tardive dyskinesia were comparable for both drugs with parkinsonism occurring in over 50% of the patients [60]. Significant EPS decreases have been reported in elderly patients treated with risperidone in an open-label study [61].

There are few data available on the effects on subtypes of EPS seen with risperidone treatment. Caroff et al. [40] suggest in their review that this is due to the fact that most original trials focused on overall changes in EPS ratings, not on specific movement disorders, but that occurrence of EPS subtypes at risperidone doses of less than 6 mg per day were comparable to placebo in the studies reviewed above, with rates of EPS subtype occurrence significantly lesser than those seen with haloperidol. In an observational study of patients with TD by Lohr et al. [62], rigidity scores were found to be lowered with risperidone use, but no effect was seen on TD, tremor, or akathisia.

Tardive dyskinesia

Long-term trial data suggest that the risk of developing TD from risperidone per year of treatment is one-fifth to one-tenth of that associated with haloperidol use in equivalent doses, even in elderly patients [49, 63–66]. Two studies specifically examining patients with TD to date have found significant decreases in dyskinesia ratings with risperidone [50, 52, 67], although in the case of the first study, which compared risperidone to haloperidol, these effects were significant only at doses of 6 mg per day or higher [50, 67]. A small study of mentally retarded adults who had been chronically treated with typical neuroleptics also found a reduction in TD following treatment with risperidone [68]. An open-label study found stabilization of TD after 12 months of risperidone treatment in elders [61]. Jeste et al. [64] reported a lower incidence of TD following risperidone treatment compared with haloperidol administration (5% vs. 30%, respectively) in a prospective, longitudinal study of elders. In contrast to these positive effects of risperidone on TD, another group found no differences in dyskinesia ratings when comparing of risperidone with haloperidol; only haloperidol showed significant amelioration of TD in this study [53]. The observational study of patients with TD found no effects on TD associated with risperidone treatment [62]. Finally, several cases of TD occurring in patients not previously exposed to standard neuroleptics have been reported with risperidone therapy [69, 70].

Neuroleptic malignant syndrome

Limited data are available on the rate and characteristics of NMS associated with risperidone use. Caroff and colleagues reported on 21 cases of NMS associated with risperidone obtained either from literature searches or from the Neuroleptic Malignant Syndrome Information Service database. Risperidone induced NMS was similar to classic NMS in presentation and symptomatology, except that NMS associated with risperidone tended not to produce extreme hyperthermia [40]. Recurrence of NMS has been reported with risperidone rechallenge in a small number of patients [40] similar to that seen with standard neuroleptic.

Parkinson's disease

Risperidone has shown some efficacy in treatment of hallucinations and psychosis in PD, however, at the cost of worsening of motor symptoms. In the first study, low-dose (mean dose 0.67 mg/day) risperidone was reported to improve hallucinations in a small series of PD patients [71], but this was followed by another report of six PD patients where "substantial worsening" of motor symptoms was seen with a mean dose of 1.5 mg per day [72]. Since then several open-label series have demonstrated consistently that the drug worsens motor features of PD [73]. One double-blind study compared clozapine and risperidone in 10 PD patients. The study demonstrated similar efficacy in both treatment groups for psychiatric symptoms; there was nonsignificant worsening of motor symptoms in the risperidone treatment group but an improvement in the clozapine group [74].

Comparison with other atypicals

There were several head-to-head comparison trials of risperidone and other atypical antipsychotics in schizophrenia patients. Two double-blind, randomized trials found similar effects with respect to EPS for risperidone and clozapine [75, 76]. Four other studies comparing these two agents reported a more favorable EPS profile for clozapine, which would seem more likely based on their pharmacology [77–80]. It should be noted that only one of these studies was a double-blind design [80]. Comparisons of risperidone with olanzapine found similar EPS profiles in two studies, the latter of which was a double-blind, randomized trial [81, 82]. Decreased EPS liability with olanzapine compared to risperidone was reported in two others, the first of which was double-blind [83, 84]. The one comparison of risperidone with quetiapine to date found a more favorable EPS profile with quetiapine [85].

Olanzapine

Olanzapine, a thienobenzodiazepine derivative, was the next atypical antipsychotic agent introduced after risperidone in 1996. When olanzapine treatment was compared with chlorpromazine and haloperidol in schizophrenia populations, reductions in acute EPS, dropout rates, and use of concomitant anticholinergic agents were all significantly reduced, including in treatment refractory patients [86–92]. Both parkinsonism and akathisia were found to be significantly reduced with olanzapine treatment compared with haloperidol in a study of first-episode patients by Sanger et al. [91]. In a meta-analysis on clinical safety of olanzapine in patients previously treated with typical agents Beasley et al. [93] found improvements in EPS from baseline compared to those treated with haloperidol. Caroff et al. [40] noted in their extensive review that olanzapine is associated with lower incidence of sedation and hypersalivation compared with clozapine, which can by itself result in lower ratings of bradykinesia and parkinsonism. A dose-dependent increase in EPS has been seen with olanzapine, especially with respect to akathisia [88].

Tardive dyskinesia

In a large-scale, long-term study comparing olanzapine and haloperidol Beasley et al. [94] found the 1-year risk of TD to be 0.52% for patients treated with olanzapine and 7.45% for those in the haloperidol group. Beasley et al. [94] and Tollefson et al. [95] have estimated that the rate of TD occurrence with olanzapine is one-twelfth of that associated with haloperidol use. Preliminary studies by Kinon et al. [96] found that olanzapine reduced dyskinesia ratings in patients with TD and that 70% of patients with TD no longer had symptoms following 8 months of olanzapine treatment [97]. Positive effects on TD ratings following olanzapine treatment in elderly patients have also been found in small open-label or prospective studies [98, 99], respectively).

Neuroleptic malignant syndrome

A review by Kontaxakis et al. [100] found 17 cases of possible NMS associated with olanzapine, including four definite cases with olanzapine monotherapy. NMS has been described in neuroleptic-naïve patients receiving olanzapine indicating a clear cause-and-effect relationship [101]. Rechallenge with olanzapine following NMS has been associated with recurrence [40]. There are no data to date on the incidence of NMS associated with olanzapine use.

Parkinson's disease

As with risperidone, olanzapine has been shown to worsen motor function in patients with PD. This was initially demonstrated in several open-label studies [73] and then confirmed in three double-blind studies [102–104]. In one of the double-blind, randomized studies comparing olanzapine and clozapine for hallucinations in PD patients, safety stopping rules were invoked after a significant decline in motor function was seen in the olanzapine-treated patients. UPDRS motor scores worsened by 12 points with olanzapine but improved by 6 points with clozapine. The authors of this study recommended that olanzapine not be used for PD patients [102]. They propose that the higher D2 receptor occupancy seen in positron emission tomography studies of olanzapine and risperidone compared to clozapine may explain the unfavorable side effect profile seen in both medications when used to treat PD patients [5].

Comparisons with other atypicals

As noted above, olanzapine has been compared in head-to-head trials with risperidone with similar [81, 82] or more favorable EPS liability reported [83, 84]. Direct comparison of olanzapine and clozapine in treatment-resistant schizophrenic patients found no differences with respect to acute EPS between the two agents [105].

Quetiapine

Quetiapine is a dibenzothiazepine compound that was developed specifically to have a profile similar to clozapine with respect to EPS, without the risk of hematopathology. It was approved for use in the United States in 1998. As with the other atypical antipsychotics, the use of quetiapine has been associated with reduction of EPS on objective ratings in schizophrenic patients, and also in significant decreases in both patient dropouts from treatment trials and use of concomitant anticholinergic medications, when compared with typical antipsychotic agents [106–114]. One of the studies cited above did find a similar rate of usage for anticholinergic medications between the quetiapine treatment group and those treated with a typical neuroleptic (chlorpromazine, in this case). However, the quetiapine group was found to have a lower incidence of adverse events, and a lower incidence of EPS during treatment, compared with the chlorpromazine group.

Tardive dyskinesia

In the few studies that exist to date, it has been reported that rates of TD seen with quetiapine are similar to those seen with olanzapine, that is, one-twelfth of that associated with haloperidol [114–117]. Tariot et al. [118] did not find a clear effect on TD in elders treated with quetiapine for 1 year in an open-label trial.

Neuroleptic malignant syndrome

There are several case studies associating NMS with quetiapine use [119–123]. In the two rechallenge cases published thus far, one developed NMS following resumption of quetiapine while the other did not [124, 125].

Parkinson's disease

At this time, quetiapine is considered by many to be the first-line treatment of hallucinations or psychosis in PD. Targum and Abbot [126] found quetiapine to be efficacious and fairly well tolerated in an open-label study of 11 PD patients with hallucinations and psychosis. Other small open-label studies have found similar results, without worsening of motor symptoms [73, 127]. More recently, several larger studies have indicated that about 80% of PD patients with psychosis improve but 13–30% demonstrate a worsening of motor symptoms. In most cases the worsening is mild and of little consequence as compared to olanzapine and risperidone [128, 129]. Low doses (12.5 mg QD may be sufficient in some patients) should be tried to minimize side effects, since there have been case reports of motor symptom exacerbation with quetiapine [130]. On average most patients require 50–100 mg per day. A randomized, double-blind, comparison between quetiapine and clozapine has yet to be made in this patient population. Despite this it is often the treatment of first choice because of ease of use, lack of compulsory blood monitoring, and consistently positively results in open-label studies.

Ziprasidone

Ziprasidone, a benzothiazolyl piperazine derivative, is the newest atypical agent to be introduced in the United States in 2001. In the limited number of studies to date, the use of ziprasidone has been associated with significant reductions in acute EPS, EPS ratings, patient dropouts, and concomitant use of anticholingergic agents in schizophrenic patients [131–135]. Data thus far suggest that ziprasidone may be associated with increases in EPS risk with higher doses [7]. A placebo-controlled study of ziprasidone for schizophrenia and schizoaffective disorder found higher rates of anticholinergic medication usage in the ziprasidone treatment group compared to those patients in the placebo-controlled group, although this difference was not significant [133].

Reduction of all EPS subtypes were seen with ziprasidone use in the studies cited above; further clinical and study data are needed to determine whether ziprasidone is associated with superior efficacy for particular EPS symptoms.

Tardive dyskinesia

Ziprasidone has not been in use long enough at this time for significant data to have been collected on TD associated with its use.

Neuroleptic malignant syndrome

As with TD, ziprasidone has not been used widely enough for there to be data on the incidence of NMS associated with its use. One case of NMS associated with ziprasidone use has been described [136].

Parkinson's disease

There are no data on the use of ziprasidone for treatment of psychiatric symptoms in PD.

Summary and conclusions

Compared with the high incidence of iatrogenic abnormal involuntary movements seen with the use of standard neuroleptics, the risk of acute EPS, and perhaps some other drug-induced movement disorders, has been reduced with the introduction of atypical agents. However, atypicals are not free of these side effects. Based on the studies reviewed above, the risk of acute EPS is best represented as risperidone > olanzapine = ziprasidone > quetiapine > clozapine. These differences become most obvious in sensitive populations such as elders and those with Parkinson's disease and related conditions. EPS liability increases at the higher end of the dosing range with risperidone and olanzapine, and probably with ziprasidone, although this may not be fully apparent until this medication is in wider use.

Based on the above data, it appears highly likely that atypical antipsychotic use significantly lowers risk of TD and may suppress symptoms in patients who have already developed this side effect (see Chapter 12). Utility of individual atypicals for suppression of particular EPS subtypes is still under investigation. The probable occurrence of spontaneous dyskinesias in untreated schizophrenics can make side effects of any medication in this population difficult to assess, as can other risk factors for TD and prior exposure to standard neuroleptics. Risk of NMS may be diminished in patients who are treated with atypicals compared to standard neuroleptics, but the relatively rare occurrence of NMS makes differences in risk difficult to ascertain, especially with the newer agents such as quetiapine and ziprasidone. Physicians should not discount the possibility of NMS in patients treated with these agents.

The limited studies to date suggest that elderly patients benefit from a decrease in drug-induced movements with the use of atypical agents. Improvement in TD may also be seen. With respect to treatment of hallucinations in Parkinson's disease and related disorders, some atypicals have an advantageous EPS profile compared with standard neuroleptics. Clozapine and quetiapine, often in very low doses, have been identified as those agents that are least likely to worsen motor symptoms in these sensitive patients. Risperidone and olanzapine are not recommended for use in PD patients due to their propensity to worsen motor function. Too few data are available to allow for recommendations for the use of ziprasidone to treat psychiatric symptoms in PD patients.

Atypical antipsychotics can be extremely helpful in the treatment of numerous conditions, including psychosis, aggression, and mood disorders. They have been shown to decrease the incidence of EPS, and perhaps of TD. They are the medications of choice for treating populations with known sensitivity to standard neuroleptics, including elders and PD patients. As more data become available, especially with respect to long-term use of these agents, firmer conclusions can be made with respect to the risk of drug-induced movement disorders associated with their use. Clinicians must use these agents judiciously, and at the lowest clinically effective doses, to further minimize the risk of movement disorders associated with their use.

References

1. Glazer WM. Extrapyramidal side effects, tardive dyskinesia, and the concept of atypicality. J Clin Psychiatry 2000; 61(suppl 3): 16–21.
2. Synder S, Greenberg D, Yamamura H. Antischizophrenic drugs and brain cholinergic receptors. Arch Gen Psychiatry 1974; 31: 58–61.
3. Rubovits R, Klawans HL Jr. Implications of amphetamine-induced stereotyped behavior as a model for tardive dyskinesia. Arch Gen Psychiatry 1972; 27: 502–507.
4. Peacock L, Gerlach J. A reanalysis of the dopamine theory of tardive dyskinesia: the hypothesis of dopamine D1/D2 imbalance. In Yassa R, Nair NPV, Jeste DV (eds) Neuroleptic Induced Movement Disorders. New York, Cambridge University Press, 1997, 141–160.
5. Kapur S, Zipursky RB, Remington G. Clinical and theoretical implications of 5HT2 and D2 receptor occupancy of clozapine, risperidone, and olanzapine in schizophrenia. Am J Psychiatry 1999; 156: 286–293.
6. Tandon R, Milner K, Jibson MD. Antipsychotics from theory to practice: integrating clinical and basic data. J Clin Psychiatry 1999; 60(suppl 8): 21–28.
7. Jibson MD, Tandon R. Treatment of schizophrenia. Psychiatr Clin N Am, Ann Drug Ther 2000; 7: 83–113.
8. Meltzer HY, Alphs LD, Bastani B, et al. Clinical efficacy of clozapine in the treatment of schizophrenia. Pharmacopsychiatry 1991; 24(2): 44–45.
9. Baldessarini RJ, Frankenburg FR. Clozapine: a novel antipsychotic agent. N Eng J Med 1991; 324: 746–754.
10. Tariot PN, Ismail MS. Use of quetiapine in elderly patients. J Clin Psychiatry 2002; 63(suppl 13): 21–26.
11. Keck PE, Nelson EB, McElroy SL. Advances in the pharmacologic treatment of bipolar depression. Biol Psychiatry 2003; 53(8): 671–679.
12. Thase ME. What role do atypical antipsychotic drugs have in treatment resistant depression? J Clin Psychiatry 2002; 63(2): 95–110.
13. Saltz BL, Woerner MG, Kane JM, et al. Prospective study of tardive dyskinesia incidence in the elderly. JAMA 1991; 266: 2402–2406.
14. Jeste DV, Caligiuri MP, Paulsen JS, et al. Risk of tardive dyskinesia in older patients: a prospective longitudinal study of 266 patients. Arch Gen Psychiatry 1995; 52: 756–765.
15. Chatterjee A, Chakos M, Koreen A, et al. Prevalence and clinical correlates of extrapyramidal signs and spontaneous dyskinesia in never-medicated schizophrenic patients. Am J Psychiatry 1995; 152: 1724–1729.
16. Morgenstern J, Glazer WM. Identifying risk factors for tardive dyskinesia among long-term outpatients maintained with neuroleptic medications: results of the Yale Tardive Dyskinesia Study. Arch Gen Psychiatry 1993; 50: 723–733.
17. Puri BK, Barnes TRE, Chapman MJ, et al. Spontaneous dyskinesia in first episode schizophrenia. J Neurol Neurosurg Psychiatry 1999; 66: 76–78.

18. Fenton WS. Prevalence of spontaneous dyskinesia in schizophrenia. J Clin Psychiatry 2000; 61 (Suppl) 4: 10–4.
19. Kane J, Honigfeld G, Singer J, et al. Clozapine for the treatment-resistant schizophrenic. Arch Gen Psychiatry 1988; 45: 789–796.
20. Casey DE. Clozapine: neuroleptic-induced EPS and tardive dyskinesia. Psychopharmacology (Berl) 1989; 99: S47-S53.
21. Matz R, Rick W, Thompson H, et al. Clozapine: potential antipsychotic agent without extrapyramidal manifestations. Curr Ther Res Clin Exp 1974; 16: 687–695.
22. Fischer-Cornelssen KA, Ferner UJ. An example of European multicenter trials: multispectral analysis of clozapine. Psychopharmacol Bull 1976; 12: 34–39.
23. Polvessen UJ, Noring U, Fog R, et al. Tolerability and therapeutic effect of clozapine: a retrospective investigation of 216 patients treated with clozapine for up to 12 years. Acta Psychiatr Scand 1985; 71: 176–185.
24. Claghorn J, Honigfeld G, Abuzzahab FS, et al. The risks and benefits of clozapine versus chlorpromazine. J Clin Psychopharmacol 1987; 7: 377–384.
25. Naber D, Holzbach R, Perro C, et al. Clinical management of clozapine patients in relation to efficacy and side effects. Br J Psychiatry 1992; 160(suppl 17): 54–59.
26. Gerlach J, Peacock L. Motor and mental side effects of clozapine. J Clin Psychiatry1994; 55 (suppl B): 107–109.
27. Kurz M, Hummer M, Oberbauer H, et al. Extrapyramidal side effects of clozapine and haloperidol. Psychopharmacology (Berl) 1995; 118: 52–56.
28. Rosenheck R, Cramer J, Xu W, et al. A comparison of clozapine and haloperidol in hospitalized patients with refractory schizophrenia. N Eng J Med 1997; 337: 809–815.
29. Tandon R, Jibson MD. Extrapyramidal side effects of antipsychotic treatment: scope of problem and impact on outcome. Ann Clin Psychiatry 2002; 14(2): 123–129.
30. Cohen BM, Keck PE, Sattlin A, et al. Prevalence and severity of akathisia in patients on clozapine. Biol Psychiatry 1991; 29: 1215–1219.
31. Chengappa KNR, Shelton MD, Baker RW, et al. The prevalence of akathisia in patients receiving stable doses of clozapine. J Clin Psychiatry 1994; 55: 142–145.
32. Wirshing WC, Phelan CK, Van Putten TV, et al. Effects of clozapine on treatment resistant akathisia and concomitant tardive dyskinesia. J Clin Psychopharmacol 1990; 10: 371–373.
33. Kane JM, Woerner MG, Pollack S, et al. Does clozapine cause tardive dyskinesia? J Clin Psychiatry 1993; 54: 327–330.
34. Tamminga C, Thaker G, Moran M, et al. Clozapine in tardive dyskinesia: observations from human and animal model studies. J Clin Psychiatry 1994; 55(9, suppl B): 102–106.
35. Simpson GM, Lindenmayer JP. Extrapyramidal symptoms in patients treated with risperidone. J Clin Psychopharmacol 1997; 17(3): 194–201.
36. Lieberman JA, Saltz BL, Johns CA, et al. The effects of clozapine on tardive dyskinesia. Br J Psychiatry. 1991; 158: 503–510.
37. Trugman JM, Leadbetter R, Zalis ME, et al. Treatment of severe axial tardive dystonia with clozapine. Case report and hypothesis. Mov Disord 1994; 9: 441–446.
38. Friedman JH. Clozapine treatment of psychosis in patients with tardive dystonia: Report of 3 cases. Mov Disord 1994; 9: 321–324.
39. Sachdev P, Kruk J, Kneebone M, et al. Clozapine-induced neuroleptic malignant syndrome: review and report of new cases. J Clin Psychopharmacol 1995; 15(5): 365–371.
40. Caroff SN, Mann SC, Campbell EC, Sullivan KA. Movement disorders associated with atypical antipsychotic drugs. J Clin Psychiatry 2002; 63(Suppl 4): 12–19.
41. Factor SA, Molho ES, Podskalny GD, Brown D. Parkinson's disease: drug-induced psychiatric states. Adv Neurol 1995; 65: 115–138.

42. Fenelon G, Mahieux F, Huon R, Ziegler M. Hallucinations in Parkinson's disease: prevalence, phenomenology and risk factors. Brain 2000; 123: 733–745.
43. Factor SA, Friedman JH. The emerging role of clozapine in the treatment of movement disorders. Mov Disord 1997; 12(4): 483–496.
44. Parkinson's Study Group. Low dose clozapine for the treatment of drug-induced psychosis in Parkinson's disease. N Engl J Med 1999, 340(10): 757–763.
45. Factor SA, Friedman JH. The emerging role of clozapine in the treatment of movement disorders. Mov Disord 1997; 12: 483–496.
46. French Clozapine Parkinson Study Group. Clozapine in drug-induced psychosis in Parkinson's Disease. Lancet 1999; 353: 2041–2042.
47. Castelao JF, Ferreira L, Gelders YG, et al. The efficacy of the D2 and 5-HT2 antagonist risperidone (R 64,766) in the treatment of chronic psychosis. An open dose-finding study. Schizophr Res 1989; 2(4–5): 411–415.
48. Peuskens J. Risperidone in the treatment of patients with chronic schizophrenia: a multinational, multi-centre, double-blind, parallel-group study versus haloperidol. Risperidone Study Group. Br J Psychiatry 1995; 166(6): 712–726, 727–733.
49. Lemmens P, Brecher M, Van Baelen B. A combined analysis of double-blind studies with risperidone vs. placebo and other antipsychotic agents: factors associated with extrapyramidal symptoms. Acta Psychiatr Scand 1999; 99(3): 160–170.
50. Chouinard G, Arnott W. Clinical review of risperidone. Can J Psychiatry 1993; 38 (Suppl) 3: S89–95.
51. Marder SR, Meibach RC. Risperidone in the treatment of schizophrenia. Am J Psychiatry 1994; 151(6): 825–835.
52. Jeste DV, Klausner M, Brecher M, et al. A clinical evaluation of risperidone in the treatment of schizophrenia: a 10-week, open-label, multicenter trial. ARCS Study Group. Assessment of Risperdal in a Clinical Setting. Psychopharmacology (Berl) 1997; 131(3): 239–247.
53. Claus A, Bollen J, De Cuyper H, et al. Risperidone versus haloperidol in the treatment of chronic schizophrenic inpatients: a multicentre double-blind comparative study. Acta Psychiatr Scand 1992; 85(4): 295–305.
54. Hoyberg OJ, Fensbo C, Remvig J, et al. Risperidone versus perphenazine in the treatment of chronic schizophrenic patients with acute exacerbations. Acta Psychiatr Scand 1993; 88(6): 395–402.
55. Min SK, Rhee CS, Kim CE, et al. Risperidone versus haloperidol in the treatment of chronic schizophrenic patients: a parallel group double-blind comparative trial. Yonsei Med J. 1993; 34(2): 179–190.
56. Malla AK, Norman RM, Scholten DJ, et al. A comparison of long-term outcome in first-episode schizophrenia following treatment with risperidone or a typical antipsychotic. J Clin Psychiatry 2001; 62(3): 179–184.
57. Kopala LC, Good KP, Honer WG. Extrapyramidal signs and clinical symptoms in first-episode schizophrenia: response to low-dose risperidone. J Clin Psychopharmacol 1997; 17(4): 308–313.
58. Simpson GM, Lindenmayer JP. Extrapyramidal symptoms in patients treated with risperidone. J Clin Psychopharmacol 1997; 17: 194–201.
59. Coley KC, Carter CS, DaPos SV, et al. Effectiveness of antipsychotic therapy in a naturalistic setting: a comparison between risperidone, perphenazine and haloperidol. J Clin Psychiatry 1999; 60(12): 850–856.
60. Rosebush RI, Mazurek MF. Neurological side effects in neuroleptic naive patients treated with haloperidol or risperidone. Neurology 1999; 52: 781–785.

61. Davidson M, Harvey PD, Vervecke J, et al. A long-term multicenter, open-label study of risperidone in elderly patients with psychosis. Int J Geriatr Psychiatry 200; 15: 506–514.

62. Lohr JB, Caligiuri MP, Edson R, et al. Treatment predictors of extrapyramidal side effects in patients with tardive dyskinesia: results from Veterans Affairs Cooperative Study 394. J Clin Psychopharmacol 2002; 22(2): 196–200.

63. Jeste DV, Okamoto A, Napolitano J, et al. Low incidence of persistent tardive dyskinesia in elderly patients with dementia treated with risperidone. Am J Psychiatry 2000; 157: 1150–1155.

64. Jeste DV, Lacro JP, Palmer B, et al. Incidence of tardive dyskinesia in early stages of low-dose treatment with typical neuroleptics in older patients. Am J Psychiatry 1999; 156: 309–311.

65. Katz IR, Jeste DV, Mintzer JE, et al. (Risperidone Study Group). Comparison of risperidone and placebo for psychosis and behavioral disturbances associated with dementia: a randomized, double-blind trial. J Clin Psychiatry 1999; 60: 107–115.

66. De Deyn PP, Rabheru K, Rassmussen A, et al. A randomized trial of risperidone, placebo and haloperidol for behavioral symptoms of dementia. Neurology 1999; 53: 946–955.

67. Chouinard G. Effects of risperidone in tardive dyskinesia: an analysis of the Canadian multicenter risperidone study. J Clin Psychopharmacol 1995; 15(suppl): 36S–44S.

68. Khan BU. Risperidone for severely disturbed behavior and tardive dyskinesia in developmentally disabled adults. J Autism Dev Disord 1997; 27: 479–489.

69. Friedman JH. Risperidone induced tardive dyskinesia ("Fly catchers tongue") in a neuroleptic naive patient. Med Health 1998; 81(8): 271–272.

70. Saran BM. Risperidone induced tardive dyskinesia. J Clin Psychiatry 1998; 59: 29–30.

71. Meco G, Alessandria A, Bonifati V, et al. Risperidone for hallucinations in levodopa-treated Parkinson's disease patients [letter]. Lancet 1994; 2: 1370–1371.

72. Ford B, Lynch T, Greene P. Risperidone in Parkinson's disease [letter]. Lancet 1994; 1: 344: 681.

73. Molho ES, Factor SA. Parkinson's disease: the treatment of drug-induced hallucinations and psychosis. Clin Neurol Neurosci Rep 2001; 1: 320–328.

74. Ellis T, Cudkowitz ME, Sexton PM, Growdon JH. Clozapine and risperidone treatment of psychosis in Parkinson's disease. J Neuropsychiatry Clin Neurosci 2000, 12(3): 364–369.

75. Klieser E, Lehman E, Kinzler E, et al. Randomized, double-blind, controlled trial of risperidone versus clozapine in patients with chronic schizophrenia. J Clin Psychopharmacol 1995; 15(suppl 1): 45S–51S.

76. Bondolfi G, Dufour H, Patris M, et al. Risperidone versus clozapine in treatment-resistant chronic schizophrenia: a randomized double-blind study. Am J Psychiatry 1998; 155: 499–504.

77. Lindenmayer J-P, Iskander A, Park M, et al. Clinical and neurocognitive effects of clozapine and risperidone in treatment-refractory schizophrenic patients: a prospective study. J Clin Psychiatry 1998; 59: 521–527.

78. Breier AF, Malhotra AK, Su TP, et al. Clozapine and risperidone in chronic schizophrenia: effects on symptoms, parkinsonian side effects, and neuroendocrine response. Am J Psychiatry 1999; 156: 294–298.

79. Miller CH, Mohr F, Umbricht D, et al. The prevalence of acute extrapyramidal signs and symptoms in patients treated with clozapine, risperidone, and conventional antipsychotics. J Clin Psychiatry 1998; 59: 69–75.

80. Azorin JM, Spiegel R, Remington G, et al. A double-blind comparative study of clozapine and risperidone in the management of severe chronic schizophrenia. Am J Psychiatry 2001; 158: 1305–1313.

81. Ho B-C, Miller D, Nopoulos P, et al. A comparative effectiveness study of risperidone and olanzapine in the treatment of schizophrenia. J Clin Psychiatry 1999; 60: 658–663.
82. Conley RR, Mahmoud R. A randomized double-blind study of risperidone and olanzapine in the treatment of schizophrenia or schizoaffective disorder. Am J Psychiatry 2001; 158: 765–774.
83. Tran PV, Dellva MA, Tollefson GD, et al. Extrapyramidal symptoms and tolerability of olanzapine versus haloperidol in the acute treatment of schizophrenia. J Clin Psychiatry 1997; 58: 205–211. Correction 1997; 58: 275.
84. Dossenbach MRK, Kratky P, Schneidman M, et al. Evidence for the effectiveness of olanzapine among patients nonresponsive and/or intolerant to risperidone. J Clin Psychiatry 2001; 62(suppl 2): 28–32.
85. Reinstein M, Bari M, Ginsberg L, et al. Quetiapine and risperidone in outpatients with psychotic disorders: results of the QUEST trial. In: New Research Programs and Abstracts of the 152nd Annual Meeting of the American Psychiatric Association, May 20, 1999; Washington, DC, Abstract NR630; 246.
86. Beasley CM Jr, Tollefson G, Tran PV, et al. Olanzapine versus placebo and haloperidol: acute phase results of the North American double-blind olanzapine trial. Neuropsychopharmacology 1996; 14: 111–123.
87. Tollefson GD, Beasley CM, Tran PV, et al. Olanzapine versus haloperidol in the treatment of schizophrenia and schizoaffective and schizophreniform disorders: results of an international collaborative trial. Am J Psychiatry 1997; 154: 457–465.
88. Beasley CM Jr. Hamilton SH, Crawford AM. Olanzapine versus haloperidol: acute phase results of the international double-blind olanzapine trial. Eur Neuropsychopharmacol 1997; 7: 125–137.
89. Tran PV, Hamilton SH, Kuntz AJ, et al. Double-blind comparison of olanzapine versus risperidone in the treatment of schizophrenia and other psychotic disorders. J Clin Psychopharmacol 1997; 17: 407–418.
90. Conley RR, Tamminga CA, Bartko JJ, et al. Olanzapine compared with chlorpromazine in treatment-resistant schizophrenia. Am J Psychiatry 1998; 155: 914–920.
91. Sanger TM, Lieberman JA, Tohen M, et al. Olanzapine versus haloperidol treatment in first episode psychosis. Am J Psychiatry 1999; 156: 79–87.
92. Costa e Silva JA, Alvarez N, Mazzoti G, et al. Olanzapine as alternative therapy for patients with haloperidol-induced extrapyramidal symptoms: results of a multicenter, collaborative trial in Latin America. J Clin Psychopharmacol 2001; 21: 375–381.
93. Beasley CM Jr. Tollefson GD, Tran PV, et al. Safety of olanzapine. J Clin Psychiatry 1997; 58(suppl 10): 13–17.
94. Beasley CM Jr, Dellva MA, Tamura RN, et al. Randomized double-blind comparison of the incidence of tardive dyskinesia in patients with schizophrenia during long-term treatment with olanzapine or haloperidol. Br J Psychiatry 1999; 174: 23–30.
95. Tollefson GD, Beasley CM, Tamura RN, et al. Blind, controlled, long-term study of the comparative incidence of treatment-emergent tardive dyskinesia with olanzapine or haloperidol. Am J Psychiatry 1997; 154: 1248–1254.
96. Kinon BJ, Basson BR, Stauffer VL, et al. Effect of chronic olanzapine treatment on the course of presumptive tardive dyskinesia. Schizophrenia Res 1999; 36: 363.
97. Kinon BJ, Stauffer VL, Wang L, et al. Olanzapine improves tardive dyskinesia in patients with schizophrenia: results of a controlled prospective study. Presented at the 53rd Institute on Psychiatric Services; October 2001; Orlando, Florida.
98. Sajatovic M, Perez D, Brescan D, Ramirez LF. Olanzapine therapy in elderly patients with schizophrenia. Psychopharmacol Bull 1998; 34: 819–823.

99. Madhusoodanan S, Brenner R, Suresh P, et al. Efficacy and tolerability of olanzapine in elderly patients with psychotic disorders: a prospective study. Ann Clin Psychiatry 2000; 12: 11–18.

100. Kontaxakis VP, Havaki-Kontaxaki BJ, Christodoulou, et al. Olanzapine-associated neuroleptic malignant syndrome. Progr Neuropsychopharmacol Biol Psychiatry 2002; 26(5): 897–902.

101. Hall KL, Taylor WH, Ware MR. Neuroleptic malignant syndrome due to olanzapine. Psychopharmacol Bull 2001; 35(3): 49–54.

102. Goetz CG, Blasucci LM, Leurgans S, Pappert EJ. Olanzapine and clozapine. Comparative effects on motor function in hallucinating PD patients. Neurology 2000, 55(6): 789–794.

103. Ondo WG, Levy JK, Vuong KD, Hunter C, Jankovic J. Olanzapine treatment for dopaminergic induced hallucinations. Mov Disord 2002; 17: 1031–1035.

104. Breier A, Sutton VK, Feldman PD, et al. Olanzapine in the treatment of dopaminomimetic induced psychosis in patients with Parkinson's disease. Biol Psychiatry 2002; 52; 438–445.

105. Tollefson GD, Birkett MA, Kiesler GM, et al. Double-blind comparison of olanzapine versus clozapine in schizophrenic patients clinically eligible for treatment with clozapine. Biol Psychiatry 2001; 49: 52–63.

106. Fabre LF, Arvantis L, Pultz J, et al. ICI 204,636, a novel, atypical antipsychotic: early indication of safety and efficacy in patients with chronic and subchronic schizophrenia. Clin Ther 1995; 17: 366–378.

107. Borison RL, Arvantis LA, Miller BG, et al. ICI 204,636, an atypical antipsychotic: efficacy and safety in a multicenter, placebo-controlled trial in patients with schizophrenia. J Clin Psychopharmacol 1996; 16: 158–169.

108. Small JG, Hirsch SR, Arvantis LA, et al. Quetiapine in patients with schizophrenia: a high and low dose double-blind comparison with placebo. Arch Gen Psychiatry 1997; 54: 549–557.

109. Arvanitis LA, Miller BG, and the Seroquel Trial 13 Study Group. Multiple fixed doses of Seroquel (quetiapine) in patients with acute exacerbation of schizophrenia: a comparison with haloperidol and placebo. Biol Psychiatry 1997; 42: 233–246.

110. Peuskens J, Link CGG. A comparison of quetiapine and chlorpromazine in the treatment of schizophrenia. Acta Psychiatr Scand 1997; 96: 265–273.

111. Meats P. Quetiapine (Seroquel) an effective and well-tolerated atypical antipsychotic. Int J Psychiatry Clin Pract 1997; 1: 231–239.

112. McManus DQ, Arvantis LA, Kowalcyk BB, et al. Quetiapine, a novel antipsychotic: experience in elderly patients with psychotic disorders. J Clin Psychiatry 1999; 60: 292–298.

113. Emsley RA, Raniwalla J, Bailey PJ, et al. A comparison of the effects of quetiapine (Seroquel) and haloperidol in schizophrenic patients with a history of and a demonstrated partial response to conventional antipsychotic treatment. Int Clin Psychopharmacol 2000; 15: 121–131.

114. Copolov DL, Link CGG, Kowalcyk B. A multicenter, double-blind, randomized comparison of quetiapine (ICI 204,636, "Seroquel") and haloperidol in schizophrenia. Psychol Med 2000; 30: 95–106.

115. Glazer WM, Morgenstern H, Pultz JA, et al. Incidence of tardive dyskinesia is lower with quetiapine treatment than with typical antipsychotics in patients with schizophrenia and schizoaffective disorder. Schizophr Res 2000; 41: 206–207.

116. Yeung PP, Liu S. Low incidence of persistent tardive dyskinesia with quetiapine. Presented at the 52nd Institute on Psychiatric Services; 2000 Philadelphia, PA.

117. Jeste DV, Lacro JP, Bailey A, et al. Lower incidence of tardive dyskinesias with risperidone compared with haloperidol in older patients. J Am Geriatr Soc 1999; 47: 716–719.

118. Tariot PN, Salzman C, Yeung PP, Pulz J, Rak IW. Long-term use of quetiapine in elderly patients with psychotic disorders. Clin Ther 2000; 22: 1068–1084.

119. Whalley N, Diaz P, Howard J. Neuroleptic malignant syndrome associated with the use of quetiapine [abstract]. Can J Hosp Pharm 1999; 52: 112.

120. Al-Waneen R. Neuroleptic malignant syndrome associated with quetiapine. Can J Psychiatry 2000; 45: 764–765.

121. Stanley AK, Hunter J. Possible neuroleptic malignant syndrome with quetiapine [letter]. Br J Psychiatry 2000; 176: 497.

122. Bourgeois JA, Babine S, Meyerovich M, et al. A case of neuroleptic malignant syndrome with quetiapine. J Neuropsychiatry Clin Neurosci 2002 14(1): 87.

123. Karagianis J, Phillips L, Hogan K, et al. Neuroleptic malignant syndrome associated with quetiapine. Can J Psychiatry 2001; 46(4): 370–371.

124. Hatch CD, Lund BC, Perry PJ. Failed challenge with quetiapine after neuroleptic malignant syndrome with conventional neuroleptics. Pharmacotherapy 2001; 21: 1003–1006.

125. Manhedran R, Winslow M, Lim D. Recurrent neuroleptic malignant syndrome. N Z J Psychiatry 2000; 34; 698–699.

126. Targum SD, Abbot JL. Efficacy of quetiapine in Parkinson's patients with psychosis. J Clin Psychopharmacol 2000, 20(1): 54–60.

127. Parsa MA, Bastani B. Quetiapine (Seroquel) in the treatment of psychosis in patients with Parkinson's disease. J Neuropsychiatry Clin Neurosci 1998; 10: 216–219.

128. Fernandez HH, Trieschmann ME, Burke MA, Jacques C, Friedman JH. Long term outcome of quetiapine use for psychosis among Parkinsonian patients. Mov Disord 2003; 18: 510–514.

129. Reddy S, Factor SA, Molho ES, Feustel PJ. The effect of quetiapine on psychosis and motor function in Parkinsonian patients with and without dementia. Mov Disord 2002; 17: 676–681.

130. Sommor BR. Quetiapine-induced extrapyramidal side effects in patients with Parkinson's disease: case report. J Geriatric Psychol Neurol 2001, 14(2): 99–100.

131. Goff DC, Posever T, Herz L, et al. An exploratory haloperidol-controlled dose-finding study of ziprasidone in hospitalized patients with schizophrenia or schizoaffective disorder. J Clin Psychopharmacol 1998; 18: 296–304.

132. Keck PE Jr., Buffenstein A, Ferguson J, et al. Ziprasidone 40 and 120 mg/day in the acute exacerbation of schizophrenia and schizoaffective disorder: a 4-week placebo-controlled trial. Psychopharmacology (Berl) 1998; 140: 173–184.

133. Daniel DG, Zimbroff DL, Potkin SG, et al. Ziprasidone 80 mg/day and 160 mg/day in the acute exacerbation of schizophrenia and schizoaffective disorder. A 6 week placebo controlled trial. Ziprasidone Study Group. Neuropsychopharmacology 1999; 20: 491–505.

134. Carnahan RM, Lund BC, Perry PJ. Ziprasidone, a new atypical antipsychotic drug. Pharmacotherapy 2001; 21: 717–730.

135. Lesem MD, Zajecka JM, Swift RH, et al. Intramuscular ziprasidone, 2 mg versus 10 mg, in the short term management of agitated psychotic patients. J Clin Psychiatry 2001; 62: 12–18.

136. Murty RG, Mistry SG, Chacko RC. Neuroleptic malignant syndrome with ziprasidone. J Clin Psychopharmacol 2002; 22(6): 624–626.

137. Jeste DV. Tardive dyskinesia in older patients. J Clin Psychiatry 2000; 61(suppl 4): 27–32.

138. Woerner MG, Alvir JMJ, Saltz BL, et al. Prospective study of tardive dyskinesia in the elderly: rates and risk factors. Am J Psychiatry 1998; 155: 1521–1528.

CHAPTER 12

Commentary: is tardive dyskinesia disappearing?

James B. Lohr

Is tardive dyskinesia (TD) disappearing? It is an optimistic question and, in my experience, one of the most commonly asked about TD. It also reflects a commonly held set of assumptions, which I believe can be summarized as follows:

1. TD is due to antipsychotic treatment.
2. Newer antipsychotics do not cause TD.
3. All patients requiring antipsychotics will eventually be treated with the newer agents.
4. TD will disappear.

Most disturbing, however, is that occasionally there is an additional concluding link added to this chain of reasoning:

5. Therefore, TD is no longer of much clinical concern.

In this chapter I would like to examine some of the problems associated with the concept that TD is disappearing, and whether the evidence really supports such a concept.

What does the "disappearance of TD" mean? Disappearance implies that at some point TD will cease to exist, that is, its prevalence will drop until it reaches 0%. Although this may seem like a straightforward determination to make, in practice it is plagued with difficulties.

One of the problems concerns inconsistency in the reports of the prevalence of TD over time and across studies. Prior to 1965, the estimated prevalence was 5%, but increased to 25% in 1980 [1, 2]. In the early 1990s the prevalence was considered to be in the range of 15% to 20%, but rates anywhere from 0.5% to over 50% have been reported [3]. In older patients, the prevalence has been reported to be much higher than in younger patients, in the range of 50% to 75% [4–8]. TD prevalence has also been reported to be higher in patients with mood disorders, being in the range of 9% to 64% [9–11]. In one direct comparison study of TD in schizophrenia and bipolar disorder the prevalence in schizophrenia was 25% and in bipolar disorder it was 42% [9].

Another problem is that some patients with psychosis manifest dyskinesias unrelated to treatment, which have sometimes been termed "spontaneous dyskinesias" (see Chapter 3). The point prevalence of these has often been estimated to be in the range of approximately 4% to 7% [4, 13], but in fact widely varying prevalence rates in antipsychotic-naïve patients with schizophrenia have been reported, from 0% to 77% [14–16]. Some of this variability may be accounted for by age, with increasing age of patients being associated with a higher rate of spontaneous dyskinesia. For example, Fenton [16] estimated that the prevalence rate of spontaneous dyskinesia in first-episode patients with schizophrenia may be about 4%, increasing to 12% in patients under 30 years who have been ill for several years, 25% in patients between age 30 and 50 years, and 40% in patients over 60 years. Some have argued that we can infer the disappearance of TD when the prevalence of TD matches that of spontaneous dyskinesias [17], but this is problematic too, for spontaneous dyskinesias have been poorly studied and inconsistently described, and they unquestionably vary with diagnosis, having been studied almost exclusively in schizophrenia. To confuse matters further, there is also a form of nonantipsychotic dyskinesias that emerge with advancing age (so-called senile dyskinesias) [18–20]. Because TD is a clinical diagnosis, based on the appearance of abnormal movements, and there is no known laboratory or other diagnostic test for it, it cannot be clearly discriminated from these other dyskinesias. This means that it will always be difficult to determine if and when TD disappears as a clinical phenomenon.

The fluctuating nature of TD is another problem [7, 21]. Patients with TD can suppress the movements voluntarily for periods of time, making assessment difficult. Even when the movements are clearly evident, they may not be recognized by clinicians, and underdiagnosis of TD has always been a significant clinical problem [22–24]. Patients themselves frequently do not notice the movements, and often do not complain about them, which further contributes to underrecognition [25–28].

Thus, there are problems determining the prevalence of TD at any given time. Is there, nevertheless, evidence to suggest that the prevalence may be declining? Of particular importance to answer, this question would be prevalence studies that have taken place in the last 5 years, when the newer, second-generation antipsychotic medications have become the most widely prescribed in the world. There have been a handful of studies since 1996 that have addressed the issue of prevalence of TD.

In 1997 Van Os et al. [29] reported that 17% of patients had TD over a 4-year follow-up period. In 1998 Van Harten and colleagues [30] reported a TD prevalence of 36% in patients who suffered primarily from schizophrenia. Two reports from 1999 [11, 31] gave TD prevalence rates of 16% and 18%, respectively, while a third report from 1999 [32] suggested a higher prevalence rate for men (21%) than women (11%) in patients who were under the age of 65 years. Schulze et al. [33], in a study from 2001, reported a prevalence rate of TD of 43%. In terms of older patients, a study of Woerner et al. [34] from 1998 reported a cumulative TD rate of 53% in patients treated for 3 years, and a study of Byne et al. [6] reported a rate of 60% in chronically institutionalized patients with schizophrenia over the age of 65 years. These prevalence or cumulative incidence rates are not different from those reported prior to the mid-1990s.

However, in none of these studies was the issue of second-generation medications addressed, so we do not know how many patients were on these newer drugs, nor what impact they may have had on the rates of TD.

Two studies, however, addressed the issue of second-generation medications directly. In a comparison of 1996 versus 1981 data, Kelly et al. [35] determined that more patients in the Nithsdale schizophrenia surveys had TD in 1996 than in 1981 (41% vs. 20%), and although when 97 matched pairs were examined, the differences were fewer (26% vs. 20%). In the same study, a comparison of patients on second-generation drugs (risperidone and sulpiride) versus first-generation drugs in 1996 revealed that 24% on second-generation medications had TD compared to 38% on first-generation, but the second-generation group was also younger (42 years vs. 51 years of age), and had a shorter duration of illness (13 years vs. 20 years), thus making it impossible to say if there was actually a reduced prevalence of TD in this group. More recently, Modestin et al. [36] determined that the point prevalence of TD in 200 patients treated with antipsychotic medications was 22%. Of these, 46 patients had been treated with clozapine for a prolonged time period (3 years or more), with no clear decrease in prevalence of TD (in fact, the prevalence was higher in the clozapine group). In 11 patients, TD appeared to have become manifest during the course of clozapine treatment.

Thus, there is currently no direct evidence that the prevalence of TD has declined or is declining, or that second-generation medications have impacted the prevalence of TD. So, where is this hopefulness for the disappearance of TD coming from? The optimism appears to be related to incidence studies that have been performed with some of the second-generation antipsychotics. These studies have shown a reduced incidence of TD with second-generation agents in comparison with first-generation drugs such as haloperidol over the time frames of the trials performed (generally only a few years). Yearly incidence rates for second-generation drugs are in the range of one-sixth to one-twelfth that of the first-generation antipsychotic haloperidol, in samples of both younger and older patients [37–43].

It is a problem to draw conclusions about prevalence from incidence studies. We know that a large proportion of patients with TD due to first-generation medications have a reduction or improvement in TD over time, even when the patients are continued on those medications. The remission rate of patients *continued* on first-generation medications over 5 to 10 years has been reported to be 25% to 50% or more [44–46]. In terms of patients for whom first-generation medications are *discontinued*, one estimate is that only 20% of patients with TD would show significant dyskinesia after 5 years [47]. Robinson and McCreadie [48] have suggested that it is this truly persistent TD, that is, that which is detectable on all occasions, which is the best index of TD outcome.

Although the incidence of TD is probably less with second-generation drugs, when it does occur we know nothing about its long-term course, which, for all we know, may be much more persistent than TD associated with first-generation agents. Suppose, for example, that the yearly incidence of TD with first-generation agents is 5%, and that with second-generation agents it is 0.5% (one-tenth). However, if permanent TD occurs in only one-fifth of the TD cases with first-generation drugs, but in all TD cases with first-generation drugs, then the incidence of permanent TD with second-generation drugs (0.5%) would still be half that of second-generation drugs (1%). At a 0.5% yearly incidence of permanent TD, then over a 20-year period of treatment the prevalence of TD would be 10%, which, although less than that observed with first-generation drugs, is still clinically significant. This discussion is speculative but in some ways that is the point – the fact that we do not have data on which to base firm convictions.

Another problem concerning the issue of TD disappearance is that certain groups of patients may be at high risk for TD, and it is not at all clear what the future of TD in these groups will be with the new drugs. We have already discussed the increased risk for TD in older patients, and, while the yearly incidence of TD with second-generation drugs in this group appears to be less than with first-generation drugs (3% vs. 25%), it is actually similar to that of first-generation drugs in younger patients (4–5%). Another high-risk group of patients is that with mood disorders. This group is of considerable concern, because the second-generation agents are showing important mood-stabilizing properties, and are being increasingly used for this purpose [49–51]. In the future, it appears that second-generation antipsychotics will be used more and more for the chronic treatment of bipolar disorder. Also, with the imminent appearance of long-acting injectable second-generation agents, these too will probably become commonly used for patients with bipolar illness. We simply have no idea what the long-term consequences of second-generation antipsychotics will be in bipolar patients. The studies of incidence of TD with these newer agents have been performed in schizophrenia and schizoaffective disorder and not mood disorders. Even if the second-generation drugs have a reduced incidence of TD overall, if they are used chronically in a much larger population of patients than first-generation drugs (a population including bipolar patients and others), then the number of patients who develop TD may still be substantial.

Given the difficulties in determining the prevalence of TD, the fact that recent prevalence studies of TD show rates that are similar to those reported in the past, the problems of interpreting incidence studies, and the growing importance of high-risk groups, optimism that the demise of TD may be close at hand should be tempered. I am concerned that, on the basis of a few short-term studies demonstrating a reduced incidence of TD with second-generation agents essentially only in schizophrenia and schizoaffective disorder, the medical world may be too eager to erase TD from the list of clinical concerns. Already, I am beginning to see clinicians give diagnoses of spontaneous dyskinesia or senile dyskinesia to patients receiving second-generation antipsychotic drugs, because of the assumption that it cannot be TD, since these drugs do not cause TD.

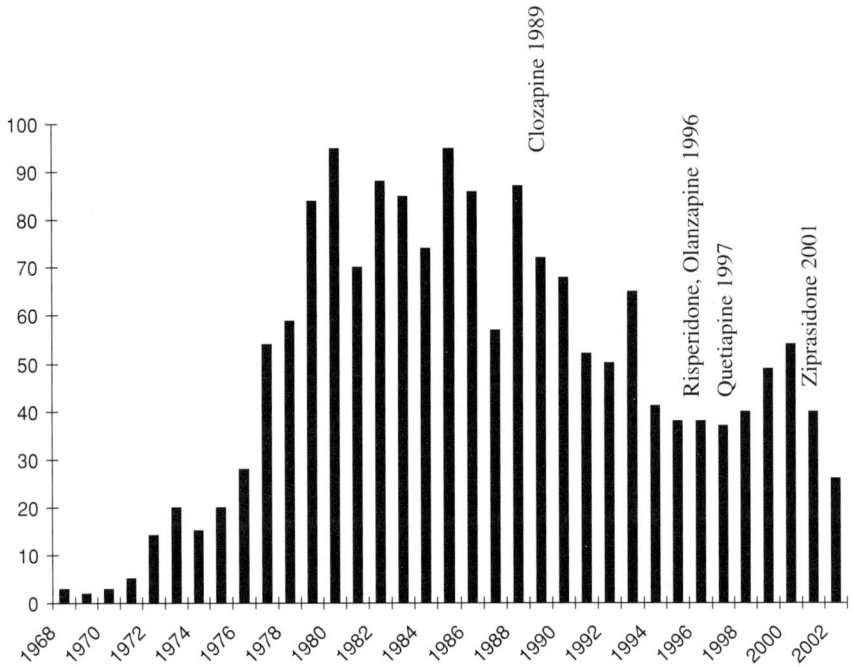

Figure 12.1 Numbers of English-language articles published per year with tardive dyskinesia or tardive dystonia in their titles, as determined by a search of PubMed with key words "tardive dyskinesia." The years of FDA approval for the second-generation antipsychotic agents are also shown. Note that data for the year 2002 only represent studies published through September.

So, the question arises, are we witnessing not so much a decline in TD, as a premature decline in *interest* in TD? Although difficult to answer, I decided to address the question by performing a search on the number of articles published on TD per year for the past several decades. I have plotted by year the number of articles drawn from a PubMed search of English language articles with the key words "tardive dyskinesia," which have the words tardive dyskinesia or tardive dystonia in their titles. This is shown in Fig. 12.1. I have also added the dates of FDA approval of the various second-generation antipsychotic agents. Although far from a definitive proof, it is of concern to note the drop-off in publications beginning in the early 1990s, shortly after the introduction of clozapine. This is considerably before the other agents were introduced, and certainly long before there was good evidence of even a reduction in incidence of TD with the newer agents.

In summary, it is premature to say that TD is disappearing. Although it would make sense that the prevalence of TD should decline over time, considering the lower incidence of TD with second-generation agents and the widespread and growing use of these drugs, there are no actual data to support the notion that TD is declining in prevalence. On the other hand, there does appear to be evidence that *interest* in TD is declining, and this is very troublesome, because it may mean fewer studies will be performed to address these very important issues.

References

1. Jeste DV, Wyatt RJ. Changing epidemiology of tardive dyskinesia: an over view. Am J Psychiatry 1981; 138: 297–309.
2. Kane JM, Smith JM. Tardive dyskinesia: prevalence and risk factors, 1959 to 1979. Arch Gen Psychiatry 1982; 39: 473–481.
3. American Psychiatry Association. Tardive dyskinesia: A task force report of the American Psychiatric Association. American Psychiatric Association, Washington DC, 1992.
4. Lieberman J, Kane J, Woerner M, et al. Prevalence of tardive dyskinesia in elderly samples. Psychopharmacol Bull 1984; 29: 22–26.
5. Jeste DV, Caligiuri MP, Paulsen JS, et al. Risk of tardive dyskinesia in older patients: a prospective longitudinal study of 266 patients. Arch Gen Psychiatry 1995; 52: 756–765.
6. Byne W, White L, Parella M, et al. Tardive dyskinesia in a chronically institutionalized population of elderly schizophrenic patients: prevalence and association with cognitive impairment. Int J Geriatr Psychiatry 1998; 13: 473–479.
7. Glazer WM. Review of incidence studies of tardive dyskinesia associated with typical antipsychotics. J Clin Psychiatry 2000; 61(suppl 4): 15–20.
8. Caligiuri MP, Jeste DV, Lacro JP. Antipsychotic-induced movement disorders in the elderly: epidemiology and treatment recommendations. Drugs Aging 2000; 17: 363–384.
9. Yassa R, Nair V, Schwartz G. Tardive dyskinesia and the primary psychiatric diagnosis. Psychosomatics 1984; 25: 135–138.
10. Mukherjee S, Rosen AM, Caracci G, et al. Persistent tardive dyskinesia in bipolar patients. Arch Gen Psychiatry 1986; 43: 342–346.
11. Akbostanci MC, Atbasoglu EC, Balaban H. Tardive dyskinesia, mild drug-induced dyskinesia, and drug-induced parkinsonism: risk factors and topographic distribution. Acta Neurol Belg 1999; 99: 176–181.
12. Keck PE, Jr, McElroy SL, Strakowski SM, et al. Antipsychotics in the treatment of mood disorders and risk of tardive dyskinesia. J Clin Psychiatry 2000; 61(suppl 4): 33–38.
13. Casey DE. Spontaneous and tardive dyskinesia: clinical and laboratory studies. J Clin Psychiatry 1985; 46: 42–47.
14. Fenton WS, Wyatt RJ, McGlashan TH. Risk factors for spontaneous dyskinesia in schizophrenia. Arch Gen Psychiatry 1994; 51: 643–650.
15. Fenton WS, Blyler CR, Wyatt RJ, McGlashan GH. Prevalence of spontaneous dyskinesia in schizophrenic and non-schizophrenic psychiatric patients. Br J Psychiatry 1997; 171: 265–268.
16. Fenton WS. Prevalence of spontaneous dyskinesia in schizophrenia. J Clin Psychiatry 2000; 61(suppl 4): 10–14.
17. Quinn NP. Prevalence of abnormal movement disorders associated with neuroleptics. Am J Psychiatry 1992; 149: 1123–1124.
18. Delwaide PJU, Desseilles M. Spontaneous buccolinguofacial dyskinesia in the elderly. Acta Neurol Scand 1977; 56: 256–262.
19. Weiner WJ, Klawans HL. Lingual-facial-buccal movements in the elderly. J Am Geriatr Soc 1973; 21: 314–317.

20. Lohr JB, Bracha HS. Association of psychosis and movement disorders in the elderly. Psychiatr Clin N Am 1988; 11: 61–81.
21. Caligiuri MP, Lohr JB, Vaughan RM, et al. Fluctuation of tardive dyskinesia. Biol Psychiatry 1995; 38: 336–339.
22. Brown P, Funk SC. Tardive dyskinesia: barriers to the professional recognition of an iatrogenic disease. J Health Soc Behav 1986; 27: 116–132.
23. Weiden PJ, Mann J, Haas G, et al. Clinical nonrecognition of neuroleptic-induced movement disorders: a cautionary study. Am J Psychiatry 1987; 144: 1148–1153.
24. Hansen TE, Brown WL, Weigel RM, et al. Underrecognition of tardive dyskinesia and drug-induced parkinsonism by psychiatric residents. Gen Hosp Psychiatry 1992; 14: 340–344.
25. Alexopoulos GS. Lack of complaints in schizophrenics with tardive dyskinesia. J Nerv Ment Disord 1979; 167: 125–127.
26. Myslobodsky MS, Tomer R, Holden T, et al. Cognitive impairment in patients with tardive dyskinesia. J Nerv Ment Disord 1985; 173: 156–160.
27. Lohr JB, Lohr MA, Wasli E, et al. Self-perception of tardive dyskinesia and neuroleptic-induced parkinsonism: a study of clinical correlates. Psychopharmacol Bull 1987; 23: 211–214.
28. Chong SA, Remington G, Mahendran R, et al. Awareness of tardive dyskinesia in Asian patients with schizophrenia. J Clin Psychopharmacol 2001; 21(2): 235–237.
29. Van Os J, Fahy T, Jones P, et al. Tardive dyskinesia: who is at risk? Acta Psychiatr Scand 1997; 96: 206–216.
30. Van Harten PN, Hoek HW, Matroos GE, et al. Intermittent neuroleptic treatment and risk for tardive dyskinesia: Curacao extrapyramidal syndromes study III. Am J Psychiatry 1998; 155: 565–567.
31. Muscettola G, Barbato G, Pampallona S, et al. Extrapyramidal syndromes in neuroleptic-treated patients: prevalence, risk factors, and association with tardive dyskinesia. J Clin Psychopharmacol 1999; 19: 203–208.
32. Van Os J, Walsh E, Van Horn E, et al. Tardive dyskinesia in psychosis: are women really more at risk? Acta Psychiatr Scand 1999; 99: 288–293.
33. Schulze TG, Muller DJ, Krauss H, et al. Affective symptomatology in schizophrenia: a risk factor for tardive dyskinesia? Eur Psychiatry 2001; 16: 71–74.
34. Woerner MG, Alvir JMJ, Saltz BL, et al. Prospective study of tardive dyskinesia in the elderly: rates and risk factors. Am J Psychiatry 1998; 155: 1521–1528.
35. Kelly C, McCreadie T, MacEwan T, et al. Nithsdale schizophrenia surveys. 17. Fifteen year review. Br J Psychiatry 1998; 172: 513–517.
36. Modestin J, Stephan PL, Erni T, et al. Prevalence of extrapyramidal syndromes in psychiatric inpatients and the relationship of clozapine treatment to tardive dyskinesia. Schizophr Res 2000; 42: 223–230.
37. Tollefson GD, Beasley CM, Tamura RN, et al. Blind, controlled, long-term study of the comparative incidence of treatment-emergent tardive dyskinesia with olanzapine or haloperidol. Am J Psychiatry 1997; 154: 1248–1254.
38. Jeste DV, Lacro JP, Bailey A, et al. Lower incidence of tardive dyskinesia with risperidone compared with haloperidol in older patients. J Am Geriatr Soc 1999; 47: 716–719.
39. Beasley CM, Dellva MA, Tamura RB, et al. Randomised double-blind comparison of the incidence of tardive dyskinesia in patients with schizophrenia during long-term treatment with olanzapine or haloperidol. Br J Psychiatry 1999; 174: 23–30.
40. Glazer WM. Expected incidence of tardive dyskinesia associated with atypical antipsychotics. J Clin Psychiatry 2000; 61(suppl 4): 21–26.

41. Glazer WM, Morgenstern H, Pultz JA, et al. Incidence of tardive dyskinesia is lower with quetiapine treatment than with typical antipsychotics in patients with schizophrenia and schizoaffective disorder. Schizophr Res 2000; 41: 206–207.

42. Jeste DV, Okamoto A, Napolitano J, et al. Low incidence of persistent tardive dyskinesia in elderly patients with dementia treated with risperidone. Am J Psychiatry 2000; 157: 150–1155.

43. Caroff SN, Mann SC, Campbell EC, et al. Movement disorders associated with atypical antipsychotic drugs. J Clin Psychiatry 2002; 63(suppl 4): 12–19.

44. Yassa R, Nair V. Mild tardive dyskinesia: an 8-year follow-up study. Acta Psychiatr Scand 1989; 81: 139–140.

45. Richardson MA, Casey DE, Lin S. Tardive dyskinesia: resolving persisting, new cases – demographics and treatment [abstract]. Biol Psychiatry 1989; 25(7A, suppl): 161A.

46. Gardos G, Casey DE, Cole JO, et al. Ten-year outcome of tardive dyskinesia. Am J Psychiatry 1994; 151: 836–841.

47. Wyatt RJ, Khot V. Reply to Quinn NP. Am J Psychiatry 1992; 149: 1124.

48. Robinson ADT, McCreadie RG. The Nithsdale schizophrenic survey, V: follow-up of tardive dyskinesia after $3^1{}_2$ years. Br J Psychiatry 1986; 149: 621–623.

49. Frye MA, Ketter TA, Altshuler LL, et al. Clozapine in bipolar disorder: treatment implications for other atypical antipsychotics. J Affect Disord 1998; 48: 91–104.

50. Strakowski SM, DelBello MP, Adler CM. Comparative efficacy and tolerability of drug treatments for bipolar disorder. CNS Drugs 2001; 15: 701–718.

51. Kusumakar V. Antidepressants and antipsychotics in the long-term treatment of bipolar disorder. J Clin Psychiatry 2002; 63(suppl 10): 23–28.

PART 3

Dopaminomimetic drugs

Dyskinesia induced by levodopa and dopamine agonists in patients with Parkinson's disease

John G. Nutt and Matthew Brodsky

History

The seminal report of Cotzias, Van Woert, and Schiffer, published in 1967, described how chronically administered oral D-levodopa ameliorated the signs and symptoms of Parkinson's disease but included the observation that athetoid movements were induced in some patients by the drug [1]. This was an unexpected side effect of the drug because the earlier report from Birkmeyer and Hornykiewicz on the acute effects of D-levodopa administered intravenously to patients with parkinsonism had not described the production of involuntary movements [2]. A subsequent report from Cotzias et al. in 1969 indicated the magnitude of the problem; 50% of the patients receiving D-levodopa or levodopa developed dyskinesia [3]. The rapid acceptance of levodopa as the therapy of choice for parkinsonism resulted in a number of clinical reports in the early 1970s, many of which emphasized the high prevalence of levodopa-induced dyskinesia [4–6]. In the mid-to-late 1970s, distinctive patterns of dyskinesia were recognized, including "peak dose" dyskinesia [7, 8], "diphasic dyskinesia" [8, 9], and "off" dystonia [10, 11].

Apomorphine, a dopamine D-1 and D-2 agonist, was the first agonist to be tried in Parkinson's disease, the initial investigations antedating the introduction of levodopa. Schwab, Amador, and Lettvin [12] found that small subcutaneous or oral doses produced modest improvement in the parkinsonism and no dyskinesia. The interest in apomorphine was revived by Cotzias, who noted a more dramatic effect of the drug on parkinsonism as well as the fact that it would induce dyskinesia in some patients in whom dyskinesia had appeared during chronic levodopa therapy [13]. Chronic oral administration of apomorphines was shown to produce dyskinesia that was very similar to that induced in the patients by levodopa [14].

Bromocriptine, a dopamine D-2 agonist, introduced by Calne in 1974, was also found to induce dyskinesia in patients who had developed dyskinesia from levodopa [15]. Other orally effective direct-acting dopamine D-2 agonists (pergolide, lisuride, PHNO, mesulergine) also induced dyskinesia. However, patients treated only with bromocriptine from the initiation of dopaminergic therapy and unexposed to levodopa, rarely developed dyskinesia [16, 17]. These observations focused interest on the factors important for the induction of dyskinesia in Parkinson's disease and resulted in the introduction of two new agonists, pramipexole and ropinirole, with an indication for early parkinsonism. This indication for dopamine agonists is backed by randomized clinical trials showing that these agonists are associated with considerably less potential for inducing dyskinesia than is levodopa [18, 19].

Another important development in the history of levodopa and dopamine agonist-induced dyskinesia was the introduction of the MPTP-treated monkey as a model of parkinsonism [20] that developed dyskinesia with repeated dosing with dopaminergic agents [21]. Physiological and pharmacological investigations of this model have yielded insight into the physiology and pharmacology of drug-induced dyskinesia in parkinsonian patients and allowed separation of drug- and disease-related factors.

Stereotaxic surgery, both ablative lesions and deep brain high frequency stimulation, and their effects on levodopa-induced dyskinesia have provided evidence for the neural circuits responsible for dyskinesia in humans. Positron emission tomography has provided another way by which to investigate the circuitry underlying dyskinesia. Finally, grafting of fetal dopamine neurons into parkinsonian subjects has revealed a new form of dyskinesia, so-called "run-away dyskinesia" or "off-drug dyskinesia," which may persist when antiparkinsonian medications are completely withdrawn [22, 23]. This observation may require revisions to our theories of the causes of dyskinesia.

Clinical features

Forms of levodopa-induced involuntary movements
Choreoathetosis

Choreoathetosis is the most common pattern of involuntary movement induced by levodopa and dopamine agonists. This form of dyskinesia often begins with very subtle rocking movements of the trunk, nodding movements of the head, or sinuous movements of the fingers, ankles, or toes. The choreoathetosis may become very severe and may affect any skeletal muscle group. This levodopa-induced dyskinesia may be indistinguishable from the movements of Huntington's disease or tardive dyskinesia. Choreoathetosis may be as disabling as the parkinsonism, but in most patients it produces modest disability and most patients prefer choreoathetosis to the parkinsonian state.

Dystonia

Dystonia is the second most common pattern for levodopa-induced dyskinesia. Dystonia in patients with parkinsonism need not be related to the use of dopaminergic drugs. Some patients have dystonia, particularly of the foot, as an early manifestation of their parkinsonism and before any drug therapy is started [24]. Most commonly, dystonia in Parkinson disease (PD) is related to the long-term use of dopaminergic drugs. Dystonia is often brought out by movement or use of the affected muscle group. It may affect any part of the body. Dystonia affecting the cranial musculature may interfere with speech and swallowing. A patient with this type of dystonia may appear relatively normal when sitting quietly although the corners of the mouth may be excessively retracted. On attempting to speak, involuntary contractures of facial, lingual, and masticatory muscles become apparent and may disrupt speech, chewing, and swallowing. Dystonic posturing of the ankle and toes, often accompanied with pain when the patient is "off" is a distinctive pattern in patients receiving levodopa chronically.

Dystonia often coexists with choreoathetosis in the same patient. Both may appear concurrently, with the dyskinesia being a mixture of choreic and dystonic movements, or there may be dystonic movements at one time and choreoathetotic movements at another time.

Ballism

Levodopa-induced involuntary movements can be extremely severe in some patients, producing wild, flinging, ballistic movements of the limbs that are very disabling and may result in injury.

Stereotyped movements

Stereotyped movements may occur with chronic levodopa therapy. These may take the form of stepping or kicking movements of the legs, particularly as the patient passes from "off" to "on" [25]. Peculiar patterns of gait may be seen, most commonly a tendency to lift one leg too high to give the patient a gait sometimes characterized as a "hemi-goose-step march." Occasionally, stereotyped movements could be characterized as tics, but it is rare for tics to be the only manifestation of levodopa-induced involuntary movements with an absence of other choreoathetotic movements.

Myoclonus

Myoclonus may be seen in parkinsonian patients treated chronically with levodopa [26]. It may occur in the setting of cognitive impairment and psychiatric symptoms and be a sign of a metabolic encephalopathy. However, myoclonus may also be induced by levodopa as an "on" phenomenon [25]. It is uncommon that the myoclonus is so severe as to produce disability itself or to require treatment.

Tremor

Tremor is, of course, part of the parkinsonism triad. However, it is worth noting that the tremor of Parkinson's disease may be augmented by levodopa. This tends to be a transitory phenomenon during each dose cycle. The tremor tends to be of lower amplitude when the patient is more severely "off" and to become more pronounced just as the patient begins to turn "on" and even be transiently mixed with choreoathetotic dyskinesia. The tremor may also be exaggerated as the patient turns "off."

Akathisia

Akathisia is the subjective sensation of the need to move not caused by other sensory complaints or anxiety. It is generally manifested by restlessness and fidgety movements. Restlessness is a rather nonspecific symptom. In the absence of the compulsion to move, this should not be termed akathisia. Akathisia may be seen in untreated Parkinson's disease but more commonly occurs in patients receiving dopaminergic drugs. A relationship to the dopaminergic drug cycle may be present in some patients; in some, the drugs appear to relieve the symptoms and, in others, they appear to induce them [27].

Temporal patterns of dyskinesia

Peak dose dyskinesia

Peak dose dyskinesia is dyskinesia occurring when the effects of levodopa on the parkinsonism are most apparent [28]. For this reason, it is sometimes called "on" dyskinesia. Although also termed "peak dose" dyskinesia, the dyskinesia often does not directly relate to plasma peaks of levodopa, as is also true for the improvement in parkinsonism [29]. The dyskinesia is commonly choreoathetotic but may be dystonic, ballistic, or stereotyped. This form of dyskinesia tends to be present throughout the period of time the patient is experiencing a reduction in the parkinsonian symptomatology (sometimes referred to as a "square-wave" response) [30]. This is the most commonly observed pattern of levodopa-induced dyskinesia [25].

Dyskinesia need not appear in all body parts simultaneously after a dose of levodopa [25]. For example, some patients will note that dyskinesia appears in the arms while the legs are still very parkinsonian. Alternatively, the legs may develop dyskinesia while a typical parkinsonian rest tremor persists in the arms. This mixture of "on" dyskinesia and parkinsonism often appears to be in a transient state when presumably striatal dopamine is near critical level. As striatal dopamine concentrations rise, only dyskinesia is present, and when levodopa is withheld for several hours, only parkinsonian bradykinesia and tremor are present. It is less common to see a marked side-to-side dissociation with, for example, one arm dyskinetic and the other tremulous. However, occasionally, the mixture of dyskinesia and tremor may be complex; for example, dyskinesia in the shoulder and elbow and tremor in the hand. Similarly, mixtures of parkinsonism and dyskinesia occur simultaneously in some neuroleptic-treated patients.

Diphasic dyskinesia

Diphasic dyskinesia refers to choreoathetotic, dystonic, stereotyped, or ballistic movements that appear as levodopa begins to take effect and as the drug effects wane [7, 9, 25, 31, 32]. Thus, the patient may have bursts of dyskinesia as the drug begins to produce an antiparkinsonism effect succeeded by another burst of dyskinesia as the drug effects wear off. In between these periods of exaggerated dyskinesia, there may be good antiparkinsonism effects with less dyskinesia. This diphasic pattern of dyskinesia is not always apparent with each dose cycle and often is manifest only by exacerbation of dyskinesia at the end of some dose cycles. Diphasic dyskinesias can be extremely severe with ballistic movements accompanied by marked sweating, hypertension, and tachycardia. Sudden death has occurred during these episodes, presumably related to cardiac arrhythmias [28]. This severe form of diphasic dyskinesia is, luckily, uncommon.

Diphasic dyskinesia in a less severe form, however, may be extremely common. Stereotyped, repetitive leg movements commonly have a diphasic pattern. Many patients will have an exacerbation of their tremor just before they begin to turn on, immediately followed by dyskinesia. The dyskinesia and tremor may even be mixed or alternate for several minutes. The dyskinesia may then partially remit and the patient is left with a milder degree of dyskinesia but good control of the parkinsonism until the effects of the medicine begin to wear off when the sequence is repeated [33]. A diphasic pattern of dyskinesia has also been seen in monkeys with MPTP-induced parkinsonism treated with levodopa or apomorphine [34].

"Off" dystonia
Dystonia, generally affecting the legs and frequently painful, occurs when dopaminergic drug levels are low, such as when the patients have been without medicine overnight or as the effects of a dose wear off [10, 11, 25, 32, 35, 36]. Because of the predisposition for it to occur in the morning, it also is termed "early morning dystonia" [10]. Commonly, the dystonia produces flexion or extension of the toes, inversion, or plantar flexion of the ankles, and internal rotation of the leg. However, dystonia may affect the trunk and arms, although this is less common. Cramping pain is almost always present with "off" dystonia. As implied by the term "off," dystonia is present when the parkinsonism is more apparent, that is, when the antiparkinsonian effects of the drug have dissipated or the patient is "off." The dystonia is frequently precipitated when the patient attempts to walk or becomes anxious. "Off" dystonia can generally be clinically differentiated from "peak dose" or "diphasic" dystonic dyskinesias by the timing of the dyskinesia in relation to the dose cycle and by the presence of cramping pain.

"Runaway dyskinesia"
This new pattern of dyskinesia has been described only in patients that have received embryonic midbrain grafts and have been followed for one or more years [22, 23]. The dyskinesia is unrelated to the dosing cycle and persists even if dopaminergic drugs are completely stopped. It may be so severe as to require deep brain stimulation or pallidotomy for control of the dyskinesia.

Spatial patterns of dyskinesia
Dyskinesia is worse on the side most affected by parkinsonism
Idiopathic parkinsonism is often asymmetrical, the tremor, rigidity, and bradykinesia appearing in one arm or leg first and spreading over months to years to involve the other limbs. The asymmetry in severity of parkinsonism at presentation may persist throughout the course of the disease. Peak dose dyskinesia as well as "off" dystonia are generally first apparent on this more affected side of the body and may be more severe on the more affected side throughout the course of the illness [37].

Somatic musculature affected by dyskinesia
Peak dose and diphasic dyskinesia commonly affect cranial, trunk, and limb musculature. Extraocular muscles are usually spared, although there are occasional cases in which dyskinesia affects the extraocular muscles [38, 39]. Patients with Parkinson's disease and levodopa-induced fluctuations in motor function may have respiratory complaints, particularly dyspnea. Sometimes, dyspnea is associated with dyskinetic movements of the respiratory muscles [40, 41]. However, dopaminergic drugs may induce dyspnea without obvious dyskinesia of chest or abdominal musculature. It has been postulated that dyskinesia of the diaphragm or upper airway musculature may be responsible or that there is a direct effect on medullary respiratory centers [41, 42]. Dyspnea may also be an "off" symptom, perhaps related to chest wall rigidity, involuntary movements of the upper airway, or anxiety [43].

Severity of dyskinesia
Effects of emotion, stress, and concentration
The severity of dyskinesia waxes and wanes throughout the day and even during a single-dose cycle. One clear contributing factor to this is the emotional state of the patient. Stress will often exacerbate dyskinesia [30]. However, stress may sometimes completely abolish the dyskinesia and concomitantly turn the patient "off." Both effects may be seen in the same patient at different times and presumably the effects of stress depend on whether the brain dopamine levels are well above threshold (stress then increasing dyskinesia) or close to threshold (stress turning the patient "off"). Concentration on mental tasks also brings out dyskinesia [44].

Effects of activity
Dyskinesia lessens when the patient is sitting or lying quietly and disappears or is greatly reduced if the patient is asleep. Conversely, dyskinesia is often brought out by motor activity [30, 44]. To some extent, this increase in dyskinesia resembles mirror movements or "motor overflow." For example, when the patient begins to use one hand in a motor task, dyskinesia will appear in the other limbs. Even talking is sufficient to bring out dyskinesia in many patients.

Effects of dopaminergic drug dose

Peak dose dyskinesias are generally considered to be dose-responsive, that is, dyskinesia is more severe with larger doses of drug [28]. However, most studies find that the severity of dyskinesia is not very dose-related, although the duration of the dyskinesia is related to the size of the dose or the peak plasma levodopa levels [29, 45]. This means that if the patient has dyskinesia, it is generally either present or absent without a gradient of severity [30].

It is also assumed that, at least initially, there is a therapeutic window and that more drug is required to produce dyskinesia than to produce the antiparkinsonian effects [28, 46, 47]. It is for these reasons, that is, to keep the plasma concentrations within the therapeutic window, that many physicians reduce the dose of levodopa and increase the frequency of dosing when dyskinesia appears. However, the evidence for a therapeutic window is based on evidence from very few patients. The majority of patients either have no dyskinesia at all or have dyskinesia that coincides with the antiparkinsonian effects [46]. Studies with intravenous infusions of levodopa have not found a consistent therapeutic window where the antiparkinsonian effects can be obtained without dyskinesia [29, 30]. Oral dosing with the associated peaks and troughs in plasma concentrations makes a therapeutic window problematic.

Natural history
Appearance of dyskinesia

Dyskinesia is not apparent with the first doses of levodopa or dopamine agonists at the initiation of long-term therapy with levodopa. However, dyskinesia may appear during the first month of chronic treatment with levodopa and successively more patients develop it over the ensuing months [4–6]. This delay in emergence of dyskinesia indicates that dyskinesia is not determined by severity of dopaminergic denervation but is somehow induced by repeated exposure to levodopa. In other words, dyskinesia represents sensitization or priming to levodopa or to other dopaminergic agents. Repeated dosing with levodopa is also required to induce dyskinesia in monkeys with MPTP-induced parkinsonism, a presumably nonprogressive dopaminergic lesion. The first doses of dopaminergic drugs do not induce dyskinesia, but repeated administration over days to weeks is required [34, 48–50].

Dyskinesias first appear as very subtle, fidgety movements that may be difficult to separate from normal extraneous movements. The fact that the movements are dyskinesia may become obvious if the patient is seen at another time when they have had no dopaminergic drugs for hours or overnight and the movements are absent. The patient and family are generally unaware of these subtle dyskinesias. Thus the emergence of dyskinesia may go undetected for some time. In a longitudinal study, dyskinesias were observed in 8 of 18 subjects after the first 6 months of levodopa therapy; only one of whom was aware of the dyskinesias. After 4 years, 13 of the 18 subjects had dyskinesia and 10 of those 13 were aware of their dyskinesia [51]. These observations must be considered when incidence of dyskinesia is an endpoint in clinical studies.

The relationship of development of "on" dyskinesia to the appearance of the fluctuating response ("wearing off" and "on-off") is problematic. There is evidence that a short-duration response (a motor fluctuation) to levodopa may be seen with the first doses of the drug but that these fluctuations are so subtle as to escape the patient's and physician's notice under most circumstances [52, 53]. The appearance of dyskinesia intermittently throughout the day may therefore offer the first evidence, recognized by patient and physician, that motor function varies during the day. Although the emergence of motor fluctuations and dyskinesia may occur at about the same time [54], there is no absolute requirement for motor fluctuations before dyskinesia appears. However, the fact that dyskinesia tends to occur in patients with a good antiparkinson response to levodopa suggests that there may be a relation and raises the question, considered below, of whether the therapeutic benefit of levodopa can be separated from dyskinesia.

"Off" dystonia also appears with chronic levodopa therapy and at first is infrequent and minor but may increase in severity to dominate the patient's complaints. "Off" dystonia is generally seen in patients treated with levodopa for years rather than months [10, 11, 35]. Many patients have both "on" dyskinesia and "off" dystonia but there is no recognized connection between these two forms of dyskinesia except that both are related to long-term therapy with levodopa [25].

Changes in severity of dyskinesia during chronic therapy

With continued levodopa therapy, the severity of the dyskinesia increases [51] and the initially subtle movement becomes more clearly choreic, dystonic, or stereotypic. Initially, dyskinesia may be present only in the most affected limb or just in the face, neck, or trunk. With continued therapy, the dyskinesia may spread to involve other body parts although it sometimes remains localized. The same pattern of increase in severity of dyskinesia and gradual involvement of more muscle groups is seen in parkinsonian monkeys treated with levodopa [34, 48–50].

Variations in severity during the day

The patient's dyskinesia is generally related to the dose cycle. This pattern may not be identical with each dose, perhaps because of the inter-dose variability in absorption and blood-to-brain transport of levodopa. Many patients notice that the control of the parkinsonism is not as good in the afternoon, and paradoxically, the afternoons may be associated with more dyskinesia. This may be partially due to poorer absorption of levodopa in the afternoon and increasing plasma amino acid concentrations [55]. However, a pharmacokinetics explanation is not adequate to explain all the diurnal patterns in motor fluctuations and dyskinesia [56].

Withdrawal of dopaminergic agents

Withdrawal of levodopa or dopamine agonists will generally cause an immediate disappearance of peak dose and diphasic dyskinesia. The "off" dystonia will also disappear within approximately 24 hours [35]. The consequence, of course, is that the patient is left in a state of parkinsonism. Very rarely, patients will have "on" dyskinesia when they have been overnight without antiparkinsonian medications [36]. In our experience, this dyskinesia is associated with less parkinsonism than is generally present when the patient is fully "off" and is self-limited, lasting minutes to a couple of hours. It may be related to sleep benefit [57]. Another exception to the clinical dictum that withdrawal of levodopa stops all dyskinesia has emerged in the studies of fetal midbrain grafting in PD. Patients receiving the grafts have developed intractable "on" dyskinesia, termed "runaway" dyskinesia, several years after the grafting procedure. The dyskinesia persists even when antiparkinsonian medications are withdrawn [22, 23]. The etiology of this phenomenon is unknown, but perhaps is due to elevated striatal levels of extracellular dopamine from the graft. A recent PET study of five transplanted patients with runaway dyskinesia revealed modest increases in levodopa uptake in left dorsal posterior and ventral putamen compared to that in transplanted subjects without dyskinesia [58].

Epidemiology

Prevalence of dyskinesia in levodopa-treated patients

Estimates of prevalence of levodopa-induced dyskinesias from the literature are hampered by a number of factors. First, the criteria for diagnosis of levodopa-induced dyskinesias are often not explicitly defined. Second, dyskinesia appears gradually, making it difficult to draw the line between vague fidgety movements and definite dyskinesia. Third, "on" dyskinesia, diphasic dyskinesia, and "off" dystonia are often not differentiated. Fourth, most studies describing prevalence of dyskinesia do not indicate whether the presence of dyskinesia is based on direct observation or on the patient's history. Patients' histories are notoriously unreliable because patients often cannot differentiate tremor, dyskinesia, and cramps. The chances of the physician observing and characterizing dyskinesia depend upon whether the patient is seen throughout one or more dose cycles and whether the patient is put through activating procedures such as carrying out motor and mental tasks. These considerations become particularly important when dyskinesia is an important endpoint, such as in studies comparing the effects of various treatment regimens in previously untreated patients. Finally, the presence of dyskinesia does not necessarily indicate a deterioration in quality of life, and differentiating nontroublesome and troublesome dyskinesia is worthwhile [59].

The prevalence of dyskinesia reported by early investigators was remarkably similar. Barbeau et al. reported that 49% of their series of 100 patients exhibited dyskinesia at 3 months [4]. The percentage rose during the ensuing 2 years, but this was partially because of dropout of nonresponding patients as well as an increase in the percentage of treated patients with dyskinesia. Markham found that 21% of 100 patients had chorea at 3 months and 38% at 1 year [6]. In the same group of patients, 68% showed a 50% or more improvement in the parkinsonism at 1 year. Mones et al. reported that 3 or more months of levodopa improved 74% of the patients and induced dyskinesia in 44% of these improved patients [5]. Lesser et al. found dyskinesia in 43% of levodopa-treated patients with idiopathic parkinsonism attending a movement disorder clinic [60]. Dyskinesia was noted in only one of the nonresponding patients. It should be noted that these early patient series, shortly after the introduction of levodopa as a therapy for PD, included much more severely affected patients than would be typical for patients beginning levodopa therapy now [59]. More recent studies have suggested a 40% prevalence after 4 to 6 years of levodopa therapy [59]. Prospective 5-year studies of early PD patients placed on levodopa in randomized, controlled trials found a prevalence of 22% in a comparison of immediate and controlled release carbidopa/levodopa [61] and 45% in a comparison of levodopa to ropinirole [18].

The prevalence of dyskinesia with continuation of levodopa therapy differs in various patient series. Sweet and McDowell [62] noted that prevalence peaked in their patient series at 57% after 3 years of treatment and fell to 49% after 5 years of treatment. Barbeau found that dyskinesia was present in 66% of a series of 80 patients after 1 year of treatment, in 55% after 6 years, and 33% after 11 years [63]. Rajput found dyskinesia in 16% of autopsy-proven idiopathic PD cases after 2.5 years and 31% after 6 years of levodopa treatment but 62% demonstrated dyskinesia eventually [64]. A more recent community-based study found a prevalence of dyskinesia of 28% in levodopa-treated patients [65]. The percentage of patients with dyskinesia in these series with longer follow-ups is confounded by (1) dropout of the patients with poor or no response to the drug, patients who rarely develop dyskinesia, (2) loss of patients from other causes, and (3) changes in treatment strategies.

Age and sex as risk factors

It is a widely held clinical impression, bolstered by clinical series, that individuals with younger age of onset of PD have a higher prevalence of levodopa-induced dyskinesia. Quinn et al. found that dyskinesias were particularly common in patients with young-onset Parkinson's disease (onset between ages 21 and 40 years) [66]. Of their 51 patients, 15.7% had developed dyskinesias within 1 week of beginning levodopa. At 1, 3, and 6 years of treatment, the percentages of patients with dyskinesias were 55%, 75%, and 100%, respectively. A recent re-review of this series of patients plus young onset patients added since the original report again emphasized the high prevalence of dyskinesia in young onset PD; 92% after 5 years of levodopa treatment [67]. However, age alone may not be entirely responsible for this difference. Young onset individuals have a good response to levodopa, tolerate higher doses, and often need or want the best control of their parkinsonism. These variables, promoting use of higher doses of levodopa, rather than age itself, may be partially responsible for younger onset patients having a greater frequency and severity of levodopa-induced dyskinesia.

Estrogens may affect basal ganglia function and parkinsonian symptomatology [68–70], and one might expect that the sex of the patient could be a risk factor for developing dyskinesia. Dyskinesia has been reported to occur more frequently in women in a retrospective analysis of a large clinic database [71]. This difference in prevalence of dyskinesia is not necessarily related to sex hormones. The increased prevalence of levodopa-induced dyskinesia in women has been attributed to the lower body weights in women and consequently, relatively higher doses of levodopa in women than in men [72].

Parkinsonism as a risk factor

Levodopa-induced dyskinesia is generally associated with idiopathic Parkinson's disease. Markham [6] and Mones et al. [5] reported that levodopa did not induce dyskinesia in normal humans nor in patients with dystonia, Huntington's disease, torticollis, or other miscellaneous diseases. Similarly, Chase et al. found no dyskinesia in patients with motor neuron disease treated with levodopa [73]. Long-term therapy with levodopa for years did not produce dyskinesia in essential tremor patients [74]. These observations in humans were, for many years, thought to be consistent with studies in nonhuman primates. Levodopa will induce hyperactivity and stereotyped movements in normal monkeys, but these motor patterns are different from the choreoathetosis and dystonia induced in the MPTP-induced parkinsonian monkey [75]. Two recent studies, however, have indicated that dyskinesia can be induced in normal monkeys [76, 77]. This finding has been questioned [78]. The fact that dyskinesia can be induced in normal monkeys suggests that parkinsonism may affect the threshold for induction of dyskinesia but is not an absolute requirement for the appearance of dyskinesia.

Sometimes dyskinesia can be induced by levodopa therapy in other movement disorders. Barbeau noted that levodopa could augment the dyskinesias of dystonia musculum deformans, Huntington's disease, Wilson's disease, and induce it in progressive supranuclear palsy [4]. Klawans found that levodopa could induce chorea in people at risk for Huntington's disease and suggested levodopa challenge as a presymptomatic test for the disease [79]. Levodopa-induced dyskinesia and motor fluctuations occur in patients with MPTP-induced parkinsonism [80], parkinsonism secondary to obstructive hydrocephalus [81] and spinocerebellar ataxias type 2 (SCA 2) and 3 (SCA 3) presenting as parkinsonism [82, 83]. Patients with parkinsonism secondary to parkin mutations have young-onset parkinsonism that is very responsive to levodopa, which is commonly associated with dyskinesia [84]. Dyskinesias as well as other features of motor fluctuations occasionally occur in patients with multiple system atrophy, including oliovpontocerebellar atrophy [27] and striatonigral degeneration [85], and less frequently in other parkinsonism-plus disorders such as progressive supranuclear palsy [86] and corticobasal degeneration [87]. Dyskinesia with multiple system atrophy, if it occurs, tends to affect cranial musculature preferentially and is often predominantly dystonic. Nevertheless, the vast majority of patients with the parkinsonism-plus syndromes such as progressive supranuclear palsy, multiple system atrophy, or corticobasal degeneration receives little therapeutic benefit from dopaminergic agents and, similarly, rarely develops dyskinesia. Induction of dyskinesia by levodopa is generally a reliable indication that the patient has idiopathic parkinsonism and not a parkinsonism-plus syndrome. This conclusion is similar to Cotzias' conclusion that PD patients receiving the greatest benefit from levodopa were the most likely to develop dyskinesia [3].

Severity of parkinsonism as a risk factor

Mones et al. noted a tendency for levodopa-induced dyskinesia to appear in patients more severely affected with parkinsonism [5]. Furthermore, Langston and Ballard [80] found that dyskinesia appeared very early in the severely parkinsonian individuals who developed the syndrome after taking MPTP. Although the evidence from various clinical series is not overwhelming that disease severity is a major risk factor for the development of dyskinesia, the fact that it generally occurs first on the side most severely affected by parkinsonism argues for severity of disease as an important risk factor for the development of dyskinesia [37]. In monkeys with MPTP-induced parkinsonism, levodopa induces dyskinesia in monkeys with more severe depletion of striatal dopamine [50], supporting the importance of disease severity. However, nigrostriatal damage probably lowers the threshold but is not required for levodopa-induced dyskinesia because dyskinesia can be induced in normal monkeys [76, 77].

Levodopa responsiveness as a risk factor

Cotzias et al. noted that dyskinesia appeared in those patients who enjoyed the most improvement in motor function with levodopa [1, 3]. This observation was verified by many subsequent investigators [5, 6]. Conversely, patients who receive little therapeutic benefit from levodopa are at low risk to develop dyskinesia, regardless of the severity of the parkinsonism. Many of these individuals do not have idiopathic Parkinson's disease at autopsy.

Type of antiparkinson medication as a risk factor

Drug-induced dyskinesia in parkinsonism is almost exclusively found in patients treated with levodopa. Although nondopaminergic agents have been occasionally reported to produce dyskinesia (see Chapter 12), this is decidedly rare. The concomitant use of anticholinergics, antihistimics, or amantadine has not been linked with increased risk to develop dyskinesia in patients treated with levodopa.

The dopamine D-2 agonist, bromocriptine, infrequently induces dyskinesia in patients who have never received levodopa [16, 88], although bromocriptine will induce dyskinesia in patients in whom dyskinesia has previously been induced by chronic levodopa therapy. The same is true in nonhuman primates with MPTP-induced parkinsonism. Bromocriptine will relieve the parkinsonism but will not induce dyskinesia unless the monkey has been previously treated with levodopa [49]. The newer dopamine D-2/D-3 agonists, pramipexole and ropinirole, have been studied in randomized clinical trials for their ability to induce dyskinesia in never-treated PD subjects. The findings are consistent with the clinical impression with bromocriptine; monotherapy with dopamine D-2/D-3 agonists in *de novo* PD patients rarely induces dyskinesia [18, 19]. It should be noted, however, that the dopamine agonists were less efficacious against parkinsonian disability in *de novo* patients than was levodopa.

An important question about the dopamine D-2/D-3 agonists is whether the decreased incidence of dyskinesias in *de novo* subjects continues when levodopa is added to the agonist as is almost invariably necessary as the disease progresses. Only one retrospective study has examined this question, finding that ropinirole did not protect the patient from developing dyskinesia when levodopa was added to ropinirole therapy [89].

Dopamine D-1 agonists have been difficult to develop and there is little experience with them in humans. The D-1 agonist, ABT-431, produced a similar amount of dyskinesia and antiparkinsonian effect as did levodopa in an acute study in subjects with established dyskinesia [90]. This was unexpected as D-1 agonists produced less dyskinesia in monkeys with MPTP-induced parkinsonism [91]. D-1 agonists have not been studied as initial therapy in *de novo* subjects.

Cumulative dose as a risk factor

There is a general impression that emergence of dyskinesia in levodopa-treated patients is related to the total daily dose or cumulative exposure [4, 60]. This has been invoked as a reason to delay initiating levodopa and to keep levodopa doses as low as possible [92]. Indeed, Poewe, Lees, and Stern [93] found that patients treated for 6 years with the maximum tolerated dose of levodopa had a prevalence of dyskinesia of 88% versus 54% in a group treated with low-dose levodopa. However, the observation that dyskinesia can occur in a significant portion of patients within the first months of therapy [4–6, 53] makes the cumulative dose unlikely to be a major risk factor in the development of dyskinesia. Similarly, the lack of correlation between early and late levodopa initiation and prevalence of dyskinesia is evidence against a cumulative dose as an important factor [94]. The size of individual doses may, however, be important in the induction of dyskinesia as suggested by the ELLDOPA study in which higher levodopa doses were associated with increased prevalence of dyskinesia in the first 9 months of therapy [95].

Summary of risk factors

Young, more severely affected patients with idiopathic Parkinson's disease, who have a good therapeutic response to levodopa, are at high risk for developing dyskinesia. Patients with other neurological diseases or with parkinsonism

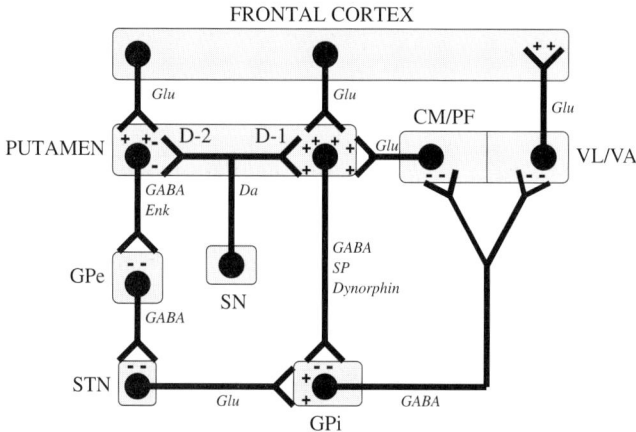

Figure 13.1 Model of neuronal connections and their neurotransmitters of basal ganglia, thalamus and motor cortex. CM/PF = nucleus centromedian and parafascicularis nuclei of thalamus, GPe = globus pallidus externa, GPi = globus pallidus interna, SN = substantia nigra, STN = subthalamic nucleus, VA and VL = nucleus ventral anterior and ventral lateral of thalamus. Neurotransmitters are, DA = dopamine, ENK = enkephalin, GLU = glutamic acid, SP = substance P, GABA = gamma amino-butyric acid. Pluses (excitation) and minuses (inhibition) indicate strength of projections.

that is not responsive to levodopa are at low risk. Patients treated only with dopamine agonists, anticholinergics, or amantadine rarely develop dyskinesia.

Pathophysiology

Model of basal ganglia function and dysfunction

Studies of the anatomical and neurotransmitter interconnections among the basal ganglia, their alterations in various disease states, and physiological studies in monkeys with MPTP-induced parkinsonism have produced a working hypothesis for the pathophysiology of parkinsonism and involuntary movements [96–100]. The major pathways and their neurotransmitters are indicated in Figure 13.1. According to the model, the loss of the dopaminergic input from the substantia nigra pars compacta (SNc) and resultant parkinsonism is related to increased firing of the principal output projections of the basal ganglia to the thalamus from the globus pallidus interna (GPi) and the substantia nigra pars reticulata (SNr) (Fig. 13.2). Involuntary movements such as chorea, dystonia, and ballism result from a decreased firing of GPi and SNr (Fig. 13.3). The rate of firing of the GPi and SNr is controlled by the balance between a direct putaminal-pallidal GABAergic pathway with substance P and dynorphin as cotransmitters and an indirect GABAergic pathway with enkephalin as a cotransmitter from putamen to the globus pallidus externa (GPe). GPe, in turn, projects via another GABAergic pathway to the subthalamic nucleus (STN). The STN

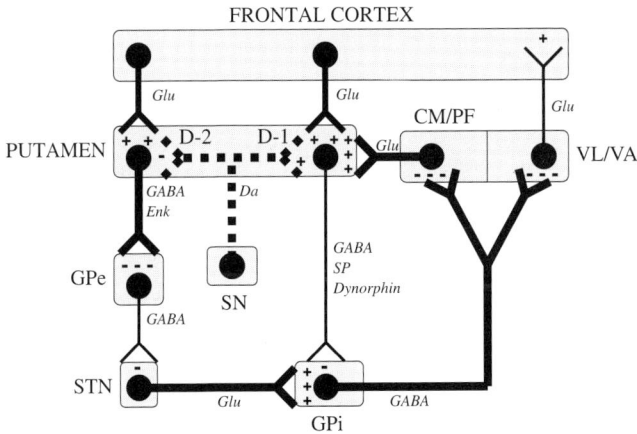

Figure 13.2 Model of basal ganglia function producing parkinsonism. Reduced dopaminergic input to the putamen results in a predominance of excitatory input to GPi from subthalamic nucleus. Abbreviations are the same as Figure 13.1.

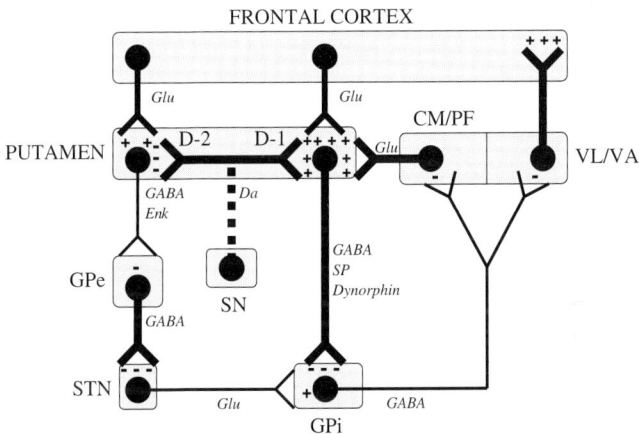

Figure 13.3 Model of basal ganglia function producing levodopa-induced dyskinesia in a parkinsonian subject. Levodopa, converted to dopamine in the putamen, reverses the balance of excitation and inhibition in the GPi by augmenting the direct inhibitory input while reducing the indirect excitatory input. This reduces or abolishes the parkinsonism but concomitantly induces dyskinesia. Abbreviations as in Figure 13.1.

has a glutamergic projection to the GPi and SNr. The loss of the dopaminergic nigrostriatal pathway in parkinsonism increases the excitation mediated by the indirect pathway from putamen to GPi via STN because of decreased inhibition of the putamen-GPe projection by dopamine D-2 receptors and reduces the inhibition mediated by the direct pathway because of loss of dopamine D-1 excitation on this projection (Fig. 13.2). In support of this model, lesions or high-frequency stimulation of the STN reverse many of the signs of parkinsonism in monkeys with MPTP-induced parkinsonism [101, 102]. In hyperkinetic disorders, there appears to be a preponderance of the direct pathway effects and reduced activity in the indirect pathway, which in turn leads to reduced output from the GPi and SNr (Fig. 13.3). Dyskinesia does not immediately appear with initiation of levodopa. Thus, levodopa treatment may progressively shift the preponderance of input to the GPi from the indirect pathway mediated through the STN to the direct pathway, clinically manifest by increasing improvement of parkinsonism accompanied by dyskinesia [103]. In patients whose parkinsonism does not respond to levodopa, striatal or pallidal pathology limits the ability of the drug to reduce activity in the indirect pathway, resulting in no clinical improvement but also no dyskinesia.

Biochemical changes associated with levodopa-induced dyskinesia

The search for the critical biochemical alterations leading to dyskinesia is ongoing. Induction of immediate early genes, *c-fos* and their transcription factors, has been described in the striata of 6-hydroxydopamine-treated rats developing abnormal movements during chronic levodopa treatment [104, 105]. Upregulation of preproenkephalin is also present in the striata of this rat model as well as in the MPTP monkey model [106] and dyskinetic PD patients coming to autopsy [107]. Prodynorphin is also reported to be upregulated in the rat model [105]. These changes in the opioid precursor mRNAs are of interest as they are markers for the direct and indirect pathways in the model of basal ganglia circuitry [96]. There are also reductions in opioid receptor binding in the striatum in dyskinetic rats suggesting compensation for the upregulation of the opioid peptide precursors [108]. This finding has been extended to humans. A PET study found decreased striatal binding of 11C-diprenorphine, an opioid receptor ligand, in patients with levodopa-induced dyskinesias as compared to nondyskinetic PD subjects [109] Of course, the changes in opioid gene expression are just a few of the many genes whose expression is altered in the dopamine denervated striatum that is exposed to dopaminergic drugs [110]. This observation suggests that dyskinesia may be a consequence of multiple changes within the basal ganglia circuitry; no single change will be sufficient to account for dyskinesia.

Physiological changes associated with dyskinesia

Parkinsonism is associated with an increase in the firing rate of GPi neurons in monkeys and in humans [100, 111]. Dopamine agonists, and presumably levodopa, reduce the GPi neuronal firing rate, which may correlate with improvement of parkinsonism [103, 112, 113]. The onset of dyskinesia has been associated with marked reduction in the firing rate and changes in firing patterns and bursting in monkeys [103, 114] but more subtle changes have been observed in humans [113]. Exactly what the abnormal firing patterns do to motor function is uncertain although it has recently been suggested that it may lead to abnormalities in force production. As opposed to PD patients without dyskinesia, dyskinetic PD patients show marked increases in force on a simple motor task, grasping and lifting a light weight [115]. This overshoot in force may have correlations in neuroimaging studies. SPECT measurements of cerebral blood flow demonstrated that levodopa increased blood flow in the supplementary motor cortex and the primary motor cortex bilaterally in dyskinetic PD patients carrying out a unilateral motor task more than in nondyskinetic PD patients. This observation is consistent with the idea that in dyskinesia there is overactivation of the frontal cortical regions via the disinhibited pallidal-thalamo-cortical projections [116]. Another contributor to abnormal force generation may be abnormal activation of the cerebellum. Even in nondyskinetic PD patients, there is evidence of cerebellar activation that correlates with spatial errors in a reaching task [117].

Neural circuitry underlying dyskinesia

The understanding of the neural circuitry underlying dyskinesia has increased in the past decade due to the wider use of stereotaxic surgery for the treatment of advanced PD and to positron emission tomography (PET) studies. The widely used model of the basal ganglia (Fig. 13.1), despite many criticisms, remains the working model for the development of therapies for PD and dyskinesias [100, 118]. It is interesting to look at where in this model prodyskinetic and antidyskinetic effects may be elicited. High-frequency electrical stimulation of the dorsal GPi or, more likely, the adjacent ventral GPe, can produce dyskinesia [119, 120]. Acute lesions in this region may also produce dyskinesia [121]. Similarly, stimulation of the subthalamic nucleus commonly induces dyskinesia [122]. Ablative lesions of posterior ventral GPi or high-frequency stimulation of the inferior portion of the posterior GPi has an antidyskinetic effect [119, 120, 123].

A ventrolateral thalamotomy, in addition to its effects on tremor, will sometimes reduce or abolish contralateral levodopa-induced dyskinesia [5, 124]. This effect has been inconsistent and is not attributed to lesioning of the Vim nucleus but to adjacent nuclei. Narabayashi and Ohye have suggested that if the Vim lesion extends rostrally into the ventralis oralis nucleus, which receives pallidal output, dyskinesia will be suppressed [124, 125]. This dyskinesia-suppressing effect of anterior ventrolateral thalamic lesions was also reported in MPTP-treated monkeys with levodopa-induced dyskinesia [126]. Capparros-Lefebvre has suggested that placement of the Vim-targeted electrode posteriorly, inferiorly, and medially into the vicinity of the centromedian/parafasicular nuclear complex was responsible for the reduction in dyskinesia seen with thalamic stimulation [127, 128]. There is insufficient experience with these thalamic targets to recommend them for clinical use. However, these observations of the effect of thalamic lesions on levodopa-induced dyskinesia emphasize that we do not completely understand the circuitry underlying dyskinesia and that there are probably more potential surgical targets for treatment of dyskinesia.

Pharmacological mechanisms
Dopaminergic denervation predisposes but is not required
Levodopa and the dopamine agonists very rarely induce dyskinesia in patients who do not have parkinsonism. This suggests that dopaminergic denervation is necessary for levodopa-induced dyskinesias. Studies in monkeys reinforce this concept. Extremely large doses of levodopa can produce hyperactivity and stereotyped movements in normal primates but requires doses that are often associated with toxicity including death (Sassin 1972, Mones 1973, Paulson 1973, Ng 1973 [75]). These movements appear to be qualitatively different from the choreiform and dystonic dyskinesia that occurs in monkeys with MPTP-induced parkinsonism [75, 97]. However, it is now apparent that dopaminergic denervation is not required; dyskinesia can be induced in normal monkeys [76, 77]. Thus, the extent of dopaminergic denervation may be just one factor that determines the susceptibility to levodopa-induced dyskinesia [129].

The effect of dopaminergic denervation is to reduce the dopamine reuptake capacity of the striatum and therefore swings in extracellular dopamine will be larger [130, 131]. Microdialysis studies in rats demonstrate that levodopa raises extracellular concentrations of dopamine in the dopaminergically denervated striatum much more than in normal striatum [132]. PET studies using displacement of raclopride binding as a measure of synaptic dopamine suggest higher extracellular concentrations of dopamine in more severely affected PD subjects, those most likely to have dyskinesia [133]. Thus dopaminergic denervation will enhance the effects of levodopa by increasing the effective dose administered.

Repeated dosing necessary
Dyskinesia does not appear with the initial administration of levodopa in patients or in monkeys with MPTP-induced parkinsonism. Repeated dosing is necessary. Thus, dyskinesia is not simply explicable by dopaminergic stimulation of a dopaminergically denervated, supersensitive striatum. Some alteration of the drug response is induced by repeated dosing with levodopa; that is, sensitization occurs.

Changes in dyskinesia dose-response curves to levodopa
One question is what changes during chronic therapy to allow the emergence of levodopa-induced dyskinesia? Two pharmacological hypotheses are invoked. The first is that the threshold for dyskinesia is lowered during levodopa therapy, narrowing the therapeutic window between antiparkinsonian effects and dyskinetic effects [46]. This is equivalent to a shift of the dose-response curve to the left. However, pharmacokinetic-pharmacodynamic modeling of the dyskinesia response to levodopa has not demonstrated a reduction in the effective concentration producing 50% of the response (EC50) as predicted by this model of increased sensitivity or leftward shift of the dyskinesia dose-response curve [134, 135].

An alternative hypothesis is that the severity of dyskinesia (E_{max}) dose-response curve increases from zero (no clinically apparent dyskinesia) without a change in EC50. That model fit the development of dyskinesia in 18 PD subjects followed for the first 4 years of levodopa therapy [51].

Dopamine receptor subtypes and dyskinesia

Dopamine D-2 agonists will only rarely induce dyskinesia in patients who have not been previously or are not concurrently treated with levodopa [16, 18, 19]. This could be explained by the fact that dopamine D-2 agonists rarely produce the antiparkinsonian effects that can be achieved with levodopa. However, in the monkey with MPTP-induced parkinsonism, doses of bromocriptine that produce as much improvement in the signs of parkinsonism as does levodopa, still did not induce dyskinesia [49]. However, another D-2 agonist, PHNO, can induce dyskinesia in monkeys with MPTP-induced parkinsonism who had not been primed with levodopa [136]. Once dyskinesia has been induced by levodopa, dopamine D-2 agonists can induce dyskinesia in humans but the dyskinesia is generally mild and transient. In fact, if patients with severe levodopa-induced dyskinesia can be switched from levodopa to dopamine D-2 agonists, dyskinesia can be markedly reduced or stopped [137]. Dopamine D-2 agonists induce dyskinesia in levodopa-primed parkinson monkeys [138].

The dopamine D-1 agonists can induce dyskinesia in the monkey with MPTP-induced parkinsonism that has not received levodopa previously [139]. Dopamine D-1 agonists have not been used in drug-naïve human PD patients to assess their ability to induce dyskinesias. In patients with levodopa-induced dyskinesias, dopamine D-1 agonists can induce dyskinesia that is similar in nature and severity to that induced by levodopa [90]. In parkinson monkeys with levodopa-induced dyskinesias, dopamine agonists D-1 appeared to produce less dyskinesia than a comparable antiparkinson dose of levodopa [91].

There is evidence that dopamine D-3 receptor supersensitivity is responsible for levodopa-induced dyskinesia; D-3 receptor binding increases in levodopa-treated animal models of parkinsonism [140, 141]. Not all findings support the importance of dopamine D-3 receptor in levodopa-induced dyskinesia. Dopamine D-3 receptors were not increased in marmosets with levodopa-induced dyskinesia as opposed to those without dyskinesia [142]. A putative dopamine D-3 agonist produced similar antiparkinson effects and dyskinesia as did the dopamine D-1 and D-2 agonist, apomorphine, in levodopa-primed parkinson monkeys [143]. There are no studies that have tested selective dopamine D-3 agonists in humans although the mixed dopamine D-2 and D-3 agonists, pramipexole and ropinirole, do not appear to be qualitatively different from dopamine D-2 agonists without D-3 activity.

Temporal pattern of drug administration and dyskinesia

The temporal pattern of drug administration is important in determining whether animals will develop tolerance or sensitization to subsequent drug administration. Continuous administration of dopaminergic agents tends to reduce the response to subsequent doses [144–148]. Intermittent administration, which may be closer to the clinical situation in humans, results in sensitization [145, 148–150]. These findings suggest that the manner in which levodopa is administered may be critical to the development of dyskinesia in humans.

The evidence that dyskinesia is a result of sensitization and the appreciation that sensitization in the dopaminergic system is related to pulsatile dopaminergic stimulation suggests that reducing the peaks and valleys in dopaminergic stimulation that is a necessary consequence of orally administered antiparkinson medications would reduce dyskinesia [151] or prevent its development [152]. Attempts to blunt the high and low concentrations of levodopa with controlled release carbidopa/levodopa and thereby prevent the development of dyskinesia in *de novo* PD patients were unsuccessful in a large randomized and blinded clinical trial [153]. The best evidence that continuous dopaminergic stimulation might benefit levodopa-induced dyskinesia comes from studies of continuous subcutaneous administration of the dopamine agonists, apomorphine or lisuride in PD patients with levodopa-induced dyskinesia. In these unblinded studies, approximately 50% reduction of dyskinesia severity and duration has been reported [154–156].

The emergence of off-phase or "runaway" dyskinesia in PD patients receiving fetal midbrain grafts [22, 23] could be construed as a blow against the hypothesis that continuous dopaminergic stimulation is more physiological. Although the grafts would be expected to release dopamine into the surrounding extracellular areas, there may be many other changes induced by the grafts that promote the development of this complication of neural grafting. Understanding "runaway" dyskinesias will be important for the field of neural transplantation and for understanding the pathogenesis of levodopa-induced dyskinesia.

Dissociation of antiparkinson effects and dyskinesia
Once dyskinesia develops, can dyskinesia and antiparkinson effects be dissociated? The relationship between the dose or plasma levels of levodopa that produce dyskinesia and those that reduce parkinsonism are controversial. There is some evidence that initially the threshold for inducing dyskinesia is much higher than the threshold for inducing the improvement in parkinsonism [3, 46, 47]. This would suggest that when dyskinesia appears, smaller doses of the drug could be administered to produce the antiparkinsonian effects without eliciting dyskinesia. In practice, this therapeutic window is elusive, if it exists at all.

Other investigators have felt that once dyskinesia appears, it is generally present when the antiparkinsonian effect is apparent [29, 30, 45]. This implies that there is no therapeutic window and full therapeutic efficacy of levodopa will be accompanied by dyskinesia in those patients in whom dyskinesia has developed. This formulation suggests that reducing the dose of levodopa will not separate the antiparkinsonian effects and dyskinetic effects of the drug.

The paragraphs above address the dissociation of the short-duration antiparkinson response and the attendant dyskinesia. The long-duration response is rarely associated with dyskinesia and could be viewed as a dissociation between the beneficial effects of levodopa and dyskinesia [157].

It has proven very difficult to separate "on" dyskinesia and antiparkinson effects of levodopa by addition of other therapies; most strategies that reduce dyskinesia also reduce the antiparkinson response [25, 157]. There are some apparent exceptions. Amantadine, reduces dyskinesia without worsening parkinsonism [159, 160]. This effect can also be seen in monkeys although amantadine also reduces the antiparkinson effect under some conditions in monkeys [161].

Pallidotomy almost always reduces or abolishes dyskinesia contralateral to the lesion and may concomitantly improve parkinsonism [123, 162, 163]. However, it is now recognized that the antidyskinesia and antibradykinesia effects are elicited from different areas within the globus pallidus interna [119, 120]. Thus the combination of improving dyskinesia and parkinsonism with pallidotomy or pallidal stimulation probably represents lesions or stimulation that affect distinct areas within the GPi that have different effects, prodyskinesia and antidyskinesia as well as antibradykinesia and probradykinesia.

Other neurotransmitters and dyskinesia

A variety of neurotransmitters other than dopamine have been implicated in dyskinesia by studies in animals, suggesting a number of drugs that might suppress levodopa-induced dyskinesias. The challenge is to find an antidyskinetic therapy without impairing antiparkinsonian efficacy of other medications or worsening the cardinal symptoms of parkinsonism. Five neurotransmitter systems have been studied.

1. Drugs acting on glutamate receptors: The increased synaptic efficacy of NMDA receptors expressed on basal ganglia neurons may play a role in the pathophysiology of levodopa-induced dyskinesias [164]. Protein phosphorylation serves as a major regulatory mechanism for NMDA receptors and an increased phosphorylation state of the NMDA receptor is related to enhanced synaptic efficacy [165]. As a result, the corticostriatal glutamatergic input is amplified, leading to altered striatal GABAergic output, which in turn might give rise to the expression of dyskinesia.

Both NMDA and AMPA receptor antagonists have been reported to reduce levodopa-induced dyskinesia in monkeys [166–168]. In humans, the putative NMDA antagonist, amantadine, has antidyskinetic actions in PD patients without significantly altering the antiparkinsonian action of levodopa [159]. Dextromethorphan, another NMDA antagonist, modestly suppressed dyskinesia in a subset of PD subjects [169]. A third NMDA antagonist, remacemide, had no effect on dyskinesia in a small multicenter randomized trial [170] nor did memantine, an analog of amantadine that is also a NMDA antagonist [171].

2. Drugs acting on serotonergic systems: The serotonergic system may modify dopamine transmission. Serotonin 5HT-1A receptors are postulated to modify dopamine and serotonin release from serotonin terminals and have been suggested as a pharmacological target for ameliorating levodopa-induced dyskinesia [172]. Sarizotan, a 5HT1A agonist, reduced levodopa-induced dyskinesias in both 6-hydroxydopamine lesioned rats and MPTP-lesioned primates [172]. Clinical trials are underway with sarizotan although the results will be clouded by the fact that this drug also has weak dopamine D-2 receptor antagonist properties. Buspirone, another 5HT1A agonist, has similarly been demonstrated to reduce levodopa-induced dyskinesia in a small crossover trial [173]. Fluoxetine, a selective serotonin reuptake inhibitor, decreased dyskinesia triggered by an acute apomorphine challenge in an open pilot study [174].

3. Drugs acting on noradrenergic systems: Drugs that block alpha-2 noradrenergic receptors in the brain have demonstrated antidyskinetic properties. The mechanism has been speculated to be an increase in noradrenergic transmission secondary to blockade of alpha-2 presynaptic autoreceptors; or alternatively reduction of alpha-2 postsynaptic effects. Yohimbine, an alpha-2 antagonist, reduces LIDs without affecting levodopa's antiparkinsonian response [175]. Idazoxan, another alpha-2 antagonist, reduced levodopa-induced dyskinesia in MTPT monkeys [176]. In a placebo-controlled study in 18 PD subjects with levodopa-induced dyskinesias, idazoxan reduced dyskinesia to test doses of levodopa. This effect was not dose related and did not reach significance [177].

4. Drugs acting on opiate systems: The upregulation of opioid peptide precursors by levodopa treatment and downregulation of opioid binding in animal models of parkinsonism and humans with PD and dyskinesia suggests a role for the endogenous opioids in the development of dyskinesia and makes the opioid systems a natural pharmacological target. Naloxone, an opioid antagonist, reduces levodopa-induced dyskinesias in MPTP-primed primates [178, 179]. A 1-month treatment with the opiate antagonist, naltrexone, was ineffective in eight dyskinetic PD subjects [180]. There is always the concern that naloxone or naltrexone may not have the ideal opiate receptor subtype affinities to produce an antidyskinetic effect.

5. Drugs acting on GABA systems: A number of pathways within the basal ganglia use GABA as a neurotransmitter (see Fig. 13.1) with the result that GABAergic agents may have relatively nonspecific or nonselective properties. However, the GABAergic neurons can be divided into subpopulations identified by their cotransmitters. For example, GABAergic neurons projecting from the putamen directly to the GPi, the direct pathway, have substance P and dynorphin as a cotransmitters; the GABAergic neurons projecting from the putamen to the GPe have enkephalin as a cotransmitter. Pharmacological methods of selectively influencing these subpopulations of GABAergic neurons by taking advantage of the cotransmitter specificity and the receptor profiles may prove useful in manipulating basal ganglia function.

The adenosine A2a receptor is highly localized to cell bodies of striatal-GPe indirect pathway and to striatal cholinergic interneurons [181]. These receptors may thus influence GABA release in the indirect pathway directly and indirectly. In MPTP-treated marmosets, the A2a antagonist KW-6002 reversed parkinsonism [182]. Furthermore, KW-6002 improved parkinsonism without evoking dyskinesia in marmosets that exhibited dyskinesia with levodopa dosing [182]. These effects are postulated to result from reducing the overactivity of the indirect pathway.

Stimulation of cannabinoid receptors in the globus pallidus reduces GABA reuptake and enhances GABA transmission and may thereby reduce dyskinesia [183]. MPTP marmosets that were coadministered nabilone, a cannabinoid receptor agonist, and levodopa had significantly less dyskinesia than marmosets administered levodopa alone, with no reduction in antiparkinsonian action of levodopa [184]. Single doses of nabilone significantly reduced levodopa-induced dyskinesia in a randomized double-blind, placebo-controlled crossover trial [185]. This result needs confirmation in a subacute study as relaxation could produce this effect as well.

These results demonstrate that a large number of drugs have been reported to reduce dyskinesia. Many of these studies have been in MPTP primates and await trials in humans. Others have been used in pilot trials in humans, often as acute doses and in small numbers of subjects. Most have not been subjected to randomized clinical trials.

Treatment

Determining pattern of dyskinesia

To treat dyskinesia, one obviously needs to know what pattern of dyskinesia the patient experiences. The patient's history and diaries are the primary way to obtain this information. However, the pattern of dyskinesia is often very difficult to obtain from the patient because the patient has difficulty in differentiating tremor, "off" dystonia, "on" dystonia, and choreoathetosis. In addition, patients with dyskinesia generally have fluctuations in motor response to further complicate the patient's interpretation of their motor state. It is important to understand the fluctuations in control of parkinsonism symptoms (wearing off, on-off) as well because any changes in the medical regimen will affect this as well as the dyskinesia. If the history or diaries are not perfectly clear, and the physician has not observed the dyskinesia described by the patient, it is worthwhile having the patient stay in the clinic through one or two dose cycles so that the various forms of dyskinesia as well as the fluctuation in the parkinsonism can be observed. Having the family video the patient during the dose cycle to document the phenomenon described by the patient but not seen in the clinic is another useful tactic. Be aware that the dyskinesia described by the patient may actually be nonmotor manifestations of fluctuations.

Monitoring the plasma levels of levodopa while monitoring motor signs may help delineate the relationship between plasma levels of drug and clinical responses [186]. However, it is important to recall that clinical response and plasma levels do not directly correlate [29]; striatal dopamine concentrations, and not plasma dopa, are the important parameter. The relationships among plasma levodopa levels and levodopa-induced rise in dopamine concentration in the vicinity of the striatal dopamine receptors and clinical response remain unclear. For plasma levodopa levels to be of assistance in managing a patient, plasma levels and clinical ratings at 30- to 60-minute intervals through one or more dose cycles are necessary. If the oral test dose of levodopa is taken in the morning on an empty stomach and when the patient is off, the relation between plasma levels and clinical response can generally be inferred without actually measuring plasma levodopa.

Peak dose ("on") dyskinesia

The first step in managing "on" dyskinesia is to examine the patient's drug regimen and determine if there are drugs that may enhance dyskinesia without adding much to the antiparkinson effects of the regimen. Selegiline promotes dyskinesia although it has weak symptomatic effects [187] and therefore stopping selegiline is sometimes sufficient to reduce dyskinesia. Although anticholinergics rarely can induce dyskinesia [188, 189], reducing anticholinergics rarely alters dyskinesia although there may be other good reasons to eliminate anticholinergics from the drug regimen.

The next step is to examine the adjunct agents and controlled release preparations. Catechol-O-methyltransferase inhibitors enhance the antiparkinson actions and dyskinesia in levodopa-treated patients [190]. Whether the enhanced dyskinesia is out of proportion to the antiparkinson effects has not been determined. However, reduction of COMT inhibitors should be considered. Controlled release preparations may also be associated with more dyskinesia, particularly late in the day and their use should also be assessed in the dyskinetic patient.

Orally administered dopamine D-2 agonists also enhance the dyskinetic effects of levodopa, and simply adding them to levodopa will increase dyskinesia [190]. In patients receiving both dopamine agonists and levodopa, the dyskinesia tends to occur in relation to the levodopa administration and not the dopamine agonist administration. If the levodopa dose can be significantly decreased by the addition of dopamine agonists, dyskinesia can be markedly reduced [137]. The difficulty of this strategy is that the dopamine agonists are less effective antiparkinsonian agents than levodopa and it is rarely possible to switch patients entirely over to oral dopamine agonists. The exception is subcutaneously administered agonists, which may largely or completely substitute for levodopa [154, 156]. Whether it is this reduction in the levodopa dose or the continuous dopaminergic stimulation that is responsible for the improvement in dyskinesia is not known.

The third step is to examine levodopa dosing. The most common strategy to try to reduce levodopa-induced dyskinesia is to give smaller doses of levodopa more frequently, trying to keep the levodopa plasma levels within the controversial therapeutic window. This change will, at a minimum, shorten the duration of dyskinesia with each dose of medication, which in itself may make the dyskinesia more acceptable to the patient. However, concomitantly, the duration of the antiparkinsonian effect of the drug is also shortened and the response to each dose of the drug may become more unpredictable because the plasma drug concentrations produced by the smaller doses are closer to the minimum effective concentration [191]. Nevertheless, this strategy is worth trying, particularly in patients who are taking very large doses of levodopa (greater than 1500 mg/day) although it benefits only a minority of patients. The reduction should be gradual to avoid suddenly worsening the parkinsonism and losing the patients' cooperation with this strategy.

A final pharmacological step is to consider adding a drug to reduce dyskinesia. The only agent available at this time is amantadine, thought to suppress dyskinesia through its action at the NMDA receptor [159]. Withdrawal of levodopa for days to a couple of weeks to "resensitize" patients to levodopa, a so-called "drug holiday" [192] has fallen out of favor because of the uncertainty of its value and its recognized physical and psychological risks [193].

The most important advance in the treatment of various forms of dyskinesia has been stereotaxic surgery of the basal ganglia. If pharmacological control of the dyskinesias and parkinsonism is not possible, surgical options should be considered. Pallidotomy, ablation of the posterior ventral GPi, is very effective against contralateral dyskinesia and somewhat reduces ipsilateral dyskinesia as well [123, 162, 163]. The problem is that bilateral pallidotomies often cause difficulties with speech, swallowing, and balance so that bilateral procedures are rarely recommended. Nevertheless, unilateral pallidotomy can be a very effective procedure in selected patients. Even if the dyskinesia is bilateral, abolishing it unilaterally will markedly improve a patient's function.

Deep brain stimulation (DBS) of the GPi is also an effective treatment of dyskinesia [194–197] but rarely as efficacious as pallidotomy. However, DBS can be done bilaterally and tends to be a more effective antiparkinson treatment than pallidotomy. Although less well documented, DBS of the GPi can reduce "off" dystonia as well.

Subthalamic nucleus (STN) stimulation is more complicated. STN stimulation can induce dyskinesia or exacerbate levodopa-induced dyskinesia [122]. However, STN DBS often allows reduction of the levodopa dose and this effect may reduce "on" dyskinesia [195, 197, 198]. Moreover, STN DBS is also effective against biphasic dyskinesia and "off" dystonia [199]. Deep brain stimulation at either site is a more "reversible" procedure, in that the implanted electrodes may be removed or stimulators may be turned off at any point in the future. Pallidotomy involves making a larger lesion that is irreversible. This consideration becomes particularly relevant as newer therapies for advanced Parkinson's disease become available.

Diphasic dyskinesia

Diphasic dyskinesia, dyskinesia that occurs at the beginning and the end of each dose cycle, is generally most prominent as the effects of a dose wear off. A mild diphasic pattern is seen in many patients although clinicians often use the term only for patients with a marked diphasic pattern. Utilizing larger doses of levodopa or scheduling the doses closer together can prevent the inter-dose exacerbation of dyskinesia until the end of the day when the patient stops or reduces levodopa intake [9]. Although this strategy clearly works in the short run, most investigators have found that it is ineffective over the long haul because of increasing peak dose dyskinesia, repeated dosage adjustments, or other toxicity [28, 32]. Furthermore, there is the impression that if the patients are kept "on" and free of the diphasic swings throughout the day, the dyskinesia may be even more severe as they "come down" at the end of the day than if it occurred with each dose throughout the day. Dopamine agonists may be of some benefit in reducing the severity of the diphasic dyskinesia but rarely completely control it [32]. Surprisingly, continuous infusions of levodopa will not control diphasic dyskinesia that continues to reappear despite progressive increases in the infusion rate [200]. The same pattern of breakthrough of the dyskinesia is described with subcutaneous apomorphine [201, 202]. If this pattern of dyskinesia is disabling, surgery is the best method of treating it.

"Off" dystonia

"Off" dystonia is more prominent in the morning when the patient has been without medication overnight, and it is the reason that "off" dystonia was initially described as "early morning dystonia" [10]. It frequently is precipitated by the patient trying to get out of bed and walk to the bathroom. Pharmacologically, it behaves as though it is due to some intermediary level of dopaminergic stimulation and either increasing dopaminergic stimulation with dopaminergic agents or decreasing it with dopamine receptor antagonists will improve "off" dystonia [25, 35]. The rate at which levodopa levels decline is not important to production of "off" dystonia, suggesting that it is the intermediate concentration that is critical [203].

Timing of the first dose of the day of levodopa may prevent or reduce painful "off" dystonia. Some patients find that if they have the medicine at the bedside, take it upon awakening, and wait for 15 to 30 minutes before getting out of bed, they may avoid the dystonia. A dose of drug taken during the night or controlled release preparations of carbidopa/levodopa taken at bedtime, which provide more sustained plasma levels of levodopa, will also reduce "off" dystonia. Dopamine agonists are also frequently efficacious in reducing "off" dystonia both in the morning and throughout the day if it is occurring at other times when levodopa levels are low. Other treatments that have been claimed to be of benefit include lithium and baclofen. Botulinum toxin injections into dystonic muscles may sometimes prove effective in persistent "off" dystonia. Finally, pallidotomy and DBS may effectively reduce "off" dystonia.

Future trends

Manipulation of other pathways within the basal ganglia

The models of normal and disordered basal ganglia function (Figs. 13.1–13.3) suggest that manipulation of other neurotransmitter systems and pathways within the basal ganglia may compensate for the loss of the dopaminergic nigrostriatal tract activity. Thus one can imagine that it may be possible to correct the parkinsonism without inducing dyskinesia or to suppress dyskinesia without reducing the antiparkinsonian actions of therapy [204].

The possibility of finding neurotransmitter systems susceptible to pharmacological modification or pathways that may be influenced by stereotaxic ablation or stimulation has been discussed. Manipulation of selected subpopulations of neurons in the basal ganglia using various neurotrophic factors may also provide therapeutic benefit [205].

It should be noted that there are other reentrant loops within the basal ganglia and thalamus, such as through the pedunculopontine nucleus or through the centromedian/parafasicular nucleus of the thalamus, for which no function is recognized but which conceivably may be as important as the substantia nigra compacta or the subthalamic nucleus in modulating basal ganglia function. These loops may be targets for pharmacological or surgical manipulation. Exploration of the basal ganglia and some of the more mysterious associated structures, such as the zona incerta, with electrical stimulation in the MPTP-treated monkey model of parkinsonism and humans with implanted DBS electrodes is likely to discover other targets.

Preventing induction of dyskinesia

The fact that dyskinesia does not occur with the first doses of levodopa but is induced by chronic treatment with levodopa suggests that it may be possible to avoid the development of dyskinesia. This presumably would be accomplished by preventing the sensitization to levodopa that is thought to underlie the development of dyskinesia. Although the antiparkinsonian actions of levodopa may be evident with the first dose of levodopa, often the antiparkinsonian effects of levodopa are mild at the initiation of therapy and increase with continued therapy, suggesting that the antiparkinsonian effect of levodopa may be augmented by sensitization as well [51]. Thus sensitization may have benefits as well as drawbacks during long-term levodopa therapy.

Determining how repeated exposure to dopaminergic agents gradually augments the antiparkinson and dyskinetic response to each dose of medication will be an important area of investigation. It seems likely that the changes will be throughout the basal ganglia circuitry and not be a single molecular mechanism. These changes will be in the transduction of dopamine receptor occupancy into changes in postsynaptic neuronal function and changes in multineuronal functional loops in basal ganglia and frontal cortex. The clinical observations that dyskinesias can result from lesions that are "down stream" from the dopaminergic system such as in Huntington's disease, basal ganglia strokes or subthalamic stimulation are evidence for this network concept underlying dyskinesia.

There is growing evidence that sensitization may be very dependent upon the degree of dopaminergic denervation of the striatum, the profile of dopamine receptor subtype activation produced by the drug, and the

interdose intervals [164]. Defining the contribution of these variables to induction of dyskinesia may have a very important impact on the manner in
which dopaminergic drugs are used in patients. Clinically, studies are underway to see if more continuous dopaminergic stimulation via controlled release
preparations, and stimulation of different combinations of dopamine receptor
subtypes by various agonists will alter the induction of dyskinesia [152, 206].

Dyskinesia is associated with the short-duration response to levodopa –
the rapid rise and fall of plasma and brain levels of levodopa or dopamine
agonists that produces an improvement of parkinsonism for minutes to hours.
However, the clinical benefit from the long-duration response to levodopa that
builds up over days to weeks, may be as large as the short-duration response
and is not associated with dyskinesia. Understanding this response may offer
ways to improve parkinsonism without dyskinesia [207, 208].

There is one other manner in which the problem of dyskinesia may be
averted; prevent parkinsonism altogether. If the intense research push for neuroprotective therapies is successful, dyskinesia may disappear before we fully
understand the problem. In the meantime, we have increasing numbers of
strategies to explore to ameliorate dyskinesia.

Acknowledgments

We thank Lynn Storey for her assistance in preparing the manuscript and
figures. Supported in part by VA Parkinson's Disease Research, Education
and Clinical Center (PADRECC), National Parkinson Foundation and NIH
(NINDS).

References

1. Cotzias GC, Van Woert MH, Schiffer LM. Aromatic amino acids and modification of parkinsonism. N Engl J Med 1967; 276: 374–379.
2. Birkmeyer W, Hornykiewicz O. The effect of L-3,4-dihydroxyphenylalanin (DOPA) on
akinesia in Parkinson's syndrome. Wein Klin Wochenschr 1961; 73: 787–788.
3. Cotzias GC, Papavasiliou PS, Gellene R. Modification of parkinsonism: chronic treatment
with L-dopa. N Engl J Med 1969; 280: 337–345.
4. Barbeau A, Mars H, Gillo-Joffroy L. Adverse clinical side effects of levodopa therapy. In
McDowell FH, Markham CH (eds) Recent Advances in Parkinson's Disease. Philadelphia:
F.A. Davis, 1971, 204–237.
5. Mones RJ, Elizan TS, Siegel GJ. Analysis of L-dopa induced dyskinesia in 51 patients with
Parkinsonism. J Neurol Neurosurg Psychiatry 1971; 34: 668–673.
6. Markham CH. The choreoathetoid movement disorder induced by levodopa. Clin Pharmacol Ther 1971; 12(pt 2): 340–343.
7. Tolosa ES, Martin WE, Cohen HP, et al. Patterns of clinical response and plasma dopa
levels in Parkinson's disease. Neurology 1975; 25(2): 177–183.
8. Muenter MD, Tyce GM. L-DOPA therapy of Parkinson's disease: plasma L-DOPA concentration, therapeutic response, and side effects. Mayo Clin Proc 1971; 46: 231–239.

9. Lhermitte F, Agid Y, Signoret JL. Onset and end-of-dose levodopa-induced dyskinesias. Possible treatment by increasing the daily doses of levodopa. Arch Neurol 1978; 35(5): 261–263.

10. Melamed E. Early-morning dystonia: a late side effect of long-term levodopa therapy in Parkinson's disease. Arch Neurol 1979; 36: 308–310.

11. Nausieda PA, Weiner WJ, Klawans HL. Dystonic foot response of parkinsonism. Arch Neurol 1980; 37: 132–136.

12. Schwab RS, Amador LV, Lettvin JY. Apomorphine in Parkinson's disease. Trans Am Neurol Assoc 1951; 76: 251–253.

13. Cotzias GC, Papavasilious PS, Fehling C, et al. Similarities between neurologic effects of L-DOPA and of apomorphine. N Engl J Med 1970; 282: 31–33.

14. Cotzias GC, Papavasilious PS, Tolosa ES, et al. Treatment of Parkinson's disease with aporphines. N Engl J Med 1976; 294: 567–572.

15. Calne DB, Teychenne PF, Leigh PN, et al. Treatment of parkinsonism with bromocriptine. Lancet 1974; 2(7893): 1355–1356.

16. Lees AJ, Stern GM. Sustained bromocriptine therapy in previously untreated patients with Parkinson's disease. J Neurol Neurosurg Psychiatry 1981; 44: 1020–1023.

17. Rinne UK. Combined bromocriptine-levodopa therapy early in Parkinson's disease. Neurology 1985; 35: 1196–1198.

18. Rascol O, Brooks DJ, Korczyn AD, et al. A five-year study of the incidence of dyskinesia in patients with early Parkinson's disease who were treated with ropinirole or levodopa. 056 Study Group. N Engl J Med 2000; 342(20): 1484–1491.

19. Pramipexole vs levodopa as initial treatment for Parkinson disease: a randomized controlled trial. Parkinson Study Group. JAMA 2000; 284(15): 1931–1938.

20. Burns RS, Phillips JM, Chuang CC, et al. The MPTP-treated monkey model of Parkinson's disease. In Markey SP, Castagnoli N, Trevor AJ, Kopin IJ (eds) MPTP: A Neurotoxin Producing a Parkinsonian Syndrome. New York, Academic Press, 1986.

21. Clarke CE, Boyse S, Sambrook MA, et al. Timing of levodopa therapy: evidence from MPTP-treated primates. Lancet 1987; 2: 625.

22. Freed CR, Greene PE, Breeze RE, et al. Transplantation of embryonic dopamine neurons for severe Parkinson's disease. N Engl J Med 2001; 344(10): 710–719.

23. Hagell P, Piccini P, Bjorklund A, et al. Dyskinesias following neural transplantation in Parkinson's disease. Nat Neurosci 2002; 5(7): 627–628.

24. Purves SJ. Paralysis agitans: with an account of a new symptom. Lancet 1889; 2: 1258–1260.

25. Luquin MR, Scipioni O, Vaamonde J, et al. Levodopa-induced dyskinesias in Parkinson's disease: clinical and pharmacological classification. Mov Disord 1992; 7: 117–124.

26. Klawans HL, Goetz C, Bergen D. Levodopa-induced myoclonus. Arch Neurol 1975; 32(5): 330–334.

27. Lang AE, Johnson K. Akathisia in idiopathic Parkinson's disease. Neurology 1987; 37(3): 477–481.

28. Marsden CD, Parkes JD, Quinn N. Fluctuations of disability in Parkinson's disease - clinical aspects. In: Marsden CD, Fahn S, editors. Neurology 2: Movement Disorders. London, Butterworth Scientific, 1981, pp. 96–122.

29. Nutt JG, Woodward WR. Levodopa pharmacokinetics and pharmacodynamics in fluctuating parkinsonian patients. Neurology 1986; 36: 739–744.

30. Hardie RJ, Lees AJ, Stern GM. On-off fluctuations in Parkinson's disease: A clinical and neuropharmacological study. Brain 1984; 107: 487–506.

31. Muenter MD, Sharpless NS, Tyce GM, et al. Patterns of dystonia ("I-D-I" and "D-I-D") in response to L-Dopa therapy for Parkinson's disease. Mayo Clin Proc 1977; 52: 163–174.

32. Fahn S. Fluctuations of disability in Parkinson's disease: pathophysiology. In: Marsden CD, Fahn S (eds) Neurology 2: Movement Disorders. London, Butterworth Scientific, 1981, pp. 123–145.

33. Marconi R, Lefebvre-Caparros D, Bonnet A-M, et al. Levodopa-induced dyskinesia in Parkinson's disease: phenomenology and pathophysiology. Mov Disord 1994; 9: 2–12.

34. Clarke CE, Boyce S, Robertson RG, et al. Drug-induced dyskinesia in primates rendered hemiparkinsonian by intracarotid administration of 1-methyl-4-phenyl-1,2,3,6- tetrahydropyridine (MPTP). J Neurol Sci 1989; 90: 307–314.

35. Poewe WH, Lees AJ, Stern GM. Dystonia in Parkinson's disease: clinical and pharmacological features. Ann Neurol 1988; 23: 73–78.

36. Cubo E, Gracies JM, Benabou R, et al. Early morning off-medication dyskinesias, dystonia, and choreic subtypes. Arch Neurol 2001; 58(9): 1379–1382.

37. Horstink MWIM, Zijlmans JCM, Pasman JW, et al. . Severity of Parkinson's disease is a risk factor for peak-dose dyskinesia. J Neurol Neurosurg Psychiatry 1990; 53: 224–226.

38. LeWitt PA. Conjugate eye deviations as dyskinesias induced by levodopa in Parkinson's disease. Mov Disord 1998; 13(4): 731–734.

39. Linazasoro G, Van Blercom N, Lasa A, et al. Levodopa-induced ocular dyskinesias in Parkinson's disease. Mov Disord 2002; 17(1): 186–187.

40. Weiner WJ, Goetz CG, Nausieda PA, et al. Respiratory dyskinesias: extrapyramidal dysfunction and dyspnea. Ann Intern Med 1978; 88(3): 327–331.

41. Zupnick HM, Brown LK, Miller A, et al. Respiratory dysfunction due to L-dopa therapy for parkinsonism: diagnosis using serial pulmonary function tests and respiratory inductive plethysmography. Am J Med 1990; 89(1): 109–114.

42. Rice JE, Antic R, Thompson PD. Disordered respiration as a levodopa-induced dyskinesia in Parkinson's disease. Mov Disord 2002; 17(3): 524–527.

43. Vincken WG, Gauthier SG, Dollfuss RE, et al. Involvement of upper-airway muscles in extrapyramidal disorders. A cause of airflow limitation. N Engl J Med 1984; 311(7): 438–442.

44. Durif F, Vidailhet M, Debilly B, et al. Worsening of levodopa-induced dyskinesias by motor and mental tasks. Mov Disord 1999; 14(2): 242–245.

45. Metman LV, van den Mundkhof P, Klaassen AAG, et al. Effects of supra-threshold levodopa doses on dyskinesia in advanced Parkinson's disease. Neurology 1997; 49: 711–713.

46. Mouradian MM, Juncos JL, Fabbrini G, et al. Motor fluctuations in Parkinson's disease: Central pathophysiological mechanisms, part II. Ann Neurol 1988; 24: 372–378.

47. Mouradian MM, Heuser IJE, Baronti F, et al. Pathogenesis of dyskinesia in Parkinson's disease. Ann Neurol 1989; 25: 523–526.

48. Boyce S, Clarke CE, Luquin R, et al. Induction of chorea and dystonia in Parkinsonian primates. Mov Disord 1990; 5: 3–7.

49. Bedard PJ, Di Paolo T, Falardeau P, et al. Chronic treatment with L-DOPA, but not bromocriptine induced dyskinesia in MPTP-parkinsonian monkeys. Brain Res 1986; 379: 294–299.

50. Schneider JS. Levodopa-induced dyskinesias in Parkinsonian monkeys: Relationship to extent of nigrostriatal damage. Pharmacol Biochem Behav 1989; 34: 193–196.

51. Nutt JG, Carter JH, Lea ES, et al. Evolution of the response to levodopa during the first 4 years of therapy. Ann Neurol 2002; 51(6): 686–693.

52. Gancher ST, Nutt JG, Woodward WR. Response to brief levodopa infusions in parkinsonian patients with and without motor fluctuations. Neurology 1988; 38: 712–716.

53. Nutt JG, Carter JH, Van Houten L, et al. Short- and long-duration responses to levodopa during the first year of levodopa therapy. Ann Neurol 1997; 42: 349–355.

54. McColl CD, Reardon KA, Shiff M, et al. Motor response to levodopa and the evolution of motor fluctuations in the first decade of treatment of Parkinson's disease. Mov Disord 2002; 17(6): 1227–1234.

55. Nutt JG, Woodward WR, Carter JH, et al. Influence of fluctuations of plasma large neutral amino acids with normal diets on the clinical response to levodopa. J Neurol Neurosurg Psychiatry 1989; 52: 481–487.

56. Nutt JG, Carter JH, Lea ES, et al. Motor fluctuations during continuous levodopa infusions in patients with Parkinson's disease. Mov Disord 1997; 12: 285–292.

57. Hogl BE, Gomez-Arevalo G, Garcia S, et al. A clinical, pharmacologic, and polysomnographic study of sleep benefit in Parkinson's disease. Neurology 1998; 50: 1332–1339.

58. Ma Y, Feigin A, Dhawan V, et al. Dyskinesia after fetal cell transplantation for parkinsonism: a PET study. Ann Neurol 2002; 52(5): 628–634.

59. Ahlskog JE, Muenter MD. Frequency of levodopa-related dyskinesias and motor fluctuations as estimated from the cumulative literature. Mov Disord 2001; 16(3): 448–458.

60. Lesser RP, Fahn S, Snider SR, et al. Analysis of the clinical problems in parkinsonism and the complications of long-term levodopa therapy. Neurology 1979; 29: 1253–1260.

61. Koller WC, Hutton JT, Tolosa E, Capilldeo R, Carbidopa/Levodopa Study Group. Immediate-release and controlled-release carbidopa/levodopa in PD: a 5-year randomized multicenter study. Neurology 1999; 53: 1012–1019.

62. Sweet RD, McDowell FH. Five years' treatment of Parkinson's disease with levodopa: therapeutic results and survival of 100 patients. Ann Intern Med 1975; 83: 456–463.

63. Barbeau A. High-level levodopa therapy in severely akinetic parkinsonian patients: Twelve years later. In Rinne UK, Klinger M, Stamm G (eds) Parkinson's disease: Current progress, problems and management. Amsterdam, New York, Elsevier, 1980, pp. 229–239.

64. Rajput AH, Fenton ME, Birdi S, et al. Clinical-pathological study of levodopa complications. Mov Disord 2002; 17(2): 289–296.

65. Schrag A, Quinn N. Dyskinesias and motor fluctuations in Parkinson's disease. A community-based study. Brain 2000; 123(Pt 11): 2297–2305.

66. Quinn N, Critchley P, Marsden CD. Young onset Parkinson's disease. Mov Disord 1987; 2(2): 73–91.

67. Schrag A, Ben-Shlomo Y, Brown R, et al. Young-onset Parkinson's disease revisted – Clinical features, natural history and mortality. Mov Disord 1998; 13: 885–894.

68. Quinn NP, Marsden CD. Menstrual-related fluctuations in Parkinson's disease. Mov Disord 1986; 1: 85–87.

69. Tsang KL, Ho SL, Lo SK. Estrogen improves motor disability in parkinsonian postmenopausal women with motor fluctuations. Neurology 2000; 54(12): 2292–2298.

70. Gomez-Mancilla B, Bedard PJ. Effect of estrogen and progesterone on L-dopa induced dyskinesia in MPTP-treated monkeys. Neurosci Lett 1992; 135(1): 129–132.

71. Lyons KE, Hubble JP, Troster AI, et al. Gender differences in Parkinson's disease. Clin Neuropharmacol 1998; 21(2): 118–121.

72. Zappia M, Crescibene L, Arabia G, et al. Body weight influences pharmacokinetics of levodopa in Parkinson's disease. Clin Neuropharmacol 2002; 25(2): 79–82.

73. Chase TN, Holden EM, Brody JA. Levodopa-induced dyskinesias: comparison in Parkinsonism-dementia and amyotrophic lateral sclerosis. Arch Neurol 1973; 29: 328–330.
74. Rajput AH, Fenton M, Birdi S, et al. Is levodopa toxic to human substantia nigra? Mov Disord 1997; 12(5): 634–638.
75. Boyce S, Rupniak NMJ, Steventon MJ, et al. Characteriztion of dyskinesia induced by L-dopa in MPTP-treated squirrel monkeys. Psychopharmacology 1990; 102: 21–27.
76. Togasaki DM, Tan L, Protell P, et al. Levodopa induces dyskinesias in normal squirrel monkeys. Ann Neurol 2001; 50: 254–257.
77. Pearce RK, Heikkila M, Linden IB, et al. L-dopa induces dyskinesia in normal monkeys: behavioural and pharmacokinetic observations. Psychopharmacology (Berl) 2001; 156(4): 402–409.
78. Weiner WJ Levodopa induced dyskinesias in normal squirred monkeys. Ann Neural 2002; 51: 531–532.
79. Klawans HL, Jr., Paulson GW, Ringel SP, et al. Use of L-dopa in the detection of presymptomatic Huntington's chorea. N Engl J Med 1972; 286(25): 1332–1334.
80. Langston WJ, Ballard P. Parkinsonsim induced by 1-methyl-4-phenyl-1,2,3,6- tetrahydropyridine (MPTP): implications for treatment and the pathogenesis of Parkinsons disease. Can J Neurol Sci 1984; 11: 160–165.
81. Lang AE, Meadows JC, Parkes JD, et al. Early onset of the "on-off" phenomenon in children with symptomatic Parkinsonism. J Neurol Neurosurg Psychiatry 1982; 45(9): 823–825.
82. Payami H, Nutt J, Gancher S, et al. SCA2 may present as levodopa-responsive parkinsonism. Mov Disord 2003; 18(4): 425–429.
83. Tuite PJ, Rogaeva EA, St.George-Hyslop PH, et al. Dopa-responsive parkinsonism phenotype of Machado-Joseph Disease: confirmation of 14q CAG expansion. Ann Neurol 1995; 38: 684–687.
84. Lucking CB, Durr A, Bonifati V, et al. Association between early-onset Parkinson's disease and mutations in the Parkin gene. N Engl J Med 2000; 342: 1560–1567.
85. Fearnley JM, Lees AJ. Striatonigral degeneration. A clinicopathological study. Brain 1990; 113(Pt 6): 1823–1842.
86. Kim JM, Lee KH, Choi YL, et al. Levodopa-induced dyskinesia in an autopsy-proven case of progressive supranuclear palsy. Mov Disord 2002; 17(5): 1089–1090.
87. Frucht S, Fahn S, Chin S, et al. Levodopa-induced dyskinesias in autopsy-proven corticalbasal ganglionic degeneration. Mov Disord 2000; 15(2): 340–343.
88. Rinne UK. Early combination of bromocriptine and levodopa in the treatment of Parkinson's disease: A 5-year followup. Neurology 1987; 37: 826–828.
89. Rascol O, Brooks DJ, Clarke CE, et al. The development of dyskinesia in Parkinson's disease patients receiving ropinirole and given supplementary levodopa [abstract]. Parkinsonism Rel Disord 2001; 7(suppl): 226.
90. Rascol O, Nutt JG, Blin O, et al. Induction by dopamine D1 receptor agonist ABT-431 of dyskinesia similar to levodopa in patients with Parkinson disease. Arch Neurol 2001; 58(2): 249–254.
91. Grondin R, Bedard PJ, Britton DR, et al. Potential therapeutic use of the selective dopamine D-1 receptor agonist, A-86929: An acute study in parkinsonian levodopa-primed monkeys. Neurology 1997; 49: 421–426.
92. Fahn S, Calne DB. Considerations in the management of parkinsonism. Neurology 1978; 28(1): 5–7.
93. Poewe WH, Lees AJ, Stern GM. Low-dose L-DOPA therapy in Parkinson's disease: A 6-year follow-up study. Neurology 1986; 36: 1528–1530.

94. Cedarbaum JM, Gandy SE, McDowell FH. "Early" initiation of levodopa treatment does not promote the development of motor response fluctuations, dyskinesias, or dementia in Parkinson's disease. Neurology 1991; 41: 622–629.
95. Fahn S, Parkinson Study Group. Results of the ELLDOPA (earlier vs. later levodopa) study [abstract]. Mov Disord 2002; 17(suppl. 5): S13–S14.
96. Albin RL, Young AB, Penney JB. The functional anatomy of basal ganglia disorders. TINS 1989; 12: 366–375.
97. Crossman AR. A hypothesis on the pathophysiological mechanism that underlie levodopa- or dopamine agonist-induced dyskinesia in Parkinson's disease: Implications for future strategies in treatment. Mov Disord 1990; 5: 100–108.
98. Alexander GE, Crutcher MD. Functional architecture of basal ganglia circuits: neural substrates of parallel processing. TINS 1990; 13: 266–271.
99. DeLong MR. Primate models of movement disorders of basal ganglia origin. TINS 1990; 13: 281–289.
100. Wichmann T, DeLong MR. Functional pathophysiological models of the basal ganglia. Curr Opin Neurobiol 1996; 6: 751–758.
101. Bergman H, Wichmann T, DeLong MR. Reversal of experimental parkinsonism by lesions of the subthalamic nucleus. Science 1990; 249: 1436–1438.
102. Limousin P, Pollak P, Benazzouz A, et al. Effect on parkinsonian signs and symptoms of bilateral subthalamic nucleus stimulation. Lancet 1995; 345: 91–95.
103. Boraud T, Bezard E, Bioulac B, et al. Dopamine agonist-induced dyskinesias are correlated to both firing pattern and frequency alterations of pallidal neurones in the MPTP-treated monkey. Brain 2001; 124(Pt 3): 546–557.
104. Mura A, Mintz M, Feldon J. Behavioral and anatomical effects of long-term L-dihydroxyphenylalanine (L-DOPA) administration in rats with unilateral lesions of the nigrostriatal system. Exp Neurol 2002; 177(1): 252–264.
105. Winkler C, Kirik D, Bjorklund A, et al. L-DOPA-induced dyskinesia in the intrastriatal 6-hydroxydopamine model of Parkinson's disease: relation to motor and cellular parameters of nigrostriatal function. Neurobiol Dis 2002; 10(2): 165–186.
106. Calon F, Grondin R, Morissette M, et al. Molecular basis of levodopa-induced dyskinesias. Ann Neurol 2000; 47(4 suppl 1): S70–S78.
107. Calon F, Birdi S, Rajput AH, et al. Increase of preproenkephalin mRNA levels in the putamen of Parkinson disease patients with levodopa-induced dyskinesias. J Neuropathol Exp Neurol 2002; 61(2): 186–196.
108. Johansson PA, Andersson M, Andersson KE, et al. Alterations in cortical and basal ganglia levels of opioid receptor binding in a rat model of l-DOPA-induced dyskinesia. Neurobiol Dis 2001; 8(2): 220–239.
109. Piccini P, Weeks RA, Brooks DJ. Alterations in opioid receptor binding in Parkinson's disease patients with levodopa-induced dyskinesias. Ann Neurol 1997; 42(5): 720–726.
110. Berke JD, Paletzki RF, Aronson GJ, et al. A complex program of striatal gene expression induced by dopaminergic stimulation. J Neurosci 1998; 18: 5301–5310.
111. Filion M, Tremblay L. Abnormal spontaneous activity of globus pallidus neurons in monkeys with MPTP-induced parkinsonism. Brain Res 1991; 547: 142–151.
112. Filion M, Tremblay L, Bedard PJ. Effects of dopamine agonists on the spontaneous activity of globus pallidus neurons in monkeys with MPTP-induced parkinsonism. Brain Res 1991; 547: 152–161.
113. Hutchison WD, Levy R, Dostrovsky JO, et al. Effects of apomorphine on globus pallidus neurons in parkinsonian patients. Ann Neurol 1997; 42: 767–775.

114. Papa SM, Desimone R, Fiorani M, et al. Internal globus pallidus discharge is nearly suppressed during levodopa-induced dyskinesias. Ann Neurol 1999; 46: 732–738.
115. Wenzelburger R, Zhang BR, Pohle S, et al. Force overflow and levodopa-induced dyskinesias in Parkinson's disease. Brain 2002; 125(Pt 4): 871–879.
116. Rascol O, Sabatini U, Brefel C, et al. Cortical motor overactivation in parkinsonian patients with L-dopa-induced peak-dose dyskinesia. Brain 1998; 121 (Pt 3): 527–533.
117. Feigin A, Ghilardi MF, Fukuda M, et al. Effects of levodopa infusion on motor activation responses in Parkinson's disease. Neurology 2002; 59(2): 220–226.
118. Levy R, Hazrati L-N, Herrero M-T, et al. Re-evaluation of the functional anatomy of the basal ganglia in normal and parkinsonian states. Neuroscience 1997; 76: 335–343.
119. Bejjani B, Damier P, Arnulf I, et al. Pallidal stimulation for Parkinson's disease: Two targets? Neurology 1997; 49: 1564–1569.
120. Krack P, Pollak P, Limousin P, et al. Opposite motor effects of pallidal stimulation in Parkinson's disease. Ann Neurol 1998; 43: 180–192.
121. Merello M, Cammarota A, Betti O, et al. Involuntary movements during thermolesion predict a better outcome after microelectrode guided posteroventral pallidotomy. J Neurol Neurosurg Psychiatry 1997; 63: 210–213.
122. Limousin P, Pollak P, Hoffmann D, et al. Abnormal involuntary movements induced by subthalamic nucleus stimulation in parkinsonian patients. Mov Disord 1996; 11: 231–235.
123. Jankovic J, Lai E, Ben Arie L, et al. Levodopa-induced dyskinesias treated by pallidotomy. J Neurol Sci 1999; 167(1): 62–67.
124. Narabayashi H, Yokochi F, Nakajima Y. Levodopa-induced dyskinesia and thalamotomy. J Neurol Neurosurg Psychiatry 1984; 47(8). 831–839.
125. Ohye C, Shibazaki T. Lesioning the thalamus for dyskinesia. Stereotact Funct Neurosurg 2001; 77(1–4): 33–39.
126. Page RD, Sambrook MA, Crossman AR. Thalamotomy for the alleviation of levodopa-induced dyskinesia: experimental studies in the 1-methyl-4-phenyl-1,2,3,6-tetrahydropyridine-treated parkinsonian monkey. Neuroscience 1993; 55(1): 147–165.
127. Caparros-Lefebvre D, Blond S, Vermersch P, et al. Chronic thalamic stimulation improves tremor and levodopa induced dyskinesias in Parkinson's disease. J Neurol Neurosurg Psychiatry 1993; 56: 268–273.
128. Caparros-Lefebvre D, Blond S, Feltin MP, et al. Improvement of levodopa induced dyskinesias by thalamic deep brain stimulation is related to slight variation in electrode placement: possible involvement of the centre median and parafascicularis complex. J Neurol Neurosurg Psychiatry 1999; 67(3): 308–314.
129. Di Monte DA, McCormack A, Petzinger G, et al. Relationship among nigrostriatal denervation, parkinsonism, and dyskinesias in the MPTP primate model. Mov Disord 2000; 15(3): 459–466.
130. Chase TN, Baronti F, Fabbrini G, et al. Rationale for continuous dopaminomimetic therapy of Parkinson's disease. Neurology 1989; 39(suppl 2): 7–10.
131. Chase TN. Levodopa therapy: consequences of the nonphysiologic replacement of dopamine. Neurology 1998; 50(5 suppl 5): S17–S25.
132. Abercrombie ED, Bonatz AE, Zigmond MJ. Effects of L-DOPA on extracellular dopamine in striatum of normal and 6-hydroxydopamine-treated rats. Brain Res 1990; 525: 36–44.
133. Tedroff J, Pedersen M, Aquilonius S-M, et al. Levodopa-induced changes in synaptic dopamine in patients with Parkinson's disease as measured by [11C]raclopride displacement and PET. Neurology 1996; 46: 1430–1436.

134. Contin M, Riva R, Martinelli P, et al. Relationship between levodopa concentration, dyskinesias and motor effect in Parkinsonian patients: a 3-year followup. Clin Neuropharmacol 1997; 20: 409–418.

135. Harder S, Baas H. Concentration-response relationship of levodopa in patients at different stages of Parkinson's disease. Clin Pharmacol Ther 1998; 64: 183–191.

136. Luquin MR, Laguna J, Obeso JA. Selective D2 receptor stimulation induces dyskinesia in parkinsonian monkeys. Ann Neurol 1992; 31(5): 551–554.

137. Facca A, Sanchez-Ramos J. High-dose pergolide monotherapy in the treatment of severe levodopa-induced dyskinesia. Mov Disord 1996; 11: 327–341.

138. Blanchet P, Bedard PJ, Britton DR, et al. Differential effect of selective D-1 and D-2 dopamine receptor agonists on levodopa-induced dyskinesia in 1-methyl-4-phenyl-1,2,3,6-tetrahydropyridine-exposed monkeys. J Pharmacol Exp Ther 1993; 267: 275–279.

139. Blanchet PJ, Grondin R, Bedard PJ. Dyskinesia and wearing-off following dopamine D1 agonist treatment in drug-naive 1-methyl-4-phenyl-1,2,3,6-tetrahydropyridine-lesioned primates. Mov Disord 1996; 11: 91–94.

140. Bordet R, Ridray S, Carboni S, et al. Induction of dopamine D3 receptor expression as a mechanism of behavioral sensitization to levodopa. Proc Natl Acad Sci USA 1997; 94(7): 3363–3367.

141. Bordet R, Ridray S, Schwartz JC, et al. Involvement of the direct striatonigral pathway in levodopa-induced sensitization in 6-hydroxydopamine-lesioned rats. Eur J Neurosci 2000; 12(6): 2117–2123.

142. Zeng BY, Pearce RK, MacKenzie GM, et al. Chronic high dose L-dopa treatment does not alter the levels of dopamine D-1, D-2 or D-3 receptor in the striatum of normal monkeys: an autoradiographic study. J Neural Transm 2001; 108(8–9): 925–941.

143. Blanchet PJ, Konitsiotis S, Chase TN. Motor response to a dopamine D3 receptor preferring agonist compared to apomorphine in levodopa-primed 1-methyl-4-phenyl-1,2,3,6-tetrahydropyridine monkeys. J Pharmacol Exp Ther 1997; 283(2): 794–799.

144. Post RM. Intermittent versus continuous stimulation: effect of time interval on the development of sensitization or tolerance. Life Sci 1980; 26: 1275–1282.

145. Castro R, Abreu P, Calzadilla CH, et al. Increased or decreased locomotor response in rats following repeated administration of apomorphine depends on dosage interval. Psychopharmacology 1985; 85: 333–339.

146. Winkler JD, Weiss B. Effect of continuous exposure to selective D1 and D2 dopainergic agonists on rotational behavior in supersensitive mice. J Pharmacol Exp Ther 1989; 249: 507–516.

147. Gancher ST, Nutt JG, Woodward WR. Time-course of tolerance to apomorphine in parkinsonism. Clin Pharmacol Ther 1992; 52: 504–510.

148. Blanchet PJ, Calon F, Martel JC, et al. Continuous administration decreases and pulsatile administration increases behavioral sensitivity to a novel dopamine D2 agonist (U-91356A) in MPTP-exposed monkeys. J Pharmacol Exp Ther 1995; 272: 854–859.

149. Juncos JL, Engber TM, Raisman R, et al. Continuous and intermittent levodopa differentially affect basal ganglia function. Ann Neurol 1989; 25: 473–478.

150. Morelli M, Di Chiara G. Agonist-induced homologous and heterologous sensitization to D-1 and D-2 dependent contraversive turning. Eur J Pharmacol 1987; 141: 101–107.

151. Chase TN. The significance of continuous dopaminergic stimulation in the treatment of Parkinson's disease. Drugs 1998; 55(suppl 1): 1–9.

152. Olanow W, Schapira AH, Rascol O. Continuous dopamine-receptor stimulation in early Parkinson's disease. Trends Neurosci 2000; 23(10 suppl): S117–S126.

153. Koller WC, Hutton JT, Tolosa E, et al. Immediate-release and controlled-release carbidopa/levodopa in PD: a 5-year randomized multicenter study. Carbidopa/Levodopa Study Group. Neurology 1999; 53(5): 1012–1019.

154. Manson AJ, Turner K, Lees AJ. Apomorphine monotherapy in the treatment of refractory motor complications of Parkinson's disease: long-term follow-up study of 64 patients. Mov Disord 2002; 17(6): 1235–1241.

155. Kanovsky P, Kubova D, Bares M, et al. Levodopa-induced dyskinesias and continuous subcutaneous infusions of apomorphine: results of a two-year, prospective follow-up. Mov Disord 2002; 17(1): 188–191.

156. Stocchi F, Ruggieri S, Vacca L, et al. Prospective randomized trial of lisuride infusion versus oral levodopa in patients with Parkinson's disease. Brain 2002; 125(Pt 9): 2058–2066.

157. Nutt JG, Carter JH, Woodward WR. Long duration response to levodopa. Neurology 1995; 45: 1613–1616.

158. Manson AJ, Schrag A, Lees AJ. Low-dose olanzapine for levodopa induced dyskinesias. Neurology 2000; 55(6): 795–799.

159. Verhagen L, Del Dotto P, van den Mundkhof P, et al. Amantadine as treatment for dyskinesias and motor fluctuations in Parkinson's disease. Neurology 1998; 50: 1323–1326.

160. Del Dotto P, Pavese N, Gambaccini G, et al. Intravenous amantadine improves levodopa-induced dyskinesias: an acute double-blind placebo-controlled study. Mov Disord 2001; 16: 515–520.

161. Blanchet PJ, Konitsiotis S, Chase TN. Amantadine reduces levodopa-induced dyskinesia in parkinsonian monkeys. Mov Disord 1998; 13: 798–802.

162. Barron MS, Vitek JL, Bakay RAE, et al. Treatment of advanced Parkinson's disease by posterior GPi pallidotomy: 1-year results of a pilot study. Ann Neurol 1996; 40: 355–366.

163. Samii A, Turnbull IM, Kishore A, et al. Reassessment of unilateral pallidotomy in Parkinson's disease: a 2-year follow-up study. Brain 1999; 122: 417–425.

164. Chase TN, Oh JD. Striatal dopamine- and glutamate-mediated dysregulation in experimental parkinsonism. Trends Neurosci 2000; 23(10 suppl): S86–S91.

165. Dunah AW, Wang Y, Yasuda RP, et al. Alterations in subunit expression, composition, and phosphorylation of striatal N-methyl-D-aspartate glutamate receptors in a rat 6-hydroxydopamine model of Parkinson's disease. Mol Pharmacol 2000; 57(2): 342–352.

166. Greenamyre JT, Eller RV, Zhang Z, et al. Antiparksonian effects of remacemide hydrochloride, a glutamate antagonist, in rodent and primate models of Parkinson's disease. Ann Neurol 1994; 35: 655–661.

167. Blanchet PJ, Konitsiotis S, Whittemore ER, et al. Differing effects of N-methyl-D-aspartate receptor subtype selective antagonists on dyskinesias in levodopa-treated 1-methyl-4-phenyl-tetrahydropyridine monkeys. J Pharmacol Exp Ther 1999; 290(3): 1034–1040.

168. Konitsiotis S, Blanchet PJ, Verhagen L, et al. AMPA receptor blockade improves levodopa-induced dyskinesia in MPTP monkeys. Neurology 2000; 54(8): 1589–1595.

169. Verhagen ML, Blanchet PJ, van den MP, et al. A trial of dextromethorphan in parkinsonian patients with motor response complications. Mov Disord 1998; 13(3): 414–417.

170. Parkinson Study Group Evaluation of dyskinesias in a pilot, randomized, placebo-controlled trial of remacemide in advanced Parkinson disease. Arch Neurol 2001; 58(10): 1660–1668.

171. Merello M, Nouzeilles MI, Cammarota A, et al. Effect of memantine (NMDA antagonist) on Parkinson's disease: A double-blind crossover randomized study. Clin Neuropharmacol 1999; 22: 273–276.

172. Bibbiani F, Oh JD, Chase TN. Serotonin 5-HT1A agonist improves motor complications in rodent and primate parkinsonian models. Neurology 2001; 57(10): 1829–1834.
173. Bonifati V, Fabrizio E, Cipriani R, et al. Buspirone in levodopa-induced dyskinesia. Clin Neuropharmacol 1994; 17: 73–82.
174. Durif F, Vidailhet M, Bonnet A-M, et al. Levodopa-induced dyskinesias are improved by fluoxetine. Neurology 1995; 45: 1855–1858.
175. Gomez-Mancilla B, Bedard PJ. Effect of nondopaminergic drugs on L-dopa-induced dyskinesias in MPTP-treated monkeys. Clin Neuropharmacol 1993; 16(5): 418–427.
176. Henry B, Fox SH, Peggs D, et al. The alpha2-adrenergic receptor antagonist idazoxan reduces dyskinesia and enhances anti-parkinsonian actions of L-dopa in the MPTP-lesioned primate model of Parkinson's disease. Mov Disord 1999; 14(5): 744–753.
177. Rascol O, Arnulf I, Peyro-Saint PH, et al. Idazoxan, an alpha-2 antagonist, and L-DOPA-induced dyskinesias in patients with Parkinson's disease. Mov Disord 2001; 16(4): 708–713.
178. Henry B, Fox SH, Crossman AR, et al. Mu- and delta-opioid receptor antagonists reduce levodopa-induced dyskinesia in the MPTP-lesioned primate model of Parkinson's disease. Exp Neurol 2001; 171(1): 139–146.
179. Klintenberg R, Svenningsson P, Gunne L, et al. Naloxone reduces levodopa-induced dyskinesias and apomorphine-induced rotations in primate models of parkinsonism. J Neural Transm 2002; 109(10): 1295–1307.
180. Rascol O, Fabre N, Blin O, et al. Naltrexone, an opiate antagonist, fails to modify motor symptoms in patients with Parkinson's disease. Mov Disord 1994; 9(4): 437–440.
181. Richardson PJ, Kase H, Jenner PG. Adenosine A2A receptor antagonists as new agents for the treatment of Parkinson's disease. Trends Pharmacol Sci 1997; 18(9): 338–344.
182. Kanda T, Jackson MJ, Smith LA, et al. Adenosine A2A antagonist: a novel antiparkinsonian agent that does not provoke dyskinesia in parkinsonian monkeys. Ann Neurol 1998; 43(4): 507–513.
183. Brotchie JM. CB(1) cannabinoid receptor signalling in Parkinson's disease. Curr Opin Pharmacol 2003; 3(1): 54–61.
184. Fox SH, Henry B, Hill M, et al. Stimulation of cannabinoid receptors reduces levodopa-induced dyskinesia in the MPTP-lesioned nonhuman primate model of Parkinson's disease. Mov Disord 2002; 17(6): 1180–1187.
185. Sieradzan KA, Fox SH, Hill M, et al. Cannabinoids reduce levodopa-induced dyskinesia in Parkinson's disease: a pilot study. Neurology 2001; 57(11): 2108–2111.
186. Sage JI, Mark MH, McHale DM, et al. Benefits of monitoring plasma levodopa in Parkinson's disease patients with drug-induced chorea. Ann Neurol 1991; 29: 623–628.
187. Shoulson I, Oakes D, Fahn S, et al. Impact of sustained deprenyl (selegiline) in levodopa-treated Parkinson's disease: a randomized placebo-controlled extension of the deprenyl and tocopherol antioxidative therapy of parkinsonism trial. Ann Neurol 2002; 51(5): 604–612.
188. Hauser RA, Olanow CW. Orobuccal dyskinesia associated with trihexyphenidyl therapy in a patient with Parkinson's disease. Mov Disord 1993; 8(4): 512–514.
189. Linazasoro G. Anticholinergics and dyskinesia. Mov Disord 1994; 9(6): 689.
190. Tolcapone Study Group. Efficacy and tolerability of tolcapone compared with bromocriptine in levodopa-treated parkinsonian patients. Mov Disord 1999; 14: 38–44.
191. Nutt JG. Levodopa-induced dyskinesia: review, observations and speculations. Neurology 1990; 40: 340–345.
192. Kaye JA, Feldman RG. The role of L-DOPA holiday in the long-term management of Parkinson's disease. Clin Neuropharmacol 1986; 9: 1–13.

193. Mayeux R, Stern Y, Mulvey K, et al. Reappraisal of temporary levodopa withdrawal ("drug holiday") in Parkinson's disease. N Engl J Med 1985; 313: 724–733.

194. Krause M, Heck A, Bonsanto M, et al. Deep brain stimulation for the treatment of Parkinson's disease: subthalamic nucleus versus globus pallidus internus. J Neurol Neurosurg Psychiatry 2001; 70: 464–470.

195. Burchiel KJ, Anderson VC, Favre J, et al. Comparison of pallidal and subthalamic nucleus deep brain stimulation for advanced Parkinson's disease: results of a randomized, blinded pilot study. Neurosurgery 1999; 45: 1375–1384.

196. Volkmann J, Strum V, Weiss P, et al. Bilateral high-frequency stimulation of the internal globus pallidus in advanced Parkinson's disease. Ann Neurol 1998; 44: 953–961.

197. Deep-brain stimulation of the subthalamic nucleus or the pars interna of the globus pallidus in Parkinson's disease. N Engl J Med 2001; 345(13): 956–963.

198. Fraix V, Pollak P, Van Blercom N, et al. Effect of subthalamic nucleus stimulation on levodopa-induced dyskinesia in Parkinson's disease. Neurology 2000; 55: 1921–1923.

199. Krack P, Pollak P, Limousin P, et al. From off-period dystonia to peak-dose chorea. The clinical spectrum of varying subthalamic nucleus activity. Brain 1999; 122 (Pt 6): 1133–1146.

200. Quinn N, Parkes JD, Marsden CD. Control of on/off phenomenon by continuous intravenous infusion of levodopa. Neurology 1984; 34: 1131–1136.

201. Lees AJ. The on-off phenomenon. J Neurol Neurosurg Psychiatry 1989; (suppl): 29–37.

202. Durif F, Deffond D, Dordain G, et al. Apomorphine and diphasic dyskinesia. Clin Neuropharmacol 1994; 17(1): 99–102.

203. Bravi D, Mouradian MM, Roberts JW, et al. End-of-dose dystonia in Parkinson's disease. Neurology 1993; 43(10): 2130–2131.

204. Bezard E, Brotchie JM, Gross CE. Pathophysiology of levodopa-induced dyskinesia: potential for new therapies. Nat Rev Neurosci 2001; 2(8): 577–588.

205. Iravani MM, Costa S, Jackson MJ, et al. GDNF reverses priming for dyskinesia in MPTP-treated, L-DOPA-primed common marmosets. Eur J Neurosci 2001; 13(3): 597–608.

206. Olanow CW, Obeso JA. Preventing levodopa-induced dyskinesias. Ann Neurol 2000; 47(4 suppl 1): S167–S176.

207. Zappia M, Bosco D, Plastino M, et al. Pharmacodynamics of the long-duration response to levodopa in PD. Neurology 1999; 53: 557–560.

208. Nutt JG. Response to L-DOPA in PD: the long and short of it. Neurology 2000; 54: 1884–1885.

CHAPTER 14

Movement disorders and dopaminomimetic stimulant drugs

Anthony E. Munson, Juan Sanchez-Ramos, and William J. Weiner

Introduction

This chapter will focus on movement disorders induced by stimulant drugs that affect dopaminergic activity within the central nervous system. The four agents reviewed are amphetamine, methylphenidate, pemoline, and cocaine. We will focus the discussion on the pharmacologic activities of these drugs, and that will be followed by a review of reports regarding both the ability of these drugs to induce movement disorders in the "normal" individual as well as in patients with a variety of preexisting disorders such as Parkinson's disease, choreiform disorders, tic disorders, and dystonia.

Cocaine had been used for centuries by the inhabitants of the highlands of Peru primarily to induce a sense of well-being. In the late 19th century, the medical profession recognized that cocaine had local anesthetic properties. Freud was particularly impressed by its CNS actions, and his overenthusiasm for the drug has been widely publicized. In the late 1970s, recreational cocaine use began to rise dramatically, and the introduction of the alkalose form ("crack" cocaine) in 1983, brought even more awareness of the neurologic effects of the drug. In 1997, it was estimated that thirty million Americans had used cocaine at least once, and five million of these people were using cocaine on a daily basis.

Cocaine is a potent psychostimulant and can induce a sense of increased wakefulness and alertness, a decreased sense of fatigue, elevation of mood, increased initiative, confidence and concentration, elation, and euphoria. These effects are mediated in the central nervous system by several mechanisms, including the competitive blockade of dopamine uptake at dopaminergic nerve terminals. This results in a hyperdopaminergic state. This effect seems to occur, in particular, in cells that originate in the ventral tegmentum and project to the nucleus accumbens, ventral pallidum, and the frontal cortex. This affects the dopaminergic mesocortical, mesolimbic, and mesostriatal pathways. Other actions of cocaine include local anesthesia and sympathomimetic effects, most apparent as potent vasoconstriction (including intracranial vasculature).

Amphetamine was first synthesized in 1887 but, it was not until the 1930s that it was introduced into clinical practice as a nasal decongestant inhaler and as an appetite suppressant. Reports of self-stimulation and abuse began in the same decade. The therapeutic effects of amphetamine were noted to include elevated mood, a sense of alertness, reduced fatigue, and decreased appetite. Additional consequences of its use include agitation, dysphoria, and in higher doses, paranoia, delusions, hallucinations, and seizures.

The CNS stimulant effects of amphetamine are primarily related to release of biogenic amines from storage sites in nerve terminals. Amphetamine affects the dopaminergic system by releasing newly synthesized cytoplasmic dopamine, inhibiting dopamine reuptake, and at high doses, inhibiting monoamine oxidase (MAO). Amphetamine's ability to induce repetitive behaviors is thought to be related to the release of newly synthesized dopamine from storage sites in the striatum. The drug also acts by increasing the release of norepinephrine at nerve terminals as well as altering the serotonergic and endogenous opiate systems.

Another closely related compound, 3,4-methylenedioxymetamphetamine (MDMA), has received considerable attention because of increased street use ("Ecstacy"). This drug has CNS stimulant effects similar to amphetamine but has a higher predilection for causing hallucinations. It is thought that this difference is due to the greater impact on the serotonergic system by MDMA in comparison to amphetamine.

Methylphenidate is a piperidine derivative that is structurally related to amphetamine. It is recognized as a mild CNS stimulant with more prominent effects on mental rather that motor activities. As with amphetamine, these actions are mediated by the release of dopamine from storage vesicles. Experimental evidence indicates that, unlike amphetamine, its dopamine effect is blocked by reserpine but not by alphamethylparatyrosine. This suggests that methylphenidate does not release dopamine from the newly synthesized dopamine pool. Methylphenidate is widely used in the United States for treatment of attention deficit hyperactivity disorder (ADHD).

Pemoline is another medication used in the treatment of ADHD. It is a central CNS stimulant whose effect is also related to the release of dopamine from storage vesicles. The use of pemoline for ADHD has dropped dramatically over the past decade due to concern over hepatic toxicity, and it is no longer considered a first-line agent for this condition.

Amphetamine-induced movement disorders

Amphetamine, as is the case with many drugs of abuse, enjoyed a period where it was prescribed and championed by the medical establishment as a treatment for a wide variety of ailments. It was, at that time, considered safe and effective. It was not until the 1960s that information on patterns of abuse surfaced in the medical literature [1]. Since then, there have been many reports of motor-related symptoms during both drug use and abuse. Amphetamine has a wide range of actions on the central nervous system, and in people who abuse it, a variety of syndromes have been reported. The effects of amphetamine on both the intact and diseased motor system will be discussed.

Stereotyped behavior

Single high doses or repeated low doses of amphetamine administered to various animals produce a motor phenomenon called amphetamine-induced stereotyped behavior. The stereotyped behavior produced is species specific; for example, a chewing, gnawing behavior occurs in guinea pigs, strange head movements occur in cats, and repetitive pecking is seen in pigeons. Amphetamine induces this stereotyped behavior through dopaminergic mechanisms in the basal ganglia. In humans, the response to amphetamine with regard to the induction of stereotyped behavior is much more varied. In fact, in an extensive review of the effects of amphetamine in humans, no definite mention is made of this phenomenon when the result of a single standard dose of amphetamine is considered. However, this review suggests that doses exceeding an individual's tolerance do produce intoxication syndromes that may be accompanied by stereotyped behavior [2]. Whether this is really an intoxication effect or a dose-response relationship is unclear and perhaps semantic.

Stereotyped behavior is considered to be present in animals when certain behavioral repertoires are repeated over and over again without any obvious goal or reinforcement. In more extreme instances, a single behavior or activity is performed continuously and dominates the animal's behavior. In guinea pigs with fully developed amphetamine-induced stereotyped behavior, the animals will chew repeatedly at the bars or grid of the cage without moving, and often even loud noises will not interrupt this activity. This type of stereotyped behavior occurs in unlesioned intact animals receiving high doses.

It has been shown in several studies that amphetamine-like stimulants increase extracellular dopamine in the nucleus accumbens and caudate-putamen, and evidence suggests that these changes are important for the stereotypy produced by these drugs [3]. In one study, it was found that the acute phase of the amphetamine response appeared to be associated with an upregulation of both D1 and D2 dopamine receptors in mice [3]. Another study demonstrated increased D1 receptor concentrations in the nucleus accumbens of methamphetamine users [4].

In human beings who are intravenous amphetamine abusers, certain abnormalities resembling stereotyped behaviors have been noted. These behaviors have been described extensively and include compulsive shoe shining, nail polishing to the point of producing finger ulcerations, repetitive sorting of objects in a handbag, manipulation of the interiors of a watch, days and nights spent rebuilding a car with unrelated parts, and hours spent trying to disassemble and repair items that are in perfect working order. Additional descriptions of this behavior include cleaning drawers and rooms, washing dishes, perpetual hair dressing, distinctive and repetitive walking patterns, and sitting in a tub and bathing all day long [5]. This behavior has been called "punding." Attempts to disrupt this stereotyped behavior often elicit anxiety, and despite its inane quality, amphetamine users often describe the behavior as pleasurable. Punding is usually not recognized by abusers as a sign worth mentioning, and a history of its occurrence has to be specifically sought. Some have suggested that these disorganized and perseverative behaviors are exaggerations of individual personality characteristics. However, in almost every patient who develops punding, paranoid symptoms occur sooner or later. Individuals exhibiting this behavior have also been described as withdrawn, giving the impression of absentmindedness. It has also been noted that the punding act appears consistent and the same for each amphetamine addict. In fact, witnessed observations of addict "punding" have also included descriptions of questionable psychotic behavior at the time, such as visual and tactile hallucinations and paranoid delusions [5, 6]. Fernandez et al. [7] described punding in three patients on levodopa therapy for Parkinson's disease, supporting the belief that this is a dopaminergic phenomenon. Similar behaviors have been described in children treated with either racemic amphetamine or d-amphetamine for various behavioral disorders. One report describes undesirable side effects of these drugs to include "accentuation of tic-like motor activities such as nail biting, hair pulling, nose picking, and the like " [8].

This stereotyped behavior was noted in earlier reports as well. Tatetsu et al. [9] described two patients admitted for amphetamine psychosis who, shortly after admission, were noted to make "incomprehensible, odd, and very unnatural movements." The movements were further described in terms almost identical to later reports of stereotyped behavior, with a repetitious, energetic quality. These abnormal movements were exaggerated by IV methylphenidate.

There is not much evidence available on the development of stereotyped behavior in human beings in the absence of preexisting factors such as psychosis. Despite this, there is also no evidence that preexisting disease need be present for stereotyped behaviors to arise in the setting of amphetamine abuse. Given the animal data available on stereotyped behavior induced by high-dose amphetamine, it appears likely that amphetamine alone is sufficient to induce these behaviors in human subjects.

Dyskinesias

Amphetamine administration is also associated with the induction of various dyskinesias, particularly chorea (Table 14.1). There may be individuals who are "predisposed" to this phenomenon because they develop dyskinesias after a single dose. These individuals may have preexisting damage to the basal ganglia (e.g., birth injury, viral infection, anoxia associated with anesthesia), which is not severe enough to produce clinical signs but which alters the response of the caudate and putamen to stimulants capable of affecting the dopaminergic system. In addition, chronic high-dose amphetamine use alone can cause dyskinesias (Table 14.1). These subjects presumably were "normal" (i.e., no prior neurological findings or history) prior to the use of stimulants and did not

Table 14.1 Amphetamine and dyskinesias

References	Age	Sex	Previous neurological history	Previous abnormal movements	Psychosis associated	Type of movement	Pattern of use	Outcome
49	21	Female	0	0	Yes	Choreoathetoid	Chronic intermittent	Resolved in 24 hours
49	25	Female	0	0	No	Choreoathetoid	Intermittent, needle tracks seen	Resolved in 6 hours
49	30	Male	0	0	No	Rolling of arms, tongue protrusions, writhing of body	Chronic long term	Resolved in 3 hours
50	27	Male	0	0	No	Chorea – face and extremities	High dose IV	Persistent abnormal movements despite abstinence
50	20	Male	0	0	No	Chorea – head and neck, ballismus – arms	High dose IV, chronic	Resolved
50	30	Male	0	0	No	Chorea – generalized	High dose IV, chronic	Resolved
50	35	Male	0	0	No, but stereotyped behavior present	Chorea – generalized	Chronic oral	Movements decreased but not resolved
51	8	Male	Organic brain syndrome, mixed seizures, hyperactivity	0	No	Choreoathetoid – mouth, tongue, and extremities	Oral 15 mg b.i.d. for 8 weeks	Resolved
53	8	Male	Learning disability, hyperkinetic	Mild choreoathetoid	No	Increased choreoathetoid	Oral 5 mg b.i.d. for 3 months	Resolved in 12 hours
53	3	Female	Seizure disorder, mental retardation	0	No	Choreoathetoid – generalized	Oral 2.5 mg b.i.d for 1 week	Resolved in 12 hours
53	5	Male	Temper tantrums, short attention span, hyperactivity	0	No	Grimacing, dyskinetic movements	Oral 1 dose 5 mg	Resolved in 8 hours
53	51	Female	Narcolepsy	0	No	Spasmodic torticollis	Oral 20 mg per day for years	Resolved when medication discontinued

respond acutely with the development of a movement disorder. However, the chronic use of stimulants (particularly amphetamine) resulted in choreoathetoid movements. This raises the possibility that chronic amphetamine administration may alter subsequent dopaminergic behavioral response (e.g., as in amphetamine-induced stereotyped behavior in animals) and eventually result in chorea. In fact, chronic use of high doses of amphetamine has been reported to produce a long-lasting depletion of dopamine in the caudate nucleus [10]. Given the extensive use of amphetamine at various times in the population and the rarity of case reports of amphetamine-induced chorea, this probably is an infrequent occurrence.

Amphetamine, cocaine, methylphenidate, and pemoline in patients with a history of movement disorders

Parkinson's disease

The symptoms of Parkinson's disease are known to be the result of dopamine depletion in the basal ganglia. Since amphetamine has dopaminergic activity, there has been substantial investigation to determine if amphetamine would be of use in treating this disease.

In the late 1930s, there were several reports that suggested that benzedrine, 20 to 60 mg per day, alone and in combination with atropine, provided significant improvement in the condition of Parkinson's disease patients. Most of these reports suggested that the positive changes were in the "subjective" sphere. Patients described increased energy, decreased fatigue, decreased somnolence, and increased well-being. These reports include the description of a bedridden patient who, when treated with amphetamine, was able to dress himself, and of another "helpless" patient who was able to feed himself again. Most of the reports were unable to document much if any objective changes, although there are descriptions of decreased tremor, decreased rigidity, and decreased salivation. These papers suggest that positive changes were seen in 50% to 93% of patients with postencephalitic parkinsonism treated with amphetamine. It is of interest that the authors also commented that oculogyric crises were improved or abolished in almost all of the patients [11, 12]. In 1961, based on the effect of methylphenidate on the dopaminergic system, Halliday and Nathan [13] reported on its use in the treatment of Parkinson's disease. They noted that some patients had increased freedom of movement and decreased rigidity, but that tremor was unaffected. However, they concluded that only one-half of the patients felt better and that they were unsure that this "feeling better" was related to methylphenidate's antiparkinsonism effects.

In 1975, Parkes et al. [14] examined the effect of both L- and D-amphetamine in Parkinson's disease. These patients continued to take their antiparkinsonism medications including levodopa, amantadine, and anticholinergics, and were started on L- or D-amphetamine as outpatients. Both L- and D-amphetamine produced slight (17–20%) reduction in total disability, tremor, akinesia, and rigidity. As a result of side effects induced by amphetamine and because of the modest nature of clinical improvement, it was concluded that neither isomer was of value in routine treatment.

The failure of amphetamine and methylphenidate to improve the disability of Parkinson's disease is not surprising when considering the mechanism of action of these medications. In Parkinson's disease, there is a net decrease in dopamine production and storage in the affected areas of the basal ganglia. Amphetamine has mechanisms of action that include blockade of dopamine reuptake mechanisms, but more importantly, induction of the release of stored and newly synthesized dopamine. This latter mechanism of action is probably ineffective in Parkinson's disease. The action of methylphenidate is linked to the release of stored dopamine without the blockade of reuptake, and therefore would be expected to have even less efficacy in the treatment of Parkinson's disease.

Amphetamine and methylphenidate are almost never employed in the treatment of Parkinson patients today. The beneficial motor effects are minimal, and the unfavorable side effect profile (anorexia, possible encephalopathic changes) makes these medications of questionable use in this patient population.

Choreiform disorders

Choreiform movements of diverse etiologies are thought to be directly related to excess activity of the nigrostriatal dopaminergic system. In this regard, stimulation of dopamine receptors is thought to enhance chorea, and central dopamine blockade or depletion is thought to reduce choreiform movements [15].

Amphetamine has been reported to enhance chorea in a variety of conditions including Sydenham's chorea, Huntington's disease, and chorea associated with systemic lupus erythematosus. In all of these patients, some preexisting dysfunction of the striatum can be assumed from their diagnosis. The lack of chorea in "normal" controls after amphetamine administration would seem to indicate that a prior neurologic insult or preexisting abnormality is required for amphetamine to produce chorea. For example, amphetamine reproduced abnormal movements in a patient with a history of Sydenham's chorea whose symptoms had resolved years prior to presentation [16]. Effects like this have been seen over a variety of time periods, usually in the acute setting, and represent a different process than the punding or stereotyped behaviors seen with chronic amphetamine use noted earlier in this chapter.

There have been several case reports of methylphenidate-induced chorea. Palatucci [17] reported the case of a 19-year-old male who developed choreiform dyskinesias after a single dose of methylphenidate in the setting of several weeks of neuroleptic use. One hour after methylphenidate administration, the patient developed dyskinesias that did not resolve for the next 30 hours. A second case involved a 55-year-old woman on chronic neuroleptics and lithium who had discontinued them prior to abusing methylphenidate. The patient developed a choreoathetoid movement disorder shortly thereafter

[18]. The chronic use of neuroleptics is believed to affect dopamine receptor mechanisms, and it is possible that the prior exposure to neuroleptics may have presensitized these patients to the dopaminergic effects of methylphenidate.

Millichap et al. [19] noted one patient in a study of hyperkinetic behavior and learning disorders who developed difficulty in speaking, difficulty in moving the lips, and twitching movements of the face. The symptoms appeared to be proportional to the dose of methylphenidate, and improved when the dose was decreased. Of the 30 patients in the study, 29 had a diagnosis of minimal brain disease, and it is unclear if this patient had carried this diagnosis or was the exception. In another patient, Weiner et al. [20] described the onset of chorea that persisted for 2 years following a dose escalation of methylphenidate for hyperactivity. In both of these patients, a preexisting abnormality was present that likely predisposed these individuals to methylphenidate-induced choreiform movements.

In guinea pigs, chronic administration of methylphenidate alters dopaminergic response [20]. Specifically, it progressively lowers the threshold to elicit stereotyped responses. Alterations in the dopamine receptors due to chronic methylphenidate use have been postulated to cause the development of chorea noted in some patients after small escalations in their dose.

Pemoline-induced chorea has rarely been reported. In two case reports, patients were treated with neuroleptics prior to the administration of pemoline [21, 22]. As noted with methylphenidate, chronic neuroleptic-induced changes in the dopamine response could be the underlying mechanism.

In patients without prior neuroleptic use or a preexisting condition, the ability of pemoline to induce chorea remains unclear. Stork and Cantor [23] reported 3-year-old twins with the diagnosis of attention deficit hyperactivity disorder (ADHD) who presented with choreoathetoid movements of the face and extremities after a pemoline overdose. The patients had been treated with methylphenidate prior to what was to be their first day of pemoline therapy. No history of movement disorders is reported before or during therapy with methylphenidate. Given the diagnosis of ADHD, however, there may be an underlying predilection for abnormal responses to dopaminergic stimulants, as well as potential complications related to the prior use of methylphenidate and its potential chronic effects. Nausieda et al. [24] reported the case of a 2-year-old who overdosed on pemoline and developed encephalopathy accompanied by a choreiform movement disorder. This consisted of buccal facial dyskinesias, tongue protrusions, and brief movements of the hands and feet. Symptoms resolved over 36 hours. There was no known history of movement disorder or ADHD in this child. Despite this, there appears to be little evidence of pemoline-induced choreiform disorder in patients without a history of a movement disorder except in cases of significant overdose.

Daras et al. [25] reported seven additional patients observed to have cocaine-induced movements. Two of these patients had a history of remote or recent neuroleptic use, and one patient was known to have AIDS, but the remaining four patients were without known history of neurodegenerative disorder or neuroleptic use. All seven patients presented with choreoathetoid movements of the extremities and the majority also had facial or head involvement. In all seven cases, symptoms resolved over 3–6 days in the hospital. At least three of the patients without predisposing factors noted similar events in the past related to crack cocaine use. The authors noted the presence of a slang term for this phenomenon ("crack dancing") as well as for buccolingual dyskinesias ("boca torsida" or "twisted mouth"), and that the presence of these terms may indicate that these phenomena are much more prevalent in the population but underreported due to the transient nature of the symptoms.

Tic disorders

There has been much debate regarding the effect on amphetamine and methylphenidate on tic disorders. Attention deficit hyperactivity disorder (ADHD), the primary indication for use of these medications in children, has a strong association with the Gilles de la Tourette syndrome (GTS). Although a wide variety of genes and neurotransmitters are involved in the pathogenesis of both ADHD and GTS [26], the motor components of GTS (motor and vocal tics) are thought to be related to abnormalities of the dopaminergic system. There has been concern that treatment of ADHD with amphetamine and methylphenidate may carry a risk of inducing motor tics or even the full syndrome of GTS. More recent studies have brought into question the concept that these drugs exacerbate tics. Black [27] reported that six patients with GTS given an acute dose of levodopa reported significant decrease in the severity of their tics. This was confirmed by a blinded observer using videotapes. If tics were caused solely by excess dopaminergic activity, they would have worsened with levodopa administration. In addition, a recent study has demonstrated that pergolide, a dopamine agonist, also improved tics [28]. It remains plausible that the dopaminergic system is involved in GTS, but the exact mechanism is unclear.

Several early case reports and studies were published reporting patients who developed increased tics or GTS seemingly secondary to stimulant medication administered for hyperkinetic behavior. In 1973, Meyerhoff and Snyder [29] described an increase in tics in a GTS patient treated with amphetamine. The following year, Golden [30] described a case of new "full-blown" GTS in a 9-year-old being treated (with good effect) for hyperkinetic behavior. The tic disorder resolved when methylphenidate was discontinued. Denckla et al. [31] examined data on 1520 patients with minimal brain dysfunction treated with methylphenidate. They reported 20 cases (1.3% of the patients) of tics related to the treatment, 14 of which were new onset and 6 of which were exacerbations of preexisting tics. It was noted, however, that reliance on phone interviews by the investigators may have underestimated the prevalence. The authors concluded that only a small percentage of patients experience exacerbation of tics by methylphenidate. Additional studies were also published regarding the ability of methylphenidate to exacerbate or induce motor and vocal tics in GTS [32, 33] including an additional case of new full-blown GTS in a child with ADHD [34].

Several larger case series support the link between stimulant treatment and exacerbation of tics in GTS. Golden [35] reported a case review of 32 GTS patients who had been exposed to amphetamine or methylphenidate, 17 of whom developed marked exacerbation of their tic symptoms. Lowe et al. [36] described 15 GTS patients with exacerbation of their tics out of 100 patients treated with stimulant medication. This series made the observation that many of these 15 patients had a family history of GTS or tic disorder, which may have predisposed them to exacerbation when exposed to stimulants. Several other case series were published with similar findings, with percentages of patients experiencing exacerbation of tics ranging from 22% to 33% [37, 46]. It is of interest that several patients were actually noted to have a decrease in tic severity while on stimulant medication. One common finding was that many of the children did not develop the tics for weeks to months after starting stimulants, and, in fact, several had discontinued the stimulant medications prior to the development or exacerbation of the tics. This observation raised the possibility that exacerbation in GTS patients or new tics seen in ADHD children may, in fact, represent the natural progression of these patients in the development or course of their GTS, rather than a medication effect.

Price et al. [38] reported on six pairs of monozygotic twins with GTS. In each twin set, both developed the disease, but there was complete discordance regarding time of onset and severity in relation to prior stimulant use. Although the number of patients is small, these data suggest that stimulants are not a factor in GTS phenotype expression. Lipkin et al. [39] looked at risk factors for the development of tic disorder in patients with ADHD on stimulant medications. They reported tic prevalence of 9% in 122 children treated with stimulants. There was no relation between personal or family tic history, medication selection, or dosage and the development or exacerbation of tic disorder.

More recently, several controlled studies have shown no effect of stimulant therapy on tics. In 1995, Gadow et al. [40] conducted a double-blind, placebo-controlled study of 34 children with ADHD and tic disorder, each treated with three doses of methylphenidate and placebo for 2 weeks each. The children showed no evidence of worsening in severity of tics on any dose of methylphenidate in comparison to placebo in evaluations by physician, teacher, or parent. Efron et al. [41] performed a double-blind, crossover trial of methylphenidate and dexamphetamine in 125 children with ADHD. Overall, the prevalence and severity of tics showed a statistically significant decrease during stimulant treatment compared to baseline, leading the authors to conclude that tics are not a symptom exacerbated by stimulant use. In 2002, a randomized controlled trial of 136 patients with tic disorder and ADHD found that the proportion of individuals reporting worsening of tics as an adverse effect of methylphenidate was no higher than placebo [42]. The measured tic severity in these same patients actually decreased compared to placebo. The authors concluded that concerns about worsening of tics with stimulant medications were not supported by their data and that methylphenidate and clonidine are effective for treatment of ADHD with comorbid tic disorders. Two other recent studies showing the effectiveness of methylphenidate treatment on symptoms of ADHD also note the absence of increased tic frequency or severity over 15 and 24 months of treatment in 62 and 34 patients, respectively [43, 44].

The American Academy of Child and Adolescent Psychiatry issued practice parameters in 2002 that stated "controlled studies have not found that [methylphenidate] worsens motor tics in Tourette's syndrome, nor does it increase motor tics in children with ADHD without Tourette's syndrome" [45]. In every study listed above and in most case reports, the symptoms of ADHD that were being treated were significantly improved (inattention, behavioral issues). The recent large randomized, placebo-controlled trials show no effect or even improvement in tic disorders with methylphenidate. The risk of exacerbation or induction of tics in this population seems almost nonexistent. At the same time, significant benefits of treatment of ADHD with stimulants have been demonstrated.

Pemoline has also been implicated, in several cases, of exacerbating or causing tic disorders. As pemoline is also used primarily to treat ADHD, it is not surprising that the reported cases are of a similar nature to those regarding methylphenidate. Bachman [46] reported a 9-year-old child who developed tics when he began treatment with pemoline. The pemoline was discontinued after 2 months, with no change in the tics. He had a fluctuating course over the next few years of both motor and verbal tics, sufficient to support the diagnosis of GTS. While the child had not evidenced these tics before treatment, it seems likely that the patient actually had incipient GTS and the pemoline treatment precipitated the appearance of the characteristic symptoms.

Mitchell and Matthews [47] and Sleator [48] each reported a child who developed new motor tics when started on pemoline for hyperactivity. In both cases, the child had no prior history of movement disorder, but it is notable that both children had previously been treated with thioridazine. These children had improvement of symptoms after discontinuing pemoline therapy. When one of the children was rechallenged with pemoline, the tics recurred, again resolving after pemoline was withdrawn. The common history of thioridazine use in both children could represent an underlying etiology, likely sensitizing the dopaminergic neurons and predisposing the patients to tics when exposed to pemoline.

Regarding cocaine and tic disorders, there have been several case reports of cocaine exacerbating or inducing tics. Mesulam [49] and Factor et al. [50] describe two patients with preexisting GTS whose tics grew more severe with the use of cocaine. Pascaul-Leone and Dhuna [51] reported four patients who had cocaine-induced worsening or onset of tics. Two of the patients had a prior diagnosis of GTS, and their response to crack cocaine consisted of increased severity of both motor and vocal tics. It is notable that the exacerbation in tic severity lasted for 4 days in one patient. The other two patients were without a prior history of tics or other movement disorder, and there was no family history of tics. These patients experienced new onset of multifocal motor tics during binge periods of cocaine use. Both patients had prolonged recovery over weeks to months. The possibility that they had undiagnosed conditions prior to presentation or subtle predisposing factors cannot be completely excluded, but an extensive hospital evaluation including imaging was otherwise normal. If these patients were indeed "normal" prior to cocaine use, it would imply that cocaine alone is sufficient to induce tics, possibly through dopaminergic supersensitivity as demonstrated in animal models of stereotyped behavior.

Dystonia

In the last decade, there have been several case reports and two case series describing acute dystonic reactions with cocaine abuse (Table 14.2). Kumor et al. [52] reported that six of seven cocaine abusers administered haloperidol in a research setting developed an acute dystonic reaction. These patients had not used cocaine for at least 10 days prior to the administration of haloperidol. The acute dystonia developed within 22 hours of the first haloperidol dose in four patients and within 3 hours of the second haloperidol dose in the other two patients. The resultant dystonia was so severe as to require administration of intravenous diphenhydramine or benztropine after which the dystonia quickly resolved. Choy-Kwong and Lipton [53] noted in a study of consecutive patients admitted to a psychiatric hospital and treated with neuroleptics that prior history of cocaine abuse was associated with a threefold increased risk of dystonic reactions. Kumor [54] described a single patient who first developed an acute dystonic response to haloperidol and who, when administered cocaine 5 days later, once again had onset of dystonia. van Harten et al. [55] conducted a prospective study to examine the matter. The subjects consisted of 29 males aged 17–45 years who had received high-potency neuroleptics after admission to a hospital psychiatric unit. None of the patients had a known neurodegenerative disease or had been exposed to anticholinergic medications or benzodiazepines, and the patients were followed for 7 days. The results indicated a significantly increased risk (RR = 4.4) for cocaine users versus nonusers. They concluded that cocaine-using patients requiring high-potency neuroleptics should be administered an anticholinergic medication for the first 7 days of neuroleptic administration. These studies have served to alert clinicians that prior history of cocaine abuse may predispose to acute neuroleptic-induced dystonia, and these patients must be carefully observed.

There have also been a number of case reports involving cocaine-induced acute dystonic reactions in patients without known predisposing risk factors. One patient developed focal dystonic movements lasting approximately 45 minutes shortly after cocaine use [56], and a second patient, a 15-year-old girl admitted to the psychiatry unit developed an acute dystonic reaction 16 hours after her last known use of cocaine without receiving neuroleptic medication [57]. Neither patient was known to have a prior history of a movement disorder. Farrell [58] reported a case of a 29-year-old man who developed spasm of his masseter muscles and inability to open his jaw 3 days after cocaine use. The patient admitted to a similar episode after cocaine use years earlier and proceeded to have a third episode with cocaine use several months after discharge.

Fines et al. [59] described two patients who presented to the emergency department with dystonic reactions after using cocaine. In both cases, symptoms quickly resolved after treatment with intravenous diphenhydramine. Catalano et al. [60] reported a similar case of a 34-year-old woman with acute facial dystonia after heavy crack cocaine use the night prior to presentation. Again, in all three cases, no history of movement disorder or prior neuroleptic use was found.

Bartzokis et al. [61] conducted a study of 71 cocaine-dependent subjects to evaluate if there was a difference in severity of choreoathetoid movement in cocaine-using individuals compared to the general population. The patients were evaluated using the Abnormal Involuntary Movement Scale. The cocaine-dependent subjects showed a significantly increased nonfacial (limbs plus body) AIMS subscore. The nine amphetamine-dependent patients in the study showed similar findings. The effect was most pronounced in the youngest age group. This was also the only group to show a significant difference in facial AIMS subscore compared to controls.

Another related movement disorder noted in two patients is opsoclonus-myoclonus. Scharf [62] reported a 26-year-old woman with a history of chronic intermittent cocaine abuse who developed opsoclonus-myoclonus the morning after she had used intranasal cocaine. The patient awoke with severe myoclonic jerks involving both trunk and limbs, and complained of the inability to keep her eyes still. The symptoms resolved over 4 months, and at 12-month follow-up she was completely normal. Elkardoudi-Pijnenburg and Van Vliet [63] reported a case of a 29-year-old man with opsoclonus, myoclonus, and ataxia after taking cocaine, resolving over 4 weeks. In both cases, well-known causes of opsoclonus-myoclonus were absent, and the temporal relation indicates cocaine as the likely etiology.

Recently, there has been evidence that cocaine can induce or predispose patients to more chronic movement disorders. Weiner et al. [64] described a 34-year-old woman with choreiform movements that had been persistent for 14 months despite abstinence from cocaine during that period. These movements had appeared during her period of abuse, improved with cocaine use, but gradually worsened to the point that they were constantly present. No improvement was noted over a 6-month follow-up.

There is a growing body of evidence that chronic cocaine use leads to significant changes in the human brain. Wilson et al. [65] demonstrated decreased levels of striatal dopamine and dopamine transporter in the autopsied brains of 12 chronic cocaine abusers, and further studies have shown decreased levels of calcium-stimulated phsopholipase A2 [66] and decreased activity of phosphatidylcholine cytidyltransferase in the putamen of chronic users [67]. Pascual-Leone et al. demonstrated cerebral atrophy in chronic cocaine abusers

Table 14.2 Cocaine-related dystonic reactions

References	Age	Sex	Previous neurological history	Pattern of use	Form and route of administration	Time from last use	Type of movement	Outcome
54	15	Female	0	Intermittent	IV	16 hours	Generalized dystonia, torticollis, and extensor posturing	Resolved immediately with IV diphenhydramine
55	29	Male	0	Intermittent	Crack cocaine	3 days	Masseter spasm, jaw clenched	Repeat episode with next use
56	34	Female	0	Daily chronic	Crack cocaine	<1 day	Choreoathetoid – extremities, lip smacking, eye blinking	Resolved over 4 days
56	24	Female	0	Intermittent	Crack cocaine	<1 day	Choreoathetoid – head, extremities, trunk	Resolved over 4 days
56	21	Female	Methylphenidate use age 9–11 years	Daily for 5 years	Crack cocaine	3 hours	Rapid chorea of head and arms, ataxic gait	Resolved over 3 days
56	29	Female	Neuroleptic use 10 years prior	Unknown	Crack cocaine	Unknown, urine positive for cocaine metabolites	Akathisia	Resolved over 5 days with one dose of diphenhydramine
56	58	Female	Neuroleptic use 2 months prior	Unknown	Crack cocaine	<1 day	Choreoathetoid – extremities, buccolingual dyskinesias	resolved over 4 days
56	38	Male	HIV/AIDS	Chronic	Crack cocaine	<1 day	Limb rigidity, inability to walk	Resolved over 6 days

No.	Age	Sex	History	Pattern of use	Route	Duration	Movement disorder	Outcome
56	46	Male	0	Chronic	Crack cocaine	<1 day	Rotations of shoulders, constant movement of hands and feet	Resolved over 3 days
57	32	Male	0	Weekly for 1 year	Intranasal	Unspecified	Opisthotonos	Resolved with diphenhydramine
57	19	Male	0	Weekly for 1 year	Intranasal	6 hours	Torticollis	Resolved with diphenhydramine
58	34	Female	0	Unknown	Crack cocaine	<1 day	Acute facial dystonia	Resolved immediately with IV diphenhydramine
59	26	Female	0	Intermittent "binge" use	Intranasal	<1 day	Opsoclonus – myoclonus	Resolved over 4 months
60	29	Male	Migraine headaches	Intermittent use for several years	Unknown	18 days, although symptoms began "shortly after use"	Opsoclonus –myoclonus, ataxia	Resolved over 4 weeks
61	34	Female	0	Chronic, multi-drug	Intranasal, IV, crack cocaine	Progressive since last use 14 months prior	Choreodystonic dyskinesias	Persistent

by planimetric CT. Most notably, there was a significant correlation between the length of time the individual had been using cocaine, and the degree of atrophy as measured on CT scan. Positron emission tomography (PET) demonstrated a reduction in cerebral blood flow that is most notable in the anterior brain regions, even in patients with minimal abnormalities on neurologic or neuropsychological testing [68]. Another study using PET revealed reduced rates of frontal metabolism in cocaine abusers, despite 3 months abstinence and the lack of gross neurologic abnormalities on exam [69]. While these changes may not be sufficient to induce movement disorders in their own right, they could predispose these individuals to the development of other conditions such as obsessive-compulsive [70] behavior or tremor disorders.

Tremor

Bauer [71] examined the effect of cocaine dependency on postural and kinetic hand tremor. All subjects were abstinent from cocaine for 1–5 months. Sixty-two subjects were evaluated and divided into the following subgroups: cocaine use only, cocaine and opiate dependence, cocaine and alcohol dependence, and alcohol dependence only. All three groups with cocaine history exhibited significantly more postural hand tremor than the alcohol only and control groups. Further analysis showed that severity of tremor appeared to be proportional to the amount of past abuse and inversely proportional to the amount of time they were abstinent.

It is written in several textbooks and drug manuals that stimulants can cause increased postural tremor in patients without preexisting movement disorders and Kramer et al. [72] reported that amphetamine abusers noted severe tremors as a sign to end a "run" or binge period of abuse. However, there is little evidence to support the role of the dopaminergic system in tremor exacerbation, and enhancement of physiologic postural tremor could be an effect of sympathomimetic effects of stimulants on peripheral adrenergic receptors.

Conclusion

Amphetamine, methylphenidate, pemoline, and cocaine all have a variety of effects on the central nervous system, one of the most prominent being an alteration of the dopaminergic system. Although some differences in mechanism of action are present, all four drugs appear to acutely increase dopaminergic mechanisms.

Although much evidence on the acute effects of stimulant medications has been accumulated, the long-term effects of chronic stimulant use are just now being investigated. Recent studies using brain imaging and neurochemical tracers have begun to elucidate changes that occur over time, which may account for stereotyped behaviors in chronic amphetamine abusers, and movement disorders caused by cocaine. Despite these new data, the mechanism through which these medications cause long-term changes in the brain are still unclear and merits further investigation.

The remaining question that has yet to be answered is whether stimulant medications can cause movement disorders in "normal" patients. In most of the reported cases, the patients were known to have a significant history of a disorder with motor components or shown to have structural or biochemical changes in the brain or were treated with neuroleptics. Based on the prevalence of the use of stimulants and the few reported cases of movement disorders in otherwise normal individuals, we continue to favor the hypothesis that stimulant-induced movement disorders occur in a subset of people, consisting of those with either subtle or preclinical movement disorders that are exacerbated by stimulants or in people with preexisting apparent or unapparent CNS alterations.

References

1. Connell PH. Clinical manifestation and treatment of amphetamine type of dependence. JAMA 1966; 196: 718–723.
2. Gunne LM. Effects of amphetamine in humans. In Martin WR (ed) Drug Addiction 2: Amphetamine, Psychogenic, and Marijuana Dependents. Berlin, Springer-Verlag, 1977, pp. 247–275.
3. Kuczenski R, Segal DS, Aizenstein ML. Amphetamine, fencafamine, and cocaine: relationships between locomotor and stereotypy response profiles and caudate and accumbens dopamine dynamics. J Neurosci 1991; 11: 2703–2712.
4. Worsley JN, Moszczynska A, Falardeau P. Dopamine D1 receptor protein is elevated in nucleus accumbens of human, chronic methamphetamine users. Molec Psychiatry 2000; 5(6): 664–672.
5. Lees AJ. Tics and Related Disorders, Edinburgh, Churchill Livingstone, 1985.
6. Schiorring E. Changes in individual and social behavior induced by amphetamine and related compounds in monkeys and man. In Ellenwood EH, Kilbey MM (eds) Cocaine and Other Stimulants. New York, Plenum Press, 1977, pp. 481–522.
7. Fernandez HH, Friedman JH. Punding on L-Dopa. Mov Disord 1999; 14: 836–838.
8. Bradley C. Benzdrine and dexedrine in the treatment of children's behavior disorders. Pediatrics 1950; 5: 24-37.
9. Tatetsu S, Goto A, Fujiwara T. The Methamphetamine-Psychosis (Kakuseizai Cudohku). Tokyo, Igaku Shoin, 1956.
10. Ellinwood EH, Jr. Amphetamine/anorectics. In Dupont RL, Goldstein A, O'Donnell J (eds) Handbook on Drug Abuse. Washington, DC, National Institute on Drug Abuse, U.S. Government Printing Office, 1979, pp. 221–231.
11. Davis PL, Stewart WB. The use of Benzedrine sulfate in postencephalitic parkinsonism. JAMA 1938; 110: 1890–1892.
12. Solomon P, Mitchell RS, Prinzmetal M. The use of benzedrine sulfate in postencephalitic Parkinson's disease. JAMA 1937; 108: 1765–1770.
13. Halliday AM, Nathan PW. Methylphenidate in parkinsonism. Br Med J 1961; 1: 1652–1655.
14. Parkes JD, Tarsy D, Marsden CD, et al. Amphetamines in the treatment of Parkinson's disease. J Neurol Neurosurg Psychiatry 1975; 38: 232–237.
15. Weiner WJ, Lang AE. Movement Disorders: A Comprehensive Survey. Mt. Kisco, NY, Futura Publishing, 1989.

16. Klawans HL, Weiner WJ. The effect of d-amphetamine on choreiform movement disorders. Neurology 1974; 24: 312–318.
17. Palatucci DM. Iatrogenic dyskinesias: a unique reaction to parental methylphenidate. J Nerv Mental Dis 1974; 159: 73–76.
18. Extein I. Methylphenidate-induced choreoathetosis. Am J Psychiatry 1979; 135: 252–253.
19. Millichap JG, Aymat F, Sturgis LH, Larsen KW, Egan RA. Hyperkinetic behavior and learning disorders. Am J Dis Child 1968; 116: 235-244.
20. Weiner WJ, Nausieda PA, Klawans HL. Methylphenidate-induced chorea: case report and pharmacologic implications. Neurology 1978; 28: 1041–1044.
21. Bonthala CM, West A. Pemoline-induced chorea and Gilles de la Tourette's syndrome. Br J Psychiatry 143: 300–302.
22. Singh BK, Singh A, Chusid E. Chorea in long-term use of pemoline. Ann Neurol 1983; 13: 218.
23. Stork CM, Cantor R. Pemoline induced acute choreoathetosis: case report and review of the literature. Clin Toxicol 1997; 35(1): 105–108.
24. Nausieda PA, Koller WL, Weiner WJ, Klawans HL. Pemoline-induced chorea. Neurology 1981; 31: 356–360.
25. Daras M, Koppel BS, Atos-Radzion E. Cocaine-induced choreoathetoid movements ("crack dancing"). Neurology 1994; 44: 751–752.
26. Comings DE. Clinical and molecular genetics of ADHD and Tourette syndrome: two related polygenic disorders. Ann N Y Acad Sci 2001; 931: 50–83.
27. Black MJ, Mink JW. Response to levedopa challenge in Tourette's syndrome. Mov Disord 2000; 15(6): 1194–1198.
28. Gilbert DL, Dure L, Sethuraman G, Raab D, Lane J, Sallee FR. Tic reduction with pergolide in a randomized controlled trial in children. Neurology 2003; 60: 606–611.
29. Meyerhoff JH, Snyder SH. Gilles de la Tourette's disease and minimal brain dysfunction: amphetamine isomers reveal catecholamine correlate in an affected patient. Psychopharmacologia 1973; 29: 211–220.
30. Golden GS. Gilles de la Tourette's syndrome following methylphenidate administration. Dev Med Child Neurol 1974; 16: 76–78.
31. Denckla MB, Bemporad JR, Mackey MC. Tics following methylphenidate administration. JAMA 1976; 235: 1349–1351.
32. Pollack MA, Cohen NL, Friedhoff AJ. Gilles de la Tourette's syndrome: Familial occurrence and precipitation by methylphenidate therapy. Arch Neurol 1977; 34: 630–632.
33. Fras I, Karlavage J. The use of methylphenidate and imipramine in Gilles de la Tourette's disease in children. Am J Psychiatry 1977; 134: 195–197.
34. Bremness AB, Sverd J. Methylphenidate-induced Tourette's syndrome: case report. Am J Psychiatry 1979; 136: 1334–1335.
35. Golden GS. The effect of CNS stimulants on Tourette's syndrome. Ann Neurol 1977; 2: 69–70.
36. Lowe TL, Cohen DJ, Detlor J, Kremenitzer MW, Shaywitz BA. Stimulant medications precipitate Tourette's syndrome. JAMA 1982; 247: 1729–1731.
37. Erenberg G, Cruse RP, Rothner AD. Gilles de la Tourette's syndrome: effects of stimulant drugs. Neurology 1985; 35: 1346–1348.
38. Price RA, Leckman JF, Pauls DL, Cohen DJ, Kidd KK. GTS: tics and CNS stimulants in twins and non-twins. Neurology 1986; 36: 232–237.
39. Lipkin PH, Goldstein IJ, Adesman AR. Tics and dyskinesias associated with stimulant treatment in attention-deficit hyperactivity disorder. Arch Pediatr Adolesc Med 1994; 148: 859–861.

40. Gadow KD, Sverd J, Sprafkin J, Nolan EE, Ezor SN. Efficacy of Methylphenidate for attention-deficit hyperactivity disorder in children with tic disorder. Arch Gen Psychiatry 1995; 52(6): 444–455.

41. Efron D, Jarman F, Barker M. Side effects of methylphenidate and dexamphetamine in children with attention deficit hyperactivity disorder: a double-blind, crossover trial. Pediatrics 1997; 100(4): 662–666.

42. The Tourette's Syndrome Study Group. Treatment of ADHD in children with tics: a randomized controlled trial. Neurology 2002; 58(4): 527–536.

43. Gadow KD, Sverd J, Sprafkin J, Nolan EE, Grossman S. Long-term methylphenidate therapy in children with comorbid attention-deficit hyperactivity disorder and chronic multiple tic disorder. Arch Gen Psychiatry 1999; 56(4): 330–336.

44. Gillberg C, Melander H, von Knorring Al, et al. Long-term stimulant treatment of children with attention-deficit hyperactivity disorder symptoms. A randomized, double-blind placebo-controlled trial. Arch Gen Psychiatry 1997; 54(9): 857–864.

45. Greenhill LL, Pliszka S, Dulcan MK, et al. Practice parameter for the use of stimulant medications in the treatment of children, adolescents, and adults. J Am Acad Child Adolesc Psych 2002; 41(2)(suppl): 26S–49S.

46. Bachman DS. Pemoline-induced Tourette's disorder: a case report. Am J Psychiatry 1981; 138: 1116–1117.

47. Mitchell E, Mathews KL. Gilles de la Tourette's disorder associated with pemoline. Am J Psychiatry 137: 979–985.

48. Sleator EK. Deleterious effects of drugs used for hyperactivity on patients with Gilles de la Tourette syndrome. Clin Pediatr 1980; 19: 453–454.

49. 49. Mesulam MM. Cocaine and Tourette's syndrome. N Engl J Med 1986; 315: 398.

50. Factor SA, Sanchez-Ramos JR, Weiner WJ. Cocaine and Tourette's syndrome. Ann Neurol 1988; 23: 423–424.

51. Pascaul-Leone A, Dhuna A. Cocaine-associated multifocal tics. Neurology 1990; 40: 999–1000.

52. Kumor K, Sherer M, Jaffe J. Haloperidol-induced dystonia in cocaine addicts. Lancet 1986; 2(8519): 1341–1342.

53. Choy-Kwong M, Lipton RB. Cocaine withdrawal dystonia. Neurology 1990; 40:863–864.

54. Kumor K. Cocaine withdrawal dystonia. Neurology 1990; 40: 863.

55. van Harten PN, van Trier JC, Horwitz EH, Matroos GE, Hoek HW. Cocaine as a risk factor for neuroleptic-induced acute dyskinesia. J Clin Psychiatry 1998; 59(3): 128–130.

56. Merab J. Acute dystonic reaction to cocaine. Am J Med 1988; 84: 564.

57. Choy-Kwong M, Lipton RB. Dystonia related to cocaine withdrawal: A case report and pathogenic hypothesis. Neurology 1989; 39: 996–997.

58. Farrell PE, Diehl AK. Acute dystonic reaction to crack cocaine. Ann Emerg Med 1991; 20:322.

59. Fines RE, Brady WJ, DeBehnke DJ. Cocaine-associated dystonic reaction. Am J Emerg Med 1997; 15(5): 513–515.

60. Catalano G, Catalano MC, Rodriguez R. Dystonia associated with crack cocaine use. South Med J 1997; 90(10): 1050–1052.

61. Bartzokis G, Beckson M, Wirshing DA, et al. Choreoathetoid movements in cocaine dependence. Biol Psychiatry 1999; 45(12): 1630–1635.

62. Scharf D. Opsoclonus-myoclonus following the intranasal usage of cocaine. J Neurol Neurosurg Psychiatry 1989; 52: 1447–1448.

63. Elkardoudi-Pijnenburg Y, Van Vliet AG. Opsoclonus, a rare complication of cocaine misuse. J Neurol Neurosurg Psychiatry 1996; 60(5): 592.

64. Weiner WJ, Rabinstein A, Levin B, Weiner C, Shulman LM. Cocaine-induced persistent dyskinesias. Neurology 2001; 56: 964–965.

65. Wilson JM, Levey AI, Bergeron C, Kalasinsky K, Ang L, et al. Striatal dopamine, dopamine transporter, and vesicular monoamine transporter in chronic cocaine users. Ann Neurol 1996; 40(3): 428–439.

66. Ross BM, Moszczynska A, Kalasinsky K, Kish SJ. Phospholipase A2 activity is selectively decreased in the striatum of chronic cocaine users. J Neurochem 1996; 67(6): 2620–2623.

67. Ross BM, Moszczynska A, Peretti FJ, et al. Decreased activity of brain phospholipid metabolic enzymes in human users of cocaine and methamphetamine. Drug Alcohol Depend 2002; 67(1): 73–79.

68. Volkow ND, Mullani N, Gould KL, Adler S, Krajewski K. Cerebral blood flow in chronic cocaine users: a study with positron emission tomography. Br J Psychiatry 1988; 151: 641–648.

69. Volkow ND, Hiyzemann R, Wang G-J, et al. Long-term frontal brain metabolic changes in cocaine abusers. Synapse 1992; 11: 184–190.

70. Crum RM, Anthony JC. Cocaine use and other suspected risk factors for obsessive-compulsive disorder: a prospective study with data from the Epidemiologic Catchment Area surveys. Drug Alcohol Depend 1993; 31: 281–295.

71. Bauer LO. Resting hand tremor in abstinent cocaine-dependent, alcohol-dependent, and polydrug-dependent patients. Alcohol Clin Exp Res 1996; 20(7): 1196–1201.

72. Kramer JC, Fischman VS, Littlefield DC. Amphetamine abuse: patterns and effects of high doses taken intravenously. JAMA 1967; 201: 305–309.

PART 4

Other drugs

CHAPTER 15

Antidepressants

Maria L. Moro-de-Casillas and David E. Riley

Introduction

The treatment of depression interacts with movement disorders in two distinct and complementary ways. On one hand, movement disorders may be induced by drugs during the course of the treatment of depression, and on the other, antidepressant therapies can alter preexisting movement disorders. Both of these relationships will be explored in this review.

In this chapter, the scope of antidepressant therapy will be limited to treatments directed against the affective component of depressive illnesses (Table 15.1). Drugs used for psychotic symptoms, particularly the neuroleptics, have been discussed in the Chapters 4–12. Selegiline will not however be discussed; this review will include lithium, which is technically used more for manic than depressive symptoms, because of the clear association between mania and depressive disorders. Fluvoxamine is approved for use in the United States only for obsessive-compulsive disorder, but it clearly belongs with the serotonin-selective reuptake inhibitors and it will be discussed.

There are four major categories of therapy for affective disorders (Table 15.1); three consist of drugs, and the other is electroconvulsive therapy (ECT). The most commonly used pharmacological agents for depression may be collectively referred to as the monoamine reuptake (MARU) inhibitors. Acknowledging that inhibition of reuptake of catecholamines may not be the only mechanism by which they exert their antidepressant effect [1], this is nevertheless the shared biochemical property by which they are most readily identified.

The original MARU inhibitor, imipramine, is a phenothiazine derivative that was relatively ineffective as an antipsychotic but was serendipitously found to have pronounced antidepressant effects. Many analogs were formulated, and collectively came to be known as *tricyclic antidepressants* (TCAs) because of a common three-ring molecular structure. Conventional TCAs increase the synaptic availability of serotonin and norepinephrine by blocking their uptake by the presynaptic neuron. The tertiary amines (imipramine, amitriptyline, trimipramine, clomipramine, and doxepin) are more potent inhibitors of serotonin reuptake, whereas nortriptyline and desipramine (secondary amines) are more potent norepinephrine reuptake inhibitors (Table 15.2) [2].

With generally fewer side effects than TCAs, the serotonin-selective reuptake inhibitors(SSRIs)(Table 15.1) have become the most widely prescribed

Table 15.1 Antidepressant therapies

---

1. Monoamine reuptake Inhibitors
   A. *Norepinephrine-reuptake inhibitors:*
   Tertiary-amine tricyclic antidepressants
   Trimipramine (Surmontil)
   Clomipramine (Anafranil)
   Amitriptyline (Elavil)
   Doxepin (Sinequan)*
   Imipramine (Tofranil)
   Secondary-amine tricyclic antidepressants
   Amoxapine (Asendin)
   Desipramine (Norpramin)
   Protriptyline (Vivactil)
   Nortriptyline (Pamelor)
   B. *Serotonin-selective reuptake inhibitors:*
   Citalopram (Celexa)*
   Fluoxetine (Prozac)*
   Fluvoxamine (Luvox)
   Paroxetine (Paxil, Paxil CR)[†,*]
   Sertraline (Zoloft)*
   Escitalopram (Lexapro)
   C. *Atypical antidepressants:*
   Bupropion (Wellbutrin, Wellbutrin SR)[†]
   Mirtazapine (Remeron)[§]
   Nefazodone (Serzone)
   Trazodone (Desyrel)
   Venlafaxine (Effexor, Effexor XR)[†]

2. Monoamine oxidase inhibitors
   I. Nonselective MAO inhibitors
   A. *Hydrazine:*
   Phenelzine (Nardil)
   Isocarboxazid (Marplan)
   B. *Nonhydrazine:*
   Tranylcypromine (Parnate)
   II. Preferential MAO-A inhibitor moclobamide (Manerix)

3. Electroconvulsive therapy

4. Lithium (Eskalith, Lithobid)[†]

---

* = Agents available in liquid forms.
[†] = Agents available in slow-release forms.
[§] = Agent available in orally-disintegrating tablet.

antidepressants. SSRIs block the reuptake of serotonin into presynaptic nerve terminals, thereby enhancing serotonin neurotransmission. This presumably results in their antidepressant effect [3]. Although this common mechanism of action predominates, each SSRI has a somewhat different pharmacology, resulting in a distinct profile of clinical activity, side effects, and drug interactions.

Antidepressants with less well-defined neuropharmacology are often lumped together under the term *atypical antidepressants* [4]. *Venlafaxine* is a

Table 15.2 Relative potencies of monoamine reuptake inhibitors on major monoamine systems

Drugs	Norepinephrine	Serotonin	Dopamine
Trimipramine	5	5*	5
Clomipramine	3	1*	5
Amitriptyline	3	2*	5
Doxepin	3	3*	6
Imipramine	3	2*	5
Amoxapine	3*	3	5
Desipramine	1*	3	5
Protriptyline	2*	3	5
Nortriptyline	2*	3	5
Citalopram	5	2*	6
Fluoxetine	4	1*	5
Fluvoxamine	5	2*	5
Paroxetine	3	1*	4
Sertraline	4	1*	3
Escitalopram	5	1*	6
Venlafaxine	5	2*	5
Bupropion	6	5	4*
Mirtazapine	5*	6	6
Nefazodone	3*	4	4
Trazodone	5	4*	5

Numerical values reflect a descending potency from 1 to 6, as follows: the inhibitor constant for 1 = less than 1 nM, 2 = 1–10 nM, 3 = 10–100 nM, 4 = 100–1,000 nM, 5 = 1, 000–10,000 nM, 6 = greater than 10,000 nM.
*The drug's greatest potency for reuptake inhibition is in this neurotransmitter.
Source: Data adapted from [4, 266]

nonselective serotonin, norepinephrine, and dopamine reuptake blocker [5]. *Trazodone* and *nefazodone* have inhibitory actions on serotonin transport [4]. Nefazodone may also modulate the norepinephrine transport system, and has a strong direct antagonistic effect on 5-HT$_{2A}$ receptors. These structurally related drugs may inhibit presynaptic 5-HT$_1$ subtype autoreceptors, and have partial agonist effects on postsynaptic 5-HT$_1$ receptors. Through these actions, they enhance neuronal release of serotonin [6]. Trazodone also blocks cerebral α_1-adrenergic and H$_1$-histamine receptors [4]. *Bupropion* and its amphetamine-like active metabolites modulate dopamine and norepinephrine transport [7]. The atypical antidepressant *mirtazapine* has potent antagonistic effects at several postsynaptic serotonin receptor types and can produce gradual downregulation of 5-HT$_{2A}$ receptors [6]. Through actions that limit the effectiveness of inhibitory α_2-adrenergic heteroreceptors on serotonergic neurons as well as inhibitory α_2-autoreceptors, and 5-HT$_{2A}$ heteroreceptors on noradrenergic neurons, mirtazapine may enhance the release of both amines, contributing to its antidepressant effect. Mirtazapine is also a potent histamine H$_1$-receptor antagonist with sedating effects [4].

MAO inhibitors were introduced in the mid-1950s and were the first clinically successful modern antidepressants [8]. Although not fully established, the antidepressant effect of MAO inhibitors is usually attributed to inhibition of catabolism of monoamine neurotransmitters in the CNS, increasing their availability. Even though MAO inhibition occurs rapidly, the usual delay of clinical benefit by several weeks may reflect secondary adaptations, including downregulation of α_2-adrenergic and β-adrenergic receptors [4, 9].

ECT has been in continuous use as a treatment for severe psychiatric illnesses since 1938, but the mechanism of its powerful antidepressant effect is still unclear. ECT is an important alternative to pharmacotherapy for major depression, mania, and mixed affective states. The exact mechanism of action of ECT remains obscure. Investigators have hypothesized that its effectiveness may be related to increases of brain norepinephrine, dopamine, and serotonin together with downregulation of adrenergic receptors. Alternatively, ECT may work by enhancing transmission of inhibitory neurotransmitters and neuropeptides (e.g., GABA and endogenous opioid concentrations) [10]. Other effects of ECT on neurochemical mechanisms include enhanced responsiveness of serotonin receptors, induction of dopamine receptor supersensitivity, and a modest downregulation of muscarinic cholinergic receptors [11]. Finally, a multitude of brain effects resulting from electrically induced seizures, including changes in cerebral blood flow, oxygen and glucose metabolism, blood-brain barrier permeability, and protein synthesis, may play roles [12–16].

Lithium carbonate was introduced into psychiatry in 1949 for the treatment of mania. The biochemical mechanism by which lithium stabilizes mood is unknown. It is probable that lithium alters the distribution of cations in the central nervous system, and modulates the metabolism of biogenic monoamines involved in the pathophysiology of mood disorders. Lithium may also affect "second messengers" and other intracellular molecular mechanisms involved in signal transduction, and cell and gene regulation. These complex actions are thought to stabilize neuronal activities, support neural plasticity, and provide neuroprotection [17–21].

Movement disorders induced by antidepressant therapy

Incorporation of the category, "Medication-Induced Movement Disorders Not Otherwise Specified," in the Diagnostic and Statistical Manual of Mental Disorders [22], has allowed physicians to formally recognize that drugs other than neuroleptics, including antidepressants, can result in the development of movement disorders [22, 23]. However, to provide a perspective regarding the epidemiological importance of the disorders to be discussed in this section, it should be stated that the frequency of movement disorders associated with antidepressant therapy (Table 15.3) is considerably lower than that of disorders related to antidopaminergic drugs. Although antidepressants are widely used, the associations described here are often drawn from anecdotal

Table 15.3 (Part A) Movement disorders caused by antidepressants

Movement disorder	Causative agents	
Parkinsonism	Amoxapine	Bupropion
	Fluoxetine	Trazodone
	Sertraline	Venlafaxine
	Paroxetine	Phenelzine
	Citalopram	Lithium
	Fluvoxamine	ECT
Tremor	MARU inhibitors (many)	Lithium
	MAO inhibitors	
Myoclonus	Tricyclic antidepressants	MAO inhibitors
	Sertraline	Lithium
	Fluvoxamine	Paroxetine
	Fluoxetine	
	Trazodone	
Dystonia/dystonic reactions	Amitriptyline	Fluoxetine
	Amoxapine	Sertraline
	Imipramine	Trazodone
	Clomipramine	Bupropion
	Doxepin	Mirtazapine
	fluvoxamine	Tranylcypromine
	Paroxetine (oculogyric crises)	
	ECT (oculogyric crises)	
	Lithium (oculogyric crises)	

Note: See text for references.
Movement disorders represented here are only the most common.
Refer to text for more information.

evidence provided by individual case reports. Furthermore, the degree of familiarity with movement disorders appears to vary greatly among authors, with consequently disparate terminology and ability to provide sufficient relevant descriptive detail. In short, the existence of many of these drug-induced movement disorder associations could be challenged on both clinical and epidemiological grounds. Since the first edition of this text, there has been a noticeable improvement in the quality of case reports in this field, and recent references appear to be more reliable. An important alternative explanation in some cases, especially those with unusual or bizarre types of abnormal movements, is a psychogenic movement disorder that is more common in patients with underlying depression.

Monoamine reuptake inhibitors

Tricyclic antidepressants
A rapid, low-amplitude action, *tremor*,can be found in up to 50% or more patients receiving various TCAs, and represents one of the most common adverse events in virtually all clinical trials of these drugs. This side effect is thought

Table 15.3 (Part B) Movement disorders caused by antidepressants

Movement disorder	Causative agent	
Chorea	Imipramine	Lithium
	Amitriptyline	Paroxetine
	Sertraline	
Dyskinesias/tardive dyskinesia	Imipramine	Bupropion
	Amitriptyline	Trazodone
	Amoxapine	ECT
	Doxepin	Fluvoxamine
	Clomipramine	Sertraline
	Fluoxetine	Paroxetine
Neuroleptic malignant syndrome	Desipramine	Lithium
	Fluoxetine	Venlafaxine
Bruxism	Fluoxetine	Venlafaxine
	Sertraline	Paroxetine
	Citalopram	
Serotonin syndrome	SSRI's	Mirtazapine
	Trazodone	Venlafaxine
Akathisia	Nortriptyline	Mirtazapine
	Fluvoxamine	Sertraline
	Paroxetine	Fluoxetine
	Tranylcypromine	

Note: See text for references.
Movement disorders represented here are only the most common.
Refer to text for more information.

to represent an "enhanced physiological tremor" [24]. The mechanism of the enhancement is unknown, but Raethjen and colleagues [25] have hypothesized that an increase in centrally driven coupling between antagonistic muscles is the basis for the development of amitriptyline-induced tremor. The tremor may respond to propranolol [26], and it will disappear with dosage reduction or discontinuation of the drug.

Acute dystonic reactions have been reported with amitriptyline, doxepin, imipramine, and clomipramine [2, 27]. In general, dystonic reactions are believed to occur because of a sudden and marked dopamine receptor antagonism in the nigrostriatal tract [28]. Amoxapine is the TCA that retains the closest ties to its phenothiazine roots, so much so that investigators continue to tout its neuroleptic effects [29]. Amoxapine has induced acute dystonia [30], akathisia [31], parkinsonism [32], and tardive dyskinesia [33]. Thus amoxapine has been associated with virtually all of the major neurological syndromes produced by antipsychotic drugs. This is most likely related to its metabolite 7-hydroxyamoxapine, which has potent dopamine receptor blocking ability [34]. Discontinuation of clomipramine was associated with acute cervical dystonia, tremulousness, and sensory ataxia in one case. The dystonia resolved with parenteral promethazine, and the other symptoms subsided with fluoxetine therapy. The authors proposed a cholinergic rebound mechanism and a hyperdopaminergic state as an explanation for the dystonic reaction [35].

A variety of *orofacial dyskinesias* have been reported with most TCAs. Fornazzari and coworkers [36] observed the "rabbit syndrome," characterized by repetitive chewing movements, in a woman who had been treated with imipramine (125–150 mg daily) for 4 years. The abnormal perioral movements ceased within 2 days of discontinuation of the antidepressant. Single-photon emission computed tomography (SPECT) demonstrated reduced basal ganglia perfusion while orofacial dyskinesia was present. Normal perfusion was restored after resolution of the movements. Treatment with amitriptyline has also been associated with reversible orofacial dyskinesias in two patients [37]. The authors interpreted these cases as examples of a tricyclic antidepressant causing "tardive dyskinesia," but there was no tardive relationship to the medication. They may represent a reaction to the anticholinergic properties of amitriptyline. However, numerous cases typical of tardive dyskinesia have emerged during the course of treatment with TCAs other than amoxapine (amitriptyline, imipramine, doxepin, and clomipramine), in patients with little or no exposure to neuroleptics [2, 38].

Chorea is an extremely rare manifestation of acute tricyclic antidepressant poisoning, but it has been well documented in two cases [39]. In both, the chorea was temporarily relieved by intravenous physostigmine, suggesting that it resulted from the anticholinergic effects of the antidepressant.

Myoclonus is a common manifestation of acute toxicity of MARU inhibitors [40]. The association of myoclonus with tricyclic antidepressants in normal therapeutic doses was studied prospectively by Garvey and Tollefson [41]. They found that treatment with such agents led to "clinically significant myoclonus" in 9 of 98 patients. In four patients the myoclonus took the form of a peculiar sudden unsustained jaw closure that interfered with speech. Three patients had disabling upper limb myoclonus; the other two developed severe nocturnal myoclonus. All experienced remission upon discontinuation of the offending agent, and the five who subsequently restarted the same drug all had a recurrence of the myoclonus. Thirty other patients noted less severe lower limb jerking, yielding an overall incidence of drug-induced myoclonus of 40% [41]. MARU inhibitor-induced myoclonus has been associated with reversible increases in somatosensory evoked potential amplitudes, suggesting cortical excitation or disinhibition as a pathogenetic mechanism [42]. The neurochemical action of MARU inhibitors that can most readily be implicated in the production of myoclonus is the potentiation of serotonin.

Clomipramine was reported to induce vocal and motor *tics* in a young patient with obsessive-compulsive disorder and schizoid personality. These symptoms disappeared after discontinuation of the drug [43].

Two cases link *akathisia* to nortriptyline administration. One patient developed akathisia after a dose increase from 50 to 100 mg per day. The second patient developed symptoms described as "feeling racy and spacey" a few days after starting therapy with nortriptyline (25 mg/day). When the daily dose was increased to 100 mg, she experienced panic, which persisted when nortriptyline was changed to fluoxetine. Both patients responded to propranolol with no depressive effects noted [44].

Baca and Martinelli [45] reported one case of *neuroleptic malignant syndrome* (NMS) in a woman taking desipramine with no previous or concurrent exposure to neuroleptics. The patient developed the classic manifestations of NMS including hyperthermia, muscular rigidity, altered mentation, tremor, elevated creatine phosphokinase, and autonomic instability. She responded to aggressive supportive care, dantrolene, and bromocriptine. NMS may be the result of the imbalance in the central nervous system ratio of norepinephrine to dopamine (NE/DA) [46]. Baca and Martinelli [45] hypothesized that, in their case, desipramine promoted the activity of norepinephrine, increasing the NE/DA ratio.

Serotonin-selective reuptake inhibitors (SSRIs)

The status of SSRIs as "drugs of choice" for depression has been accompanied by increased reports of adverse events associated with their use including a wide variety of movement disorders [23].

Tremor is the most common movement disorder caused by SSRIs, as is true of TCAs. Tremor occurs as a dose-related side effect of all SSRIs in approximately 10% of individuals. Tremor may also complicate treatment with SSRIs as a component of the serotonin syndrome [47], or as a manifestation of withdrawal [48].

Acute dystonic reactions have been associated with fluoxetine [49, 50], paroxetine [51], and sertraline [52, 53]. Meltzer et al. [54] reported a man with severe bipolar depression who developed acute torticollis, jaw stiffness, and loss of gait fluidity after 4 days of fluoxetine monotherapy. The patient's serum prolactin concentration increased markedly and the cerebrospinal fluid (CSF) homovanillic acid concentration decreased. The acute dystonic reaction and the parkinsonian symptoms responded well to trihexyphenidyl. After 2 days, the anticholinergic treatment was withdrawn and no extrapyramidal symptoms returned, despite continued fluoxetine treatment. The clinical and biochemical findings suggested that a significant interaction between the central serotoninergic and dopaminergic systems resulted in the dystonic reaction. Oculogyric crisis and generalized chorea occurred in one patient 14 hours after a single dose of 20 mg of paroxetine, and resolved with anticholinergic treatment [51]. Delayed mandibular dystonia occurred during fluvoxamine treatment in one patient after 1 month [55], and in a second patient after 2 months [56]. In both cases, the dystonia resolved with discontinuation of the drug.

Akathisia has been reported with fluoxetine [28], paroxetine [28], sertraline [57], and fluvoxamine [2]. Lipinski et al. [58] proposed that fluoxetine induces akathisia through serotoninergic inhibition of dopaminergic neurons of the ventral tegmental area. Bauer and colleagues [59] described two patients with refractory depression treated with a combination of nortriptyline, high-dose thyroxine, and thioridazine. Failure of response in one patient, and anticholinergic side effects in the other, led to replacement of nortriptyline with fluoxetine up to a dose of 80 mg per day. Both patients developed akathisia, which resolved with discontinuation of the fluoxetine. Subsequent administration of paroxetine was well tolerated without recurrence of akathisia.

Drug-induced parkinsonism has been reported with the use of fluoxetine [60], sertraline [61, 62], paroxetine [63], citalopram [64], and fluvoxamine [65]. Di Rocco et al. [62] suggested that sertraline has a direct effect on dopamine metabolism in the striatum, resulting in a parkinsonian syndrome. After reporting a patient with parkinsonism induced by sertraline, they conducted a small trial in which sertraline or placebo was administered to two groups of six normal rats. In animals pretreated with sertraline, the dopamine metabolites, homovanillic acid (HVA) and dihydroxyphenylacetic acid (DOPAC), and the serotonin metabolite 5-hydroxyindoleacetic acid (5-HIAA), were significantly decreased compared to control animals.

Tardive dyskinesia, classically associated with neuroleptics, has been described in relation to fluoxetine [2], sertraline [2], and paroxetine [66] use. Many cases reported as examples of tardive dyskinesias did not document a tardive relationship between the treatment and the involuntary movements.

A single case of *neuroleptic malignant syndrome* occurring 5 days after initiation of fluoxetine has been reported [67].

Myoclonus has been associated with the use of sertraline [68], fluvoxamine [69], and a combination of fluoxetine and trazodone [70]. Lauterbach [71] described a 61-year-old man with Pick's disease who developed "intermittent rhythmic myoclonus" when treated with fluoxetine. The author advised caution when prescribing fluoxetine to patients with degenerative dementias as degeneration of the dorsal raphe nucleus, and depletion of telencephalic serotonin, may unduly sensitize serotonin receptors.

Tics were also reported in single cases with the use of fluvoxamine [72] and fluoxetine [73]. In both patients the tics disappeared once the medication was discontinued.

Reversible dyskinesias, including lingual-facial-buccal dyskinesias, choreiform movements, and limb-truncal choreoathetoid movements have been described in multiple patients with the use of fluoxetine, fluvoxamine, sertraline, and paroxetine [2]. Generalized chorea was noted 3 days after a sertraline dosage increase in an 86-year-old woman with prolonged prior exposure to haloperidol without dyskinesias. The chorea resolved with withdrawal of sertraline and treatment with lorazepam [74].

Although not traditionally considered a movement disorder, the *serotonin syndrome* often features myoclonus and may additionally include tremor, ataxia, and muscle spasms [47]. The association of serotonin syndrome with a combination of SSRIs and selegiline in patients with PD is rare [75], but may be fatal [76].

Nocturnal *bruxism* has been reported with the use of fluoxetine [77], sertraline [77], and citalopram [78]. Romanelli et al. [79] described a patient who complained of "gritting" of her teeth and "tenseness" in her jaw each morning 5 months after starting paroxetine treatment for depression. The etiology of SSRI-induced bruxism remains unclear, but several theories have been proposed, including the effects of these medications on sleep, dopaminergic-serotoninergic imbalance, and activation of anxiety [77, 80].

Atypical antidepressants

Lu et al. [81] reported a 63-year-old man who developed upper extremity dystonia 10 days after he started mirtazapine (15 mg/day). His symptoms resolved completely once the medication was discontinued. Bupropion has also been associated with dose-related dystonic reactions, described as bilateral trismus, inability to rotate the head laterally, and spontaneous left temporomandibular joint dislocation [82]. Acute *akathisia* developed in two patients while taking mirtazapine. In one patient the akathisia responded well to clonazepam. In the second, symptoms disappeared with discontinuation of the medication, but reappeared when mirtazapine was reintroduced [83].

Two cases of trazodone-induced *parkinsonism* have been reported [84, 85]. Venlafaxine was also reported to induce dose-related and reversible parkinsonism [86]. Szuba and colleagues [87] reported two elderly patients who developed difficulty in walking and falling backward while on bupropion. One also displayed a paucity of movement, and a shuffling, "magnetic" gait. Symptoms resolved after discontinuing bupropion. The authors hypothesized that this side effect may be mediated through dopaminergic effects in the basal ganglia. A 45-year-old man with severe depression and anxiety developed tremor, nausea, micrographia, and shuffling gait, when bupropion was added to his therapy with nefazodone. These symptoms resolved over 10 days, once bupropion was discontinued [88].

A single dose of venlafaxine was also reported to precipitate a *neuroleptic malignant syndrome* in a patient receiving trifluoperazine [89].

Trazodone has been linked to a reaction consisting of *oromandibular and lingual dyskinesias*, and dystonic posturing of the limbs [90]. The movement disorder began after 2 months of gradually increasing the dosage of trazodone to 400 mg per day, and resolved 2 weeks after cessation of trazodone therapy.

The use of bupropion was associated with intermittent attacks of *"ballism"* in a 42-year-old woman [91]. These movements consisted of involuntary gross axial flexion and slapping of the hands and legs. These episodes lasted 5–10 seconds, and occurred 10 to 15 times per hour. When bupropion was discontinued, and haloperidol and oxazepam were given, the movements diminished.

Mirtazapine-induced *restless legs syndrome* has also been described [92].

In one reported case [93], trazodone was associated with *serotonin syndrome*, manifested by muscular rigidity, myoclonic jerking, and pronounced resting tremor. The tremor and rigidity resolved when trazodone was discontinued, but a parkinsonian gait, frequent falls, fluctuating disorientation, and visual hallucinations persisted. Mirtazapine has also been associated with serotonin syndrome, including oral dyskinesias, generalized tremors and ataxia, after titration from 7.5 mg to 15 mg daily in one patient. Withdrawal of the drug resulted in rapid resolution with only residual hypertonia after 2 weeks. The hypothesized pathophysiologic mechanism was overstimulation of serotonin-type IA receptors in the brainstem and spinal cord [94]. A patient developed serotonin syndrome when he received a single dose of venlafaxine, 16 days after selegiline was discontinued [95].This case highlights the importance of the "washout period" recommended for conventional MAO inhibitors (typically 14 days), after which it is assumed that an antidepressant with serotonergic properties can be safely prescribed. Under certain circumstances, not yet defined, the washout period might need to be of greater length.

Nocturnal *bruxism* has been described with the use of venlafaxine, in which case it responded to gabapentin [96].

Monoamine oxidase (MAO) inhibitors

Tremor is a common complication of treatment with MAO inhibitors. Evans and colleagues [97] prospectively analyzed the side effects in 41 patients given phenelzine for depression. They found a 15% incidence of tremor, which was roughly comparable to the 21% incidence detected in another group treated with imipramine. The mechanism for the production of tremor is unknown. Two cases of *parkinsonism* that resolved upon discontinuation, have been associated with trials of phenelzine [98, 99].

Zubenko et al. [100] described a case of tranylcypromine-induced *akathisia* in a 32-year-old woman with dysthymic disorder.

Tranylcypromine was reported to produce truncal *dystonia* within 3 days of initiation of treatment in one patient [101]. The dystonia did not resolve with intramuscular benztropine, but did upon discontinuation of the MAO inhibitor, and then recurred after a rechallenge with tranylcypromine. However, the same patient had a truncal dystonic reaction to propranolol, and so the specificity of the response to MAO inhibition must be questioned.

Lieberman and colleagues [102] reviewed the subject of *myoclonus* induced by MAO inhibitors. They concluded that this was a common side effect that was chiefly manifested as twilight or nocturnal myoclonus, but daytime myoclonus (i.e., during full alertness) occurred as well. Myoclonus may be brought out by adding the serotonin precursor L-tryptophan to MAO inhibitor therapy [103, 104]. However, this combination may also have antimyoclonic properties when given to patients with postanoxic action myoclonus. Further evidence of the role of serotoninergic mechanisms in MAO inhibitor-induced myoclonus comes from a case report where methysergide, a serotonin antagonist, brought relief of symptoms [105].

Concomitant administration of tranylcypromine and lithium was associated with the development of *buccolingual-masticatory syndrome* in two patients with no prior history of neuroleptic use [106].

Electroconvulsive therapy

ECT was associated with the development of persistent *tardive dyskinesia* in three patients with ongoing or recent neuroleptic use [107]. In three patients with little, no, or only remote exposure to antidopaminergic drugs, ECT brought out orofacial dyskinesias that resolved spontaneously in 2 weeks to 6 months [108]. ECT has been identified as a risk factor for tardive dystonia [109], but this association was based on particularly meager data. ECT used as adjunctive therapy for schizophrenia has actually been associated with a lower prevalence of tardive dyskinesia, possibly by sparing patients from higher doses of neuroleptics [110].

Contrary to its usually beneficial effect in PD, a patient with schizoaffective disorder and neuroleptic-induced parkinsonism manifested a marked increase of parkinsonian symptoms plus dystonia after ECT [111].

Brief post-ECT *asterixis* in one patient led to a search for metabolic disorders and an eventual diagnosis of primary hyperparathyroidism [112]. Given their relative rarity, post-ECT movement disorders should prompt a careful review of the preanesthetic and anesthetic drugs employed.

Lithium

Lithium carbonate is a standard therapy for the treatment of acute mania as well as bipolar disorders. Potential side effects are common, largely because of its narrow therapeutic window [113]. At concentrations exceeding 1.5 mmol/L, patients may become ataxic, hypertonic, hyperreflexic, dysarthric, and confused. At lithium concentrations greater than 3 mmol/L, clinical deterioration may progress to seizures, coma, and irreversible brain damage. The most common causes of lithium intoxication are deliberate ingestion while attempting suicide, and acute water and electrolyte disturbance in a patient undergoing long-term treatment [114].

Like the *tremor* induced by TCAs, that associated with lithium use, is thought to represent an enhancement of physiological tremor. Its occurrence rate and severity increase with higher serum levels of lithium. Estimates of its incidence vary because of differing doses used or because of coadministration of other tremor-producing drugs, but generally fall in the range of 33% to 65% [115]. The mechanism of tremor amplification may involve β_2-adrenergic hyperactivity, as suggested by the greater response of the tremor to metoprolol given at nonselective doses, and to propranolol given at β_1-receptor-selective doses [116]. Lithium-induced tremor may improve in response to a variety of beta-blockers or from dosage reduction. In a double-blind study, Zaninelli et al. [117] assessed tremor in lithium-maintained patients during treatment of major depression with either paroxetine or amitriptyline. The authors found that tremor increased significantly during therapy to a comparable degree with either antidepressant.

Patients have experienced permanent neurological deficits after episodes of lithium intoxication [113, 118]. The clinical picture includes encephalopathy, memory loss, hypokinesia, rigidity, mutism, muscular twitches, ataxia, nystagmus, scanned speech, and hyperreflexia. Unfortunately, in most of the cases reported the patients were concomitantly receiving different antipsychotics, including haloperidol or chlorpromazine. Apte and Langston [113] described a 38-year-old man with depression on no other psychoactive medication who took an overdose of lithium leading to markedly elevated serum lithium levels. He developed parkinsonism accompanied by athetosis and later *ataxia*. An athetotic cerebellar syndrome persisted during 18 months of observation. A 71-year-old man with mania suffered a lithium-induced encephalopathy that responded to chlorpromazine. Later, lithium was restarted with close serum level monitoring. After remaining fairly stable for 7 years, he developed dysarthria, masked fascies, drooling of saliva, a stooped posture, increased muscle tone, hyperreflexia, and a coarse tremor. Postmortem examination revealed significant cerebellar cortical atrophy, with marked loss of Purkinje cells and astrocytic proliferation, but no basal ganglia abnormalities. The authors suggested that the cerebellar degeneration could be directly attributed to the toxic effect of high lithium levels on the central nervous system [119]. Schou [120] has demonstrated in adult albino rats that concentrations of lithium in the brain are higher than in the serum within 24 hours of initiation of treatment.

Several other cases of parkinsonism due to lithium have been documented [121, 122]. Its occurrence may be related to the serum lithium level [122]. One case responded to pramipexole but not to levodopa [121]. Muthane et al. [123] reported a 65-year-old female treated for manic-depressive psychosis who after a brief exposure to lithium, developed persistent parkinsonism, akathisia, and orofacial dyskinesia. There was no history of neuroleptic use. Her symptoms persisted despite discontinuation of lithium, and treatment with trihexyphenidyl and amantadine. "Cogwheel rigidity" was the subject of a report associating it with lithium therapy, in which it was categorized as a form of extrapyramidal disorder [124]. The term actually represents a fusion of two distinct clinical findings, cogwheeling and rigidity. The latter is clearly a manifestation of basal ganglia disease, but the cogwheel phenomenon is a sign associated with the presence of an action tremor [125, 126]. It is commonly found in patients with essential tremor [127] who have no abnormalities of muscle tone.

Chorea has been reported as a side effect of lithium in a small number of patients, possibly as a result of anticholinergic activity. In one case, the movement disorder recurred with haloperidol treatment [128]. In another case, the patient had been treated with antidopaminergic drugs intermittently for 6 years, and the chorea persisted for 3 months after lithium was stopped [129]. Thus, there is some question whether lithium directly caused the chorea or precipitated the emergence of tardive dyskinesia. The latter conclusion conflicts with experimental evidence suggesting a protective effect of lithium against tardive dyskinesia [130]. Chorea was reported in one patient with no psychiatric history who became toxic from lithium sulfate taken as a sodium-free salt substitute [131]. Two cases of lithium poisoning [132] were interpreted elsewhere [129] as examples of chorea associated with lithium. However, the descriptions are limited to "twitches of the small muscles of the hand and face" that were accompanied by jerking of the whole limbs. There was no clear reason to have segregated these two cases from the other four in the report, all of whom evidently had myoclonus.

Lithium frequently causes *myoclonus* as a toxic manifestation or, at times, with therapeutic serum levels [133]. This is likely related to enhancement of serotoninergic activity. The myoclonus reported to occur in one patient as a result of combined treatment with TCAs and lithium was clearly related to the initiation of lithium, and its cessation was just as clearly related to discontinuation of the drug. The author's contention that the abolition of myoclonus was prompted by a switch in tricyclics ignored the prolonged excretion time of lithium (10–14 days), which was stopped 3 days earlier [134]. Caviness et al. [135] reported that lithium could be associated with cortical action myoclonus without the presence of epileptiform abnormalities on a routine electroencephalogram (EEG). Lithium aggravated nocturnal myoclonus, and restless legs syndrome in a 48-year-old woman with mania [136].

Oculogyric crises were noted in a patient who was taking lithium in addition to a longstanding regimen of haloperidol and amitriptyline [137]. Lithium therapy may be a contributing factor to the development of *neuroleptic malignant syndrome* in patients receiving antipsychotic agents, as these drugs may increase lithium levels [138]. A cross-sectional study of parkinsonism and tardive dyskinesia in lithium-treated patients with affective disorders confirmed that the combination of lithium and a neuroleptic is associated with a higher prevalence of movement disorders, including tremor and hypokinesia, than either agent alone [139]. The authors also observed the presence of dyskinetic movements in approximately 14% of lithium-treated patients more than 6 months after the discontinuation of any previous neuroleptic therapy. They suggested that lithium might exacerbate the vulnerability of patients with affective disorders to dyskinesias.

Effects of antidepressant therapy on movement disorders

Depression is a common feature of a number of basal ganglia disorders, particularly Parkinson's disease (PD) and Huntington's disease. For the most part, the management of depression is identical to that used for patients with

Table 15.4 Treatment of movement disorders with antidepressants

Treatment	Movement disorder	Results
Tricyclic antidepressants	• Parkinsonism	Improved
	• Tics	Mixed
	• Dystonia	Rare benefit
	• Dyskinesia	Improved
Serotonin-selective Reuptake inhibitors	• Parkinsonism	Mixed
	• Myoclonus	Improved
	• Tics	Improved
	• Huntington's	Mixed
Mirtazapine	• Tremor	Improved
Trazodone	• Tardive dyskinesia	Improved
Bupropion	• Parkinsonism	Improved
	• Periodic leg movements	Improved
	• Tourette syndrome	Mixed
Nefazodone	• Parkinsonism	Worsened
	• Myoclonus	Improved
Monoamine oxidase Inhibitors	• Postanoxic myoclonus	Improved
	• Huntington's chorea	Improved
Electroconvulsive therapy	• Parkinsonism	Improved
	• Tics	Improved/no effect
	• Dystonia	Improved
	• Tardive dyskinesia	Mixed
Lithium	• Parkinsonism	Mixed
	• Tourette syndrome	Mixed
	• Dystonia	Improved/mixed
	• Tardive dyskinesia	No effect/worsened
	• Huntington's	Mixed

Note: Only those movement disorders in which an effect was seen are displayed.

pure affective disorders. One important exception is the use of nonselective MAO inhibitors in PD. Although these drugs have been used in hopes of improving parkinsonism in the past, the strong potential for hypertensive crises contraindicates their application to patients treated with other dopaminergic agents.

This section will focus on the influence of antidepressant therapies on patients with established movement disorders (Table 15.4). As with the literature concerning antidepressant-induced movement disorders, a note of caution is in order. There have been very few controlled clinical trials, and there is a wide range of neurological sophistication among authors of case reports reviewed in this section.

Parkinsonism

Depression is the most frequent psychiatric complication in PD [140, 141]. The biochemical mechanisms underlying depression in this group of patients have been linked to a variety of neurotransmitter abnormalities, including dopamine and serotonin [142, 143].

Largely because of their known anticholinergic effects, it was not long after their introduction that MARU inhibitors were thought to be potentially useful for Parkinson's disease. Current data suggest that TCAs are efficacious in the treatment of depression in PD, but study designs of published trials involving TCAs have been appropriately criticized as inadequate [144]. Relief of parkinsonism by imipramine was first reported in a 1959 open-label study [145]. There were numerous confirmatory case reports, and the findings were substantiated by the results of a 1965 double-blind trial in which 63% of patients receiving imipramine improved versus 16% of placebo-treated patients [146]. The population studied included postencephalitic and "arteriosclerotic" patients, as well as those with idiopathic parkinsonism, and there was no therapeutic difference among the groups. Response to imipramine was independent of the response to depression. Desipramine was also found to have significant symptomatic benefit for PD patients in a double-blind placebo-controlled study [147]. Ten of the 16 patients improved, but it was not stated how many of them were depressed. A double-blind, crossover study involving 22 depressed patients with levodopa-treated PD found that nortriptyline was superior to placebo in treating depressive symptoms, but had little effect on motor signs [148]. Amoxapine should be avoided in PD, as one of its metabolites, 7-hydroxyamoxapine, is a potent dopamine receptor blocker and can worsen this movement disorder [149].

SSRIs have been reported to be useful in the treatment of depression in patients with PD. In this context, two principles are important. First, most SSRIs are metabolized by the cytochrome P450 enzyme system, and can interfere with the clearance and toxicity of other medications, such as tricyclic antidepressants that are metabolized through the same route [4, 144, 150]. Second, selegiline should not be used concomitantly with either SSRIs or TCAs, as it loses its selectivity at higher doses, and can induce serotonin syndrome [144, 149]. This is an extremely rare occurrence and very often selegiline has been used in combination with SSRIs in patients with PD. Multiple reports have described worsening of parkinsonian motor symptoms after the use of SSRIs [63, 151–153], but this finding has not been universal [154–156]. An open-label prospective study [155] evaluated 52 nondemented, nonfluctuating, depressed patients, with PD who were treated with SSRIs (fluoxetine, fluvoxamine, sertraline, or citalopram) for depression. There was significant improvement in depressive symptoms without deterioration in parkinsonism. A low likelihood of aggravating parkinsonism was also found in a retrospective study of 58 patients with PD treated with SSRIs, mainly sertraline [157].

The mechanism by which SSRIs might interact with motor performance is controversial. It has been suggested that depressed patients with PD may represent a subgroup of PD with a different neurochemical substrate [155]. The cerebrospinal fluid content of 5-HIAA is lower in depressed than in nondepressed patients with PD [158], and neuronal density in the dorsal raphe nucleus is more severely reduced in depressed than in nondepressed patients with PD [159]. Caley and Friedman [15] retrospectively reviewed medical records of 23 outpatients with PD who were treated with fluoxetine up to 40 mg per day. The parkinsonism of three patients worsened to a mild degree, while 20 patients experienced no worsening at all. It was not established whether the declines were due to fluoxetine treatment or to progression of the disease. A prospective open-label study [153] of 65 patients with PD and depression, treated with paroxetine (10–20 mg/day) and followed up for at least 3 months, showed overall good tolerability. Thirteen patients (20%) discontinued the medication within the first 30 days of treatment, two because of increased "off" time and exacerbation of parkinsonian tremor. This study supports a previous observation that SSRI-induced parkinsonism occurs within the first month of treatment [28]. Overall, one may conclude that SSRI-induced parkinsonism is an idiosyncratic response, and patients are most vulnerable during the first month of therapy. Citalopram was found to significantly improve bradykinesia and finger taps in patients with PD with and without depression [156]. Citalopram does not inhibit cytochrome P450 isoenzymes [160, 161], and therefore would not interfere with other drugs, including anticholinergics [156].

Comparatively little is known regarding the effects of *atypical antidepressants*. A study of 20 patients with PD given bupropion found that half experienced improvement of 30% or greater in their symptoms [162]. Mirtazapine may reduce the resting tremor of PD [163]. Mirtazapine was also reported to induce psychosis when added to chronic levodopa therapy in a patient with PD [164]. Mirtazapine induced rapid eye movement (REM) sleep behavior disorder in four patients with parkinsonism, which resolved once mirtazapine was discontinued [165]. Nefazodone reportedly aggravated PD in one patient [166].

Since early reports in the 1940s and 1950s, *ECT* has repeatedly been shown to improve the motor manifestations of PD. This benefit has stood up to double-blind random scrutiny [167]. All manifestations of PD, including tremor, appear to share equally in the effects of ECT. Levodopa-related fluctuations may be eliminated [15, 167]. In some patients the improvement appears to be transient, while in others it may last for 6 months or more [15, 168, 169]. Older patients might experience a more robust response to ECT [15, 168, 170]. Faber and Trimble [171] reviewed 27 publications, mostly case reports or case series, on ECT and PD with and without psychiatric comorbidity. The results were overall favorable with consistent descriptions of improvement in motor symptoms. The authors recommended (1) bilateral ECT (up to eight treatments) for those patients with PD who have an unsatisfactory response to conventional treatment, and (2) maintenance ECT for those patients who showed significant improvement lasting for at least 1 month. ECT should be used with caution in patients with dementia because of the potential for worsening of cognition and the risk of delirium [172].

As with the MARU inhibitors, there is some controversy regarding whether the benefit of ECT in PD is a direct result of the treatment or a secondary effect of treating depression. It has been argued that depression may worsen parkinsonism, and its treatment may thus produce relief from its manifestations [173, 174]. Differentiation between parkinsonism and the psychomotor retardation of depression may cause diagnostic confusion; yet there are several reasons to believe that ECT has a direct effect on parkinsonism. In depressed patients with PD, there is often dissociation between the effects on motor manifestations and mood. Parkinsonism may improve before depression [68, 175], or there may be a clear motor response in the absence of detectable affective benefit [176]. Manic PD patients treated with ECT have also shown improvement in their parkinsonian symptoms and signs [177, 178]. ECT may provoke dyskinesias that resolve with the reduction of antiparkinsonian medications [167, 168]. This supports a direct action on dopaminergic systems rather than an indirect effect of mood elevation.

ECT may also relieve drug-induced parkinsonism, whether administered therapeutically [179–183] or prophylactically [184]. A study of 35 neuroleptic-treated schizophrenic patients, who previously received or were receiving adjunctive bilateral ECT, suggested that it may have protective effects against neuroleptic-induced parkinsonism, and may reduce the risk for the development of tardive dyskinesias [185]. The prophylactic benefit of ECT was independent of neuroleptic dose, indicating that this was not simply due to a "sparing" effect, in contrast to the possible protective role of ECT in tardive dyskinesia. Two patients had a fine tremor of the hands and only one met the criteria for probable mild tardive dyskinesia. The authors hypothesized that in the absence of any other obvious explanation, adjunctive ECT at the initiation of neuroleptic treatment may have prevented the development of neuroleptic-induced parkinsonism. A limitation of this study was the lack of a matched control group of neuroleptic-treated patients who did not receive ECT [185]. Hanin et al. [111] described an unusual negative effect of ECT on drug-induced parkinsonism and tardive dystonia, with a worsening of these symptoms after ECT.

Both depression and parkinsonian symptoms in patients with multiple system atrophy may respond to bilateral ECT [186]. Other authors have suggested that ECT can be a safe and effective tool in the treatment of depression in MSA [187].

Theoretically, ECT could also benefit patients with progressive supranuclear palsy (PSP). Barclay et al. [188] found limited usefulness of ECT in five patients with PSP who each received nine treatments and an apomorphine challenge. One patient experienced a dramatic benefit, two improved mildly, and two were unchanged. However, the authors concluded that the long hospitalization required, and posttreatment confusion, limited the usefulness of this tool. ECT improved depression in a 68-year-old woman with PSP with no effect on her neurological symptoms [189].

Lithium was reported to reduce "off" periods by greater than 60% in four of five patients with levodopa-related fluctuations [190]. Three of these suffered increased dyskinesias. However, a trial of lithium in 12 patients with fluctuations produced improvement in only three, and this was transient [191]. Lithium was found to increase akinesia and decrease dyskinesias in two other patients [192]. A similar trial failed to show a reduction in dyskinesias [193].

In a larger study, 21 patients showed no significant change in their parkinsonism or dyskinesias [194]. Lithium has been reported to decrease painful "off"-period dystonia, verified by a double-blind placebo-controlled trial in seven patients [195].

Myoclonus

There is considerable speculation but little evidence that inhibition of serotonin reuptake by MARU inhibitors, and particularly SSRIs, may improve postanoxic action myoclonus (PAAM). Paroxetine was beneficial in one patient with PAAM [196]. In two patients with "intention" myoclonus responsive to L-5HTP and carbidopa, fluoxetine reduced the required dose of L-5HTP to approximately one third, decreasing side effects and increasing antimyoclonic activity [197]. Incidentally, nefazodone improved myoclonus in familial myoclonus-dystonia syndrome with panic attacks [198].

MAO inhibitors have been used successfully to treat PAAM. Iproniazid was reported to produce significant improvement in one case, although not as much as L-5-HTP [199]. Phenelzine has also been of benefit in one case [200]. Isocarboxazid given alone showed slight or no effects in four patients with action myoclonus, but potentiated improvement when combined with tryptophan [201]. A fifth patient with strictly spontaneous myoclonus showed no benefit from either or both drugs.

Periodic leg movement disorder improved after treatment with bupropion for ADHD in a 14-year-old girl [202].

Tremor

The widespread recognition of tremor as a side effect of MARU inhibitors has undoubtedly dimmed enthusiasm for investigating their potential therapeutic effects. A report of two patients whose essential tremor improved with *trazodone* [203] prompted a double-blind placebo-controlled investigation [204]. Ten patients experienced no significant subjective or objective amelioration of either the postural or kinetic components of their tremor. It was concluded that a serotonergic deficit probably does not play a role in the pathogenesis of essential tremor.

Mirtazapine was reported to improve resting tremor in PD, essential tremor (ET), and levodopa-induced dyskinesias in five patients [163]. The effect on tremor was confirmed in an open-label trial involving 26 patients [205].

However, of 13 patients with ET completing a double-blind crossover placebo-controlled trial, 10 were unchanged [206]. Two experienced only moderate benefit and one marked benefit from mirtazapine.

Tics and Tourette's syndrome

TCAs have been found effective in some children with Tourette's syndrome (TS). Desipramine improved both attention deficit hyperactivity disorder (ADHD) and tics in 33 patients [207]. Similar findings were reported by the same authors when studying nortriptyline [208]. A double-blind placebo-controlled trial [209] studied desipramine in 41 children and adolescents with chronic tic disorders and comorbid ADHD. Desipramine (mean total daily dose 3.4 mg/kg/day) significantly reduced motor and vocal tics and core symptoms of ADHD. However, it may alter heart rate and blood pressure, and patients should be screened for cardiovascular risk before administration of this drug [209]. Clomipramine induced a full-blown picture of TS in a 29-year-old man with schizoid personality, simple motor tics, and severe OCD. When clomipramine was discontinued, the vocal and motor tics disappeared, but the original eye blinking persisted [43].

In an 8-week open trial [210], the SSRIs, citalopram and fluvoxamine, were well tolerated in 6 children with TS. The group treated with citalopram showed a significant improvement in motor and vocal tics over time. Buckingham and Gaffney [211] reported that sertraline was efficacious in the treatment of motor and vocal tics, and obsessions, in a 15-year-old patient with TS who had failed treatment with clonidine, pimozide, and haloperidol. With less effect than fluoxetine on the cytochrome P450IID6 system, and a shorter half-life, the authors suggested that sertraline may offer certain advantages over fluoxetine in TS patients. Fluoxetine was reported to improve obsessive-compulsive symptoms, without major effects on tics in two different studies involving patients with TS [212, 213]. By contrast, there are also reports of the worsening of tics with the use of SSRIs [214]. Paroxetine exacerbated tics in a 12-year-old boy treated for depression [215].

Initial reports of the use of *bupropion* in TS suggested it might be a useful alternative tool for the treatment of ADHD, especially in patients who could not tolerate or have responded poorly to stimulants [216, 217]. However, Spencer et al. [218] reported a group of four children with ADHD and comorbid TS in whom treatment with bupropion exacerbated the tics within weeks to months.

ECT had no effect on TS in two patients [219, 220], but one patient who developed a disabling complex motor tic at the age of 59 years in association with severe depression experienced a complete resolution of both conditions following four bilateral and six unilateral treatments [221]. Similarly, Rapoport et al. [222] described a woman with preexisting TS, latent for years that was exacerbated with the onset of a major depressive episode. Both her depression and tics completely remitted after eight sessions of right unilateral ECT. Hypotheses to explain this finding included improvement of emotional stress associated with her depression that could have exacerbated her tics, and increased serotoninergic tone after ECT.

Lithium has had mixed effects on the manifestations of TS, producing improvement in some cases [223–225], but worsening in others [226].

Dystonia

In a retrospective study of patients with dystonia, only one of 25 patients was found to have a "good response" to treatment with TCAs [227]. In a questionnaire study, 200 patients with spasmodic torticollis, blepharospasm, or hemifacial spasm rated botulinum toxin as having a "good effect," and citalopram and physical therapy as having a moderate effect. All other therapies were felt to convey minimal benefit [228].

ECT was reported to induce complete remission in a patient with tardive dystonia [229], and a marked, though transient, improvement in another [230]. ECT improved parkinsonism-dystonia in one patient after nine sessions [231]. However, ECT also had negative effects in a patient with schizoaffective disorder and neuroleptic-induced parkinsonism, with marked worsening of parkinsonian symptoms and dystonia after treatment [111].

Individual cases of improvement of spasmodic torticollis or segmental dystonia with *lithium* have been reported [232–234]. However, in an unselected group of nine patients, there was no objective improvement [235]. In a group of 14 dystonia (not further qualified) patients, only one enjoyed a "good response" [227]. By contrast, lithium was found to show marked (persistent for greater than 3 months) improvement in 9 of 34 patients with cranial-cervical dystonia so treated; an unsustained benefit was noted in a further study of 17 patients [236]. The same group of investigators has found that lithium enhances the response of cranial-cervical dystonia to tetrabenazine [237]. A double-blind placebo-controlled study of six patients with various forms of dystonia found no benefit in any patients [238].

Tardive dyskinesia

Desipramine and *trazodone* reportedly improved oral-lingual-facial dyskinesias in two patients [239]. The authors proposed that antidepressants may improve dyskinesias by decreasing the number and density of beta-adrenergic receptors, which inhibit norepinephrine-stimulated release of dopamine. *Amoxapine* was found to temporarily suppress tardive orofacial dyskinesias, described as teeth grinding and blinking. However, symptoms recurred once amoxapine was discontinued [240]. This case again emphasizes the neuroleptic properties of this drug.

Korsgaard and colleagues [241] studied the effects of *citalopram* in 13 psychiatric patients with tardive dyskinesia, 11 of whom also had neuroleptic-induced parkinsonism. There was no significant benefit for dyskinesia, but no adverse effects occurred. The authors suggested that citalopram may be useful in the treatment of depressed patients who also have TD. *Trazodone* showed a possible beneficial effect in the treatment of tardive dyskinesias in a double-blind placebo-controlled trial [242].

ECT has been reported to improve [181, 243], worsen [180], or have no effect on TD [244, 245]. *Lithium* has been reported to aggravate tardive dyskinesia [246], and to attenuate the salutary effects of reserpine [247]. More often, it has been found to have a beneficial effect that may be mild [248], or marked [249, 250]. However, a double-blind, placebo-controlled study of 11 patients showed no effect of lithium on this movement disorder [251].

Huntington's disease

Fluoxetine was reported to improve obsessive-compulsive symptoms in two patients with Huntington's disease [252]. However, it has also been associated with the exacerbation of the chorea [253]. *Sertraline* improved aggressiveness and severe irritability in two patients with HD [254], and improved obsessive-compulsive symptoms in a third patient [255].

Mirtazapine successfully treated depression in a 32-year-old woman with Huntington's disease after a suicidal attempt [256].

MAO inhibitors were reported to reduce the severity of chorea in two patients with Huntington's disease, simultaneously with an improvement in their affective state [257]. The observed benefit on chorea was contrary to the expected result of using agents known to increase brain dopamine levels, and it was attributed to "a consequence of mental well-being" rather than a direct effect of the drugs.

Lithium has been used to treat the chorea of Huntington's disease. In one study [249], there was a "striking reduction of hyperkinetic symptoms" in three of six patients. In another report [258], treatment with lithium produced a 40% to 50% improvement in chorea, as measured by a " brachio-kineso-meter," in three of four patients with Huntington's disease. However, when examined in a double-blind, placebo-controlled fashion, lithium has not produced improvement in chorea [259–261]. A patient with hemichorea also failed to improve with lithium [235]. In a rat model of Huntington's disease, lithium appeared to be neuroprotective against striatal lesion formation when given 16 days prior to the infusion of quinolinic acid into the striatum [262].

ECT was shown to be beneficial for the management of chorea [263], and depression [264, 265] in patients with Huntington's disease.

Conclusion

What are we to make of this hodge-podge of mostly anecdotal reports and open-label trials? Some trends emerged from the reports reviewed here, prompting us to draw the following conclusions.

1. Reports of effects of SSRIs have mushroomed in number during the past decade, while reports related to MAO inhibitors have almost vanished. This undoubtedly reflects practice and prescription patterns; the new replaces the old. In the near future, clinicians should expect to see more patients with adverse effects from SSRIs than any other category of antidepressant treatment.

2. Tremor remains the most common movement disorder caused by antidepressant drugs, including lithium. Myoclonus is also a common side effect. Mirtazapine is the only antidepressant that does not cause or aggravate tremors. In some cases of either resting or action tremors, it may have an ameliorative effect.

3. Movement disorders commonly associated with neuroleptic treatment including acute dystonic reactions, akathisia, parkinsonism, tardive dyskinesia and neuroleptic malignant syndrome, may occur as complications of antidepressant drug therapy, but only rarely. Amoxapine should be avoided as an antidepressant because it is a much more likely offender in this regard than other MARU inhibitors.

4. Rare permanent neurologic deficits may occur as a consequence of treatment with MARU inhibitors (tardive dyskinesia) or toxic levels of lithium (cerebellar degeneration).

5. Parkinson's disease may improve as a result of treatment with ECT, or rarely with TCAs or lithium. For ECT, there is good evidence that this is a direct effect rather than mediated by alleviation of a mood disorder. Parkinsonism may be caused or aggravated by SSRIs, but the risk of this is quite low. Overall, because of other advantages, SSRIs are the first line of therapy for depression in patients with PD, as they are in those without PD.

6. Apart from Parkinson's disease, there is only anecdotal evidence that antidepressant therapies are effective treatments for movement disorders.

The frequently conflicting reports of the effects of antidepressant medications underscore the complex biochemical natures of movement disorders and the variety of neurotransmitter changes that can be brought about by a single drug. For example, lithium may cause or aggravate parkinsonism, tardive dyskinesia, or tics in some patients while ameliorating them in others. They also emphasize that we must consider that multiple pathophysiological processes underlie the expression of many movement disorders. It is hoped that study of the effects of antidepressants selective for various neurotransmitter pathways will provide keys to understanding the neurochemical bases of both depression and movement disorders, and lead to improved treatment for both patient populations.

References

1. Heninger GR, Charney DS. Mechanism of action of antidepressant treatments: implications for the etiology and treatment of depressive disorders. In Meltzer H (ed) Psychopharmacology: The Third Generation in Progress. New York, Raven Press, 1987, pp. 535–544.
2. Gill HS, DeVane CL, Risch SC. Extrapyramidal symptoms associated with cyclic antidepressant treatment: a review of the literature and consolidating hypotheses. J Clin Psychopharmacol 1997; 17: 377–389.

3. Ables AZ, Baughman OL, III. Antidepressants: update on new agents and indications. Am Fam Physician 2003; 67: 547–554.

4. Baldessarini RJ. Drugs and the treatment of psychiatric disorders. Depression and anxiety disorders. In Hardman JG, Limbird LE, Goodman M, Gilman A (eds) The Pharmacological Basis of Therapeutics, 10th edition. New York, Mc-Graw Hill, 2001, pp. 447–483.

5. Fisher AA, Davis MW. Serotonin syndrome caused by selective serotonin reuptake-inhibitors- metoclopramide interaction. Ann Pharmacother 2002; 36: 67–71.

6. Golden RN, Dawkins K, Nicholas L, et al. Trazodone, nefazodone, bupropion, and mirtazapine. In Schatzberg AF, Nemeroff CB (eds) The American Psychiatric Press Textbook of Psychopharmacology. Washington DC, American Psychiatric Press, 1998, pp. 251–259.

7. Ascher JA, Cole JO, Colin JN, et al. Bupropion: a review of its mechanism of antidepressant activity. J Clin Psychiatry 1995; 56: 395–401.

8. Healy D. The Antidepressant Era. Cambridge, MA, Harvard University Press, 1997.

9. Murphy DL, Aulakh CS, Garrick NA, et al. Monoamine oxidase inhibitors as antidepressants. In Meltzer HY (ed) Psychopharmacology: The Third Generation of Progress. New York, Raven Press, 1987, pp. 545–552.

10. Mc Donald WM, Mc Call WV, Epstein CM. Electroconvulsive Therapy: Sixty Years of Progress and a Comparison with Transcranial Magnetic Stimulation. In Davis KL, Charney D, Coyle JT, Nemeroff C (eds) Neuropsychopharmacology: The Fifth Generation of Progress. Philadelphia Lippincott Williams and Wilkins, 2002, 1097–1108.

11. Lerer B. Neurochemical and other Neurological Consequences of ECT: Implications for the Pathogenesis and Treatment of Affective Disorders. In Meltzer H (ed) Psychopharmacology: The Third Generation of Progress. New York, Raven, 1987, pp. 577–588.

12. Poewe W, Seppi K Treatment options for depression and psychosis in Parkinson's disease. J Neurol 2001; 248(suppl 3): III12–III21.

13. Nutt DJ, Glue P. The neurobiology of ECT: animal studies. In Coffey CE (ed) The Clinical Science of Electroconvulsive Therapy. Washington, DC, American Psychiatry Press, 1993 pp. 213–234.

14. Rudorfer MV, Manji HK, Potter WZ. Monoaminergic actions of ECT. Clin Neuropharmacol 1992; 15: 677A–678A.

15. Balldin J, Granerus AK, Lindstedt G, et al. Predictors for improvement after electroconvulsive therapy in parkinsonian patients with on-off symptoms. J Neural Transm 1981; 52: 199–211.

16. Bolwig TG, Hertz MM, Paulson OB, et al. The permeability of the blood-brain barrier during electrically induced seizures in man. Eur J Clin Invest 1977; 7: 87–93.

17. Manji HK, McNamara R, Chen G, et al. Signalling pathways in the brain: cellular transduction of mood stabilisation in the treatment of manic-depressive illness. Aust N Z J Psychiatry 1999; 33(suppl): S65–S83.

18. Manji HK, Lenox RH. Ziskind-Somerfeld Research Award. Protein kinase C signaling in the brain: molecular transduction of mood stabilization in the treatment of manic-depressive illness. Biol Psychiatry 1999; 46: 1328–1351.

19. Manji HK, Bebchuk JM, Moore GJ, et al. Modulation of CNS signal transduction pathways and gene expression by mood-stabilizing agents: therapeutic implications. J Clin Psychiatry 1999; 60: 27–39; discussion 40–1, 113–6.

20. Lenox RH, McNamara RK, Papke RL, et al. Neurobiology of lithium: an update. J Clin Psychiatry 1998; 59: 37–47.

21. Jope RS. Anti-bipolar therapy: mechanism of action of lithium. Mol Psychiatry 1999; 4: 117–128.

22. Association AP. Diagnostic and Statistical Manual of Mental Disorders. Washington, 2000.

23. Leo RJ. Movement disorders associated with the serotonin selective reuptake inhibitors. J Clin Psychiatry 1996; 57: 449–454.

24. Nelson JC, Jatlow PI, Quinlan DM. Subjective complaints during desipramine treatment. Relative importance of plasma drug concentrations and the severity of depression. Arch Gen Psychiatry 1984; 41: 55–59.

25. Raethjen J, Lemke MR, Lindemann M, et al. Amitriptyline enhances the central component of physiological tremor. J Neurol Neurosurg Psychiatry 2001; 70: 78–82.

26. Kronfol Z, Greden JF, Zis AP. Imipramine-induced tremor: effects of a beta-adrenergic blocking agent. J Clin Psychiatry 1983; 44: 225–226.

27. Lee HK. Dystonic reactions to amitriptyline and doxepin. Am J Psychiatry 1988; 145: 649.

28. Caley CF. Extrapyramidal reactions and the selective serotonin-reuptake inhibitors. Ann Pharmacother 1997; 31: 1481–1489.

29. Apiquian R, Ulloa E, Fresan A, et al. Amoxapine shows atypical antipsychotic effects in patients with schizophrenia: results from a prospective open-label study. Schizophr Res 2003; 59: 35–39.

30. Lydiard RB, Gelenberg AJ. Amoxapine–an antidepressant with some neuroleptic properties? A review of its chemistry, animal pharmacology and toxicology, human pharmacology, and clinical efficacy. Pharmacotherapy 1981; 1: 163–178.

31. Barton JL. Amoxapine-induced agitation among bipolar depressed patients. Am J Psychiatry 1982; 139: 387.

32. Gammon GD, Hansen C. A case of akinesia induced by amoxapine. Am J Psychiatry 1984; 141: 283–284.

33. Huang CC. Persistent tardive dyskinesia associated with amoxapine therapy. Am J Psychiatry 1986; 143: 1069–1070.

34. Cohen BM, Harris PQ, Altesman RI, et al. Amoxapine: neuroleptic as well as antidepressant? Am J Psychiatry 1982; 139: 1165–1167.

35. Duggal HS, Dutta S, Sinha VK. Clomipramine discontinuation-emergent dystonia. Aust N Z J Psychiatry 2001; 35: 696.

36. Fornazzari L, Ichise M, Remington G, et al. Rabbit syndrome, antidepressant use, and cerebral perfusion SPECT scan findings. J Psychiatry Neurosci 1991; 16: 227–229.

37. Fann WE, Sullivan JL, Richman BW. Dyskinesias associated with tricyclic antidepressants. Br J Psychiatry 1976; 128: 490–493.

38. Clayton AH. Antidepressant-induced tardive dyskinesia: review and case report. Psychopharmacol Bull 1995; 31: 259–264.

39. Burks JS, Walker JE, Rumack BH, et al. Tricyclic antidepressant poisoning. Reversal of coma, choreoathetosis, and myoclonus by physostigmine. JAMA 1974; 230: 1405–1407.

40. Noble J, Matthew H. Acute poisoning by tricyclic antidepressants: clinical features and management of 100 patients. Clin Toxicol 1969; 2: 403–407.

41. Garvey MJ, Tollefson GD. Occurrence of myoclonus in patients treated with cyclic antidepressants. Arch Gen Psychiatry 1987; 44: 269–272.

42. Forstl H, Pohlmann-Eden B. Amplitudes of somatosensory evoked potentials reflect cortical hyperexcitability in antidepressant-induced myoclonus. Neurology 1990; 40: 924–926.

43. Moshe K, Iulian I, Seth K, et al. Clomipramine-induced tourettism in obsessive-compulsive disorder: clinical and theoretical implications. Clin Neuropharmacol 1994; 17: 338–343.

44. Sabaawi M, Richmond DR, Fragala MR. Akathisia in association with nortriptyline therapy. Am Fam Physician 1993; 48: 1024-1026.
45. Baca L, Martinelli L. Neuroleptic malignant syndrome: a unique association with a tricyclic antidepressant. Neurology 1990; 40: 1797–1798.
46. Schibuk M, Schachter D. A role for catecholamines in the pathogenesis of neuroleptic malignant syndrome. Can J Psychiatry 1986; 31: 66–69.
47. Sternbach H. The serotonin syndrome. Am J Psychiatry 1991; 148: 705–713.
48. Black K, Shea C, Dursun S, et al. Selective serotonin reuptake inhibitor discontinuation syndrome: proposed diagnostic criteria. J Psychiatry Neurosci 2000; 25: 255– 261.
49. Boyle SF. SSRIs and movement disorders. J Am Acad Child Adolesc Psychiatry 1999; 38: 354–355.
50. Reccoppa L, Welch WA, Ware MR. Acute dystonia and fluoxetine. J Clin Psychiatry 1990; 51: 487.
51. Fox GC, Ebeid S, Vincenti G. Paroxetine-induced chorea. Br J Psychiatry 1997; 170: 193– 194.
52. Christensen RC, Byerly MJ. Mandibular dystonia associated with the combination of sertraline and metoclopramide. J Clin Psychiatry 1996; 57: 596.
53. Stanislav SW, Childs NL. Dystonia associated with sertraline. J Clin Psychopharmacol 1999; 19: 98–100.
54. Meltzer HY, Young M, Metz J, et al. Extrapyramidal side effects and increased serum prolactin following fluoxetine, a new antidepressant. J Neural Transm 1979; 45: 165–175.
55. George MS, Trimble MR. Dystonic reaction associated with fluvoxamine. J Clin Psychopharmacol 1993; 13: 220–221.
56. Chong SA. Fluvoxamine and mandibular dystonia. Can J Psychiatry 1995; 40: 430–431.
57. Opler LA. Sertraline and akathisia. Am J Psychiatry 1994; 151: 620–621.
58. Lipinski JF, Jr, Mallya G, Zimmerman P, et al. Fluoxetine-induced akathisia: clinical and theoretical implications. J Clin Psychiatry 1989; 50: 339–342.
59. Bauer M, Hellweg R, Baumgartner A. Fluoxetine-induced akathisia does not reappear after switch to paroxetine. J Clin Psychiatry 1996; 57: 593–594.
60. Coulter DM, Pillans PI. Fluoxetine and extrapyramidal side effects. Am J Psychiatry 1995; 152: 122–125.
61. Pina Latorre MA, Modrego PJ, Rodilla F, et al. Parkinsonism and Parkinson's disease associated with long-term administration of sertraline. J Clin Pharm Ther 2001; 26: 111– 112.
62. Di Rocco A, Brannan T, Prikhojan A, et al. Sertraline induced parkinsonism. A case report and an in-vivo study of the effect of sertraline on dopamine metabolism. J Neural Transm 1998; 105: 247–251.
63. Jimenez-Jimenez FJ, Tejeiro J, Martinez-Junquera G, et al. Parkinsonism exacerbated by paroxetine. Neurology 1994; 44: 2406.
64. Stadtland C, Erfurth A, Arolt V. De novo onset of Parkinson's disease after antidepressant treatment with citalopram. Pharmacopsychiatry 2000; 33: 194–195.
65. Wils V. Extrapyramidal symptoms in a patient treated with fluvoxamine. J Neurol Neurosurg Psychiatry 1992; 55: 330–331.
66. Botsaris SD, Sypek JM. Paroxetine and tardive dyskinesia. J Clin Psychopharmacol 1996; 16: 258–259.
67. Halman M, Goldbloom DS. Fluoxetine and neuroleptic malignant syndrome. Biol Psychiatry 1990; 28: 518–521.
68. Ghaziuddin N, Iqbal A, Khetarpal S. Myoclonus during prolonged treatment with sertraline in an adolescent patient. J Child Adolesc Psychopharmacol 2001; 11: 199–202.

69. Bauer M. Severe myoclonus produced by fluvoxamine. J Clin Psychiatry 1995; 56: 589–590.

70. Darko W, Guharoy R, Rose F, et al. Myoclonus secondary to the concurrent use of trazodone and fluoxetine. Vet Hum Toxicol 2001; 43: 214–215.

71. Lauterbach EC. Reversible intermittent rhythmic myoclonus with fluoxetine in presumed Pick's disease. Mov Disord 1994; 9: 343–346.

72. Lenti C. Movement disorders associated with fluvoxamine. J Am Acad Child Adolesc Psychiatry 1999; 38: 942–943.

73. Eisenhauer G, Jermain DM. Fluoxetine and tics in an adolescent. Ann Pharmacother 1993; 27: 725–726.

74. Madhusoodanan S, Brenner R. Reversible choreiform dyskinesia and extrapyramidal symptoms associated with sertraline therapy. J Clin Psychopharmacol 1997; 17: 138–139.

75. Richard IH, Kurlan R, Tanner C, et al. Serotonin syndrome and the combined use of deprenyl and an antidepressant in Parkinson's disease. Parkinson Study Group. Neurology 1997; 48: 1070–1077.

76. Bilbao Garay J, Mesa Plaza N, Castilla Castellano V, et al. Serotonin syndrome: report of a fatal case and review of the literature. Rev Clin Esp 2002; 202: 209–211.

77. Ellison JM, Stanziani P. SSRI-associated nocturnal bruxism in four patients. J Clin Psychiatry 1993; 54: 432–434.

78. Wise M. Citalopram-induced bruxism. Br J Psychiatry 2001; 178: 182.

79. Romanelli F, Adler DA, Bungay KM. Possible paroxetine-induced bruxism. Ann Pharmacother 1996; 30: 1246–1248.

80. Faulkner KDB. Bruxism a review of the literature. Aust Dent J 1990; 35: 266–276.

81. Lu R, Hurley AD, Gourley M. Dystonia induced by mirtazapine. J Clin Psychiatry 2002; 63: 452–453.

82. Detweiler MB, Harpold G. Bupropion-induced acute dystonia. Ann Pharmacother 2002; 36: 251–254.

83. Girishchandra BG, Johnson L, Cresp RM, et al. Mirtazapine-induced akathisia. Med J Aust 2002; 176: 242.

84. Fukunishi I, Kitaoka T, Shirai T, et al. A hemodialysis patient with trazodone-induced parkinsonism. Nephron 2002; 90: 222–223.

85. Albanese A, Rossi P, Altavista MC. Can trazodone induce parkinsonism? Clin Neuropharmacol 1988; 11: 180–182.

86. Garcia-Parajua P, Alvarez Iniesta I, Magarinos M. Reversible and dose-related parkinsonism induced by venlafaxine. Med Clin (Barc). 2003; 120: 759.

87. Szuba MP, Leuchter AF. Falling backward in two elderly patients taking bupropion. J Clin Psychiatry 1992; 53: 157–159.

88. Jerome L. Bupropion and drug-induced parkinsonism. Can J Psychiatry 2001; 46: 560–561.

89. Nimmagadda SR, Ryan DH, Atkin SL. Neuroleptic malignant syndrome after venlafaxine. Lancet 2000; 355: 289–290.

90. Kramer MS, Marcus DJ, DiFerdinando J, et al. Atypical acute dystonia associated with trazodone treatment. J Clin Psychopharmacol 1986; 6: 117–118.

91. De Graaf L, Admiraal P, van Puijenbroek EP. Ballism associated with bupropion use. Ann Pharmacother 2003; 37: 302–303.

92. Bonin B, Vandel P, Kantelip JP. Mirtazapine and restless leg syndrome: a case report. Therapie 2000; 55: 655–656.

93. Rao R. Serotonin syndrome associated with trazodone. Int J Geriatr Psychiatry 1997; 12: 129–130.

94. Ubogu E, Katirji B. Mirtazapine-induced serotonin syndrome. Clin Neuropharmacol 2003; 26: 54–57.
95. Gitlin MJ. Venlafaxine, monoamine oxidase inhibitors, and the serotonin syndrome. J Clin Psychopharmacol 1997; 17: 66–67.
96. Brown ES, Hong SC. Antidepressant-induced bruxism successfully treated with gabapentin. J Am Dent Assoc 1999; 130: 1467–1469.
97. Evans DL, Davidson J, Raft D. Early and late side effects of phenelzine. J Clin Psychopharmacol 1982; 2: 208–210.
98. Gillman MA, Sandyk R. Parkinsonism induced by a monoamine oxidase inhibitor. Postgrad Med J 1986; 62: 235–236.
99. Teusink JP, Alexopoulos GS, Shamoian CA. Parkinsonian side effects induced by a monoamine oxidase inhibitor. Am J Psychiatry 1984; 141: 118–119.
100. Zubenko GS, Cohen BM, Lipinski JF. Antidepressant-related akathisia. J Clin Psychopharmacol 1987; 7: 254–257.
101. Pande AC, Max P. A dystonic reaction occurring during treatment with tranylcypromine. J Clin Psychopharmacol 1989; 9: 229–230.
102. Lieberman JA, Kane JM, Reife R. Neuromuscular effects of monoamine oxidase inhibitors. Adv Neurol 1986; 43: 231–249.
103. Baloh RW, Dietz J, Spooner JW. Myoclonus and ocular oscillations induced by L-tryptophan. Ann Neurol 1982; 11: 95–97.
104. Pope HG, Jonas JM, Hudson JI, et al. Toxic reactions to the combination of monoamine oxidase inhibitors and tryptophan. Am J Psychiatry 1985; 142: 491–492.
105. Askenasy JJ, Yahr MD. Is monoamine oxidase inhibitor induced myoclonus serotoninergically mediated? J Neural Transm 1988; 72: 67–76.
106. Stancer HC. Tardive dyskinesia not associated with neuroleptics [letter]. Am J Psychiatry 1979; 136: 727.
107. Uhrbrand L, Faurbye A. Reversible and irreversible dyskinesia after treatment with perphenazine, chlorpromazine, reserpine and electroconvulsive therapy. Psychopharmacologia 1960; 1.
108. Flaherty JA, Naidu J, Dysken M. ECT, emergent dyskinesia, and depression. Am J Psychiatry 1984; 141: 808–809.
109. Friedman JH, Kucharski LT, Wagner RL. Tardive dystonia in a psychiatric hospital. J Neurol Neurosurg Psychiatry 1987; 50: 801–803.
110. Gardos G, Samu I, Kallos M, et al. Absence of severe tardive dyskinesia in Hungarian schizophrenic out-patients. Psychopharmacology 1980; 71: 29–34.
111. Hanin B, Lerner Y, Srour N. An unusual effect of ECT on drug-induced parkinsonism and tardive dystonia. Convuls Ther 1995; 11: 271–274.
112. Dysken MW, Halaris AE. Post-ECT asterixis associated with primary hyperparathyroidism. Am J Psychiatry 1978; 135: 1237–1238.
113. Apte SN, Langston JW. Permanent neurological deficits due to lithium toxicity. Ann Neurol 1983; 13: 453–455.
114. Goddard J, Bloom SR, Frackowiak RS, et al. Lithium intoxication. Br Med J 1991; 302: 1267–1269.
115. Vestergaard P. Clinically important side effects of long-term lithium treatment: a review. Acta Psychiatr Scand 1983; 67(suppl): 11–36.
116. Zubenko GS, Cohen BM, Lipinski JF, Jr. Comparison of metoprolol and propranolol in the treatment of lithium tremor. Psychiatry Res 1984; 11: 163–164.
117. Zaninelli R, Bauer M, Jobert M, et al. Changes in quantitatively assessed tremor during treatment of major depression with lithium augmented by paroxetine or amitriptyline. J Clin Psychopharmacol 2001; 21: 190–198.

118. Donaldson IM, Cuningham J. Persisting neurologic sequelae of lithium carbonate therapy. Arch Neurol 1983; 40: 747–750.

119. Lecamwasam D, Synek B, Moyles K, et al. Chronic lithium neurotoxicity presenting as Parkinson's disease. Int Clin Psychopharmacol 1994; 9: 127–129.

120. Schou M. Lithium studies. Distribution between serum and tissues. Acta Pharmacol Toxicol 1958; 15: 115–124.

121. Dallocchio C, Mazzarello P. A case of Parkinsonism due to lithium intoxication: treatment with pramipexole. J Clin Neurosci 2002; 9: 310–311.

122. Holroyd S, Smith D. Disabling parkinsonism due to lithium: a case report. J Geriatr Psychiatry Neurol 1995; 8: 118–119.

123. Muthane UB, Prasad BNK, Vasanth A, et al. Tardive parkinsonism, orofacial dyskinesia and akathisia following brief exposure to lithium carbonate. J Neurol Sci 2000; 176: 78–79.

124. Shopsin B, Gershon S. Cogwheel rigidity related to lithium maintenance. Am J Psychiatry 1975; 132: 536–538.

125. Lance JW, Schwab RS, Peterson EA. Action tremor and the cogwheel phenomenon in Parkinson's disease. Brain 1963; 86: 95–110.

126. Findley LJ, Gresty MA, Halmagyi GM. Tremor, the cogwheel phenomenon and clonus in Parkinson's disease. J Neurol Neurosurg Psychiatry 1981; 44: 534–546.

127. Cleeves L, Findley LJ, Koller W. Lack of association between essential tremor and Parkinson's disease. Ann Neurol 1988; 24: 23–26.

128. Shopsin B, Johnson G, Gershon S. Neurotoxicity with lithium: differential drug responsiveness. Int Pharmacopsychiatry 1970; 5: 170–182.

129. Zorumski CF, Bakris GL. Choreoathetosis associated with lithium: case report and literature review. Am J Psychiatry 1983; 140: 1621–1622.

130. Klawans HL, Weiner WJ, Nausieda PA. The effect of lithium on an animal model of tardive dyskinesia. Prog Neuropsychopharmacol 1977; 1: 53–60.

131. Peters HA. Lithium intoxication producing chorea athetosis with recovery. Wis Med J 1949; 48: 1075–1076.

132. Coats DA, Trautner EM, Gershon S. The treatment of lithium poisoning. Australas Ann Med 1957; 6: 11–15.

133. Rosen PB, Stevens R. Action myoclonus in lithium toxicity. Ann Neurol 1983; 13: 221–222.

134. Devanand DP, Sackeim HA, Brown RP. Myoclonus during combined tricyclic antidepressant and lithium treatment. J Clin Psychopharmacol 1988; 8: 446–447.

135. Caviness JN, Evidente VG. Cortical myoclonus during lithium exposure. Arch Neurol 2003; 60: 401–404.

136. Heiman EM, Christie M. Lithium-aggravated nocturnal myoclonus and restless legs syndrome. Am J Psychiatry 1986; 143: 1191–1192.

137. Sandyk R. Oculogyric crisis induced by lithium carbonate. Eur Neurol 1984; 23: 92–94.

138. Pandey GN, Goel I, Davis JM. Effect of neuroleptic drugs on lithium uptake by the human erythrocyte. Clin Pharmacol Ther 1979; 26: 96–102.

139. Ghadirian AM, Annable L, Belanger MC, et al. A cross-sectional study of parkinsonism and tardive dyskinesia in lithium-treated affective disordered patients. J Clin Psychiatry 1996; 57: 22–28.

140. Mayeux R. Depression and dementia in Parkinson's disease. In Marsden CD, Fahn S (eds) Movement Disorders. London: Butterworth, 1982, pp. 75–95.

141. Tandberg E, Larsen JP, Aarsland D, et al. The occurrence of depression in Parkinson's disease. A community-based study. Arch Neurol 1996; 53: 175–179.

142. Mayeux R, Stern Y, Cote L, et al. Altered serotonin metabolism in depressed patients with Parkinson's disease. Neurology 1984; 34: 642–646.

143. Javoy-Agid F, Agid Y. Is the mesocortical dopaminergic system involved in Parkinson disease? Neurology 1980; 30: 1326–1330.

144. Brandstadter D, Oertel WH. Depression in Parkinson's disease. Adv Neurol 2003; 91: 371–381.

145. Sigwald J, Bouttier D, Raymondeaud C, et al. Etude de l'action sur l'akinesie parkinsonienne de deux derives de l'iminodibenzyle. Presse Med 1959; 67: 1697–1698.

146. Strang RR. Imipramine in the treatkent of parkinsonism: a double-blind placebo study. Br Med J 1965; 2: 33–34.

147. Laitinen L. Desipramine in treatment of Parkinson's disease. A placebo-controlled study. Acta Neurol Scand 1969; 45: 109–113.

148. Andersen J, Aabro E, Gulmann N, et al. Anti-depressive treatment in Parkinson's disease. A controlled trial of the effect of nortriptyline in patients with Parkinson's disease treated with L-DOPA. Acta Neurol Scand 1980; 62: 210–219.

149. Cunningham LA. Depression in the medically ill: choosing an antidepressant. J Clin Psychiatry 1994; (55)(suppl A): 90–97; discussion 98–100.

150. Stoudemire A. New antidepressant drugs and the treatment of depression in the medically ill patient. Psychiatr Clin North Am 1996; 19: 495–514.

151. Ceravolo R, Nuti A, Piccinni A, et al. Paroxetine in Parkinson's disease: effects on motor and depressive symptoms. Neurology 2000; 55: 1216–1218.

152. Steur EN. Increase of Parkinson disability after fluoxetine medication. Neurology 1993; 43: 211–213.

153. Tesei S, Antonini A, Canesi M, et al. Tolerability of paroxetine in Parkinson's disease: a prospective study. Mov Disord 2000; 15: 986–989.

154. Caley CF, Friedman JH. Does fluoxetine exacerbate Parkinson's disease? J Clin Psychiatry 1992; 53: 278–282.

155. Dell' Agnello G, Ceravolo R, Nuti A, et al. SSRIs do not worsen Parkinson's disease: evidence from an open-label, prospective study. Clin Neuropharmacol 2001; 24: 221–227.

156. Rampello L, Chiechio S, Raffaele R, et al. The SSRI, citalopram, improves bradykinesia in patients with Parkinson's disease treated with L-dopa. Clin Neuropharmacol 2002; 25: 21–24.

157. Richard IH, Maughn A, Kurlan R. Do serotonin reuptake inhibitor antidepressants worsen Parkinson's disease? A retrospective case series. Mov Disord 1999; 14: 155–157.

158. Mayeux R, Stern Y, Williams JB, et al. Clinical and biochemical features of depression in Parkinson's disease. Am J Psychiatry 1986; 143: 756–759.

159. Paulus W, Jellinger K. The neuropathologic basis of different clinical subgroups of Parkinson's disease. J Neuropathol Exp Neurol 1991; 50: 743–755.

160. Greenblatt DJ, von Moltke LL, Harmatz JS, et al. Drug interactions with newer antidepressants: role of human cytochromes P450. J Clin Psychiatry 1998; 59: 19–27.

161. Brosen K. Are pharmacokinetic drug interactions with the SSRIs an issue? Int Clin Psychopharmacol 1996; 11(suppl 1): 23–27.

162. Goetz CG, Tanner CM, Klawans HL. Bupropion in Parkinson's disease. Neurology 1984; 34: 1092–1094.

163. Pact V, Giduz T. Mirtazapine treats resting tremor, essential tremor, and levodopa-induced dyskinesias. Neurology 1999; 53: 1154.

164. Normann C, Hesslinger B, Frauenknecht S, et al. Psychosis during chronic levodopa therapy triggered by the new antidepressive drug mirtazapine. Pharmacopsychiatry 1997; 30: 263–265.

165. Onofrj M, Luciano AL, Thomas A, et al. Mirtazapine induces REM sleep behavior disorder (RBD) in parkinsonism. Neurology 2003; 60: 113–115.
166. Benazzi F. Parkinson's disease worsened by nefazodone. Int J Geriatr Psychiatry 1997; 12: 1195.
167. Andersen K, Balldin J, Gottfries CG, et al. A double-blind evaluation of electroconvulsive therapy in Parkinson's disease with "on-off" phenomena. Acta Neurol Scand 1987; 76: 191–199.
168. Douyon R, Serby M, Klutchko B, et al. ECT and Parkinson's disease revisited: a "naturalistic" study. Am J Psychiatry 1989; 146: 1451–1455.
169. Moellentine C, Rummans T, Ahlskog JE, et al. Effectiveness of ECT in patients with parkinsonism. J Neuropsychiatry Clin Neurosci 1998; 10: 187–193.
170. Kellner DH, Beale MD, Pritchett JT, et al. Electroconvulsive therapy and Parkinson's disease: the case for further study. Psychopharmacol Bull 1994; 30: 495–500.
171. Faber R, Trimble MR. Electroconvulsive therapy in Parkinson's disease and other movement disorders. Mov Disord 1991; 6: 293–303.
172. Guttman M. ECT for Parkinson's? Correspondence. Can Med Assoc J 2003; 168: 1392.
173. Wilder J, Brown GL, Lebensohn ZM. Letter: Parkinsonism, depression, and ECT. Am J Psychiatry 1975; 132: 1083–1084.
174. Ward C, Stern GM, Pratt RT, et al. Electroconvulsive therapy in Parkinsonian patients with the "on-off" syndrome. J Neural Transm 1980; 49: 133–135.
175. Rasmussen K, Abrams R. Treatment of Parkinson's disease with electroconvulsive therapy. Psychiatr Clin North Am 1991; 14: 925–933.
176. Young RC, Alexopoulos GS, Shamoian CA. Dissociation of motor response from mood and cognition in a parkinsonian patient treated with ECT. Biol Psychiatry 1985; 20: 566–569.
177. Roth SD, Mukherjee S, Sackeim HA. Electroconvulsive therapy in a patient with mania, parkinsonism, and tardive dyskinesia. Convuls Ther 1988; 4: 92–97.
178. Atre-Vaidya N, Jampala VC. Electroconvulsive therapy in parkinsonism with affective disorder. Br J Psychiatry 1988; 152: 55–58.
179. Ananth J, Samra D, Kolivakis T. Amelioration of drug-induced Parkinsonism by ECT. Am J Psychiatry 1979; 136: 1094.
180. Holcomb HH, Sternberg DE, Heninger GR. Effects of electroconvulsive therapy on mood, parkinsonism, and tardive dyskinesia in a depressed patient: ECT and dopamine systems. Biol Psychiatry 1983; 18: 865–873.
181. Chacko RC, Root L. ECT and tardive dyskinesia: two cases and a review. J Clin Psychiatry 1983; 44: 265–266.
182. Goswami U, Dutta S, Kuruvilla K, et al. Electroconvulsive therapy in neuroleptic-induced parkinsonism. Biol Psychiatry 1989; 26: 234–238.
183. Hermesh H, Aizenberg D, Friedberg G, et al. Electroconvulsive therapy for persistent neuroleptic-induced akathisia and parkinsonism: a case report. Biol Psychiatry 1992; 31: 407–411.
184. Gangadhar BN, Choudhary JR, Channabasavanna SM. ECT and drug-induced parkinsonism. Indian J Psychiatry 1983; 25: 212–213.
185. Mukherjee S, Debsikdar V. Absence of neuroleptic-induced parkinsonism in psychotic patients receiving adjunctive electroconvulsive therapy. Convuls Ther 1994; 10: 53–58.
186. Hooten WM, Melin G, Richardson JW. Response of the Parkinsonian symptoms of multiple system atrophy to ECT. Am J Psychiatry 1998; 155: 1628.
187. Roane DM, Rogers JD, Helew L, et al. Electroconvulsive therapy for elderly patients with multiple system atrophy: a case series. Am J Geriatr Psychiatry 2000; 8: 171–174.

188. Barclay CL, Duff J, Sandor P, et al. Limited usefulness of electroconvulsive therapy in progressive supranuclear palsy. Neurology 1996; 46: 1284–1286.

189. Netzel PJ, Sutor B. Electroconvulsive therapy-responsive depression in a patient with progressive supranuclear palsy. J ECT 2001; 17: 68–70.

190. Coffey CE, Ross DR, Ferren EL, et al. The effect of lithium on the "on-off" phenomenon in parkinsonism. Adv Neurol 1983; 37: 61–73.

191. Lieberman A, Gopinathan G. Treatment of "on-off" phenomena with lithium. Ann Neurol 1982; 12: 402.

192. Dalen P, Steg G. Lithium and levodopa in parkinsonism. Lancet 1973; 1: 936–937.

193. Van Woert MH, Ambani LM. Lithium and levodopa in parkinsonism. Lancet 1973; 1: 1390–1391.

194. McCaul JA, Stern GM. Lithium in Parkinson's disease. Lancet 1974; 1: 1117.

195. Quinn N, Marsden CD. Lithium for painful dystonia in Parkinson's disease. Lancet 1986; 1: 1377.

196. Magnussen I, Mondrup K, Engbaek F, et al. Treatment of myoclonic syndromes with paroxetine alone or combined with 5-HTP. Acta Neurol Scand 1982; 66: 276–282.

197. Van Woert MH, Magnussen I, Rosenbaum D, et al. Fluoxetine in the treatment of intention myoclonus. Clin Neuropharmacol 1983; 6: 49–54.

198. Scheidtmann K, Muller F, Hartmann E, et al. Familial myoclonus-dystonia syndrome associated with panic attacks. Nervenarzt 2000; 71: 839–842.

199. Lhermitte F, Marteau R, Degos CF. Pharmacologic analysis of a new case of postanoxic intention and action myoclonus. Rev Neurol (Paris) 1972; 126: 107–114.

200. De Lean J, Richardson JC, Hornykiewicz O. Beneficial effects of serotonin precursors in postanoxic action myoclonus. Neurology 1976; 26: 863–868.

201. Chadwick D, Hallett M, Harris R, et al. Clinical, biochemical, and physiological features distinguishing myoclonus responsive to 5-hydroxytryptophan, tryptophan with a monoamine oxidase inhibitor, and clonazepam. Brain 1977; 100: 455–487.

202. Malek-Ahmadi P. Bupropion, periodic limb movement disorder, and ADHD. J Am Acad Child Adolesc Psychiatry 1999; 38: 637–638.

203. McLeod NA, White LE, Jr. Trazodone in essential tremor. JAMA 1986; 256: 2675–2676.

204. Koller WC. Tradozone in essential tremor. Probe of serotoninergic mechanisms. Clin Neuropharmacol 1989; 12: 134–137.

205. Gordon PH, Pullman SL, Louis ED, et al. Mirtazapine in Parkinsonian tremor. Parkinsonism Relat Disord 2002; 9: 125–126.

206. Pahwa R, Lyons KE. Mirtazapine in essential tremor: A double-blind, placebo-controlled pilot study. Mov Disord 2003; 18: 584–587.

207. Spencer T, Biederman J, Kerman K, et al. Desipramine treatment of children with attention-deficit hyperactivity disorder and tic disorder or Tourette's syndrome. J Am Acad Child Adolesc Psychiatry 1993; 32: 354–360.

208. Spencer T, Biederman J, Wilens T, et al. Nortriptyline treatment of children with attention-deficit hyperactivity disorder and tic disorder or Tourette's syndrome. J Am Acad Child Adolesc Psychiatry 1993; 32: 205–210.

209. Spencer T, Biederman J, Coffey B, et al. A double-blind comparison of desipramine and placebo in children and adolescents with chronic tic disorder and comorbid attention-deficit/hyperactivity disorder. Arch Gen Psychiatry 2002; 59: 649–656.

210. Bajo S, Battaglia M, Pegna C, et al. Citalopram and fluvoxamine in Tourette's disorder. J Am Acad Child Adolesc Psychiatry 1999; 38: 230–231.

211. Buckingham D, Gaffney G. New TS treatment. J Am Acad Child Adolesc Psychiatry 1993; 32: 224.

212. Scahill L, Riddle MA, King RA, et al. Fluoxetine has no marked effect on tic symptoms in patients with Tourette's syndrome: a double-blind placebo-controlled study. J Child Adolesc Psychopharmacol 1997; 7: 75–85.

213. Eapen V, Trimble MR, Robertson MM. The use of fluoxetine in Gilles de la Tourette syndrome and obsessive compulsive behaviours: preliminary clinical experience. Prog Neuropsychopharmacol Biol Psychiatry 1996; 20: 737–743.

214. Delgado PL, Goodman WK, Price LH, et al. Fluvoxamine/pimozide treatment of concurrent Tourette's and obsessive- compulsive disorder. Br J Psychiatry 1990; 157: 762–765.

215. Ruth U, Mayer-Rosa J, Schlamp D, et al. Tourette's syndrome and antidepressant therapy: exacerbation of nervous tics with paroxetine. Z Kinder Jugendpsychiatr Psychother 2000; 28: 105–108.

216. Wender PH, Reimherr FW. Bupropion treatment of attention-deficit hyperactivity disorder in adults. Am J Psychiatry 1990; 147: 1018-1020.

217. Simeon JG, Ferguson HB, Van Wyck Fleet J. Bupropion effects in attention deficit and conduct disorders. Can J Psychiatry 1986; 31: 581–585.

218. Spencer T, Biederman J, Steingard R, et al. Bupropion exacerbates tics in children with attention-deficit hyperactivity disorder and Tourette's syndrome. J Am Acad Child Adolesc Psychiatry 1993; 32: 211–214.

219. Araneta E, Magen J, Musci MN, Jr. et al. Gilles de la Tourette's syndrome symptom onset at age 35. Child Psychiatry Hum Dev 1975; 5: 224–230.

220. Guttmacher LB, Cretella H. Electroconvulsive therapy in one child and three adolescents. J Clin Psychiatry 1988; 49: 20–23.

221. Swerdlow NR, Gierz M, Berkowitz A, et al. Electroconvulsive therapy in a patient with severe tic and major depressive episode. J Clin Psychiatry 1990; 51: 34–35.

222. Rapoport M, Feder V, Sandor P. Response of major depression and Tourette's syndrome to ECT: a case report. Psychosom Med 1998; 60: 528–529.

223. Kerbeshian J, Burd L. Differential responsiveness to lithium in patients with Tourette disorder. Neurosci Biobehav Rev 1988; 12: 247–250.

224. Erickson HM, Goggins JE, Messiha FS. Comparison of lithium and haloperidol therapy in Gilles de la Tourette syndrome. Adv Exp Med Biol 1976; 90: 197–205.

225. Hamra BJ, Dunner FH, Larson C. Remission of tics with lithium therapy: case report. J Clin Psychiatry 1983; 44: 73–74.

226. Borison RL, Ang L, Chang S, et al. New pharmacological approaches in the treatment of Tourette syndrome. Adv Neurol 1982; 35: 377–382.

227. Greene P, Shale H, Fahn S. Experience with high dosages of anticholinergic and other drugs in the treatment of torsion dystonia. Adv Neurol 1988; 50: 547–556.

228. Birner P, Schnider P, Muller J, et al. Torticollis spasmodicus, blepharospasm and hemifacial spasm. Subjective evaluation of therapy by patients. Nervenarzt 1999; 70: 903–908.

229. Kwentus JA, Schulz SC, Hart RP. Tardive dystonia, catatonia, and electroconvulsive therapy. J Nerv Ment Dis 1984; 172: 171–173.

230. Adityanjee, Jayaswal SK, Chan TM, et al. Temporary remission of tardive dystonia following electroconvulsive therapy. Br J Psychiatry 1990; 156: 433–435.

231. Lauterbach EC, Moore NC. Parkinsonism-dystonia syndrome and ECT. Am J Psychiatry 1990; 147: 1249–1250.

232. Couper-Smartt J. Lithium in spasmodic torticollis. Lancet 1973; 2: 741–742.

233. Lippmann S, Kareus J. Lithium for spasmodic torticollis. Am J Psychiatry 1983; 140: 946.

234. Marti-Masso JF, Obeso JA, Carrera N, et al. Lithium therapy in torsion dystonia. Ann Neurol 1982; 11: 106–107.

235. McCaul JA, Stern GM. Letter: Lithium and haloperidol in movement disorders. Lancet 1974; 1: 1058.
236. Jankovic J, Ford J. Blepharospasm and orofacial-cervical dystonia: clinical and pharmacological findings in 100 patients. Ann Neurol 1983; 13: 402–411.
237. Jankovic J, Orman J. Tetrabenazine therapy of dystonia, chorea, tics, and other dyskinesias. Neurology 1988; 38: 391–394.
238. Koller WC, Biary N. Lithium ineffective in dystonia. Ann Neurol 1983; 13: 579–580.
239. el-Awar M, Freedman M, Seeman P, et al. Response of tardive and L-dopa-induced dyskinesias to antidepressants. Can J Neurol Sci 1987; 14: 629–631.
240. D'Mello DA, Nasrallah HA. Suppression of tardive dyskinesia with amoxapine: case report. J Clin Psychiatry 1986; 47: 148.
241. Korsgaard S, Noring U, Povlsen UJ, et al. Effects of citalopram, a specific serotonin uptake inhibitor, in tardive dyskinesia and parkinsonism. Clin Neuropharmacol 1986; 9: 52–57.
242. Hayashi T, Yokota N, Takahashi T, et al. Benefits of trazodone and mianserin for patients with late-life chronic schizophrenia and tardive dyskinesia: an add-on, double-blind, placebo-controlled study. Int Clin Psychopharmacol 1997; 12: 199–205.
243. Price TR, Levin R. The effects of electroconvulsive therapy on tardive dyskinesia. Am J Psychiatry 1978; 135: 991–993.
244. Rosenbaum AH, Niven RG, Hanson NP, et al. Tardive dyskinesia: relationship with a primary affective disorder. Dis Nerv Syst 1977; 38: 423–427.
245. Asnis GM, Leopold MA. A single-blind study of ECT in patients with tardive dyskinesia. Am J Psychiatry 1978; 135: 1235–1237.
246. Crews EL, Carpenter AE. Lithium-induced aggravation of tardive dyskinesia. Am J Psychiatry 1977; 134: 933.
247. Reches A, Hassan MN, Jackson V, et al. Lithium interferes with reserpine-induced dopamine depletion. Ann Neurol 1983; 13: 671–673.
248. Reda FA, Escobar JI, Scanlan JM. Lithium carbonate in the treatment of tardive dyskinesia. Am J Psychiatry 1975; 132: 560–562.
249. Dalen P. Lithium therapy in Huntington's chorea and tardive dyskinesia. Lancet 1973; 1: 107–108.
250. Ehrensing RH. Letter: Lithium and M.R.I.H. in tardive dyskinesia. Lancet 1974; 2: 1459–1460.
251. MacKay AV, Sheppard GP, Saha BK, et al. Failure of lithium treatment in established tardive dyskinesia. Psychol Med 1980; 10: 583–587.
252. De Marchi N, Daniele F, Ragone MA. Fluoxetine in the treatment of Huntington's disease. Psychopharmacology (Berl) 2001; 153: 264–266.
253. Chari S, Quraishi SH, Jainer AK. Fluoxetine-induced exacerbation of chorea in Huntington's disease? A case report. Pharmacopsychiatry 2003; 36: 41–43.
254. Ranen NG, Lipsey JR, Treisman G, et al. Sertraline in the treatment of severe aggressiveness in Huntington's disease. J Neuropsychiatry Clin Neurosci 1996; 8: 338–340.
255. Patzold T, Brune M. Obsessive compulsive disorder in Huntington disease: a case of isolated obsessions successfully treated with sertraline. Neuropsychiatry Neuropsychol Behav Neurol 2002; 15: 216–219.
256. Bonelli RM. Mirtazapine in suicidal Huntington's disease. Ann Pharmacother 2003; 37: 452.
257. Ford MF. Treatment of depression in Huntington's disease with monoamine oxidase inhibitors. Br J Psychiatry 1986; 149: 654–656.
258. Mattsson B. Huntington's chorea and lithium therapy. Lancet 1973; 1: 718–719.

259. Vestergaard P, Baastrup PC, Petersson H. Lithium treatment of Huntington's chorea. A placebo-controlled clinical trial. Acta Psychiatr Scand 1977; 56: 183–188.

260. Aminoff MJ, Marshall J. Treatment of Huntington's chorea with lithium carbonate. A double-blind trial. Lancet 1974; 1: 107–109.

261. Carman JS, Shoulson I, Chase TN. Letter: Huntington's chorea treated with lithium carbonate. Lancet 1974; 1: 811.

262. Wei H, Qin ZH, Senatorov VV, et al. Lithium suppresses excitotoxicity-induced striatal lesions in a rat model of Huntington's disease. Neuroscience 2001; 106: 603–612.

263. Beale MD, Kellner CH, Gurecki P, et al. ECT for the treatment of Huntington's disease: a case study. Convuls Ther 1997; 13: 108–112.

264. Lewis CF, DeQuardo JR, Tandon R. ECT in genetically confirmed Huntington's disease. J Neuropsychiatry Clin Neurosci 1996; 8: 209–210.

265. Ranen NG, Peyser CE, Folstein SE. ECT as a treatment for depression in Huntington's disease. J Neuropsychiatry Clin Neurosci 1994; 6: 154–159.

266. Owens MJ, Knight DL, Nemeroff CB. Second-generation SSRI's: human monoamine transporter binding profile of escitalopram and R-fluoxetine. Biol Psychiatry 2001; 50: 345–350.

CHAPTER 16

Antiepileptics

John C. Morgan and Madaline B. Harrison

Antiepileptic drugs (AEDs) have been in use since bromides were first employed to treat epilepsy in the 19th century [1]. Today, phenobarbitone (PB), phenytoin (PHT), carbamazepine (CBZ), and valproate (VPA) have become the most commonly used AEDs. While these four AEDs were introduced over a period of 120 years after bromides were first used to treat epilepsy, the armamentarium of AEDs has almost doubled in the past 10 years. Table 16.1 lists the major oral AEDs approved for use in the United States today.

With some exceptions (ataxia with PHT, tremor with VPA), movement disorders are relatively rare in patients using these drugs. While AEDs are increasingly used to treat movement disorders (e.g., primidone (PRM) in essential tremor, gabapentin (GBP) in essential tremor restless legs syndrome), it is important to recognize that movement disorders can occur during treatment with AEDs, particularly in the setting of polypharmacy. In this chapter we will focus on movement disorders associated with the use of AEDs based upon a review of the English language literature.

Ataxia

Ataxia is the most common movement disorder that occurs in patients taking AEDs. It can develop in the setting of oral or intravenous loading, as a sign of toxicity, or less commonly as a side effect of chronic treatment. Ataxia occurs most often in the setting of acute intoxication and PHT and CBZ are the two AEDs most commonly implicated. A review of 85 cases of PHT intoxication in a general hospital revealed ataxia in 88% of the cases with a median serum PHT level of 46.5 μg/mL (range 30.3–95.0) [2]. The majority of the patients was receiving increased oral doses or intravenous loading for single seizures secondary to subtherapeutic serum PHT levels [2]. While the outcome in these patients is usually good with the resolution of ataxia after the responsible drug is metabolized to nontoxic levels, some patients develop chronic complications. Prolonged treatment with high doses (or serum levels) of PHT has been associated with irreversible ataxia and cerebellar atrophy in multiple reports in both children [3, 4] and adults [5–7]. Whether ataxia and cerebellar atrophy are due to the effect of epilepsy on the cerebellum or due to PHT itself

Table 16.1 Major AEDs Approved for Use in the United States Today. A conventional abbreviation for many of the drugs is listed beside the full generic name. The year of first use or year of United States FDA approval is indicated beside each drug as well

Conventional AEDs		Approved in the last 10 years	
Phenobarbitone (PB)	1912	Felbamate (FBM)	1993
Phenytoin (PHT)	1938	Gabapentin (GBP)	1994
Primidone (PRM)	1954	Lamotrigine (LMT)	1994
Methsuximide	1957	Topiramate (TPM)	1996
Ethosuximide (ESM)	1958	Tiagabine (TGB)	1997
Diazepam (DZP)	1963	Levetiracetam (LEV)	1999
Clorazepate	1972	Zonisamide (ZNS)	2000
Carbamazepine (CBZ)	1974	Oxcarbazepine (OXC)	2000
Clonazepam	1976		
Valproate/divalproex (VPA)	1978		

is debated in the literature [8]. Hypoxia in patients who experience generalized convulsions may predispose to loss of Purkinje cells. Alternatively, pathological studies in humans have linked diffuse loss of Purkinje cells in epileptics to PHT use [9]. Addressing this issue further, there are reports of cerebellar atrophy and ataxia following acute or chronic PHT intoxication in patients without epilepsy [10, 11]. However, a recent quantitative neuropathological study in epileptics treated with PHT concluded that it is unlikely that PHT acts alone in inducing Purkinje cell loss [12].

CBZ is also commonly implicated as a cause of ataxia. Fifty-three percent of pediatric patients with CBZ toxicity demonstrated ataxia at mean serum levels of 73 μmol per liter (range 37–128) in one study [13]. In another study of 33 cases of CBZ overdose, ataxia, nystagmus, or opthalmoplegia were seen in 48% of adults with a mean overdose of 12 grams (range 1.6–45) [14]. In a case series of four patients who attempted suicide by CBZ overdose, all patients demonstrated ataxia and nystagmus 1 to 2 days after admission but none suffered permanent neurological sequelae [15]. It appears that the presence of cerebellar atrophy as seen on MRI, predisposes CBZ-treated patients to ataxia at significantly lower serum levels compared to patients without cerebellar atrophy [16]. This may also occur with GBP [17], PB and PRM.

Unlike other conventional AEDs, VPA does not typically cause ataxia or nystagmus at toxic levels but most commonly causes stupor, confusion, and coma [18, 19].

Among the newer AEDs, there is one postmarketing report of two patients developing severe ataxia on relatively low doses of GBP that resolved after discontinuation of the drug [17]. Modulation of a GBP-specific neuronal binding site in the cerebellum was the mechanism proposed by the authors in this chapter. They recommended caution when initiating GBP in patients with preexisting cerebellar dysfunction [17]. Ataxia was also quite common in

Table 16.2 Incidence of ataxia with newer AEDs versus placebo in premarketing trials. The incidence of ataxia in premarketing trials for each drug versus placebo is indicated. Most newer AEDs are indicated as adjunctive epilepsy therapy. When the drug is indicated for monotherapy in epilepsy or other conditions, the premarketing incidence of ataxia is reported as well. Information is taken directly from the product information for each drug (supplied by the manufacturer)

Drug	Adjunctive therapy	Monotherapy	Other
VPA	8% vs. 1%	<1%	Not different versus placebo in migraine prophylaxis
FBM	3.5% vs. 0% adults, 6.5% vs. 3.7% children with Lennox Gastaut	<2%	
GBP	12.5% vs. 5.6%		3.3% vs. 0% postherpetic neuralgia
LMT	10% (300 mg/day) vs. 10% 28% (500 mg/day) vs. 10%	2% vs. 0%	
TPM	16% (200–400 mg/day) vs. 14% (600–1000 mg/day) vs. 7%		
TGB	5% vs. 3% (overall) 9% (56 mg/day) vs. 6% (32 mg/day) vs. 6%		
LEV	3% vs. 1%		
ZNS	6% vs. 1%		
OXC	9% (600 mg/day) 17% (1200 mg/day) 31% (2400 mg/day) vs. 5%	5% vs. 0%	

premarketing studies of oxcarbazepine (OXC) with an incidence ranging from 9% to 31% in adjunctive trials, and this side effect resulted in discontinuing the drug in 5.2% of patients [20].

Table 16.2 lists the premarketing incidence of ataxia for many of the AEDs listed in Table 16.1 (with particular emphasis on the newer agents). Since many of the newer AEDs were studied in adjunctive epilepsy therapy trials, it is important to consider that the incidence of ataxia and other movement disorders reported in adjunctive therapy may reflect changes in serum levels for other AEDs these patients were taking. This is probably reflected in the considerably higher incidence of ataxia in patients receiving adjunctive therapy with the newer AEDs compared to patients receiving the same AED as monotherapy (see Table 16.2).

The mainstay of treatment in patients who develop ataxia with AEDs is discontinuing or reducing the dose of the responsible drug. If the patient is on more than one AED, the drug that was added most recently or that demonstrates a supratherapeutic level should be tapered or discontinued first. In cases of overdose, orogastric lavage followed by the administration of oral-activated charcoal or charcoal hemoperfusion are often recommended [13, 15, 19]. Careful hemodynamic monitoring and close observation for adverse events specific for each drug are also very important in improving patient outcomes.

Table 16.3 Incidence of tremor with newer AEDs versus placebo in premarketing trials. The incidence of tremor in premarketing trials for each drug versus placebo is indicated. Most newer AEDs are indicated as adjunctive epilepsy therapy. When the drug is indicated for monotherapy in epilepsy or other conditions, the premarketing incidence of tremor is reported as well. When AEDs were administered at varying doses, the incidence of tremor is included for each dose/dosing range. Information is taken directly from the product information for each drug supplied by the manufacturer

Drug	Adjunctive therapy	Monotherapy	Other
VPA	25% vs. 6%	57% "high dose" 19% "low dose"	9% vs. 0% in migraine prophylaxis
FBM	6.1% vs. 2.3% adults, not listed in children with Lennox Gastaut	not listed	
GBP	6.8% vs. 3.2%		Not listed in postherpetic neuralgia
LMT	4% vs. 1%, 3% vs. 0% in Lennox Gastaut patients	<2%	
TPM	9% (200–400 mg/day) vs. 9% (600–1000 mg/day) vs. 6%		
TGB	9% vs. 3% 21% (56 mg/day) vs. 14% (32 mg/day) vs. 1%		
LEV	not different versus placebo		
ZNS	not different versus placebo		
OXC	3% (600mg/day) 18% (1200 mg/day) 16% (2400 mg/day) vs. 5%	4% vs. 0%	

Tremor

Of the AEDs reported to cause tremor, VPA is by far the most common [21, 22]. VPA-induced tremor usually appears within a month of starting therapy and is typically a postural and action tremor, but occasionally the tremor is present at rest [22]. The severity of the tremor is usually mild, but can range from minimal to debilitating. Approximately 20% to 25% of patients on chronic VPA therapy develop tremor evident on accelerometric recordings; however, only half of these patients are symptomatic [22, 23]. This is much lower than the incidence of tremor in premarketing VPA/divalproex sodium monotherapy trials for epilepsy; 57% of patients receiving "high-dose" VPA experienced tremor whereas 19% of patients experienced tremor in the "low-dose" group [24] (Table 16.3), suggesting that development of VPA-induced tremor is dose dependent. The incidence of tremor is less in premarketing trials of VPA in migraine prophylaxis and as adjunctive therapy for complex partial seizures (see Table 16.3). It has been suggested that VPA may either induce tremor or unmask a preexisting, clinically silent essential tremor [23].

In one report, propranolol and amantadine were effective in treating VPA-induced tremor, but cyproheptadine, diphenhydramine, and benztropine

RESTING   INTENTION   POSTURAL

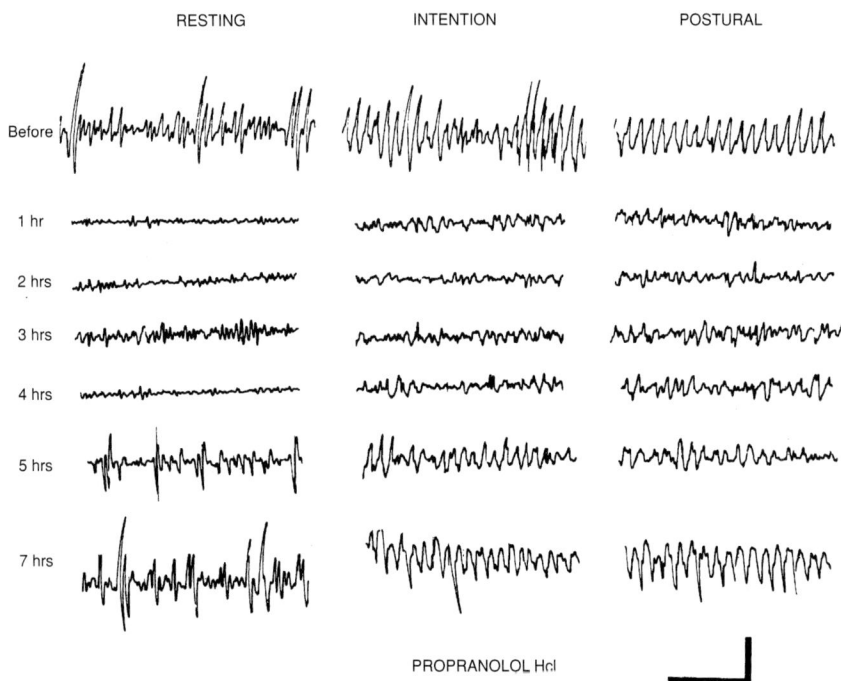

Figure 16.1 Serial accelerometric recordings in a 58-year-old man with VPA-induced tremor treated with 20 mg of propranolol. Tremor was recorded in an upper extremity while at rest, with intention and with maintenance of posture. The tremor returns as propranolol is metabolized by the patient, returning to baseline by 7 hours. Calibration is 1 second and 10 mV. [From [3], with permission from the publisher (Lippincott, Williams & Wilkins).

provided little relief [23]. Acetazolamide has also been reported to be beneficial [25]. Figure 16.1 illustrates the response of VPA-induced tremor to propranolol and return of the tremor as propranolol is metabolized [23].

The clinical features of the VPA-induced tremor and its response to beta-blockers suggest that there is perhaps a common pathophysiology for this disorder and essential tremor. Unfortunately, the etiology of essential tremor remains to be elucidated and VPA interacts with multiple neurotransmitters including serotonin, GABA, dopamine and acetylcholine [26]. However, elucidating the mechanism(s) of VPA-induced tremor may provide further insight into the pathophysiology of essential tremor.

Among the older AEDs, there is one report of mandibular tremor associated with intravenous PHT treatment and toxicity [27]. Tremor is listed as an uncommon adverse event (0.1 to 1% of patients) with CBZ [28]. We could find little information regarding tremor in patients on PB. There is no listing of tremor as an adverse event with ethosuximide (ETS), and we could find no case reports.

Table 16.3 illustrates the incidence of tremor in premarketing trials for each of the newer AEDs. Among them, tiagabine (TGB) was frequently associated with tremor in a dose-dependent manner. The incidence was highest in patients taking 56 mg per day compared to 32 mg or placebo (21%, 14%, and 1%, respectively) [29]. GBP was associated with tremor in 6.8% of treated patients compared to 3.2% on placebo in premarketing trials as adjunctive therapy for epilepsy [30]. This is interesting considering recent interest in its use in patients with essential tremor (see below). Tremor was an adverse reaction in 4% of patients on monotherapy with OXC compared to 0% on placebo in a controlled clinical trial [20]. Tremor due to this drug caused 1.8% of patients to discontinue its use [20]. Levetiracetam (LEV) was not associated with an increased incidence of tremor in adjunctive epilepsy therapy trials [31]. Lamotrigine (LMT) was associated with tremor in 4% of patients (vs. 1% of patients on placebo) in adjunctive trials; however, there was no significantly increased incidence of tremor in a placebo-controlled monotherapy trial [32]. In postmarketing experience, LMT was associated with a disabling tremor when added to VPA in one patient [33]. Tremor is listed as a frequent adverse event in patients taking ZNS (1 in 100) as adjunctive therapy; however, it was not more frequent than placebo in a premarketing controlled trial [34]. TPM was associated with tremor in 9% of patients (vs. 6% of patients on placebo) in adjunctive therapy trials [35].

There is evidence that AEDs are useful in treating essential and other forms of tremor. PRM is used extensively as a first-line treatment of essential tremor with documented benefits [36]. CBZ was effective for cerebellar tremors in a small series [37]. There are reports that GBP is effective in treating essential tremor [38–40] as well as orthostatic tremor [41, 42]. TPM, like PRM and GBP, is also used to treat essential tremor [43, 44].

Myoclonus/asterixis

Myoclonus is also frequently associated with AED treatment. Asterixis (negative myoclonus) is the most common type reported in the literature. Asterixis secondary to AEDs was first recognized in the 1970s [45–47]. PHT [45–47] was initially the most commonly implicated drug; however, PB [47], PRM [47, 48], CBZ [49, 50], and VPA [51, 52] were all subsequently found to cause this movement disorder as well.

Asterixis classically occurs with advanced hepatic disease [53]. While abnormal liver function predisposes patients to developing asterixis when administered AEDs [54], there are reports of PHT-induced asterixis with high serum levels in patients with normal liver function [55]. Asterixis was first reported as a sign of toxic PHT serum levels [45, 46]. It was present in five of eight patients studied with AED-related movement disorders in one study, four of whom were on PHT [47]. There are also patients who develop PHT-induced asterixis with serum levels in the usual therapeutic range [47]. Unilateral asterixis contralateral to the lesion has been reported in patients receiving PHT (with therapeutic levels) following thalamotomy. While the true pathophysiology for asterixis in this setting is unknown, it is thought that PHT may cause central dopaminergic blockade similar to that induced by neuroleptics [47, 56]. How this relates to onset of asterixis, which is unknown. It is interesting to note, however, that PHT has been used to successfully treat another form of myoclonus, diaphragmatic myoclonus [57].

CBZ is reported to cause asterixis in multiple clinical settings: (1) as a sign of toxicity [47, 58, 59], (2) in conjunction with hyperammonemia [50, 60], and (3) in patients on concomitant therapy with lithium [60–62]. Asterixis can occur in patients on CBZ in the setting of normal hepatic function as a dose-related effect [50] or at normal serum levels [61]. While the mechanism of CBZ-induced asterixis is unknown, some authors have suggested that CBZ causes isolated mitochondrial dysfunction/damage in patients who develop asterixis and hyperammonemia [60]. CBZ has been used to treat palatal myoclonus [63].

VPA-associated asterixis was first reported in a patient who had intractable seizures and was being treated with multiple AEDs [64]. Subsequently, two patients were reported to develop asterixis without toxic VPA serum levels or evidence of concomitant hepatic dysfunction [51]. A recent report of six patients suffering a VPA-related stupor suggested that the negative myoclonus observed in these patients was due to a cortical nonepileptic mechanism [52]. While these patients had VPA serum levels in the typical therapeutic range (less than 100 μg/mL), they did have hyperammonemia ranging from 94 to 345 μg/dl (reference range <50) [52]. Like other AEDs, VPA is frequently used to treat myoclonus of various etiologies [65, 66].

There are few reports of drug-induced asterixis among the other older AEDs. There is one report that lorazepam (a benzodiazepine) triggered myoclonus in very low birth-weight infants [67]. There is also a report of PRM-induced asterixis in a patient with moderate renal insufficiency [68].

While myoclonus is listed as a rare (fewer than 1/1000 patients treated) adverse event with GBP in premarketing studies [30], there is one report of 13 cases of myoclonus (out of 104 patients treated by the authors) associated with this drug in refractory epileptics [69]. The myoclonus was focal in three patients and multifocal in the other ten patients. Static encephalopathy was a significant risk factor for the development of multifocal myoclonus and focal myoclonus developed in patients with partial seizures and otherwise normal neurological function [69]. There is also a recent report of asterixis in a patient being treated for postherpetic neuralgia with GBP [70]. While the mechanism for GBP-induced myoclonus is unknown, some authors speculate that GBP may cause myoclonus by influencing serotonergic or GABAergic neurotransmission [69, 70]. In contrast to these reports, GBP ameliorates both posthypoxic myoclonus in a rat model [71] and opioid-related myoclonus in cancer patients [72].

Among other newer AEDs, zonisamide (ZNS) has the highest reported incidence of myoclonus (1/100) in adjunctive premarketing studies [34]. We could not identify reports of ZNS-induced myoclonus, however. ZNS is particularly effective in the treatment of myoclonic epilepsies [73]. CBZ and LMT may worsen myoclonus in myoclonic epilepsy, whereas benzodiazepines, VPA,

LMT, and ZNS may result in improvement depending on the etiology of the myoclonus [74].

Tics

Tics are common movement disorders in children and may be present but unrecognized or exacerbated by treatment with certain drugs. The diagnosis of a tic disorder frequently follows the appearance of tics while being treated with certain medications (especially stimulants), or even after the medication has been discontinued [75]. CBZ is the most common drug associated with AED-induced tics in the literature. Tics (as a group with abnormal involuntary movements) are listed as an uncommon side effect of CBZ (occurring in $\geq 0.1\%$ and $\leq 1\%$ of patients) in the package insert [28]. We identified 13 reported cases in the literature [75–80]. Eleven of the 13 reported patients were children and 6 of the 13 patients had prior tics either at baseline or on other medications. While motor tics were the most prominent, some patients developed vocal tics as well. In some patients the tics were a transient phenomenon while the patients remained on CBZ; in others they resolved when CBZ was discontinued. Patients who had a baseline tic disorder frequently required treatment with antipsychotics. While the cause of CBZ-induced tics is unknown, some authors speculate that CBZ modulates the dopaminergic systems in the brain of susceptible patients triggering onset or exacerbation of tics [75]. Certainly, CBZ is known to alter levels of dopamine in multiple brain regions in chronically treated rats [81]. Tics were also reported with PB treatment in at least six children, due to unknown mechanisms [82, 83]. There is one report of PHT-induced Tourettism in a 16-year-old patient with a history of generalized tonic-clonic seizures [84].

Among the newer AEDs, LMT is associated with tic disorders in at least two reports. LMT-induced Tourettism was first reported in three patients in 1999 [85] followed by a report of five cases of motor and vocal tic disorders [86]. In three of five patients tics resolved within 1 month after the discontinuation of LMT. Two patients had recurrence of tics when LMT was reintroduced. All patients were observed for tics on follow-up from 6 to 22 months and none had recurrence of tics once off LMT [86]. GBP was associated with tics and other dyskinesias in a 41-year-old man with generalized anxiety disorder. This patient had complete resolution of the tics and other movements within 36 hours of stopping the drug [87].

We could not identify reports of tic disorders associated with the other newer AEDs except as above. There are reports of improvement in Tourette's syndrome with benzodiazepines [88–90]. Like benzodiazepines, TPM may have some efficacy in the treatment of Tourette's syndrome [91].

Choreoathetosis

PHT is the AED most commonly associated with the development of dyskinesias, particularly chorea [92, 93]. In our review in 1993 we identified 70 patients who developed choreoathetosis while being treated with PHT [93]. Since then, additional case reports/series of PHT-induced chorea have appeared in both children and adults. In one case series three children with severe myoclonic epilepsy developed choreoathetosis as their doses of PHT were increased [94]. There was also a report of PHT-related chorea in children with deep hemispheric vascular malformations [95]. PHT also precipitated left upper extremity chorea in a 74-year-old man with a contralateral putaminal lesion [96]. Static encephalopathy is the most common predisposing condition, occurring in 39% of 77 reported cases of PHT-associated dyskinesias [93]. Only 12% of patients had an associated structural lesion [93]. Choreoathetosis can occur in PHT-treated patients at nontoxic serum levels and patients that develop choreoathetosis are often on multiple AEDs [93].

Among other older AEDs, VPA has also caused choreic movements. In one report [97] three patients were described, all of whom had severe brain damage and epilepsy. Two were on concomitant therapy with PHT. Choreic movements started within 30 minutes to 3 hours after ingestion of VPA and lasted from 30 minutes to 8 hours. The chorea resolved after discontinuing the VPA or changing to divalproex sprinkles [97]. A more recent report described a patient with a history of head trauma and secondary generalized seizures that developed generalized chorea during the second month of therapy with VPA [98]. This occurred at a dose of 1500 mg per day. Choreic movements disappeared within 2 months after discontinuing VPA [98]. In contrast, VPA has been used to treat Sydenham's chorea [99], postanoxic choreoathetosis [100], posttraumatic choreoathetosis [101], age-related chorea [102], choreoathetoid movements of kernicterus [103], and steroid-resistant chorea associated with lupus [104].

Other conventional AEDs such as CBZ have also been implicated in cases of choreoathetosis [15, 105]. Choreic movements were present in all four patients reported with CBZ overdose when serum levels declined from their peak to between 15 and 25 μg/mL [15]. Like VPA, CBZ has also been used for therapy of both hereditary and nonhereditary choreas [106–109]. ESM caused choreiform movements in a 15-year-old girl hours after she ingested 500 mg of the drug [110]. She responded quickly to intravenous diphenhydramine. A 17-year-old boy with uncontrolled epilepsy also developed choreoathetoid movements 26 days into therapy with methsuximide [111]. The movements lasted 10 days and were severe enough to cause abrasions and confinement to bed. The chorea and athetosis were unresponsive to benztropine and diphenhydramine; however, his movements resolved within a week after discontinuing the drug [111]. We identified one report in the literature where PB was identified as the offending drug in a patient with both chorea and dystonia [112]. We could find no reports linking benzodiazepines with choreoathetosis. Benzodiazepines [113] and PB [114], however, appear useful in treating some forms of chorea.

Among newer AEDs, GBP was associated with choreoathetosis in several patients in postmarketing reports. In 1996 Buetefisch et al. [115] reported a case of choreoathetosis in a 37-year-old man with severe mental retardation and epilepsy after initiation of GBP therapy. He was on FBM and PHT concurrently, but had no prior episodes of choreoathetosis. The movement disorder resolved after discontinuing the drug. Another report presented two mentally retarded, institutionalized patients who developed choreoathetosis at dosages of GBP from 1.2 to 1.8 grams per day [116]. The choreoathetosis resolved after discontinuation of the drug and one had recurrence of the movements after rechallenge [116]. These data are consistent with our findings that patients with a static encephalopathy are predisposed to develop movement disorders related to PHT therapy, particularly in the setting of treatment with multiple AEDs [93].

Among the other newer AEDS, FBM was associated with at least one reported case of choreoathetosis in a 13-year-old boy with epilepsy [117]. The choreoathetosis resolved 36 hours after his last dose of FBM. Combined treatment with LMT and PHT also precipitated chorea in three patients and it improved with tapering one of the medications [118]. There is one report of choreic movements in a child treated with ZNS who had suffered a heat stroke-like episode [119]. LEV, like several other AEDs, has been used successfully to treat paroxysmal kinesiogenic choreoathetosis [120] and we could find no reports of this medication inducing choreic movements.

Orofacial dyskinesias have been reported during treatment with AEDs, often in association with chorea. In 1993, we reported a patient with orofacial dyskinesias provoked by PHT treatment [93]. and found that 49 of 77 patients with PHT-induced dyskinesias described in the literature had orofacial dyskinesias, almost invariably in association with choreoathetosis [93]. PHT may also aggravate preexisting tardive dyskinesia [121]. PB, PRM, and CBZ have been reported to cause orofacial dyskinesias as well [47, 49, 122, 123]. Preexisting cerebral injury was associated with the development of orobuccolingual dyskinesias during treatment with PB in a child [122] as well as an adult [123]. CBZ also induced dose-related orobuccolingual dyskinesias in a 51-year-old epileptic man [49]. Among newer AEDs, orofacial dyskinesias were also reported in a 61-year-old man treated with GBP for anxiety [87]. LMT caused blepharospasm and bilateral contraction of platysma muscles in another man [124]. Clonazepam plus PB [125], VPA [126], and CBZ [127] may be effective treatments for tardive dyskinesia in animals and humans.

The mechanism(s) of AED-induced dyskinesias is(are) unknown. PHT may alter dopamine receptor subtypes or their associated second messenger systems [47, 93, 128]. The ability of PHT to potentiate neuroleptic-induced dyskinesias through mechanisms other than D2 dopamine receptors [129], however, suggests that dopamine receptor blockade/modulation is not the only mechanism involved. The anticholinergic action of PHT may also play a role [130, 131]. Some authors suggest that CBZ, like PHT, causes dyskinesias in the proper clinical setting by altering cholinergic systems [122] or by acting as a dopamine antagonist given CBZ's structural similarity to phenothiazines [133]. Future research may clarify the pathophysiology of AED-induced dyskinesias as the mechanisms of action for each AED are further elucidated.

Dystonia

Of all AEDs, dystonia has been most commonly reported in patients using PHT or CBZ. Eighteen of 77 patients (or 23%) with dyskinesias associated with PHT use experienced some form of dystonia [93]. Dystonias were not isolated movement disorders in the majority of these patients as 15 of the 18 patients suffered another movement disorder as well [93]. As with other dyskinesias, dystonia was more common in the setting of prior CNS injury.

CBZ is also commonly associated with dystonia, especially in pediatric patients [13, 133–136]. While CBZ-induced dystonia typically occurs in the setting of CNS injury combined with toxic serum levels [133], it can occur with toxic CBZ levels in normal children [13, 136] or nontoxic levels in children with brain damage [133]. Dystonia was present in 3 of 45 pediatric patients admitted to an intensive care unit for CBZ toxicity [13]. Transient dystonia was also reported in three children with multifocal epilepsy treated with CBZ [133]. These children experienced dystonic posturing in all four extremities as well as opisthotonus, which completely resolved within 2 weeks after discontinuing the drug [133]. Another child had oculogyric crisis associated with CBZ toxicity [135]. Dystonia also occurs in CBZ-treated adults [136–138,] especially in the setting of prior brain injury [138]. Three of the four adult patients reported by Jacome [138] were brain-damaged men who developed axial dystonia while on CBZ. Segmental dystonia was the sole manifestation of carbamazepine toxicity in one other reported case [139]. Most CBZ-related dystonias are transient and resolve soon after CBZ dosing is reduced or the drug is discontinued. However, there are reported cases of intermittent dystonia persisting during CBZ therapy [136]. While these cases implicate CBZ as a cause of dystonia in the proper setting, it is a drug of choice for the treatment of some paroxysmal dystonias [140].

Among other older AEDs, PB is also known to cause dystonia in children [122, 141] and adults [112]. Torticollis and blepharospasm occurred in a neurologically impaired 2-year-old boy [122] and a 36-year-old woman who took a PB overdose [112]. In a more recent report, a 2-year-old girl developed torticollis, opisthotonus, and oculogyric crises associated with initiation of PB therapy [141]. PB, unlike other AEDs, was actually shown to aggravate paroxysmal dystonia in a rodent model after chronic treatment [142]. It was suggested that this may be due to PB's activity as a GABA receptor agonist under pathological conditions [142]. There are few reports of dystonias in patients on VPA; however, camptocormia was reported in a mentally retarded 23-year-old woman with myoclonic epilepsy while on monotherapy with VPA [143]. In contrast, VPA may have some beneficial effect in some forms of dystonia such as spasmodic torticollis [144]. While there is a report in the literature of acute dystonic reactions associated with DZP ingestion [145], benzodiazepines are routinely used and sometimes quite effective in the treatment of dystonia [146, 147].

Among the newer AEDs, TGB was associated with transient dystonia in three patients who were concomitantly treated with CBZ [148]. The three patients developed a focal limb dystonia, oromandibular dystonia, and writer's cramp, respectively. Unlike many patients who develop dystonia during treatment with AEDs, these patients had normal neurological examinations and two had normal brain MRIs with one having mesial temporal sclerosis (patient with writer's cramp) [148]. All three patients had transient dystonia and remained on TGB therapy. The appearance of the dystonia did not correlate with changes in serum CBZ levels [148]. While the mechanism of TGB-induced dystonia is unknown, TGB may act via a GABAergic mechanism to cause dystonia as it inhibits GABA uptake in the CNS [149].

GBP was also associated with an acute dystonic reaction after 1 month as adjunctive therapy for intractable frontal lobe epilepsy in a 24-year-old man [150]. He experienced oculogyric crisis, opisthotonic posturing, and repetitive jaw clenching without an EEG correlate. Intravenous lorazepam aborted the movements, and there was no recurrence in 20 months of follow-up after discontinuation of GBP [150]. In contrast, GBP is known to decrease the severity of dystonia in a genetic animal model of paroxysmal dystonic choreoathetosis [151]. FBM was associated with a dystonic reaction in a 2-month old boy [117]. LMT was also associated with blepharospasm in a 51-year-old man with secondarily generalized epilepsy [124]. This may correspond with the prodystonic effects of LMT in a mutant hamster model of generalized dystonia [152]. There are no reports of dystonias associated with LEV, and LEV was shown to decrease dystonia in a similar animal paradigm [153].

Parkinsonism/akinetic rigid syndromes

While PHT was one of the first AEDs associated with parkinsonism/bradykinesia [154], VPA has emerged as the most commonly implicated cause of AED-induced parkinsonism in the literature. The first report that we could identify was by Lautin et al. in 1979 [155]. These authors presented a patient who developed an extrapyramidal syndrome associated with VPA monotherapy [155]. Reversible parkinsonism associated with VPA therapy was also reported in 1990 in abstract form [156]. In 1991, Armon et al. [157] reported on VPA-induced syndrome of dementia and parkinsonism in an epilepsy clinic population. This was later published as a full prospective study of 36 patients who had been on VPA for at least 12 months [158]. Thirty-two patients were thought to have some cognitive or motor impairment related to VPA and they were subjected to follow-up testing for at least 3 months after discontinuing VPA. Seventy-five percent of the patients in this group (27 of 36 patients) had three or more signs of parkinsonism (bradykinesia, tremor, rigidity, postural instability) [158]. Twenty-three of 24 patients or 96% improved after stopping VPA. Mean Unified Parkinson's Disease Rating Scale scores for 23 patients were 29.7 ($\pm$21.7) on VPA versus 10.1 ($\pm$12.6) off VPA (p < 0.0001). While the median age of patients was 51.5 years in this study, there are other reports of reversible parkinsonism associated with VPA therapy in a 12-year-old girl [159], and in two young men aged 20 and 26 years [160]. There was also an additional case series of levodopa-responsive parkinsonism that began after 4 years of VPA therapy in two elderly patients [161]. Their parkinsonian signs resolved less than 3 months after substitution of CBZ for VPA. Another case of parkinsonism was recently reported in a demented elderly patient treated with VPA [162]. While the mechanism of VPA-induced parkinsonism is unknown, Armon et al. [159] suggested that VPA may affect Complex I activity in the electron transport chain of mitochondria, similar to a mechanism proposed for Parkinson's disease [163, 164]. Alternatively, VPA may act through GABAergic mechanisms on the basal ganglia [158]. VPA was also reported to cause a reversible multiple system atrophy-like syndrome [165]. In this case, a 67-year-old woman developed dysarthria, impaired smooth pursuits, progressive action tremor, bradykinesia, and ataxia. Eventually, she was wheelchair bound and incontinent after 9 to 10 years of treatment with VPA for post-traumatic seizures. Within 3 months of stopping VPA, the patient had almost complete reversal of her syndrome and after 3 years of follow-up her neurological exam was normal [165].

Among other AEDs, there was also a report of reversible parkinsonism associated with hepatotoxicity following addition of CBZ to VPA [166]. In this case, a 67-year-old woman developed cogwheel rigidity, resting tremor, and bradykinesia, which recurred after rechallenge with CBZ. Most features improved in 2 days after discontinuing CBZ therapy; however, the resting tremor persisted in this patient [166], suggesting the possibility that some patients with parkinsonism associated with AEDs may have subclinical Parkinson's disease. PHT also caused parkinsonism in a 68-year-old man with generalized tonic-clonic seizures [167]. This man developed a shuffling gait, rest tremor (greater on the left), and a persistent nasopalpebral reflex that resolved with switching the patient to CBZ. After discontinuing the PHT, he was symptom free at 6 years of follow-up [167].

While we could find no reports of parkinsonism related to other AEDs, it has been reported that ZNS reduces wearing off in Parkinson's disease patients, possibly due to the drug's long-lasting activation of dopamine synthesis [168]. LMT had no antiparkinsonian activity in rat models of Parkinson's disease [169] or symptomatic benefits for Parkinson's patients in a small double-blind, placebo-controlled study [170].

Miscellaneous movement disorders

Restless legs syndrome (RLS) was reported in two patients taking methsuximide and PHT [171]; however, there is overwhelming evidence that multiple AEDs provide significant benefit for patients with RLS. CBZ [172–174] and clonazepam are effective [175, 176]. GBP was also recently well studied and effective [177–179].

While very uncommon, there are two reports of akathisia related to carbamazepine treatment [180, 181]. One patient had prior exposure to neuroleptics and was treated with CBZ for dysphoria following a left temporal lobe injury

Table 16.4 Summary of movement disorders associated with various AEDs. $+++$ = More common or significant evidence in the literature, $++$ = reported in several case series/reports or in premarketing trials, $+$ = rarely reported in premarketing studies or described in a single case series/report.

	PB	PHT	PRM	ESM	CBZ	VPA	FBM	GBP	LMT	TGB	ZNS	OXC
Ataxia	+	+++	+		+++			+				++
Tremor		+			+	+++	+	+	++	+	+	
Myoclonus	++	++	+		++	++	++				+	
Tics	++	+			+++		+	++				
Chorea	+	+++		+	++	++	+	++	+			+
Dystonia	++	+++			+++	+	+		+			
Parkinsonism		+			+	+++						
RLS		+										
Akathisia				+	++							

[180]. Two others did not have prior neuroleptic exposure and were taking CBZ for treatment of epilepsy [181]. Reducing the dose of CBZ ameliorated the symptoms [181]. There was also one case of akathisia reported in a child receiving ESM [182].

Summary

While movement disorders in patients taking AEDs are rare, it is clear from the literature that three of the most commonly used AEDs (PHT, CBZ, and VPA) are associated with the vast majority of reported cases. (See Table 16.4 for a summary of movement disorders associated with AEDs.). This probably reflects exposure of large patient populations over many years for each of these drugs. Several clinical points have emerged from a review of the cases reported in the literature: (1) patients with preexisting brain injuries have a greater risk of developing movement disorders associated with AEDs; (2) acute toxicity with many AEDs increases the likelihood of developing movement disorders; and (3) polypharmacy with multiple AEDs is frequently associated with the development of movement disorders. Avoiding polypharmacy will not only lead to improved patient compliance, it will also likely prevent the development of iatrogenic movement disorders in some patients. As the newer AEDs are administered to larger patient populations over time, reports of more AED-induced movement disorders will inevitably occur.

References

1. Locock C. In discussion: Sieveking EH. Analysis of 52 cases of epilepsy observed by author. Lancet 1857; 1: 527.
2. Murphy JM, Motiwala R, Devinsky O. Phenytoin intoxication. South Med J 1991; 84: 1199–1204.

3. Selhorst JB, Kaufman B, Horwitz SJ. Diphenylhydantoin-induced cerebellar degeneration. Arch Neurol 1972; 27: 453–455.
4. Baier WK, Beck U, Doose H, et al. Cerebellar atrophy following diphenylhydantoin intoxication. Neuropediatrics 1984; 15: 76–81.
5. Ghatak NR, Santoso RA, McKinney WM. Cerebellar degeneration following long term phenytoin therapy. Neurology 1976; 26: 818–820.
6. McLain LW Jr, Martin JT, Allen JH. Cerebellar degeneration due to chronic phenytoin therapy. Ann Neurol 1980; 7: 18–23.
7. Luef G, Burtscher J, Kresmer C, et al. Magnetic resonance volumetry of the cerebellum in epileptic patients after phenytoin overdosages. Eur Neurol 1996; 36: 273–277.
8. Ney GC, Lantos G, Barr WB, et al. Cerebellar atrophy in patients with long-term phenytoin exposure and epilepsy. Arch Neurol 1994; 51: 767–771.
9. Gessaga EC, Urich H. The cerebellum of epileptics. Clin Neuropath 1985; 4: 238–245.
10. Lindvall O, Nilsson B. Cerebellar atrophy following phenytoin intoxication. Ann Neurol 1984; 16: 258–260.
11. Tan EK, Chan LL, Auchus AP. Phenytoin cerebellopathy without epilepsy. Acta Neurol Scand 2001; 104: 61–62.
12. Crooks R, Mitchell T, Thom M. Patterns of cerebellar atrophy in patients with chronic epilepsy: a quantitative neuropathological study. Epilepsy Res 2000; 41: 63–73.
13. Tibballs J. Acute toxic reaction to carbamazepine: clinical effects and serum concentrations. J Pediatr 1992; 121: 295–299.
14. Seymour JF. Carbamazepine overdose. Features of 33 cases. Drug Saf 1993; 8: 81–88.
15. Weaver DF, Camfield P, Fraser A. Massive carbamazepine overdose: clinical and pharmacologic observations in five episodes. Neurology 1988; 38: 755–759.
16. Specht U, May TW, Rohde M, et al. Cerebellar atrophy decreases the threshold of carbamazepine toxicity in patients with chronic focal epilepsy. Arch Neurol 1997; 54: 427–431.
17. Steinhoff BJ, Herrendorf G, Bittermann HJ, et al. Isolated ataxia as an idiosyncratic side-effect under gabapentin. Seizure 1997; 6: 503–504.
18. Garnier R, Boudignat O, Fournier PE. Valproate poisoning. Lancet 1982; 2: 97.
19. Jones AI, Proudfoot AT. Features and management of poisoning with modern drugs used to treat epilepsy. Q J Med 1998; 91: 325–332.
20. Product Information, Trileptal®, Novartis.
21. Hyman NM, Dennis PD, Sinclair KG. Tremor due to sodium valproate. Neurology 1979; 29: 1177–1180.
22. Karas BJ, Wilder BJ, Hammond EJ, et al. Valproate tremors. Neurology 1982; 32: 428–432.
23. Karas BJ, Wilder BJ, Hammond EJ, et al. Treatment of valproate tremors. Neurology 1983; 33: 1380–1382.
24. Product Information, Depakote®, Abbott.
25. Lancman ME, Asconape JJ, Walker F. Acetazolamide appears effective in the management of valproate-induced tremor. Mov Disord 1994; 9: 369.
26. Perucca E. Pharmacological and therapeutic properties of valproate: a summary after 35 years of clinical experience. CNS Drugs 2002; 16: 695–714.
27. Turkdogan D, Onat F, Ture U, et al. Phenytoin toxicity with mandibular tremor secondary to intravenous administration. Int J Clin Pharmacol Ther 2002; 40: 18–19.
28. Product Information, Tegretol®, Novartis.
29. Product Information, Gabatril®, Cephalon.
30. Product Information, Neurontin®, Parke-Davis.
31. Product Information, Keppra®, UCB Pharma.
32. Product Information, Lamictal®, GlaxoSmithKline.

33. Reutens DC, Duncan JS, Patsalos PN. Disabling tremor after lamotrigine with sodium valproate. Lancet 1993; 342: 185–186.
34. Product Information, Zonegran®, Elan.
35. Product Information, Topamax®, Ortho-McNeil.
36. Louis ED. Clinical practice. Essential tremor. N Engl J Med 2001; 345: 887–891.
37. Sechi GP, Zuddas M, Piredda M, et al. Treatment of cerebellar tremors with carbamazepine: a controlled trial with long-term follow-up. Neurology 1989; 39: 1113–1115.
38. Merren MD. Gabapentin for treatment of pain and tremor: a large case series. South Med J 1998; 91: 739–744.
39. Gironell A, Kulisevsky J, Barbanoj M, et al. A randomized placebo-controlled comparative trial of gabapentin and propranolol in essential tremor. Arch Neurol 1999; 56: 475–480.
40. Ondo W, Hunter C, Vuong KD, et al. Gabapentin for essential tremor: a multiple-dose, double-blind, placebo-controlled trial. Mov Disord 2000; 15: 678–682.
41. Onofrj M, Thomas A, Paci C, et al. Gabapentin in orthostatic tremor: results of a double-blind crossover with placebo in four patients. Neurology 1998; 51: 880–882.
42. Evidente VG, Adler CH, Caviness JN, et al. Effective treatment of orthostatic tremor with gabapentin. Mov Disord 1998; 13: 829–831.
43. Galvez-Jimenez N, Hargreave M. Topiramate and essential tremor. Ann Neurol 2000; 47: 837–838.
44. Connor GS. A double-blind placebo-controlled trial of topiramate treatment for essential tremor. Neurology 2002; 59: 132–134.
45. Kooiker JC, Sumi SM. Movement disorder as a manifestation of diphenylhydantoin intoxication. Neurology 1974; 24: 68–71.
46. Murphy MJ, Goldstein MN. Diphenylhydantoin-induced asterixis. A clinical study. JAMA 1974; 229: 538–540.
47. Chadwick DD, Reynolds RH, Marsden CD. Anticonvulsant induced dyskinesias – a comparison with dyskinesias induced by neuroleptics. J Neurol Neurosurg Psychiatry 1976; 39: 1210–1218.
48. Forman MB, Chouler C, Milne FJ. Primidone-induced "uraemic flap". Lancet 1979; 2: 1250–1251.
49. Joyce RP, Gunderson CH. Carbamazepine-induced orofacial dyskinesias. Neurology 1980; 30: 1333–1334.
50. Ambrosetto G, Riva R, Baruzzi A. Hyperammonemia in asterixis induced by carbamazepine: two case reports. Acta Neurol Scand 1984; 69: 186–189.
51. Bodensteiner JB, Morris HH, Golden GS. Asterixis associated with sodium valproate. Neurology 1981; 31: 194–195.
52. Aguglia U, Gambardella A, Zappia M, et al. Negative myoclonus during valproate-related stupor. Neurophysiological evidence of a cortical non-epileptic origin. Electroencephalogr Clin Neurophysiol 1995; 94: 103–108.
53. Adams RD, Foley JD. The neurological changes in the more common types of severe liver disease. Trans Am Neurol Assoc 1949; 74: 217.
54. Sandford NL, Murray N, Keyser AJ, et al. Phenytoin toxicity and hepatic encephalopathy: simulation or stimulation? J Clin Gastroenterol 1987; 9: 337–341.
55. Chi WM, Chua KSG, Kong K-H. 2000. Phenytoin-induced asterixis – uncommon or underdiagnosed? Brain Injury 2000; 14: 847–850.
56. Duarte J, Sempere AP, Cabezas MC, et al. Postural myoclonus induced by phenytoin. Clin Neuropharmacol 1996; 19: 536–538.

57. Young CR, Clapp L, Salcedo V, et al. Diaphragmatic myoclonus: diagnosis by fluoroscopy and electromyography with response to phenytoin. South Med J 1995; 88: 1270–1273.

58. Terzano MG, Salati MR, Gemgignani F. Asterixis associated with carbamazepine. Acta Neurol Belg 1983; 83: 158–165.

59. Ng K, Silbert PL, Edis RH. Complete external opthalmoplegia and asterixis with carbamazepine toxicity. Aust NZ J Med 1991; 21: 886–887.

60. Rivelli M, El-Mallakh RS, Nelson WH. Carbamazepine-associated asterixis and hyperammonemia. Am J Psychiatry 1988; 145: 269–270.

61. Rittmannsberger H, Leblhuber F, Sommer R. Asterixis as a side effect of carbamazepine therapy. Klin Wochenschr 1991; 69: 279–281.

62. Rittmannsberger H, Leblhuber F. Asterixis induced by carbamazepine therapy. Biol Psychiatry 1992; 32: 364–368.

63. Sakai T, Murakami S. Palatal myoclonus responding to carbamazepine. Ann Neurol 1981; 9: 199–200.

64. Adams DJ, Luders H, Pippenger C. Valproic acid in the treatment of intractable seizure disorders: a clinical and electroencephalographic study. Neurology 1978; 28: 152–157.

65. Fahn S. Post-anoxic action myoclonus: improvement with valproic acid. N Engl J Med 1978; 299: 313–314.

66. Chapman AG. Valproate and myoclonus. Adv Neurol 1986; 43: 661–674.

67. Lee DS, Wong HA, Knoppert DC. Myoclonus associated with lorazepam therapy in very-low-birth-weight infants. Biol Neonate 1994; 66: 311–315

68. Forman MB, Chouler C, Milne FJ. Primidone-induced "uraemic flap". Lancet 1979; 2: 1250–1251.

69. Asconape J, Diedrich A, DellaBadia J. Myoclonus associated with the use of gabapentin. Epilepsia 2000; 41: 479–481.

70. Jacob PC, Chand RP, Omeima el-S. Asterixis induced by gabapentin. Clin Neuropharmacol 2000; 23: 53.

71. Kanthasamy AG, Vu TQ, Yun RJ, et al. Antimyoclonic effect of gabapentin in a posthypoxic animal model of myoclonus. Eur J Pharmacol 1996; 297: 219–224.

72. Mercadante S, Villari P, Fulfaro F. Gabapentin for opioid-related myoclonus in cancer patients. Support Care Cancer 2001; 9: 205–206.

73. Kyllerman M, Ben-Manachem E. Zonisamide for progressive myoclonus epilepsy: long term observations in seven patients. Epilepsy Res 1998; 29: 109–114.

74. Dulac O, Plouin P, Shewmon A. Myoclonus and epilepsy in childhood: 1996 Royaumont meeting. Epilepsy Res 1998; 30: 91–106.

75. Neglia JP, Glaze DG, Zion TE. Tics and vocalizations in children treated with carbamazepine. Pediatrics 1984; 73: 841–844.

76. Gualtieri CT, Evans RW. Carbamazepine-induced tics. Dev Med Child Neurol 1984; 26: 546–548.

77. Aguglia U, Zappia M, Quattrone A. Carbamazepine-induced nonepileptic myoclonus in a child with benign epilepsy. Epilepsia 1987; 28: 515–518.

78. Kurlan R, Kersun J, Behr J, et al. Carbamazepine-induced tics. Clin Neuropharmacol 1989; 12: 298–302.

79. Robertson PL, Garofalo EA, Silverstein FS, et al. Carbamazepine-induced tics. Epilepsia 1993; 34: 965–968.

80. Holtmann M, Korn-Merker E, Boenigk HE. Carbamazepine-induced combined phonic and motor tic in a boy with Down's syndrome. Epileptic Disord 2000; 2: 39–40.

81. Baf MH, Subhash MN, Lakshmana KM, et al. Alterations in monoamine levels in discrete regions of rat brain after chronic administration of carbamazepine. Neurochem Res 1994; 19: 1139–1143.

82. Sandyk R. Phenobarbital-induced Tourette-like symptoms. Pediatr Neurol 1986; 2: 54–55.

83. Burd L, Kerbeshian J, Fisher W, et al. Anticonvulsant medications: an iatrogenic cause of tic disorders. Can J Psychiatry 1986; 31: 419–423.

84. Drake ME, Cannon PA. Tourette syndrome precipitated by phenytoin. Clin Pediatr 1985; 24: 323.

85. Lombroso CT. Lamotrigine-induced tourettism. Neurology 1999; 52: 1191–1194.

86. Sotero de Menezes MA, Rho JM, Murphy P, et al. Lamotrigine-induced tic disorder: report of five pediatric cases. Epilepsia 2000; 41: 862–867.

87. Norton JW, Quarles E. Gabapentin-related dyskinesia. J Clin Psychopharmacol 2001; 21: 623–624.

88. Frederiks JA. Facial tics in children: the therapeutic effect of low-dosage diazepam. Br J Clin Pract 1970; 24: 17–20.

89. Gonce M, Barbeau A. Seven cases of Gilles de la Tourette's syndrome: partial relief with clonazepam: a pilot study. Can J Neurol Sci 1977; 4: 279–283.

90. Kaim B. A case of Gilles de la Tourette's syndrome treated with clonazepam. Brain Res Bull 1983; 11: 213–214.

91. Abuzzahab FS, Brown VL. Control of Tourette's syndrome with topiramate. Am J Psychiatry 2001; 158: 968.

92. Lazaro RP. Involuntary movements induced by anticonvulsant drugs. Mt Sinai J Med 1982; 49: 274–281.

93. Harrison MB, Lyons GR, Landow ER. Phenytoin and dyskinesias: a report of two cases and review of the literature. Mov Disord 1993; 8: 19–27.

94. Saito Y, Oguni H, Awaya Y, et al. Phenytoin-induced choreoathetosis in patients with severe myoclonic epilepsy in infancy. Neuropediatrics 2001; 32: 231–235.

95. Koukkari MW, Vanefsky MA, Steinberg GK, et al. Phenytoin-induced chorea in children with deep hemispheric vascular malformations. J Child Neurol 1996; 11: 490–491.

96. Shulman LM, Singer C, Weiner WJ. Phenytoin-induced focal chorea. Mov Disord 1996; 11: 111–114.

97. Lancman ME, Asconape JJ, Penry JK. Choreiform movements associated with the use of valproate. Arch Neurol 1994; 51: 702–704.

98. Gunal DI, Guleryuz M, Bingol CA. Reversible valproate-induced choreiform movements. Seizure 2002; 11: 205–206.

99. Daoud AS, Zaki M, Shakir R, et al. Effectiveness of sodium valproate in the treatment of Sydenham's chorea. Neurology 1990; 40: 1140–1141.

100. Giroud M, Dumas R. Valproate sodium in postanoxic choreoathetosis. J Child Neurol 1986; 1: 80.

101. Chandra V, Spunt AL, Rusinowitz MS. Treatment of post-traumatic choreo-athetosis with sodium valproate. J Neurol Neurosurg Psychiatry 1983; 46: 963.

102. Hoffman AS, Feinberg TE. Successful treatment of age-related chorea with sodium valproate. J Am Geriatr Soc 1990; 38: 56–58.

103. Kulkarni ML. Sodium valproate controls choreoathetoid movements of kernicterus. Indian Pediatr 1992; 29: 1029–1030.

104. Song CH, Oftadeh LC, Oh C, et al. Successful treatment of steroid-resistant chorea associated with lupus by use of valproic acid and clonidine-HCL patch. Clin Pediatr (Phila) 1997; 36: 659–662.

105. Bimpong-Buta K, Froescher W. Carbamazepine-induced choreoathetoid dyskinesias. J Neurol Neurosurg Psychiatry 1982; 45: 560.

106. Roig M, Montserrat L, Gallart A. Carbamazepine: an alternative drug for the treatment of nonhereditary chorea. Pediatrics 1988; 82: 492–495.

107. Roulet E, Deonna T. Successful treatment of hereditary dominant chorea with carbamazepine. Pediatrics 1989; 83: 1077.

108. Harel L, Zecharia A, Straussberg R, et al. Successful treatment of rheumatic chorea with carbamazepine. Pediatr Neurol 2000; 23: 147–151.

109. Genel F, Arslanoglu S, Uran N, et al. Sydenham's chorea: clinical findings and comparison of the efficacies of sodium valproate and carbamazepine regimens. Brain Dev 2002; 24: 73–76.

110. Kirschberg GJ. Dyskinesia – an unusual reaction to ethosuximide. Arch Neurol 1975; 32: 137–138.

111. Dooley J, Camfield P, Buckley D, et al. Methsuximide-induced movement disorder. Pediatrics 1991; 88: 1291–1292.

112. Lightman SL. Phenobarbital dyskinesia. Postgrad Med J 1978; 54: 114–115.

113. Peiris JB, Boralessa H, Lionel ND. Clonazepam in the treatment of choreiform activity. Med J Aust 1976; 1: 225–227.

114. Garello L, Ottonello GA, Regesta G, et al. Familial paroxysmal kinesigenic choreoathetosis. Report of a pharmacological trial in 2 cases. Eur Neurol 1983; 22: 217–221.

115. Buetefisch CM, Gutierrez A, Gutmann L. Choreoathetotic movements: a possible side effect of gabapentin. Neurology 1996; 46: 851–852.

116. Chudnow RS, Dewey RB Jr, Lawson CR. Choreoathetosis as a side effect of gabapentin therapy in severely neurologically impaired patients. Arch Neurol 1997; 54: 910–912.

117. Kerrick JM, Kelley BJ, Maister BH, et al. Involuntary movement disorders associated with felbamate. Neurology 1995; 45: 185–187.

118. Zaatreh M, Tennison M, D'Cruz O, et al. Anticonvulsants-induced chorea: a role for pharmacodynamic drug interaction? Seizure 2001; 10: 596–599.

119. Shimizu T, Yamashita Y, Satoi M, et al. Heat stroke-like episode in a child caused by zonisamide. Brain Dev 1997; 19: 366–368.

120. Chatterjee A, Louis ED, Frucht S. Levetiracetam in the treatment of paroxysmal kinesiogenic choreoathetosis. Mov Disord 2002; 17: 614–615.

121. DeVeaugh-Geiss J. Aggravation of tardive dyskinesia by phenytoin. N Engl J Med 1978; 298: 457–458.

122. Wiznitzer M, Younkin D. Phenobarbital-induced dyskinesias in a neurologically-impaired child. Neurology 1984; 34: 1600–1601.

123. Sechi GP, Piras MR, Rosati G, et al. Phenobarbital-induced buccolingual dyskinesia in oral apraxia. Eur Neurol 1988; 28: 139–141.

124. Verma A, Miller P, Carwile ST, et al. Lamotrigine-induced blepharospasm. Pharmacotherapy 1999; 19: 877–880.

125. Bobruff A, Carlos G, Tarsy D, et al. Clonazepam and phenobarbital in tardive dyskinesia. Am J Psychiatry 1981; 138: 189–193.

126. Nasrallah HA, Dunner FJ, McCalley-Whitters M. A placebo-controlled trial of valproate in tardive dyskinesia. Biol Psychiatry 1985; 20: 205–208.

127. LaHoste GJ, Wigal T, King BH, et al. Carbamazepine reduces dopamine-mediated behavior in chronic neuroleptic-treated and untreated rats: implications for treatment of tardive dyskinesia and hyperdopaminergic states. Exp Clin Psychopharmacol 2000; 8: 125–132.

128. Mendez JS, Cotzias GC, Mena I, et al. Diphenylhydantoin blocking of levodopa effects. Arch Neurol 1975; 32: 44–46.

129. Sethi KD, Hitri A, Diamond BI. Phenytoin potentiation of neuroleptic-induced dyskinesias. Mov Disord 1990; 5: 325–327.

130. Agrawal S, Bhargara V. Effect of drugs on brain acetylcholine level in the rat. Indian J Med Res 1964; 52: 1179–1182.

131. Pincus JH, Kiss A. Phenytoin, tetrodotoxin, and acetylcholine release. Exp Neurol 1986; 94: 777–781.

132. Jacome DE. Movement disorder induced by carbamazepine. Neurology 1981; 31: 1059–1060.

133. Crosley CJ, Swender PT. Dystonia associated with carbamazepine administration: experience in brain-damaged children. Pediatrics 1979; 63: 612–615.

134. Bradbury AJ, Bentick B, Todd PJ. Dystonia associated with carbamazepine toxicity. Postgrad Med J 1982; 58: 5250526.

135. Arnstein E. Oculogyric crisis: a distinct toxic effect of carbamazepine. J Child Neurol 1986; 1: 289–290.

136. Lee JW. Persistent dystonia associated with carbamazepine therapy: a case report. N Z Med J 1994; 107: 360–361.

137. Soman P, Jain S, Rajsekhar V, et al. Dystonia – a rare manifestation of carbamazepine toxicity. Postgrad Med J 1994; 70: 54–55.

138. Jacome DE. Carbamazepine induced dystonia. JAMA 1979; 241: 2263.

139. Stryjer R, Strous RD, Bar F, et al. Segmental dystonia as the sole manifestation of carbamazepine toxicity. Gen Hosp Psychiatry 2002; 24: 114–115.

140. Bhatia KP. The paroxysmal dyskinesias. J Neurol 1999; 246: 149–155.

141. Lacayo A, Mitra N. Report of a case of Phenobarbital-induced dystonia. Clin Pediatr (Phila) 1992; 31: 252.

142. Richter A, Loscher W. Paradoxical aggravation of paroxysmal dystonia during chronic treatment with phenobarbital in a genetic rodent model. Eur J Pharmacol 2000; 397: 343–350.

143. Kiuru S, Iivanainen M. Camptocormia, a new side effect of sodium valproate. Epilepsy Res 1987; 1: 254–257.

144. Sandyk R. Beneficial effect of sodium valproate and baclofen in spasmodic torticollis. A case report. S Afr Med J 1984; 65: 62–63.

145. Hooker EA, Danzl DF. Acute dystonic reactions due to diazepam. J Emerg Med 1988; 6: 491–493.

146. Ziegler DK. Prolonged relief of dystonic movements with diazepam. Neurology 1981; 31: 1457–1458.

147. Chuang C, Fahn S, Frucht SJ. The natural history and treatment of acquired hemidystonia: report of 33 cases and review of the literature. J Neurol Neurosurg Psychiatry 2002; 72: 59–67.

148. Wolanczyk T, Grabowska-Grzyb A. Transient dystonias in three patients treated with tiagabine. Epilepsia 2001; 42: 944–946.

149. Leppik IE, Gram L, Deaton R, et al. Safety of tiagabine: summary of 53 trials. Epilepsy Res 1999; 33: 235–246.

150. Reeves AL, So EL, Sharbrough FW, et al. Movement disorders associated with the use of gabapentin. Epilepsia 1996; 37: 988–990.

151. Richter A, Loscher W. Gabapentin decreases the severity of dystonia at low doses in a genetic animal model of paroxysmal dystonic choreoathetosis. Eur J Pharmacol 1999; 369: 335–338.

152. Richter A, Loschmann PA, Loscher W. The novel antiepileptic drug, lamotrigine, exerts prodystonic effects in a mutant hamster model of generalized dystonia. Eur J Pharmacol 1994; 264: 345–351.
153. Loscher W, Richter A. Piracetam and levetiracetam, two pyrrolidone derivatives, exert antidystonic activity in a hamster model of paroxysmal dystonia. Eur J Pharmacol 2000; 391: 251–254.
154. Prensky AL, DeVivo DC, Palkes MA. Severe bradykinesia as a manifestation of toxicity to antiepileptic medications. J Pediatr 1971; 78: 700–704.
155. Lautin A, Stanley M, Angrist B, et al. Extrapyramidal syndrome with sodium valproate. Br Med J 1979; 2: 1035–1036.
156. Power C, Blume WT, Young GB. Reversible parkinsonism associated with valproate therapy [abstract]. Neurology 1990; 40(Suppl 1): 139.
157. Armon C, Miller P, Carwile S, et al. Valproate-induced dementia and parkinsonism: prevalence in actively ascertained epilepsy clinic population [abstract]. Neurology 1991; 41: 1162.
158. Armon C, Shin C, Miller P, et al. Reversible parkinsonism and cognitive impairment with chronic valproate use. Neurology 1996; 47: 626–635.
159. Alvarez-Gomez MJ, Vaamonde J, Narbona J, et al. Parkinsonian syndrome in childhood after sodium valproate administration. Clin Neuropharmacol 1993; 16: 451–455.
160. Sasso E, Delsoldato S, Negrotti A, et al. Reversible valproate-induced extrapyramidal disorders. Epilepsia 1994; 35: 391–393.
161. Onofrj M, Thomas A, Paci C. Reversible parkinsonism induced by prolonged treatment with valproate. J Neurol 1998; 245: 794–796.
162. Iijima M. Valproate-induced parkinsonism in a demented elderly patient. J Clin Psychiatry 2002; 63: 75.
163. Parker WD, Boyson SJ, Parks JK. Abnormalities of the electron transport chain in idiopathic Parkinson's disease. Ann Neurol 1989; 26: 719–723.
164. Greenamyre JT, Sherer TB, Betarbet R, et al. Complex I and Parkinson's disease. IUBMB Life 2001; 52: 135–141.
165. Shill HA, Fife TD. Valproic acid toxicity mimicking multiple system atrophy. Neurology 2000; 55: 1936–1937.
166. Froomes PR, Stewart MR. A reversible parkinsonian syndrome and hepatotoxicity following addition of carbamazepine to sodium valproate. Aust NZ J Med 1994; 24: 413–414.
167. Goni M, Jimenez M, Feijo M. Parkinsonism induced by phenytoin. Clin Neuropharmacol 1985; 8: 383–384.
168. Murata M, Horiuchi E, Kanazawa I. Zonisamide has beneficial effects on Parkinson's disease patients. Neurosci Res 2001; 41: 397–399.
169. Loschmann PA, Eblen F, Wullner U, et al. Lamotrigine has no antiparkinsonian activity in rat models of Parkinson's disease. Eur J Pharmacol 1995; 284: 129–134.
170. Shinotoh H, Vingerhoets FL, Lee CS, et al. Lamotrigine trial in idiopathic parkinsonism: a double-blind, placebo-controlled, crossover study. Neurology 1997; 48: 1282–1285.
171. Drake ME. Restless legs with antiepileptic drug therapy. Clin Neurol Neurosurg 1988; 90: 151–154.
172. Telstad W, Sorensen O, Larsen S, et al. Treatment of the restless legs syndrome with carbamazepine: a double blind study. Br Med J 1984; 288: 444–446.
173. Larsen S, Telstad W, Sorensen O, et al. Carbamazepine therapy in restless legs. Discrimination between responders and non-responders. Acta Med Scand 1985; 218: 223–227.
174. Zucconi M, Coccagna G, Petronelli R, et al. Nocturnal myoclonus in restless legs syndrome effect of carbamazepine treatment. Funct Neurol 1989; 4: 263–271.

175. Boghen D, Lamothe L, Elie R, et al. The treatment of the restless legs syndrome with clonazepam: a prospective controlled study. Can J Neurol Sci 1986; 13: 245–247.

176. Saletu M, Anderer P, Saletu-Zyhlarz G, et al. Restless legs syndrome (RLS) and periodic limb movement disorder (PLMD): acute placebo-controlled sleep laboratory studies with clonazepam. Eur Neuropsychopharmacol 2001; 11: 153–161.

177. Happe S, Klosch G, Saletu B, et al. Treatment of idiopathic restless legs syndrome (RLS) with gabapentin. Neurology 2001; 57: 1717–1719.

178. Thorp ML, Morris CD, Bagby SP. A crossover study of gabapentin in treatment of restless legs syndrome among hemodialysis patients. Am J Kidney Dis 2001; 38: 104–108.

179. Garcia-Borreguero D, Larrosa O, De La Llave, et al. Treatment of restless syndrome with gabapentin: A double-blind, cross-over study. Neurology 2002; 59: 1573–1579.

180. Schwarcz G, Gosenfeld L, Gilderman A, et al. Akathisia associated with carbamazepine therapy. Am J Psychiatry 1986; 143: 1191–1192.

181. Milne IK. Akathisia associated with carbamazepine therapy. N Z Med J 1992; 105: 182.

182. Ehyai A, Kilroy A, Fenichel G. Dyskinesia and akathisia induced by ethosuximide. Am J Dis Child 1978; 132: 527–528.

Miscellaneous drug-induced movement disorders

Daniel Tarsy

Introduction

This chapter will review movement disorders caused by a variety of miscellaneous drugs not considered in other chapters. The majority of drugs causing movement disorders are either neuroleptic agents that interfere with dopamine neurotransmission or central nervous system stimulants, which potentiate dopaminergic mechanisms. By contrast, movement disorders are infrequent adverse effects of other medications and there is often no obvious mechanism to explain their occurrence. Among this group, antidepressants and anticonvulsants are more common causes and have also been addressed in separate chapters (Chapters 15 and 16). In some instances, drugs produce myoclonus or chorea together with altered mental status and other neurologic manifestations in the context of a toxic encephalopathy. For the most part, with regard to other drugs only single causes of a movement disorder have been reported and the etiologic relationship between the drug and movement disorder may be open to question. Individual vulnerabilities to medication-induced movement disorders are possible but, except for preexisting extrapyramidal disorders or genetically determined disorders of brain dopamine metabolism [1], these have not been identified for most of the miscellaneous drug-induced movement disorders.

Calcium channel blockers

Cinnarizine and flunarizine are selective calcium channel blockers that appear to be second only to antipsychotic drugs in the frequency with which they produce movement disorders. They have been widely used in Europe and Latin America for the treatment of a variety of conditions including migraine prophylaxis, vertigo, cerebrovascular and peripheral vascular disease, epilepsy, and essential tremor [2]. In addition to being calcium entry blockers, both are piperazine derivatives with mild dopamine receptor-blocking properties [3, 4]. They also have antihistaminic and serotonin-blocking effects.

The spectrum of movement disorders produced by these agents is remarkably similar to those produced by the antipsychotic drugs and includes acute dystonic reactions, akathisia, tremor, and parkinsonism. Acute dystonic reactions and akathisia occur within several hours or days of exposure while parkinsonism may appear up to several months later. Micheli et al. [5] reported on 101 patients who developed movement disorders during treatment with these agents. There were 93 patients with parkinsonism characterized by bradykinesia, rigidity, and tremor, 19 of whom had been misdiagnosed with Parkinson's disease. There were 15 patients with tardive dyskinesia, 5 with orofacial tremor, and one each with acute dystonia and acute akathisia. Although all 93 patients with parkinsonism recovered within 7 to 270 days after drug withdrawal, more recent reports indicate that 11% to 33% have persistent parkinsonism [6, 7] suggesting that these agents may unmask subclinical Parkinson's disease. Ten of the 15 patients with tardive dyskinesia improved within 8 months while 5 had persistent dyskinesia and the single cases of acute dystonia or akathisia recovered immediately. Similar to antipsychotic-induced parkinsonism, most patients were above 50 years of age, women were more commonly affected than men, and antiparkinson drugs were ineffective. Very similar results have been reported in a more recent survey of 74 patients with cinnarizine-induced parkinsonism and dyskinesia [7] and cinnarizine has also been shown to exacerbate motor signs in patients with preexisting Parkinson's disease [8].

The mechanism accounting for the movement disorders produced by these particular calcium channel blockers is uncertain but the strong similarity of their motor effect profile to that of the antipsychotic drugs suggests that dopamine receptor blockade is important. However, since their dopamine receptor-blocking effects are relatively modest, their calcium entry-blocking effects and interference with catecholamine release may also be relevant [2]. The higher incidence of movement disorders in family members of individuals affected with primary disease has raised the possibility of a genetic predisposition [9].

In contrast with cinnarizine and flunarizine, calcium channel blockers used in the United States have been associated with a much lower incidence of movement disorders with only rare cases being reported. One patient with tardive dyskinesia on lithium developed generalized chorea on verapamil, which resolved several days after stopping the verapamil [10]. Another patient developed repeated axial dystonia together with myoclonus after each of several exposures to verapamil [11]. Diltiazem has been associated with akathisia [12] and a single case of parkinsonism [13]. Amlodipine was associated with reversible parkinsonism in a single patient [14] while manidipine exacerbated parkinsonism in two patients with existing Parkinson's disease [15]. Nimodipine may inhibit dopamine synthesis and release due to its calcium-blocking action [16] but the relevance of this effect for the exceedingly rare clinical extrapyramidal reactions that occur is uncertain.

Myoclonus is a more common movement disorder associated with the latter group of calcium channel blockers. Several have been implicated in rapid onset myoclonus, which resolves in days to weeks after stopping the drug [17–20].

In one case, nifedipine was associated with a fine tremor [21] and has also been reported to increase physiologic and essential tremor [22].

Anticholinergic and antihistaminic drugs

Anticholinergic drugs such as trihexyphenidyl, benztropine, and other less frequently used agents are an uncommon but well-established cause of reversible choreiform movement disorders. The movement disorders usually occur in patients with preexisting parkinsonism or dystonia. They occasionally also occur in neurologically normal elderly individuals. Less common but similar effects are reported following treatment with tricyclic antidepressants with anticholinergic properties (see Chapter 15).

Anticholinergic drugs may cause orofacial dyskinesia or more generalized chorea in patients with Parkinson's disease, may increase the severity of levodopa-induced dyskinesia, and may exacerbate tardive dyskinesia [2]. Fahn and David [23] reported four patients above 66 years of age with orofacial and lingual dyskinesia due to anticholinergic drugs including trihexyphenidyl, ethopropazine, and procyclidine. Two had Parkinson's disease, one had torticollis with head tremor, and one had bipolar disorder and was on lithium. Dyskinesia occurred after each of two challenges with the anticholinergic agents and subsided after drug discontinuation in all cases. Mano et al. [24] reported 10 elderly patients with parkinsonism who developed orofacial and extremity dyskinesias on trihexyphenidyl, benztropine, or procyclidine. The involuntary movements disappeared with discontinuation of the drugs. Birket-Smith [25] reported six patients who developed abnormal involuntary movements following treatment with trihexyphenidyl, orphenadrine, procyclidine, ethopropazine, or biperiden. Four had Parkinson's disease while two had isolated tremor. All were female and older than 63 years of age. None was being treated with levodopa or neuroleptic drugs. Four patients had isolated orolingual dyskinesia while two also had choreic limbs and truncal dyskinesia. Dyskinesia cleared completely within several weeks of discontinuing anticholinergic treatment. In the four patients with Parkinson's disease, retreatment with a different anticholinergic was followed by the reappearance of dyskinesia within 1 to 2 weeks. Additional isolated case reports of anticholinergic-induced dyskinesia in patients with parkinsonism have been described [26, 27].

Chorea has also been reported in dystonia patients being treated with anticholinergic drugs [28, 29]. Nomoto et al. described five adults with focal dystonia who developed generalized chorea while receiving high-dose trihexyphenidyl for up to 9 years [28]. Chorea diminished or disappeared in all cases when the dose was reduced. Horn et al. reported chorea in four of 13 patients with dystonia (cervical in 11 cases), which cleared when anticholinergics were stopped [29].

The mechanism whereby anticholinergic drugs cause dyskinesia likely relates to well-established antagonistic actions of dopamine and acetylcholine in the basal ganglia. Anticholinergic drugs potentiate striatal dopaminergic effects and cholinergic agents have the opposite effect [30–32]. Clinically, dopaminergic drugs cause choreiform dyskinesia in Parkinson's disease, cholinergic agents suppress levodopa-induced dyskinesia and chorea in Huntington's disease [33, 34] and anticholinergics appear to aggravate levodopa-induced dyskinesia in Parkinson's disease [35] and tardive dyskinesia [36].

Antihistaminic drugs also possess central anticholinergic properties [2, 37, 38] and, presumably for this reason, have occasionally been associated with dyskinetic and choreiform involuntary movements. Cyclizine, pheniramine, chlorpheniramine, brompheniramine, phenindramine, and mebhydroline have all been implicated in single case reports [37–41]. Movement disorders have included orofacial dyskinesia, blepharospasm, cranial-cervical dystonia, and involuntary hand movements. However, the precise relationship of antihistamines to these reactions is obscured by the fact that several have occurred in patients also exposed to neuroleptic drugs with possible underlying tardive dyskinesia [39, 42]. Although an acute dystonic reaction has been reported after diphenhydramine [43] this is an exceedingly rare event and, in fact, antihistamines are remarkably effective in terminating acute dystonic reactions to neuroleptic drugs. Cyproheptadine combines antihistaminic, anticholinergic, and antiserotoninergic properties and has rarely been associated with akathisia and chorea [44, 45].

Very rare cases of chorea [46, 47], acute dystonia [48, 49], and tremor [50] have also been reported after the use of H2 receptor blockers such as cimetidine and ranitidine, which lack central anticholinergic effects and, in fact, have anticholinesterase activity. It has been suggested that these rare reactions are more likely related to central H2 receptor blockade than the effects on catecholamine or cholinergic mechanisms [47].

Antianxiety agents

Orofacial dyskinesias have occasionally been reported in patients treated with a variety of benzodiazepines [2]. However, in most cases, patients were already on antipsychotic drugs or antidepressants and the benzodiazepines appear to have either exacerbated a preexisting tardive dyskinesia or contributed to the unmasking of a covert dyskinesia [51–54]. Acute dystonic reactions, similar to those seen with antipsychotic drugs, have also been very rarely reported [54, 55]. Unusually high doses of benzodiazepines (140–400 mg/day of diazepam) have apparently caused drug-induced parkinsonism in patients with schizophrenia previously withdrawn from antipsychotic drugs [56]. The mechanisms whereby benzodiazepines would precipitate or exacerbate dyskinesias or parkinsonism are obscure but their interactions with GABA receptors may be relevant. It should be noted that benzodiazepines much more commonly ameliorate acute [57] or chronic dyskinesia [58] than precipitate or aggravate them.

Buspirone is an anxiolytic that is a partial agonist at 5-hydroxytryptamine 1A receptors, which also has properties as a mixed agonist-antagonist at dopamine receptors [59]. Similar to the benzodiazepines, exacerbation of pre-existing dyskinesia or dystonia has rarely been associated with this drug. In rare cases buspirone also appears to have produced akathisia [60], orofacial dyskinesia [61], dystonia [62], and myoclonus [63]. Although the relatively weak dopamine antagonist properties of buspirone may account for these effects, it has also been used to treat levodopa-induced dyskinesia in patients with Parkinson's disease without consistently exacerbating parkinsonism [64].

Oral contraceptives

Chorea has been a recognized complication of therapy with estrogen and progesterone-containing oral contraceptive agents for many years. In one of the first significant reviews of this subject, Nausieda et al. [65] reported five cases and reviewed the literature concerning 17 other previously described cases prior to 1979. Subsequent reviews of contraceptive drug-induced chorea have delineated the clinical features of this stereotyped syndrome in more detail [2, 66]. Most cases have occurred in relatively young, nulliparous women. Abnormal movements begin subacutely about 9 to 12 weeks after starting hormone therapy. In nearly all cases, chorea is the only neurological symptom; however, it has been associated with the abrupt onset of hemiparesis or personality changes in a few cases [65, 67]. The distribution of chorea is unilateral in two thirds of cases and generalized but often asymmetric in the remainder. Chorea persists as long as contraceptive treatment continues but resolves spontaneously within 8 weeks of stopping it. Reexposure to contraceptives is associated with recurrence of chorea in the majority of patients [2] and chorea has reappeared premenstrually in cyclic fashion in a small number of patients with preexisting brain injury [65].

A striking feature of contraceptive-induced chorea is the frequency with which it occurs in women who had a previous history of chorea from other causes. According to one review, rheumatic fever has previously occurred in 46% and Sydenham's chorea in 30% of cases [2]. Other patients have had antecedent chorea due to chorea gravidarum, systemic lupus erythematosis, Henoch-Schonlein purpura, cyanotic heart disease, and other forms of static encephalopathy [65]. Interestingly, the body distribution of contraceptive chorea is often similar to the distribution of antecedent chorea. It is therefore commonly thought that preexisting basal ganglia damage predisposes to the appearance of contraceptive-induced chorea.

Several proposals have been made concerning the pathophysiology of contraceptive-induced chorea. Estrogen has been cited as playing an important role in enhancing dopamine receptor sensitivity since, in early studies, oophorectomized animals treated with estrogen or progesterone showed increased sensitivity to dopamine agonists [65]. However, subsequent studies have shown that under different experimental circumstances estrogen can either enhance or suppress dopamine-mediated motor behaviors [68] leaving the effects of estrogen on dopaminergic systems uncertain. The variable effects of estrogen on dopamine function may relate to regional brain effects, timing, and dosage of hormonal administration, metabolism, and other properties of the particular experimental system being employed [2]. Occasional cases of acute hemichorea with or without hemiparesis strongly suggest an ischemic mechanism perhaps mediated by known effects of oral contraceptives on co-agulation [69]. However, this probably does not explain the more commonly occurring subacute presentations. A possible immunologic basis has also been proposed [70], possibly supported by more recent findings of antistriatal anti-bodies in patients with Sydenham's chorea [71] and the association of chorea with systemic lupus erythematosis but there is no direct evidence to support this notion.

Narcotic analgesics

Myoclonus is the most frequent movement disorder associated with narcotic drugs. In particular, meperidine may cause painful, stimulus-sensitive, and action myoclonus. Patients with chronic renal failure and cancer are particu-larly susceptible to this effect due to the accumulation of normeperidine and this should not be treated with this particular narcotic [72–74]. Myoclonus has also been reported following treatment with high-dose morphine and other narcotic analgesics but cases are rare and may be related to interaction with concomitant neuroleptics or other drugs [75–78].

Although opiates have effects on striatal dopamine mechanisms and there is an enkephalin-mediated projection between striatum and globus pallidus, narcotics have only rarely been associated with hypokinetic or hyperkinetic movement disorders. Two cases of reversible parkinsonism have been reported following treatment with meperidine [78, 79]. It is unknown whether these are related to the permanent parkinsonism that occurs after exposure to the meperidine derivative,1-methyl-4-phenyl-1,2,5,6-tetrahydropyridine (MPTP), which causes selective damage to the substantia nigra. Fentanyl treatment or withdrawal has been associated with a variety of movement disorders in very small numbers of patients including myoclonus, facial dyskinesia, muscular rigidity, tremor, and torticollis but often occurring together with seizures sug-gesting a more complex form of neurologic toxicity [80]. Transient chorea has been reported in a patient following methadone [81]. Orofacial dyskinesia, chorea, and akathisia have also been reported in a patient following oxycodone withdrawal [82].

Other drugs

There are numerous case reports of movement disorders caused by a variety of other drugs, the mechanism of which is obscure in most cases. Many of these have been tabulated and reviewed elsewhere [2, 83–85]. These include cardiac and antihypertensive drugs, antimicrobials, chemotherapeutic agents, immunosuppressive agents, and a number of miscellaneous drugs. Exaggerated physiologic tremor is a commonplace side effect of most sympathomimetic medications such as beta agonists, bronchodilators, and corticosteroids and will not be discussed.

Cardiac drugs and antihypertensives. Amiodarone is a potent cardiac antiarrhythmic used for the treatment of serious ventricular arrhythmias, which is associated with a high incidence of neurologic side effects. In one series, neurologic side effects occurred in 29 of 54 treated patients [86]. Tremor was the earliest and most common adverse effect and occurred in 21 patients. This was a 6–10 Hz postural tremor producing flexion-extension movements in the fingers, wrist, and elbows, which were indistinguishable from essential tremor. Ataxia occurred in 20 patients and included falls, gait ataxia, and limb ataxia. A small number of patients also developed peripheral neuropathy. These effects were dose dependant and appeared after several weeks to months of drug exposure. Parkinsonian rest tremors involving the legs, hands, and jaw and less frequent additional signs of parkinsonism have also been described in a small number of patients [87]. Reversibility of parkinsonian signs appears to correlate inversely with the duration of amiodarone treatment [87]. The mechanism of amiodarone's extrapyramidal toxicity is unknown but its effects on mitochondrial respiratory chain complexes I and II may be relevant [88]. Myoclonus and dyskinesia have also been described in patients on amiodarone [87]. Pindolol is an antihypertensive beta blocker with partial beta agonist effects, which has produced postural tremor [89, 90]. Isolated reports linking oromandibular dystonia to flecainide [91], parkinsonism to diazoxide or captopril [92, 93], chorea to digoxin toxicity [94], and parkinsonism or chorea to methyldopa [2, 95] have either been associated with more diffuse neurologic toxicity or are of uncertain significance because of their extreme rarity.

Antimicrobial drugs. The most common movement disorder associated with antibiotics is myoclonus. The penicillins are the most common and well-known offender and often also produce seizures, typically in the context of renal failure with breakdown of the blood-brain barrier. Isolated reports of myoclonus, tremor, or parkinsonism following cephalosporins, trimethoprim-sulfamethoxazole, and amphotericin B have typically occurred in a setting of severe infectious or neoplastic disease and are of uncertain significance [2]. Chloroquine occasionally produces acute dystonic reactions or dyskinesias similar to those produced by neuroleptic drugs.

Chemotherapeutic, immunosuppressive, and antiinflammatory agents. Cytosine and adenosine arabinoside have been associated with cerebellar ataxia and tremor, both of which appear to be dose related. There is also one case report of reversible parkinsonism in a patient treated with high-dose cytosine arabinoside [96]. Persistent cranial-cervical dystonia has been reported in four patients days to months following treatment with 5-fluorouracil and doxorubicin [97]. Cyclosporine frequently produces neurological toxicity. Postural tremor is the most common side effect, occurring in more than 20% of patients [2, 98]. Rare reports of parkinsonism following cyclosporine are difficult to interpret as they may have occurred in a background of acquired hepatolenticular degeneration [99] or in association with concomitant neuroleptic administration [100]. There are very rare reports of acute dystonic reactions after certain nonsteroidal antiinflammatory drugs such as mefenamic acid [101, 102] and azapropazone [103].

References

1. Tu JB. Psychopharmacogenetic basis of medication-induced movement disorders. Int Clin Psychopharmacol 1997; 12: 1–12.
2. Lang AE, Weiner WJ. Drug-Induced Movements Disorders. Mount Kisco, NY, Futura , 1992, pp. 339–381.
3. Fadda F, Gessa GL, Mosca E, et al. Different effects of the calcium antagonists nimodipine and flunarizine on dopamine metabolism in the rat brain. J Neural Transm 1989; 75: 195–200.
4. De Vries DJ, Beart PM. Competitive inhibition of [3H] spiperone binding to D-2 dopamine receptors in striatal homogenates by organic calcium-channel antagonists and polyvalent actions. Eur J Pharmacol 1985; 106: 133–139.
5. Micheli FE, Fernandes Pardal MM, Giannaula G, et al. Movement disorders and depression due to Flunarizine and Cinnarizine. Mov Disord 1989; 4: 139–146.
6. Garcia-Ruiz PJ, Garcia de Yebenes J, Jimenez-Jimenez SJ, et al. Parkinsonism associated with calcium channel blockers: A perspective follow-up study. Clin Neuropharmacol 1992; 15: 19–26.
7. Marti-Masso JF, Poza JJ. Cinnarizine-induced parkinsonism: ten years later. Mov Disord 1998; 13: 453–456.
8. Marti-Masso JF, Obeso JA, Carrera N, et al. Aggravation of Parkinson's disease by Cinnarizine. J Neurol Neurosurg Psychiatry 1987; 50: 804–805.
9. Negrotti A, Calzetti S, Sasso E. Calcium-entry blockers-induced parkinsonism: possible role of inherited susceptibility. Neurotoxicology 1992; 13: 261–264.
10. Helmuth B, Ljaijevic Z, Ramirez L, et al. Choreoathetosis induced by verapamil and lithium treatment. J Clin Psychopharmacol 1989; 9: 454–455.
11. Hicks CB, Abraham K. Verapamil and myoclonic dystonia. Ann Intern Med 1985; 103: 154.
12. Jacobs NB. Diltiazem and akathisia. Ann Intern Med 1983; 99: 794–795.
13. Dick RS, Barold SS. Diltiazem-induced parkinsonism. Am J Med 1989; 87: 95–96.
14. Sempere AP, Duarte J, Cabezas C, et al. Parkinsonism induced by amlodipine. Mov Disord 1995; 10: 115–116.
15. Nakashima K, Shimoda M, Kuno N, et al. Temporary symptom worsening caused by manidipine hydrochloride in two patients with Parkinson's disease. Mov Disord 1994; 9: 106–107.
16. Pileblad E, Carlsson A. In vivo effects of the Ca-antagonists nimodipine on dopamine metabolism in mouse brain. J Neural Trans 1986; 66: 171–187.
17. Caviness JN. Myoclonus. Mayo Clin Proc 1996; 71: 679–688.

18. Pedro-Botet ML, Bonal J, Caralps A. Nifedipine and myoclonic disorders. Nephron 1989; 51: 281.

19. DeMedina A, Biasini O, Frafara A, et al. Nifedipine and myoclonic dystonia. Ann Intern Med 1986; 104: 125.

20. Vadlamudi L, Wijdicks EFM. Multifocal myoclonus due to verapamil overdose. Neurology 2002; 58: 984–985.

21. Rodger C, Stewart A. Side effects of nifedipine. Br Med J 1978; 276: 1619–1620.

22. Topaktas S, Onur R, Dalkara P. Calcium channel blockers and essential tremor. Eur Neurol 1987; 27: 114–119.

23. Fahn S, David E. Oral-facial lingual dyskinesia due to anticholinergic medications. Trans Am Neurol Assoc 1972; 97: 277–279.

24. Mano T, Sobue I, Hirose K, et al. Dyskinesias induced by anticholinergic drugs. An electrophysiological analysis. X Intern Congress Neurology. Intern Congress Series No. 296. Excerpta Medica, 1973.

25. Birket-Smith SE. Abnormal involuntary movements induced by anticholinergic therapy. Acta Neurol Scand 1974; 50: 801–811.

26. Warne RW, Gubbay SS. Choreiform movements induced by anticholinergic therapy. Med J Aust 1979; 1: 465.

27. Hauser RA, Olanow CW. Orobuccal dyskinesia associated with trihexyphenidyl therapy in a patient with Parkinson's disease. Mov Disord 1993; 8: 512–514.

28. Nomoto N, Thompson PD, Sheehy NP, et al. Anticholinergic-induced chorea in the treatment of focal dystonia. Mov Disord 1987; 2: 53–56.

29. Horn S, Hinson M, Morrissey M, et al. Blinded evaluation for the frequency of chorea in dystonia patients both on and off anticholinergic medication. Mov Disord 2002 (Suppl 5); 17: S276–S277.

30. Pycock Z, Milson J, Tarsy D, et al. The effect of manipulation of cholinergic mechanisms on turning behavior in mice with unilateral destruction of the nigro-neostriatal dopaminergic system. Neuropharmacology 1978; 17: 175–183.

31. Tarsy D. Interactions between acetylcholine and dopamine in the basal ganglia. In Davis KL, Berger PA (eds) Acetylcholine and Neuropsychiatric Disease. New York, Plenum Press, 1979, pp. 395–424.

32. Weiner WJ, Klawani HL. Cholinergic-monoaminergic interactions within the striatum implications for choreiform disorders. In Butcher L (ed) Cholinergic-Monoaminergic Interaction in the Brain: Basic Mechanisms & Clinical Implications. New York, Academic Press, 1978, pp. 335–362.

33. Tarsy D, Leopold N, Sax DS. Physostigmine in choreiform movement disorders. Neurology 1974; 24: 28–33.

34. Klawans HL, Rubovits R. Central cholinergic-anticholinergic antagonism in Huntington's chorea. Neurology 1972; 22: 107–116.

35. Birket-Smith E. Abnormal involuntary movements in relation to anticholinergics and levodopa therapy. Acta Neurol Scand 1975; 52: 150–160.

36. Klawans HL. The pharmacology of tardive dyskinesias. Am J Psychiatry 1973; 130: 82–86.

37. Klawans HL, Moskovitz C. Cyclizine-induced chorea. J Neurol Sci 1977; 31: 237–244.

38. Mendelson G. Pheniramine aminosalicylate overdosage. Arch Neurol 1977; 34: 313.

39. Thach BT, Chase TN, Bosma JF. Oral facial dyskinesias associated with prolonged use of antihistaminic decongestants. N Eng J Med 1975; 293–486–487.

40. Worz R. Spate extrapyramidale hyperkinesen wahrend langzeiger einnahme zon mebhybrolin. Dtsch Med Wochenschr 1975; 98: 1071–1074.

41. Davis WA. Dyskinesia associated with chronic antihistamine use. N Engl J Med 1976; 294: 113.
42. Jones B, Lal S. Tardive dyskinesia uncovered after ingestion of Sominex, an over-the-counter drug. Can J Psychiatry 1985; 30: 370–371.
43. Lavenstein BL, Cantor FK. Acute dystonia. An unusual reaction to diphenhydramine. JAMA 1976; 236: 291.
44. Calmels JP, Sorbette F, Montastruc JL, et al. Syndromes hyperkinetique iatrogene par antihistaminique. La Nouvelle Presse Med 1982; 30: 2296–2297.
45. Samie MR, Ashton AK. Choreoathetosis induced by cyproheptadine. Mov Disord 1989; 4: 81–84.
46. Kushner MJ. Chorea and cimetidine. Ann Intern Med 1982; 96: 126.
47. Lehmann AB. Reversible chorea due to ranitidine and cimetidine. Lancet 1988; 332: 158.
48. Romisher S, Felter R, Dougherty J. Tagamet-induced acute dystonia. Ann Emerg Med 1987; 16: 1162–1164.
49. Davis BJ, Aul EA, Granner MA, et al. Ranitadine-induced cranial dystonia. Clin Neuropharmacol 1994; 17: 489–491.
50. Bateman BN, Bevan P, Longley BP, et al. Cimetidine induced postural and action tremor. J Neurol Neurosurg Psychiatry 1981; 44: 94.
51. Rosenbaum AH, De la Fuente JR. Benzodiazepines and tardive dyskinesia. Lancet 1979; 314: 900.
52. Sandyk R. Orofacial dyskinesias associated with lorazepam therapy. Clin Neuropharmacol 1986; 5: 419–421.
53. Kaplan SR, Murkofsky C. Oro-buccal dyskinesia symptoms associated with low-dose benzodiazepine treatment. Am J Psychiatry 1978; 135: 1558–1559.
54. Hooker EA, Danzl DS. Acute dystonic reaction due to diazepam. J Emerg Med 1988; 6: 491–493.
55. Stolarek IH, Ford MJ. Acute dystonia induced by midazolam and abolished by flumazenil. Br Med J 1990; 300: 614.
56. Surany-Cadotte BE, Nestoros JN, Mair NPV, et al. Parkinsonism induced by high doses of diazepam. Biol Psychiatry 1985; 20: 451–460.
57. Korczyn AD, Goldberg GJ. Intravenous diazepam and drug-induced dystonic reactions. Br J Psychiatry 1972; 121: 75–77.
58. Bobruff A, Gardos G, Tarsy D, et al. Clonazepam and phenobarbital in tardive dyskinesia. Am J Psychiatry 1981; 138: 189–193.
59. LeWitt PA, Walters A, Hening W, et al. Persistent movement disorders induced by buspirone. Mov Disord 1993; 8: 331–334.
60. Patterson JF. Akathisia associated with buspirone. J Clin Psychopharmacol 1988; 8: 296–297.
61. Strauss A. Oral dyskinesia associated with buspirone use in an elderly woman. J Clin Psychiatry 1988; 49: 322–323.
62. Boylan K. Persistent dystonia associated with buspirone. Neurology 1990; 40: 1904.
63. Ritchie EC, Bridenbaugh RH, Jabbari B. Acute generalized myoclonus following buspirone administration. J Clin Psychiatry 1988; 49: 242–243.
64. Kleedorfer B, Lees AJ, Stern GN. Buspirone in the treatment of levodopa induced dyskinesias. J Neurol Neurosurg Psychiatry 1991; 54: 376–377.
65. Nausieda PA, Koller WC, Weiner WJ, et al. Chorea induced by oral contraceptives. Neurology 1979; 29: 1605–1609.
66. Weiner WJ, Lang AE. Movement Disorders. A Comprehensive Survey. Mount Kisco, NY, Futura, 1989, pp 628–630.

67. Galamberti B. Chorea induced by the use of oral contraceptives: report of a case and review of the literature. Ital J Neurol Sci 1987; 8: 383–386.
68. Kompoliti K. Estrogen and movement disorders. Clin Neuropharmacol 1989; 22: 318–326.
69. Riddoch D, Jefferson M, Bickerstaff ER. Chorea and the oral contraceptives. Br Med J 1971; 4: 217–218.
70. Gamboa ET, Isaacs G, Harter DH. Chorea associated with oral contraceptive therapy. Arch Neurol 1971; 25: 112–114.
71. Church AJ, Cardoso F, Dale RC, et al. Anti-basal ganglia antibodies in acute and persistent Sydenham's chorea. Neurology 2002; 59: 227–231.
72. Szeto HH, Inturrisi CE, Houde R, et al. Accumulation of normeperidine, an active metabolite of meperidine, in patients with renal failure or cancer. Ann Intern Med 1977; 86: 738–740.
73. Hochman MS. Meperidine-associated myoclonus and seizures in long-term hemodialysis patients. Ann Neurol 1983; 14: 593.
74. Reutens DC, Stewart-Wynn EG. Norpethidine-induced myoclonus in a patient with renal failure. J Neurol Neurosurg Psychiatry 1989; 52: 1450–1451.
75. Potter JM, Reid DB, Shaw RJ, et al. Myoclonus associated with treatment with high doses of morphine: a role of supplemental drugs. Br Med J 1989; 299: 150–153.
76. Quinn N. Myoclonus associated with high doses of morphine. Br Med J 1989; 299: 683–684.
77. McQuay HJ, Gorman DJ, Hanks GW. Myoclonus associated with high doses of morphine. Br Med J 1989; 299: 684.
78. Lieberman AN, Goldstein M. Reversible parkinsonism related to meperidine. N Engl J Med 1985; 312: 509.
79. Olive JM, Masana L, Gonzalez J. Meperidine and reversible parkinsonism. Mov Disord 1994; 9: 115–116.
80. Petzinger G, Mayer SA, Przedborski S. Fentanyl-induced dyskinesias. Mov Disord 1995; 10: 679–680.
81. Wasserman S, Yahr MD. Choreic movements induced by the use of methadone. Arch Neurol 1980; 37: 727–728.
82. Gardos G. Dyskinesia after discontinuation of compound analgesic containing oxycodone. Lancet 1977; 309: 759–760.
83. Jimenez-Jimenez FJ, Garcia-Ruiz PJ, Antonio Molina J. Drug-induced movement disorders. Drug Safety 1997; 16: 180–204.
84. Hubble JP. Drug-induced parkinsonism. In Watts RL, Koller WC (eds) Movement Disorders. Neurologic Principles and Practice. New York, McGraw-Hill, 1997, pp. 325–330.
85. Miller LG, Jankovic J. Drug-induced dyskinesias: An overview. In Joseph AB, Young RR (eds) Movement Disorders in Neurology and Neuropsychiatry. Malden, MA, Blackwell Science, 1999, pp 5–30.
86. Charness ME, Morady F, Sheinman MM. Frequent neurologic toxicity associated with amiodarone therapy. Neurology 1984; 34: 669–671.
87. Werner EG, Olanow CW. Parkinsonism and amiodarone therapy. Ann Neurol 1989; 25: 630–632.
88. Dotti MT, Federico A. Amiodarone-induced parkinsonism: A case report and pathogenetic discussion. Mov Disord 1995; 10: 233–234.
89. Hod H, Kaplinsky N, Har-Zahav J, et al. Pindolol-induced tremor. Postgrad Med J 1980; 56: 346–347.
90. Koller WC, Orebaugh C, Lawson L, et al. Pindolol-induced tremor. Clin Neuropharmacol 1987; 10: 449–452.

91. Miller LG, Jankovic J. Persistent dystonia possibly induced by flecainide. Mov Disord 1992; 7: 62–63.
92. Neary D, Thurston H, Pohl JEF. Development of extrapyramidal symptoms in hypotensive patients treated with diazoxide. Br Med J 1973; 3: 474–475.
93. Sandyk R. Parkinsonism induced by captopril. Clin Neuropharmacol 1985; 8: 197–200.
94. Wedzicha JA, Gibb WR, Lees HA, et al. Chorea and digoxin toxicity. J Neurol Neurosurg Psychiatry 1984; 47: 419.
95. Yamadori A, Albert ML. Involuntary movement disorder caused by methyldopa. N Engl J Med 1972; 236: 609.
96. Luque FA, Selhorst JB, Petruska P. Parkinsonism induced by high-dose cytosine arabinoside. Mov Disord 1987; 2: 219–222.
97. Brashear A, Siemers E. Focal dystonia after chemotherapy: A case series. J Neuro-Oncol 1997; 34: 163–167.
98. Walker RW, Brochstein JA. Neurologic complications of immunosuppressive agents. Neurol Clin 1988; 6: 261–268.
99. Bird GLA, Meadows J, Goka J, et al. Cyclosporin-associated akinetic mutism and extrapyramidal syndrome after liver transplantation. J Neurol Neurosurg Psychiatry 1990; 53: 1068–1071.
100. Wasserstein PH, Honig LS. Parkinsonism during cyclosporine treatment. Bone Marrow Transplant 1996; 18: 649–650.
101. Kremona-Barbaro A. Extrapyramidal symptoms following mefenamic acid. J R Soc Med 1983; 76: 435.
102. Redmond AD. Dyskinesia induced by mefenimic acid? J R Soc Med 1981; 74; 558–559.
103. Wood N, Paull HS, Williams AC, et al. Extrapyramidal reactions to anti-inflammatory drugs. J Neurol Neurosurg Psychiatry 1988; 51: 731–732.

Index